Advances in Psychiatry Research

Advances in Psychiatry Research

Edited by Chase Harris

hayle
medical

New York

Hayle Medical,
750 Third Avenue, 9th Floor,
New York, NY 10017, USA

Visit us on the World Wide Web at:
www.haylemedical.com

ISBN: 978-1-63241-743-5

Cataloging-in-Publication Data

Advances in psychiatry research / edited by Chase Harris.
    p. cm.
Includes bibliographical references and index.
ISBN 978-1-63241-743-5
1. Psychiatry. 2. Psychiatry--Research. 3. Psychology, Pathological. 4. Mental health.
5. Medicine and psychology. I. Harris, Chase.
RC454 .A28 2019
616.89--dc23

Table of Contents

Preface

The medical speciality concerned with the study of mental disorders, along with their diagnosis, prevention and treatment is known as psychiatry. Problems related to mood, behavior and perception also fall under psychiatry. Psychiatric disorders include among others, schizophrenia and other psychotic disorders, bipolar disorder, anxiety disorders, dissociative disorders, personality disorders, etc. Psychological tests and physical examinations are often conducted for diagnostic purposes. Psychiatric medication and psychotherapy are two of the most common and effective ways of treating psychiatric disorders. A doctor who has specialized in the field of psychiatry is called a psychiatrist. The topics included in this book on psychiatry are of utmost significance and bound to provide incredible insights to readers. It studies, analyses and upholds the pillars of psychiatry and its utmost significance in modern times. As this field is emerging at a rapid pace, the contents of this book will help the readers understand the modern concepts and applications of the subject.

After months of intensive research and writing, this book is the end result of all who devoted their time and efforts in the initiation and progress of this book. It will surely be a source of reference in enhancing the required knowledge of the new developments in the area. During the course of developing this book, certain measures such as accuracy, authenticity and research focused analytical studies were given preference in order to produce a comprehensive book in the area of study.

This book would not have been possible without the efforts of the authors and the publisher. I extend my sincere thanks to them. Secondly, I express my gratitude to my family and well-wishers. And most importantly, I thank my students for constantly expressing their willingness and curiosity in enhancing their knowledge in the field, which encourages me to take up further research projects for the advancement of the area.

Editor

Weight changes before and after lurasidone treatment: a real-world analysis using electronic health records

Jonathan M. Meyer[1], Daisy S. Ng-Mak[2]* ⓘ, Chien-Chia Chuang[3], Krithika Rajagopalan[2] and Antony Loebel[4]

Abstract

Background: Severe and persistent mental illnesses, such as schizophrenia and bipolar disorder, are associated with increased risk of obesity compared to the general population. While the association of lurasidone and lower risk of weight gain has been established in short and longer-term clinical trial settings, information about lurasidone's association with weight gain in usual clinical care is limited. This analysis of usual clinical care evaluated weight changes associated with lurasidone treatment in patients with schizophrenia or bipolar disorder.

Methods: A retrospective, longitudinal analysis was conducted using de-identified electronic health records from the Humedica database for patients who initiated lurasidone monotherapy between February 2011 and November 2013. Weight data were analyzed using longitudinal mixed-effects models to estimate the impact of lurasidone on patient weight trajectories over time. Patients' weight data (kg) were tracked for 12-months prior to and up to 12-months following lurasidone initiation. Stratified analyses were conducted based on prior use of second-generation antipsychotics with medium/high risk (clozapine, olanzapine, quetiapine, or risperidone) versus low risk (aripiprazole, ziprasidone, first-generation antipsychotics, or no prior antipsychotics) for weight gain.

Results: Among the 439 included patients, the mean age was 42.2 years, and 69.7% were female. The average duration of lurasidone treatment across all patients was 55.2 days and follow-up duration after the index date was 225.1 days. The estimated impact of lurasidone on weight was − 0.77 kg at the end of the 1-year follow-up. Patients who had received a prior second-generation antipsychotic with medium/high risk for weight gain were estimated to lose an average of 1.68 kg at the end of the 1-year follow-up.

Conclusions: Lurasidone was associated with a reduction in weight at 1 year following its initiation in patients with schizophrenia or bipolar disorder. Stratified analyses indicated that weight reduction was more pronounced among patients who had received second-generation antipsychotics associated with a higher risk of weight gain prior to lurasidone treatment. These findings are consistent with the results of prior short- and long-term prospective studies and suggest that lurasidone is associated with low risk for weight gain in patients with schizophrenia or bipolar disorder.

Keywords: Weight change, Mental illness, Electronic health records, Lurasidone, Antipsychotic treatment

Introduction

Severe and persistent mental illnesses, such as schizophrenia and bipolar disorder, are associated with increased risk of obesity [1] compared to the general population. While over one-third of adults in the United States are obese [body mass index (BMI) ≥ 30 kg/m^2], [2, 3] the prevalence of obesity or being overweight is estimated at 40–63% among patients with schizophrenia, [4–6] and 49–68% among patients with bipolar disorder [7–10]. Evidence suggests that the presence of obesity using BMI, or central adiposity by waist circumference criteria, may negatively impact the disease course in

*Correspondence: daisy.ng-mak@sunovion.com
[2] Sunovion Pharmaceuticals Inc., 84 Waterford Drive, Marlborough, MA 01752, USA
Full list of author information is available at the end of the article

schizophrenia and bipolar disorder, and increase risks of cardiovascular disease, diabetes, and stroke in addition to reducing health-related quality of life [6, 11].

One of the contributing factors for this higher risk of overweight or obesity in patients with schizophrenia or bipolar disorder may be the use of antipsychotics. While antipsychotics are the current standard pharmacological treatment for severe mental illnesses, as a class they are associated with varying rates of adverse metabolic effects, including a propensity for weight gain [12–15]. Proposed biological mechanisms leading to weight gain in patients treated with antipsychotics include changes in leptin [16] and adiponectin [17]. Among the second-generation antipsychotic (SGA) medications with extensive historical data, clozapine, olanzapine, quetiapine, and risperidone are associated with medium and high risk for weight gain, while aripiprazole and ziprasidone have a lower risk [18, 19]. Lurasidone is an SGA associated with lower risk for inducing weight gain and other cardiometabolic abnormalities in controlled trials and long-term extension studies [15, 20–23]. In addition to the metabolic and social burden of obesity related to SGA use, patients consider the issue of weight gain as the most important treatment concern for the management of bipolar depression [24]. Weight gain is one of the primary adverse effects that lead to treatment non-adherence or discontinuation among schizophrenia patients [25–27]. Non-adherence to psychotropic medications has been found to be associated with consequent relapse and hospitalization rates, resulting in greater healthcare resource use and higher healthcare costs [25, 26, 28, 29].

Given these factors, it is important for clinicians to consider SGAs that are not only efficacious but also provide a lower or more acceptable risk of metabolic disturbance in patients with schizophrenia [30–32]. The value of switching to a lower metabolic risk SGA for patients with high metabolic risk has been reported in other studies [30, 33]. Selection of such SGAs may potentially lead to lowered metabolic risk, improved overall health-related quality of life, and reduced healthcare costs [34]. While the association of lurasidone and lower risk of weight gain has been established in short and longer-term clinical trial settings, information about lurasidone's association with weight gain in usual clinical care is limited. This study sought to assess the effect of lurasidone treatment on body weight among patients with schizophrenia or bipolar disorder in real-world settings.

Methods
Study design
This study was a retrospective, longitudinal analysis of de-identified electronic health records. The health

records were from the Humedica NorthStar™ database from February 1, 2011 to December 31, 2013.

Data source
The Humedica database contains detailed medical information from integrated claims, prescription, and practice management data on approximately 30 million individuals across 38 states in the US [35]. The de-identified data are representative of the US population in terms of distributions of age, gender, and geographical region. Humedica partners with the nation's leading medical groups, integrated delivery networks, and hospital chains to obtain data from their electronic medical records and information technology systems in real time. The data are then normalized, validated, and aggregated to generate a complete and longitudinal view of patient care [35]. The data used in this study were sourced from the Humedica analytics platform. In addition to the inclusion of standard disease diagnosis and procedure details, the Humedica database includes information of direct relevance to this study, including body weight [kilograms (kg)], body mass index [BMI (kg/m^2)], and prescription drug information obtained from each provider group's platform. While Humedica standardizes these data to ensure consistency across values (i.e., weight in kg), there is no additional logic or algorithm applied. All data used in this study were de-identified and are compliant with the Health Insurance Portability and Accountability Act (HIPAA) of 1996. The study did not require institutional review board approval.

Sample selection
Patients were included in this study if they met the following criteria: (a) had at least one prescription for lurasidone between February 1, 2011 and November 30, 2013 (first lurasidone prescription date was defined as the index date), (b) did not have prescriptions for other antipsychotics or mood-stabilizing agents at the time of the first prescription for lurasidone, (c) did not have any lurasidone prescriptions during the 12 month pre-index period, (d) were aged 18 years or older at index, (e) had ≥ 1 weight recorded during the 12 month pre-index period and ≥ 1 weight recorded during the 12 month post-index period, (f) had ≥ 1 medical encounter in the electronic health record system atleast 12 months prior to the index date, and (g) did not receive other first-generation antipsychotics (FGAs) or SGAs during the 12 month post-index period. Patients were followed for 12 months before the first lurasidone prescription (baseline period) and up to 12 months (minimum 30 days) after the index date (follow-up period).

Study variables

Demographic characteristics consisted of age at index date (first lurasidone prescription date), gender, and geographic region (Midwest, Northeast, South, West). Duration of follow-up (in days) was truncated at 365 days after the index date. Clinical characteristics included whether the patient had been diagnosed with a schizophrenia spectrum or bipolar disorder [see Appendix: Table 2 for the International Classification of Diseases, Ninth Revision, Clinical Modification (ICD-9-CM) codes], presence of selected comorbidities (i.e., major depressive disorder, substance abuse, hypertension, hyperlipidemia, diabetes, chronic obstructive pulmonary disease; see Appendix: Table 2), and the Charlson Comorbidity Index score [36]. In addition, prior use of FGAs or SGAs, and prior use of other medications (i.e., antidepressants and diuretics) were included. Presence of medication was identified based on the drug names in the electronic health records (see Appendix: Table 3). Pre-index clinical characteristics also included the most recent BMI measure prior to the index date and BMI classification (i.e., underweight < 18.5 kg/m^2, normal weight 18.5–24.9 kg/m^2, overweight 25.0–29.9 kg/m^2, and obese $\geq$ 30 kg/m^2). Characteristics of lurasidone treatment included the duration of treatment in days (defined as the number of days between the first and last prescription for lurasidone during the follow-up period), and the number of lurasidone prescriptions during the follow-up period.

The primary outcome variable for this study was patient weight (kg) during pre-index and follow-up periods. Weight observations were trimmed such that any records with extreme weight values (i.e., less than 25 kg or greater than 200 kg) were dropped. Patients were only allowed one unique weight observation per day. In cases where a patient had multiple weight measures on the same day, the first recorded weight (based on the timestamp) was selected. For patients with multiple height measures, the modal value was selected; if no modal value existed, the median result was selected as it was less affected by outliers. Height observations were trimmed so that any values less than 120 cm or greater than 220 cm were dropped from the analysis. The patient's BMI was calculated using a uniform height measure; therefore, changes in BMI over time reflected changes in weight.

Statistical analyses

Longitudinal mixed-effects modeling of patient weight trajectories over time was conducted to estimate: (a) patient weight on the index date, (b) the slope of weight change between the beginning and the end of the baseline period (i.e., up until the index date), and (c) the slope of weight change between the beginning and the end of the follow-up period (i.e., a maximum of 365 days after the index date). In addition to the analysis of the overall patient cohort, stratified analyses were conducted on subsets of the overall patient cohort. The first stratified analysis split patients into those who did or did not receive a SGA during the pre-index period. The second split the sample into those who received a SGA with a medium or high risk for weight gain (i.e., clozapine, olanzapine, quetiapine, and risperidone) versus low risk for weight gain (aripiprazole, ziprasidone, first-generation antipsychotics, or no prior antipsychotics).

Results

Of 3491 patients who received at least one lurasidone prescription, 439 patients initiated lurasidone as monotherapy, continued on lurasidone monotherapy, and had multiple weight measures (Fig. 1). Demographics and patient characteristics during the pre-index period are reported in Table 1. The mean sample age was 42.2 years, and 69.7% were female. The mean duration of follow-up after the index date was 225.1 days. At index, 65.8% of patients had a diagnosis of schizophrenia spectrum or bipolar disorder, and 34.2% had other or no diagnoses. Almost half of the patients (45.8%) had prior use of a SGA; of these, a total of 27% of patients had prior use of a SGA associated with medium or high risk for weight gain. First-generation antipsychotics were prescribed to 14.1% of patients in the year prior to lurasidone initiation. Over half of the patients had prior use of antidepressants. Psychiatric and cardiometabolic comorbidities were commonly observed at index. The mean baseline weight for patients included in this analysis was 93.9 kg, and almost two-thirds of patients were classified as obese according to their BMI at index.

The average duration of lurasidone treatment across all patients was 55.2 days, and the majority of patients (76.1%) received lurasidone for < 90 days. On average, patients received two lurasidone prescriptions during the study follow-up period. In the year prior to initiating lurasidone treatment, weight increased by a mean value of 1.64 kg. This trend was reversed after lurasidone initiation (the index date), with patients losing an average of 0.77 kg (Fig. 2a).

Stratified analyses are shown in Fig. 2b, and c. Similar to the overall findings, increases in weight prior to lurasidone initiation and reduction in weight after lurasidone use were observed in all subgroups. The average weight change after lurasidone treatment in subgroups with or without prior use of second-generation antipsychotics were − 1.50 and − 0.29 kg, respectively. The average weight changes after lurasidone treatment in the medium/high weight gain risk antipsychotic subgroups and low weight gain risk antipsychotic subgroups were − 1.68 and − 0.62 kg, respectively (Fig. 2c).

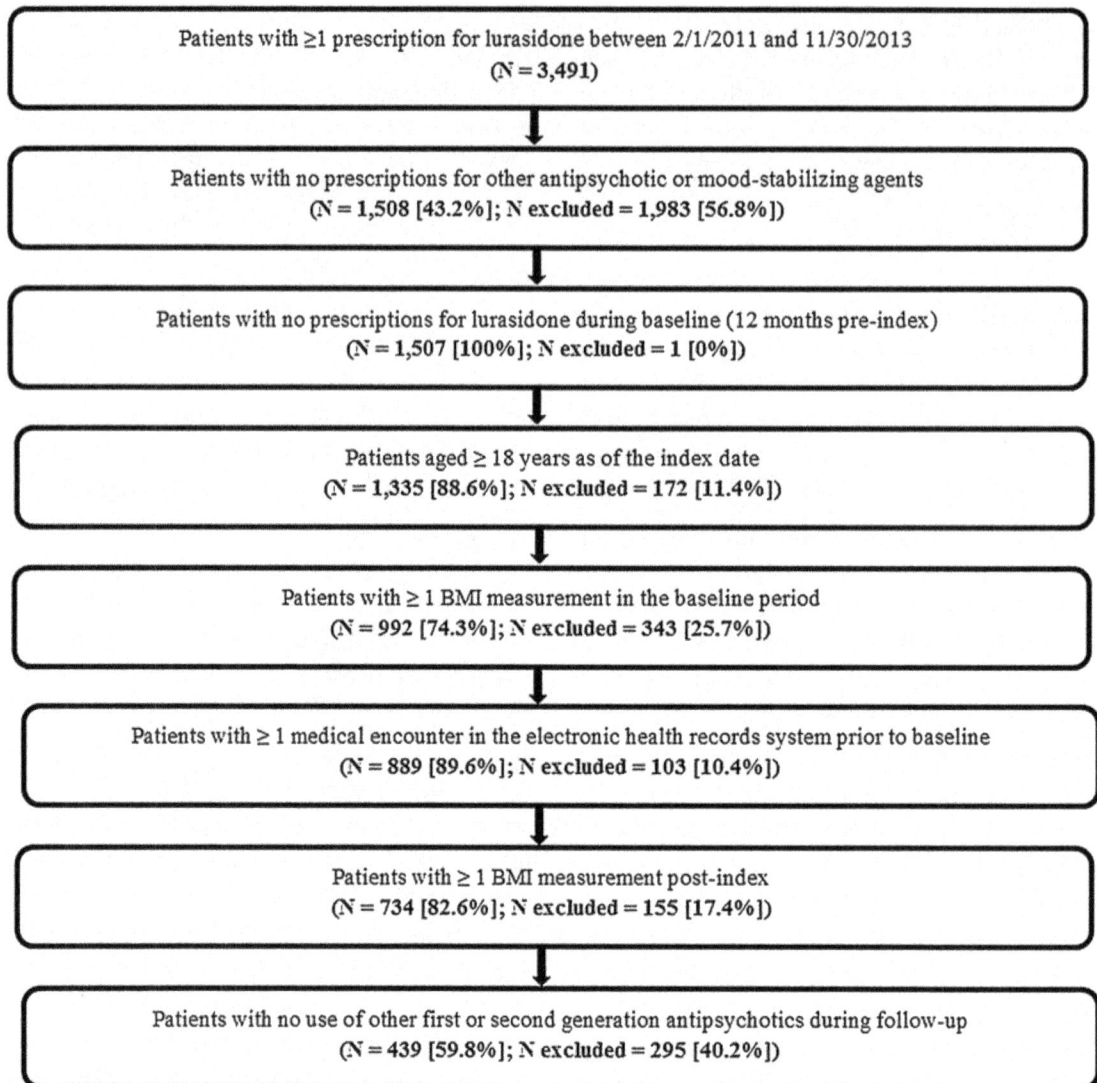

Fig. 1 Patient selection flowchart

Discussion

This retrospective, longitudinal study using electronic health records from the Humedica database for patients who initiated lurasidone monotherapy between February 2011 and November 2013 examined patterns of weight change before and after initiating lurasidone therapy in patients with schizophrenia or bipolar disorder. Our findings indicated that lurasidone was associated with a reduction in weight, with an estimated average weight loss of 0.77 kg during the 12-month follow-up period. Weight reduction associated with lurasidone was more pronounced in a subgroup of patients who had previously received SGAs with medium or high risk for weight gain.

Prior switch trials of antipsychotics among patients who changed from an antipsychotic with a higher weight

gain risk to one with lower risk have reported that weight loss occurs gradually following the medication change [33, 37]. Six-month open-label extension trials of lurasidone have demonstrated that the weight gained during 6 weeks of exposure to olanzapine can be reversed upon a switch to lurasidone, with the weight loss occurring over 3–4 months [38]. A previous analysis evaluated the effect of 12 months' treatment with lurasidone on weight in schizophrenia patients using pooled data from eight clinical trials [13]. Meyer et al. reported that weight loss of at least 7% was observed in more than twice as many patients receiving lurasidone (18.5%) than patients receiving risperidone (6.7%) or quetiapine extended release (XR) (9.1%). In addition, patients receiving lurasidone for 12 months were more likely to experience a

Table 1 Patient demographic and clinical characteristics at index

Characteristics	Lurasidone (N = 439)
Age (years), mean (SD)	42.2 (13.5)
Female, N (%)	306 (69.7%)
Follow-up duration (days), mean (SD)	225.1 (124.6)
Diagnosis of schizophrenia or bipolar disorder, N (%)	
Schizophrenia spectrum diagnosis	83 (18.9%)
Bipolar disorder diagnosis	206 (46.9%)
Other/unknown diagnosis[a]	150 (34.2%)
Prior use of any second-generation antipsychotics N (%)	201 (45.8%)
Prior use of second-generation antipsychotics associated with medium or higher risk for weight gain[b]	119 (27.1%)
Prior use of any first-generation antipsychotic, N (%)	62 (14.1%)
Prior use of other medications, N (%)	
Antidepressants	246 (56.0%)
Diuretics	90 (20.5%)
Comorbidities, N (%)	
Depression	196 (44.6%)
Substance abuse	166 (37.8%)
Hypertension	158 (36.0%)
Hyperlipidemia	155 (35.3%)
Diabetes	89 (20.3%)
Chronic obstructive pulmonary disease	85 (19.4%)
Charlson Comorbidity Index Score, mean (SD)	0.8 (1.3)
Weight[c] and BMI classification[d]	
Weight (kg), mean (SD)	93.9 (25.4)
Underweight, N (%)	4 (0.9%)
Normal, N (%)	70 (15.9%)
Overweight, N (%)	89 (20.3%)
Obese, N (%)	276 (62.9%)

[a] As lurasidone would not be prescribed for any other condition except schizophrenia and bipolar, and the lack of a diagnosis in administrative data does not indicate the lack of the disorder, the data from these patients was deemed acceptable to use in the analysis

[b] Second-generation antipsychotics associated with medium or higher risk of weight gain included clozapine, olanzapine, quetiapine, and risperidone

[c] Weight was the most recent weight observation at index (i.e., weight observation closest to and before index date)

[d] BMI classification based on the closest BMI reading prior to the index date. Underweight, BMI < 18.5 kg/m^2; normal weight, BMI $\geq$ 18.5 and < 25.0 kg/m^2; overweight, BMI $\geq$ 25.0 and < 30 kg/m^2; obese, BMI $\geq$ 30 kg/m^2

shift from a higher BMI category to a lower BMI category compared with patients treated with risperidone or quetiapine XR [13]. The results of the current study confirm and extend these prior findings by demonstrating weight loss in real-world patients with schizophrenia or bipolar disorder who were switched to lurasidone for up to 12 months.

Patients with serious mental illness have a greater risk for obesity and associated cardiovascular and metabolic diseases [6, 39]. Antipsychotic-induced weight gain may exacerbate these conditions and lead to treatment discontinuations [25, 26]. The results of this study suggest that a potential strategy to manage antipsychotic weight gain may be to switch patients to an antipsychotic with a lower risk of weight gain, such as lurasidone. In this electronic medical record analysis, patients previously treated with SGAs associated with medium/high risk for weight gain had an average weight loss of 1.68 kg within the 12 months following initiation of lurasidone. Similarly, in a lurasidone switch trial for patients with schizophrenia or schizoaffective disorder, patients lost an average of 0.2 kg at 6 weeks, and more patients had a clinically significant ($\geq$ 7%) weight loss (1.8%) than weight gain (0.9%) [40]. After 6 months of treatment, the average weight loss was 0.8 kg, with 11.8% having clinically significant weight loss. Additionally, patients previously treated with a medium/high risk SGA for weight gain [olanzapine (23.1%) quetiapine (16.7%), and risperidone (22.2%)] appeared more likely to have a clinically significant weight loss than patients who were previously

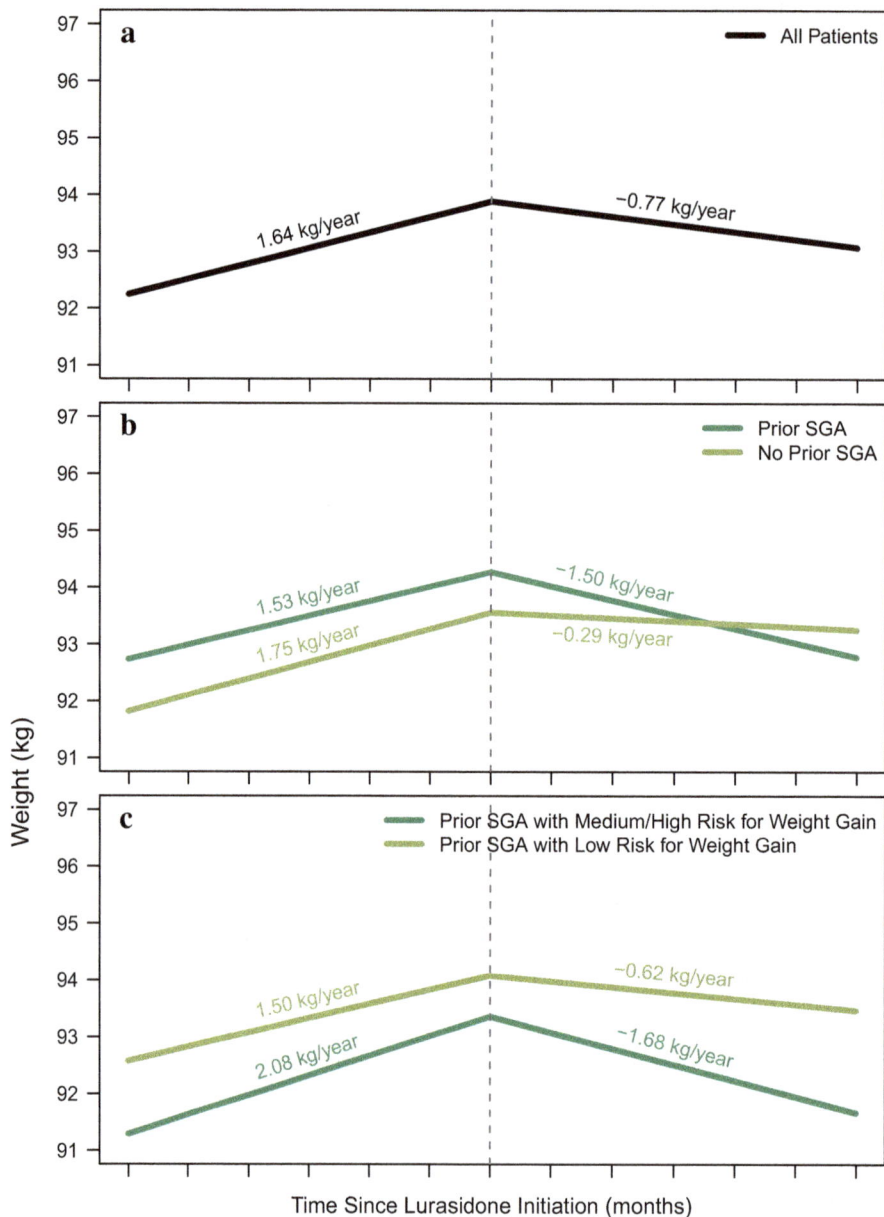

Fig. 2 Impact of lurasidone on weight (**a**) overall, and stratified by prior use of second-generation antipsychotics (**b**), and prior use of second-generation antipsychotics with medium/high risk for weight gain (**c**)

treated with a low risk SGA [aripiprazole (3.2%) or ziprasidone (16.7%)] [41]. Consistent with these findings, a recent meta-analysis of 15 different antipsychotics in patients with schizophrenia, reported significantly less weight gain in patients treated with lurasidone compared with the majority of treatments [19].

Even a relatively modest degree of weight loss (5%) has been associated with metabolic benefits [42] and savings in healthcare costs [43]. This suggests that the weight loss observed for lurasidone-treated patients in this study was meaningful from both clinical and cost perspectives.

Pairing the medication switch with a behavioral intervention may lead to an even greater weight loss [44].

The study methodology does have some limitations. The data were collected retrospectively, and other interventions for weight loss could have been implemented by patients at the same time that lurasidone was initiated. Thus, the associations between lurasidone and the reduction in weight following lurasidone initiation could also be due (in whole or in part) to other unobserved interventions such as dietary counseling or prescribed exercise. Mean lurasidone use was only 55.2 days, and weight changes associated with lurasidone were estimated at 1 year. The study was a single-group pre-post assessment and did not include a control group. Therefore, no conclusion could be drawn regarding the relative effectiveness of lurasidone for weight management compared to other antipsychotics or add-on treatments like metformin [45]. Only patients with sufficient weight measurements recorded before and after lurasidone initiation were included in this study. Therefore, this study may have been subject to selection bias towards an overweight/obese cohort whose clinicians were concerned enough to be more assiduous about monitoring weight. It is unclear whether our findings are generalizable to patients with low/normal baseline BMI [46] or to patients who did not gain weight prior to lurasidone treatment. No assessment of cardiometabolic risk factors (e.g., waist circumference or metabolic parameters) were obtained in this study. In addition, assessments of symptomatic change were not available in this study. However, lurasidone is a well-established antipsychotic treatment in patients with schizophrenia and bipolar depression [20, 22–24, 41, 47]. Although one-third of patients in this study did not have a diagnosis code, given the indications for prescribing lurasidone, it is likely that most patients in this study were being treated for schizophrenia spectrum or bipolar disorder.

Another limitation of this study was the linear weight change assumption over a 1-year follow-up period. Prior research suggests that weight change appears to be more pronounced early in treatment and levels off as time passes [38, 48, 49]. To assess the degree to which the choice of a linear model may have resulted in an overestimate of the amount of weight change, a sensitivity analysis (see Additional file 1: Appendix S1) was conducted using 6-month lurasidone data from an open-label extension study [38]. The sensitivity analysis modeled a linear longitudinal mixed-effects model and a nonlinear longitudinal mixed-effects model to test the difference in weight loss estimates. Had a nonlinear model been used in the current study, the weight change estimates may have been about two-thirds the size (see Additional file 1: Appendix S1 for details). While the weight loss estimates may differ somewhat based on whether the weight loss was linear or nonlinear, our study results suggest that lurasidone treatment resulted in statistically significant and clinically meaningful reduction in weight among patients with schizophrenia and bipolar disorder in real-world settings.

Conclusions

This retrospective, longitudinal study using electronic health records obtained from real-world treatment settings suggests that lurasidone was associated with a reduction in weight at 1 year following its initiation in patients with serious mental illness, primarily schizophrenia or bipolar disorder. Weight reduction was more pronounced among patients who had received second-generation antipsychotics associated with a higher risk of weight gain prior to lurasidone treatment. These findings are consistent with the results of prior short- and long-term prospective studies and suggest that lurasidone is associated with low risk for weight gain in patients with schizophrenia or bipolar disorder.

Abbreviations
BMI: body mass index; cm: centimeter; FGA: first-generation antipsychotic; HIPAA: Health Insurance Portability and Accountability Act; ICD-9-CM: International Classification of Diseases, Ninth Revision, Clinical Modification; kg: kilogram; SGA: second-generation antipsychotic; XR: extended release.

Authors' contributions
All authors were involved in the study conception and design, the drafting of the manuscript, and the critical revisions of the manuscript. All authors read and approved the final manuscript.

Author details
[1] Department of Psychiatry, University of California, San Diego, California, USA. [2] Sunovion Pharmaceuticals Inc., 84 Waterford Drive, Marlborough, MA 01752, USA. [3] Vertex Pharmaceuticals, Cambridge, MA, USA. [4] Sunovion Pharmaceuticals Inc., Fort Lee, NJ, USA.

Acknowledgements
Medical writing support was provided by Anita Fitzgerald of York Health Economics Consortium Ltd. and Dr. Michael Stensland of Agile Outcomes Research, Inc., and was funded by Sunovion Pharmaceuticals Inc. Statistical analytical support was provided by Dr. Robert Griffiths of Boston Health Economics which was funded by Sunovion Pharmaceuticals Inc.

Competing interests
Jonathan Meyer, MD, has received research support from Bristol-Myers Squibb, National Institutes of Health (as General Clinical Research Center support), National Institute of Mental Health, and Pfizer Inc., and speaking or advising fees from Acadia Pharmaceuticals, Alkermes, Allergan, Arbor Scientia, Bristol-Myers Squibb Company, Forum Pharmaceuticals Inc., Genentech, Neuroscience Education Institute, Neurocrine, Inc., Otsuka America Inc., Sunovion Pharmaceuticals Inc., and Teva Pharmaceuticals. Daisy Ng-Mak, Ph.D., Krithika Rajagopalan, Ph.D., and Antony Loebel, MD are employees of Sunovion Pharmaceuticals Inc. Chien-Chia Chuang, Ph.D. was an employee of Sunovion Pharmaceuticals Inc. at the time of the development and write-up of the manuscript and is currently an employee at Vertex Pharmaceuticals.

Consent for publication
Not applicable.

Funding
This research was funded by Sunovion Pharmaceuticals Inc., Marlborough, MA, USA.

Previous presentations
Ng-Mak D, Rajagopalan K, Griffiths R, Lin I, Kanevsky E, Loebel A. Patterns of weight change before and after lurasidone initiation in patients with serious mental illness. Poster presented at: College of Psychiatric and Neurologic Pharmacists (CPNP), April 19–22, 2015, Tampa, FL.
Ng-Mak D, Rajagopalan K, Griffiths R, Lin I, Kanevsky E, Loebel A. Weight changes before and after lurasidone treatment in patients with serious mental illness: real-world analysis using electronic health record (EHR). Poster presented at: Academy of Managed Care Pharmacy (AMCP), April 7–10, 2015, San Diego, CA.

Appendix
See Tables 2, 3.

Table 2 ICD-9-CM codes used to classify mental and somatic disorders

Comorbidities	ICD-9-CM codes
Schizophrenia	295.XX
Bipolar disorder	296.01, 296.02, 296.03, 296.04, 296.05, 296.06, 296.40, 296.41, 296.42, 296.43, 296.44, 296.45, 296.46, 296.50, 296.51, 296.52, 296.53, 296.54, 296.55, 296.56, 296.60, 296.61, 296.62, 296.63, 296.64, 296.65, 296.66, 296.7, 296.80, 296.89
Major depressive disorder	296.2X, 296.3X, 311.XX
Substance abuse	296.5x, 303.xx–305.xx
Hypertension	401–405
Hyperlipidemia	272.2–272.4
Diabetes	250.XX
Chronic obstructive pulmonary disease	490–496, 500–505, 506.4

ICD-9-CM The International Classification of Diseases, Ninth Revision, Clinical Modification. ICD-9-CM was the diagnostic coding available in administrative data during the period of this study

Table 3 Medications used in database query

Drug name	Drug name
First-generation antipsychotics	Chlorpromazine, fluphenazine, haloperidol, loxapine, perphenazine, pimozide, thiothixene, thioridazine, and trifluoperazine
Second-generation antipsychotics	Clozapine, olanzapine, quetiapine, risperidone, paliperidone, aripiprazole, ziprasidone, iloperidone, and asenapine
Second-generation antipsychotics that placed patients at higher risk of weight gain	Clozapine, olanzapine, quetiapine, risperidone
Antidepressants	
Diuretics	

References

1. Zhao Z, Okusaga OO, Quevedo J, Soares JC, Teixeira AL. The potential association between obesity and bipolar disorder: a meta-analysis. J Affect Disord. 2016;202:120–3.
2. Flegal KM, Kruszon-Moran D, Carroll MD, Fryar CD, Ogden CL. Trends in obesity among adults in the United States, 2005 to 2014. JAMA. 2016;315:2284–91.
3. Ogden CL, Carroll MD, Fryar CD, Flegal KM. Prevalence of obesity among adults and youth: United States, 2011–2014. NCHS Data Brief. 2015;219:1–8.
4. Catapano L, Castle D. Obesity in schizophrenia: what can be done about it? Australas Psychiatry. 2004;12:23–5.
5. Dickerson FB, Brown CH, Daumit GL, Fang L, Lijuan F, Goldberg RW, et al. Health status of individuals with serious mental illness. Schizophr Bull. 2006;32:584–9.
6. Kolotkin RL, Corey-Lisle PK, Crosby RD, Swanson JM, Tuomari AV, L'italien GJ, et al. Impact of obesity on health-related quality of life in schizophrenia and bipolar disorder. Obesity. 2008;16:749–54.
7. Fagiolini A, Frank E, Houck PR, Mallinger AG, Swartz HA, Buysse DJ, et al. Prevalence of obesity and weight change during treatment in patients with bipolar I disorder. J Clin Psychiatry. 2002;63:528–33.
8. Fagiolini A, Frank E, Scott JA, Turkin S, Kupfer DJ. Metabolic syndrome in bipolar disorder: findings from the Bipolar Disorder Center for Pennsylvanians. Bipolar Disord. 2005;7:424–30.
9. Garcia-Portilla MP, Saiz PA, Benabarre A, Sierra P, Perez J, Rodriguez A, et al. The prevalence of metabolic syndrome in patients with bipolar disorder. J Affect Disord. 2008;106:197–201.
10. McElroy SL, Frye MA, Suppes T, Dhavale D, Keck PE, Leverich GS, et al. Correlates of overweight and obesity in 644 patients with bipolar disorder. J Clin Psychiatry. 2002;63:207–13.
11. Lindenmayer JP, Khan A, Kaushik S, Thanju A, Praveen R, Hoffman L, et al. Relationship between metabolic syndrome and cognition in patients with schizophrenia. Schizophr Res. 2012;142:171–6.
12. American Diabetes Association, American Psychiatric Association, American Association of Clinical Endocrinologists, North American Association for the Study of Obesity. Consensus development conference on antipsychotic drugs and obesity and diabetes. J Clin Psychiatry. 2004;65:267–72.
13. Meyer JM, Mao Y, Pikalov A, Cucchiaro J, Loebel A. Weight change during long-term treatment with lurasidone: pooled analysis of studies in patients with schizophrenia. Int Clin Psychopharmacol. 2015;30:342–50.
14. Newcomer JW. Second-generation (atypical) antipsychotics and metabolic effects: a comprehensive literature review. CNS Drugs. 2005;19(Suppl 1):1–93.
15. Newcomer JW. Metabolic considerations in the use of antipsychotic medications: a review of recent evidence. J Clin Psychiatry. 2007;68(Suppl 1):20–7.
16. Potvin S, Zhornitsky S, Stip E. Antipsychotic-induced changes in blood levels of leptin in schizophrenia: a meta-analysis. Can J Psychiatry. 2015;60:S26–34.
17. Bartoli F, Crocamo C, Clerici M, Carrà G. Second-generation antipsychotics and adiponectin levels in schizophrenia: a comparative meta-analysis. Eur Neuropsychopharmacol. 2015;25:1767–74.
18. Muench J, Hamer AM. Adverse effects of antipsychotic medications. Am Fam Physician. 2010;81:617–22.
19. Leucht S, Cipriani A, Spineli L, Mavridis D, Orey D, Richter F, et al. Comparative efficacy and tolerability of 15 antipsychotic drugs in schizophrenia: a multiple-treatments meta-analysis. Lancet. 2013;382:951–62.
20. Citrome L. Lurasidone for schizophrenia: a review of the efficacy and safety profile for this newly approved second-generation antipsychotic. Int J Clin Pract. 2011;65:189–210.
21. Citrome L. Lurasidone in schizophrenia: new information about dosage and place in therapy. Adv Ther. 2012;29:815–25.
22. De Hert M, Yu W, Detraux J, Sweers K, van Winkel R, Correll CU. Body weight and metabolic adverse effects of asenapine, iloperidone, lurasidone and paliperidone in the treatment of schizophrenia and bipolar disorder. CNS Drugs. 2012;26:733–59.
23. Newcomer J, Tocco M, Pikalov A, Zheng H, Cucchiaro J, Loebel A. Metabolic syndrome in patients with schizophrenia receiving long-term treatment with lurasidone, quetiapine XR, or risperidone. Eur Psychiatry. 2016;33(Suppl 1):107.
24. Ng-Mak DS, Poon JL, Rajagopalan K, Kleinman L, Roberts L, Revicki DA, et al. Qualitative study of patients' preferences for bipolar depression treatment. Value Health. 2015;18:A123.
25. Weiden PJ, Kozma C, Grogg A, Locklear J. Partial compliance and risk of rehospitalization among California Medicaid patients with schizophrenia. Psychiatr Serv. 2004;55:886–91.

26. Weiden PJ, Mackell JA, McDonnell DD. Obesity as a risk factor for antipsychotic noncompliance. Schizophr Res. 2004;66:51–7.

27. Lieberman JA, Stroup TS, McEvoy JP, Swartz MS, Rosenheck RA, Perkins DO, et al. Effectiveness of antipsychotic drugs in patients with chronic schizophrenia. N Engl J Med. 2005;353:1209–23.

28. Knapp M, King D, Pugner K, Lapuerta P. Non-adherence to antipsychotic medication regimens: associations with resource use and costs. Br J Psychiatry. 2004;184:509–16.

29. Panish J, Karve S, Candrilli SD, Dirani R. Association between adherence to and persistence with atypical antipsychotics and psychiatric relapse among US Medicaid-enrolled patients with schizophrenia. J Pharm Health Serv Res. 2013;4:29–39.

30. Stroup TS, Byerly MJ, Nasrallah HA, Ray N, Khan AY, Lamberti JS, et al. Effects of switching from olanzapine, quetiapine, and risperidone to aripiprazole on 10-year coronary heart disease risk and metabolic syndrome status: results from a randomized controlled trial. Schizophr Res. 2013;146:190–5.

31. Stroup TS, McEvoy JP, Ring KD, Hamer RH, LaVange LM, Swartz MS, et al. A randomized trial examining the effectiveness of switching from olanzapine, quetiapine, or risperidone to aripiprazole to reduce metabolic risk: comparison of antipsychotics for metabolic problems (CAMP). Am J Psychiatry. 2011;168:947–56.

32. Uçok A, Gaebel W. Side effects of atypical antipsychotics: a brief overview. World Psychiatry. 2008;7:58–62.

33. Weiden PJ, Newcomer JW, Loebel AD, Yang R, Lebovitz HE. Long-term changes in weight and plasma lipids during maintenance treatment with ziprasidone. Neuropsychopharmacology. 2008;33:985–94.

34. Van Gaal LF. Long-term health considerations in schizophrenia: metabolic effects and the role of abdominal adiposity. Eur Neuropsychopharmacol. 2006;16(Suppl 3):S142–8.

35. Humedica life sciences: detailed clinical data. Humedica, Boston. 2013. http://www.optum.ca/content/dam/optum/resources/productSheets/Optum_Humedica_NorthStar_brochure.pdf. Accessed 06 Mar 2017.

36. Deyo RA, Cherkin DC, Ciol MA. Adapting a clinical comorbidity index for use with ICD-9-CM administrative databases. J Clin Epidemiol. 1992;45:613–9.

37. Tarricone I, Ferrari Gozzi B, Serretti A, Grieco D, Berardi D. Weight gain in antipsychotic-naive patients: a review and meta-analysis. Psychol Med. 2010;40:187–200.

38. Stahl SM, Cucchiaro J, Simonelli D, Hsu J, Pikalov A, Loebel A. Effectiveness of lurasidone for patients with schizophrenia following 6 weeks of acute treatment with lurasidone, olanzapine, or placebo: a 6-month, open-label, extension study. J Clin Psychiatry. 2013;74:507–15.

39. Fagiolini A, Kupfer DJ, Houck PR, Novick DM, Frank E. Obesity as a correlate of outcome in patients with bipolar I disorder. Am J Psychiatry. 2003;160:112–7.

40. McEvoy JP, Citrome L, Hernandez D, Cucchiaro J, Hsu J, Pikalov A, et al. Effectiveness of lurasidone in patients with schizophrenia or schizoaffective disorder switched from other antipsychotics: a randomized, 6-week, open-label study. J Clin Psychiatry. 2013;74:170–9.

41. Citrome L, Weiden PJ, McEvoy JP, Correll CU, Cucchiaro J, Hsu J, et al. Effectiveness of lurasidone in schizophrenia or schizoaffective patients switched from other antipsychotics: a 6-month, open-label, extension study. CNS Spectr. 2014;19:330–9.

42. Blackburn G. Effect of degree of weight loss on health benefits. Obes Res. 1995;3(Suppl 2):211s–6s.

43. Cawley J, Meyerhoefer C, Biener A, Hammer M, Wintfeld N. Savings in medical expenditures associated with reductions in body mass index among US adults with obesity, by diabetes status. Pharmacoeconomics. 2015;33:707–22.

44. Green CA, Yarborough BJH, Leo MC, Yarborough MT, Stumbo SP, Janoff SL, et al. The STRIDE weight loss and lifestyle intervention for individuals taking antipsychotic medications: a randomized trial. Am J Psychiatry. 2015;172:71–81.

45. Newall H, Myles N, Ward PB, Samaras K, Shiers D, Curtis J. Efficacy of metformin for prevention of weight gain in psychiatric populations: a review. Int Clin Psychopharmacol. 2012;27:69–75.

46. Lee CMY, Huxley RR, Wildman RP, Woodward M. Indices of abdominal obesity are better discriminators of cardiovascular risk factors than BMI: a meta-analysis. J Clin Epidemiol. 2008;61:646–53.

47. Franklin R, Zorowitz S, Corse AK, Widge AS, Deckersbach T. Lurasidone for the treatment of bipolar depression: an evidence-based review. Neuropsychiatr Dis Treat. 2015;11:2143–52.

48. Bushe CJ, Slooff CJ, Haddad PM, Karagianis JL. Weight change from 3-year observational data: findings from the worldwide schizophrenia outpatient health outcomes database. J Clin Psychiatry. 2012;73:e749–55.

49. Millen BA, Campbell GM, Beasley CM. Weight changes over time in adults treated with the oral or depot formulations of olanzapine: a pooled analysis of 86 clinical trials. J Psychopharmacol. 2011;25:639–45.

2

Psychological and somatic distress in Chinese outpatients at general hospitals

Nana Xiong[1], Jing Wei[1]*[iD], Kurt Fritzsche[2], Rainer Leonhart[3], Xia Hong[1], Tao Li[1], Jing Jiang[1], Liming Zhu[4], Guoqing Tian[5], Xudong Zhao[6], Lan Zhang[7] and Rainer Schaefert[8]

Abstract

Background: Our study aimed (1) to describe the proportion of psychological distress among Chinese outpatients at general hospitals, (2) to compare cognitive and behavioral characteristics of patients with different distress patterns, and (3) to investigate the discriminant function of the analyzed variables in indicating the affinity towards the different distress patterns.

Methods: This multicenter cross-sectional study was conducted at ten outpatient departments at Chinese general hospitals. The somatic symptom severity scale (PHQ-15), the nine-item depression scale (PHQ-9), and the seven-item anxiety scale (GAD-7) were employed to classify patients in terms of four distress patterns.

Results: A total of 491 patients were enrolled. Among them, the proportion of patients with high psychological distress was significantly higher within those with high somatic distress (74.5% vs. 25.5%, $p < .001$). Patients with psychological distress alone and mixed distress were significantly younger and with lower monthly family income, while the proportion of female patients (80.9%) was highest in the somatic distress group. Patients with mixed distress had the most negative cognitive and behavioral characteristics [highest health anxiety (5.0 ± 1.9), lowest sense of coherence (35.5 ± 10.0), the worst doctor–patient relationship from both patients' (36.0 ± 7.3) and doctors' perspectives (23.3 ± 7.0)], as well as most impaired quality of life (41.6 ± 7.4 and 31.9 ± 10.3). In addition, compared with patients with somatic distress alone, those with psychological distress alone had lower sense of coherence, worse doctor–patient relationship, and more impaired mental quality of life, but less doctor visits. Discriminant analysis showed that gender, mental quality of life, health anxiety, sense of coherence, and frequent doctor visits were significant indicators in identifying patients with different distress patterns.

Conclusions: Our study found that (1) psychological distress was not rare in the Chinese general hospital outpatients, especially in those with high somatic distress; (2) patients with psychological distress alone sought less help from doctors, despite their severe psychosocial impairment; and (3) gender, health anxiety, sense of coherence, mental quality of life, and frequent doctor visits could help to identify different distress patterns.

Keywords: China, Discriminant analysis, General hospital outpatients, Psychological distress, Somatic distress

Background

The most common mental disorders worldwide are depression, anxiety, and somatoform disorders [1–6]. A recent population-based survey on the most frequent mental disorders in Europe found the following prevalence rates: 14.0% for anxiety disorders, 6.9% for major depression, and 6.3% for somatoform disorders [7]. Among those disorders, high comorbidity rates have been observed, leading to further impairment in health-related quality of life (QoL) [8–11].

*Correspondence: weijing@pumch.cn
[1] Department of Psychological Medicine, Peking Union Medical College Hospital, Chinese Academy of Medical Sciences & Peking Union Medical College, Beijing 100730, People's Republic of China
Full list of author information is available at the end of the article

However, the prevalence of depression, anxiety, and somatoform disorders in China differed greatly under different research backgrounds. For example, the lifetime prevalence of affective disorders was only reported as 0.08% in 1998 [12]. Therefore, previously, it was believed that Chinese people are more likely to express somatic symptoms, rather than emotional distress [13, 14]. Nevertheless, more recent epidemiological studies in China have suggested that the rates of depression and anxiety disorders were comparable with those reported in Western countries [15, 16]. A recent study conducted in the Hong Kong general population detected both common somatic and psychological distress [17]. Just like the dimensions of stability and extroversion used to describe the personality types, patients were classified into four distress patterns according to their scores on both the somatic and the psychological dimensions. Even though such categorization was not as rigorous as psychiatric diagnoses, it provided a simple way to assess and distinguish clusters of symptoms among a large sample. Besides, previous research suggested that the elevated self-rated was consistent with the diagnoses of depression/anxiety/somatoform disorders by the general practitioners [1]. Therefore, inspired by the above results, we intend to clarify the proportion of psychological and somatic distress among mainland Chinese general hospital outpatients and the associated frequency of doctor visits.

In addition, a deterioration of the doctor–patient relationship (DPR) has emerged as a highly visible risk in China. As commented by the Lancet, "a third of doctors have experienced conflict and thousands have been injured; the scale, frequency, and viciousness of attacks have shocked the world" [18, 19]. Besides health-care reform and improving hospital governance, to solve the problem of patients' dissatisfaction and violence against doctors, trustful DPR needs to be rebuilt bottom–up. Therefore, it is essential to first to understand what happens in the real world and how patients with different distress patterns experience their DPR. Previous studies found that somatizing patients were less satisfied with their doctors [20], especially when they believed that they were not being understood or did not obtain clear diagnoses or explanations [21]. On the other hand, doctors also experienced more difficulties with patients with multiple somatic symptoms and comorbid mental disorders [22, 23]. However, whether the DPR differed among patients with different distress patterns remained unclear.

Furthermore, how patients understand their symptoms or illness is essential, as it influences their coping behavior [24, 25] and consecutive health outcomes [26]. In our study, we used health anxiety and sense of coherence (SOC) as key elements to reflect illness-related cognitions. Health anxiety has been found to be closely associated with somatization and hypochondriasis in both Western [27] and Chinese populations [28]. The SOC is a theoretical framework that provides an explanation of the role of distress in human functioning, considering comprehensibility, manageability, and meaningfulness when confronted with illnesses [29]. Individuals with strong SOC are capable of perceiving stressors rationally and remain healthy when facing stressful events. Previous studies conducted in China showed that lower SOC were associated with higher depression levels among patients with post-stroke depression [30], and that the SOC of patients with acquired immune deficiency syndrome (AIDS) was lower than the national norms [31]. However, studies were conducted among separate groups of patients with physical or mental illnesses, while the similarities and differences of the cognitive characteristics of patients with different distress patterns remained unclear.

Our previous research has showed that patients with high somatic distress were associated with psychobehavioral features like "catastrophising" and "illness vulnerability" [32]. Comparing with it, this secondary data analysis shifted the focus to the level of psychological distress, and its combination with different level of somatic distress. Besides, unlike the previous research, general health-related indicators were employed for comparisons, like the sense of coherence, and the doctor–patient relationship. Therefore, the aims of this research were threefold: (1) to describe the proportion of psychological distress among Chinese general hospital outpatients; (2) to compare the cognitive and behavioral characteristics patients with different distress patterns; and (3) to investigate the discriminant function of the external sociodemographic, cognitive and behavioral variables in indicating the affinity towards the different distress patterns.

Methods

Study design and setting

A detailed enrollment procedure has already been published [32]. The data was collected in a multicenter cross-sectional study conducted between February 1, 2011 and October 30, 2012 at 10 general hospital outpatient clinics in Beijing, Shanghai, Chengdu, and Kunming. The neurology and gastroenterology departments were chosen to represent the modern biomedicine model. Traditional Chinese Medicine (TCM) departments were selected to represent the traditional medicine model. Psychological medicine departments were chosen to represent the psychosomatic medicine model. On randomly selected screening days, all consecutive patients who entered one of the participating departments were informed about the study and invited to participate by research assistants.

All participants were screened using the 15-item patient health questionnaire (PHQ-15) to assess the severity of somatic symptoms. Recruitment continued until a sample size of 25 patients with high and low somatic distress was enrolled in each medical setting.

Subjects

The inclusion criteria for the study were as follows: 18 years or older, seeking treatment voluntarily for their own problems, and able to read and sign the informed consent form. The exclusion criteria included language barriers or limited writing skills in Mandarin Chinese, cognitive impairment/organic brain disorder/dementia, psychosis, and acute suicidal tendency. The named criteria were clinically assessed by both research assistants (medical students) and medical doctors.

Written informed consent was obtained from all eligible participants. For data analysis, all questionnaires were copied and sent to the study center located at the medical center of Freiburg University, where all data were entered, stored and monitored. The study was approved by the ethics committees of the two principal investigators' (XZ and KF) universities as well as the Shanghai Dong Fang Hospital and the University Medical Centre Freiburg.

Assessment instruments

The 15-item patient health questionnaire (PHQ-15)

The PHQ-15 includes 15 prevalent somatic symptoms or symptom clusters that represent over 90% of the symptoms observed in primary care [33]. Studies in both Western and Chinese populations have exhibited the satisfactory reliability and validity of the PHQ-15 [33–36]. The cut-off score of 10 points was adopted to separate patients with high or low somatic distress, since it was previously identified as optimal for predicting the diagnosis of somatoform disorder [37]. The Cronbach's alpha of the PHQ-15 was .80 in this study. An additional question was included about the symptom duration, and the responses were divided into five categories ("fewer than 4 weeks", "4 weeks to 6 months", "6 months to 1 year", "1 to 2 years" and "greater than 2 years").

The nine-item patient health questionnaire (PHQ-9)

It was used to measure the severity of depression. Respondents were asked to rate the frequency of the symptoms indicated during the past 2 weeks between 0 (not at all) and 3 (nearly every day), resulting in a total score ranging from 0 to 27. It was proved to be reliable and valid to detect major depression in Chinese patients with multiple somatic symptoms at the cut-off point of 10 (sensitivity = .77, specificity = .76) [38]. The Cronbach's alpha of the PHQ-9 was .89 in this study.

The seven-item anxiety scale (GAD-7)

The questionnaire was used to measure the severity of generalized anxiety. A meta-analysis suggested that the GAD-7 had good operating characteristics for detecting generalized anxiety, panic, social anxiety and post-traumatic stress disorder with an optimal cut-off point of 10. Using this cut-off point, the GAD-7 has demonstrated good reliability and validity in screening anxiety disorders in Chinese general hospital outpatients [39]. The Cronbach's alpha of the GAD-7 was .92 in this study.

The Whiteley-7 scale (WI-7)

The instrument was used to assess health-related anxiety by seven items, such as "do you think there is something seriously wrong with your body". It has demonstrated good sensitivity and specificity for screening DSM-IV somatization disorder and hypochondriasis in primary care samples [40, 41]. The Chinese version of the WI-7 has exhibited satisfactory reliability and internal validity in the general population [28]. The Cronbach's alpha of the WI-7 was .75 in this study.

The nine-item sense of coherence scale (SOC-9)

It was employed to assess meaningfulness, comprehensibility and manageability when confronted with illnesses, by asking "do you have the feeling that you are in an unfamiliar situation and don't know what to do", etc. Since the factorial validity of the original SOC-29 was found to be problematic [42], this brief scale was recommended to provide a single-factor solution, with higher scores reflecting a stronger SOC [43]. Our previous research showed that the Chinese version of the SOC-9 was reliable with Chinese general outpatients [44]. The Cronbach's alpha of the SOC-9 was .82 in this study.

The patient–doctor relationship questionnaire (PDRQ-9) and the difficult doctor–patient relationship questionnaire (DDPRQ-10)

They were employed to measure the DPR from patients' and doctors' perspectives, respectively. The PDRQ-9 was derived from the Helping Alliance Questionnaire [45]. Nine items, such as "my doctor helps me", are rated on a Likert-scale from 1 (not appropriate at all) to 5 (totally appropriate), with higher sum scores indicating a better DPR. The doctor-rated DDPRQ-10 was used to measure how difficult the doctor perceived the interaction to be when caring for patients, with items like "how frustrating do you find this patient". Higher sum scores indicate a poorer DPR (range 10–60) [22]. The Cronbach's alpha of the PDRQ-9 and DDPRQ-10 in this study was .93 and .84, respectively. The frequency of doctor visits in the past 12 months was also assessed, and responses were divided into five categories ("0",

"1–2 times", "3–10 times", "11–20 times", and "more than 20 times").

The 12-item short-form health survey (SF-12)

This short version of SF-36 captures practical, reliable, and valid information on health-related QoL in the previous 4 weeks [46], which produces a physical composite score (PCS) and a mental composite score (MCS). The SF-12 has been demonstrated to be reliable and valid for use with the Chinese population [47]. The Cronbach's alpha of the SF-12 was .78 in this study.

Since the SOC-9, PDRQ-9, and DDPRQ-10 were not yet available in Mandarin Chinese, they were translated and back-translated from German using a state-of-the-art test translation procedure. Following the "ITC-Test Adaptation Guidelines" (Version 2000) of the International Test Commission [48], independent translations were translated by three Chinese native speakers (one psychiatrist, one psychologist, and one an educator), who resided in Germany and were fluent in written and spoken German. Translations were discussed during the project meetings until the agreed versions were reached at for the next step. Then, they were back-translated into German and compared with the original German versions to create the final results [32].

Operationalization of the somatic and psychological distress patterns

In our study, a high level of somatic distress was defined as a PHQ-15 total score ≥ 10. High psychological distress was defined as either a PHQ-9 or a GAD-7 total score ≥ 10. Thus, similar to the study performed in Hong Kong [17], our participants were divided into four groups: (1) a low-distress group with low levels of both somatic and psychological distress; (2) a somatically distressed group with a high level of somatic and a low level of psychological distress; (3) a psychologically distressed group with a low level of somatic and a high level of psychological distress; and (4) a mixed distress group with high levels of both somatic and psychological distress.

Statistical procedures

Continuous data were presented as the means and standard deviations and compared using one-way analysis of variance (ANOVA) for the four independent groups. Analysis of covariance was employed to control for the potential bias introduced by different sociodemographic characteristics [49]. Categorical variables were described as absolute and relative frequencies and compared using Chi-square tests. Rank scaled variables were compared using the Kruskal–Wallis test. Since 12 of the 491 (2.4%) participants had missing values on the PHQ-9 and GAD-7 scales, they were replaced with the mean value of the remaining items. A p value of less than .05 (two-tailed) was considered to be significant.

Cramer's V coefficients were calculated to reflect the associations between the four distress groups and other independent variables. Discriminant analyses were employed to investigate the discriminant function of those variables in predicting the different patterns of distress. Even though the distress patterns can be judged by the PHQ-15, PHQ-9, and GAD-7 scores, the multivariate analysis can show if there are predictors beyond these determining variables for the groups. For one thing, it can provide external evidence for the validity of the grouping. For another, it can control the confounding factors during the univariate analyses. The Wilks' lambda stepwise method was adopted. A variable was entered into the model if its F value was greater than 3.84 (p value less than .05) and was removed if the F value was less than 2.71 (p value higher than .10) [50]. Statistical analyses were performed with IBM SPSS Statistics 20.0 and SAS 9.2.

Results

Study sample

Participants were recruited from the biomedical (139/243, 57.2%), TCM (148/250, 59.2%) and psychological (204/306, 66.7%) medical settings. The main reasons for not enrolling were lack of time ($n = 137$, 17.1%), lack of interest in the study ($n = 81$, 10.2%), or other reasons ($n = 38$, 4.8%), such as bad health status, lack of trust, and patients picked up prescriptions for others. Most participants were middle-aged (44.9 ± 16.4), were female (65.4%), were married (61.8%), had medical insurance (84.7%), lived in an urban area (79.6%), lived with others (87.6%), and had an education level higher than middle school (66.5%).

Psychological distress of Chinese general hospital outpatients with high and low somatic distress

According to the study design, an equal number of participants with high and low somatic distress were recruited. Therefore, 238 (48.5%) of all respondents in our study had a PHQ-15 score ≥ 10, among whom 74.5% (149/238) also had high psychological distress. The proportion of high psychological distress in patients with low somatic distress was significantly lower [25.5% (51/253), Chi square $= 91.5$, $p < .001$]. Altogether, 41.1% ($n = 202$) of the patients in our sample had low distress, 18.1% ($n = 89$) had somatic distress alone, 10.4% ($n = 51$) had psychological distress alone, and 30.3% ($n = 149$) had mixed distress.

Sociodemographic characteristics of patients with different distress patterns

As shown in Table 1, patients in both the psychologically distressed group and the mixed distress group were significantly younger. The proportion of female participants was highest in the somatic distress group. After adjustment for age and gender, the four distress groups did not differ significantly on the other sociodemographic characteristics, except that the proportion of families with a low monthly income was higher in the psychologically distressed and mixed distress groups.

In terms of illness duration, approximately 60% of somatically/psychologically distressed/mixed distress participants had been ill for at least 1 year. Among them, the illness duration of patients with mixed distress and somatic distress was significantly longer than those with low distress.

Cognitive characteristics of patients with different distress patterns

Cognitive characteristics were evaluated in terms of health anxiety and SOC. As measured by the WI-7 (see Table 2), mixed distressed patients had the severest health anxiety, whereas somatically and psychologically distressed patients had comparably moderate levels of health anxiety. As reflected by the salutogenic concept

Table 1 Sociodemographic characteristics of patients with different distress patterns ($n = 491$)

	Low-distress group ($n = 202$)	Somatically distressed group ($n = 89$)	Psychologically distressed group ($n = 51$)	Mixed distress group ($n = 149$)	F/χ^2 value	p value
Age (M ± SD)	46.5 ± 16.7[a]	47.7 ± 15.4[a]	41.2 ± 16.5[b]	42.4 ± 16.0[b]	3.6	.014
Female (%)	59.4	80.9	51.0	69.1	18.3	< .001
Insurance (yes %)	85.8	91.0	70.8	84.0	2.5	.060
Residence (%)					1.5	.219
City	82.7	84.3	78.4	73.0		
Rural	17.3	15.7	21.6	27.0		
Marital status (%)					1.0	.388
Single	18.0	11.2	26.0	25.9		
Married	64.5	68.5	48.0	58.5		
Divorced/widowed	17.5	20.2	26.0	15.6		
Life situation (%)					.8	.479
Alone	9.5	11.4	17.6	15.2		
With others	90.5	88.6	82.4	84.8		
Monthly family income (%)					3.1	.027
Less than 4000 RMB	35.6[b]	36.4[b]	52.9[a]	47.6[a]		
4000–8000 RMB	37.6	37.5	27.5	34.5		
More than 8000 RMB	26.7	26.1	19.6	17.9		
Occupation (%)					.3	.835
Employed/student	39.0	33.0	43.1	41.9		
Unemployed	37.4	38.6	27.5	29.7		
Retired	23.6	28.4	29.4	28.4		
Education (%)					2.0	.115
Elementary	10.0	13.5	6.0	11.8		
College preparatory	46.5	48.3	48.0	54.2		
University or higher	43.5	38.2	46.0	34.0		
Illness duration (%)					4.4	.004
< 4 weeks	22.3	9.0	11.8	5.4		
4 weeks–6 months	13.9	19.1	19.6	20.0		
6 months–1 year	14.9	13.5	7.8	12.8		
1–2 years	19.8	15.7	21.6	18.8		
> 2 years	29.2[b]	42.7	39.2[a]	42.3[a]		

Values with [a] were significantly higher than values with [b] in multi-group comparisons; age and gender were controlled for comparisons of other sociodemographic characteristics among the four distress groups

Italic values indicate significance of p value (p<0.05)

Table 2 Clinical characteristics, health-seeking behaviors, and health-related quality of life of patients with different distress patterns ($n = 491$)

	Low-distress group ($n = 202$)	Somatically distressed group ($n = 89$)	Psychologically distressed group ($n = 51$)	Mixed distress group ($n = 149$)	F/χ^2 value	p value
PHQ-15 total score	4.5 ± 2.6^d	12.3 ± 2.3^b	6.2 ± 2.3^c	14.6 ± 5.3^a	415.1	<.001
PHQ-9 total score	4.1 ± 2.8^c	5.7 ± 2.4^b	15.0 ± 4.8^a	15.7 ± 5.2^a	320.3	<.001
GAD-7 total score	2.7 ± 1.7^b	3.7 ± 2.8^b	11.3 ± 3.9^a	10.9 ± 4.6^a	155.6	<.001
WI-7 total score	2.6 ± 1.8^c	4.0 ± 2.0^b	4.0 ± 2.0^b	5.0 ± 1.9^a	44.2	<.001
SOC-9 total score	47.0 ± 8.1^a	46.7 ± 9.1^a	36.8 ± 10.2^b	35.5 ± 10.0^b	54.3	<.001
Doctor visits (%)					4.3	.005
0–2 times	35.6	27.0	37.3	25.5		
3–10 times	40.1	38.2	47.1	36.9		
11–20 times	9.4	10.1	5.9	18.1		
> 20 times	14.9	24.7	9.8	19.5		
PDRQ-9 total score	38.8 ± 5.7^a	38.8 ± 5.7^a	35.1 ± 7.2^b	36.0 ± 7.3^b	6.8	<.001
DDPRQ-10 total score	20.2 ± 7.3^b	19.7 ± 6.9^b	21.8 ± 6.4^a	23.3 ± 7.0^a	6.2	<.001
SF-12 PCS	46.4 ± 7.6^a	44.6 ± 6.7^a	44.7 ± 8.3^a	41.6 ± 7.4^b	13.7	<.001
SF-12 MCS	47.3 ± 8.9^a	46.3 ± 8.6^a	33.8 ± 8.7^b	31.9 ± 10.3^b	90.4	<.001

Values with [a] were significant higher than values with [b], values with [b] were significant higher than values with [c], and values with [c] were significant higher than values with [d] in multi-group comparison. F/χ^2 values and p values were controlled for age and gender

Italic values indicate significance of p value (p<0.05)

of SOC, patients with psychological or mixed distress seemed to manage their health significantly worse than those with low distress and somatic distress.

Help-seeking behavioral characteristics of patients with different distress patterns

Help-seeking behaviors were measured in terms of doctor-visiting frequency and the doctor–patient relationship. As summarized in Table 2, the doctor-visiting frequency of psychologically distressed patients was similar to or even lower than that of patients with low distress. Only 15.7% of them had visited the doctor more than ten times in the past 12 months. However, approximately 35% of the participants in the somatically distressed and mixed distress groups had visited a doctor more than ten times, and approximately 20% of them had done so more than 20 times in the past year. Multi-group comparisons showed that patients with mixed or somatic distress had visited doctors significantly more frequently in the past 12 months than those with low or psychological distress.

Regarding the doctor–patient relationship, psychologically distressed and mixed distress patients rated their DPR as significantly worse than patients with low distress or somatic distress. Interestingly, doctors reported the exact same trend. That is, psychologically distressed and mixed distress patients were considered to be significantly more difficult than their counterparts with low or somatic distress.

Health-related QoL of patients with different distress patterns

As measured by the SF-12 (see Table 2), patients with mixed distress were found to have the lowest PCS, while the other three groups of patients had similar PCS. Regarding the mental QoL, psychologically distressed and mixed distress patients were significantly more impaired than patients with low distress or somatic distress.

Associations between the distress patterns with sociodemographic, cognitive, and help-seeking behavioral characteristics and QoL

Correlation analyses showed that the four distress groups were significantly correlated with sociodemographic [including gender ($r = .193$, $p < .001$) and health insurance ($r = .145$, $p = .018$)], illness duration ($r = .144$, $p = .002$), cognitive characteristics [including total scores of WI-7 ($r = .319$, $p < .001$), and SOC-9 ($r = -.427$, $p < .001$)], and behavioral characteristics [doctor-visiting frequency ($r = .111$, $p = .032$) and patient-experienced good DPR ($r = .285$, $p = .031$)], as well as the physical ($r = .247$, $p < .001$) and mental QoL ($r = .582$, $p < .001$).

A subsequent discriminant analysis was conducted to examine how well these external variables could help to distinguish among the four distress groups. Finally, five independent variables, including gender, mental QoL, total scores of the WI-7 and the SOC-9, and frequent doctor visits remained in the model (see Table 3),

Table 3 Stepwise discriminant function analysis of patients with different distress patterns (n = 491)

	Unstandardized coefficient			Standardized coefficient		
	Function 1	Function 2	Function 3	Function 1	Function 2	Function 3
Gender	− .23	1.13	.11	− .11	.53	.05
SF-12 MCS	.07	.04	− .01	.65	.37	− .08
WI-7	− .20	.37	− .27	− .37	.69	− .50
SOC-9	.03	.02	− .02	.31	.18	− .19
Frequent doctor visits	− .25	.79	1.94	− .11	.36	.87
Constant	− 3.34	− 4.86	1.60	–	–	–
Variance explained	85.8%	13.5%	.7%			

resulting in three discriminant functions. However, the third function could be ignored, since it contributed little to the model (explaining only .7% of the variance).

As shown in Table 4, our model could correctly predict 60.7% membership of the distress patterns. However, due to the smaller group sizes of somatically distressed and psychologically distressed, there were high risks that somatically distressed participants were misclassified as with low distress (51.7%), and psychologically distressed participants were wrongly predicted as with mixed distress (64.7%).

Discussion
Psychological and somatic distress in Chinese general hospital outpatients
Since questionnaires like PHQ-15/PHQ-9/GAD-7 could only provide a one-dimensional assessment of the somatic or psychological distress, the two dimensional assessment and four distress patterns provided a more complete picture. Our study confirmed that psychological burden was not rare in the Chinese general hospital outpatients, especially among those with high somatic distress. According to Lee's study, 5.0, 15.8, and 10.0% of the general population in Hong Kong have been identified as having somatic, psychological, and mixed distress, respectively [17]. Due to our study design, the proportion of each distress pattern could not stand for its distribution in the whole sample of Chinese general

hospital outpatients. Nevertheless, our results showed that patients with mixed distress and somatic distress alone were much common. The distribution of distress patterns between mainland and Hong Kong Chinese might be different. For example, mainland Chinese could be more conservative in expressing their emotions, especially the elderly, and female patients, or patients with higher family income. Further study conducted in the general population of mainland Chinese will help to clarify. Still, this could be enlightening for Chinese clinicians that the demand for mental health service was high, even though psychosomatic medicine as part of a patient's health care is only beginning in China [51].

Somatic/psychological distress and psycho-behavioral characteristics
As evidenced by lower health anxiety and higher SOC, our study showed that patients with mixed distress were strained to the greatest extent in comprehending and managing their illnesses. Since health anxiety has been found to be closely associated with somatization in both Western [27] and Chinese populations [28], and SOC apparently is a resource that enabled people to comprehend, manage and find meaning in their suffering, we have expected that somatically distressed patients had a higher level of health anxiety and lower level of SOC. On the contrary, our study found that psychologically distressed patients had a comparable level of heath anxiety

Table 4 Classification results of the discriminant functions (n = 491)

	Predicted group membership			
	Low distress	Somatically distressed	Psychologically distressed	Mixed distressed
Low distress (n = 202)	(167) 82.7%	(14) 6.9%	(1) .5%	(20) 9.9%
Somatically distressed (n = 89)	(46) 51.7%	(19) 21.3%	(1) 1.1%	(23) 25.8%
Psychologically distressed (n = 51)	(17) 33.3%	(0)	(1) 2.0%	(33) 64.7%
Mixed distressed (n = 149)	(29) 19.5%	(7) 4.7%	(2) 1.3%	(111) 74.5%

The results were computed based on group sizes

as their somatically distressed counterparts, and a significantly lower level of SOC. Possible explanation could be that previously surveyed patients with somatoform disorders were more likely to resemble the mixed distressed patients identified in our study, instead of those with somatic distress alone. And psychological distress itself could also influence patients' cognition negatively. Similarly, a systematic review found that the SOC was strongly related to and predictive of perceived health, especially mental health [52]. Our previous research also found that SOC was correlated with somatic symptom severity as well as the level of depression and generalized anxiety, with stronger correlation coefficients being found for depression and anxiety [44].

In addition, our study revealed that patients with psychological distress visited doctors less frequently, despite their high level of health anxiety and difficulties in understanding their condition. Lee's community-based study also found that only somatic distress predicted health service utilization [17]. As the author noted, the potential reason could be that Chinese people tend not to view psychosocial complaints as a disorder and, thus, prefer to use self-help methods instead of seeking professional help. In addition, it is important to notice that mixed distress patients visited doctors more frequently. Therefore, somatic symptoms might have served as opportunities or "ticket behavior" for them to visit a doctor [53].

In terms of their doctor–patient relationship, psychologically distressed patients and their doctors rated their DPR as more difficult than those with only somatic distress. For a long time, it has been believed that patients with medically unexplained symptoms or somatoform disorders tended to be more unsatisfied with their doctor. As discussed above, it is probably that patients with somatoform disorders addressed mixed distress in our study, instead of somatic distress only. However, it is important to note that psychological distress might play a more important role in DPR than we previously hypothesized. As a previous study suggested, rather than somatic symptom severity, it is the level of depression that predicted patients' experiences of the DPR [54]. Therefore, we assume that multiple somatic symptoms could have an indirect relationship with patients' experiences of the DPR via psychological problems. However, our cross-sectional study design and exploratory research into this topic could not provide solid evidence. To better understand the interrelationships, a new data set from the longitudinal research is needed to test the model with mediation analysis.

Besides, our discriminate analysis and the classification results showed that large percentages of somatically distressed and psychologically distressed patients were misclassified. This furthered reminded us that, in terms of psycho-behavioral characteristic, psychologically distressed individuals resembled those with mixed distress. However, such classification prediction was based on the group sizes. Further studies with different samples and possibly different distribution of distress patterns are needed to examine the predictive ability of those demographic and psycho-behavioral characteristics.

Our study has several limitations. First, an equal number of participants with high and low somatic distress were recruited according to the study design, so that the proportions of different distress patterns in our study could not illustrate their distribution among Chinese general hospital outpatients. In addition, the sample only included patients from the internal medicine. Characteristics of patients from surgical and other departments remained unknown. Furthermore, to ensure the reliability of our results, patients with cognitive impairment, organic brain disorder, dementia, psychosis, and acute suicidal tendency were excluded, which could decrease the proportion of psychological distress. Second, the study was based on general hospital outpatients instead of a community population. Therefore, we did not know the characteristics of somatically or psychologically distressed patients who did not consult with a doctor. Third, only self-report questionnaires have been used to measure somatic and psychological distresses. Structured interviews and psychiatric diagnoses are needed in the future to confirm the spectrum of mental disorders of Chinese outpatients in general hospitals. Fourth, the Chinese versions of the SOC-9, PDRQ-9, and DDPRQ-10 have not been validated, even though their reliability and validity were found to be satisfactory in our study, as mentioned in the methods section. Moreover, even though the measurements have predominantly originated under Western cultural contexts. Future researches could explore the most common emotional and physical complaints of Chinese to better reflect their distress patterns.

Conclusions

In conclusion, our study found that patients with psychological burden were not rare in the Chinese general hospital outpatients, who, however, were less likely to seek help despite the severe psychosocial impairment unless they were bothered by somatic distress at the same time. Therefore, the demand and challenge for mental health service in China were high. Gender, health anxiety, sense of coherence, mental quality of life, and frequent doctor visits could help to identify different distress patterns.

Abbreviations
DDPRQ-10: the difficult doctor–patient relationship questionnaire; DPR: doctor–patient relationship; GAD-7: the seven-item anxiety scale; PDRQ-9: the patient–doctor relationship questionnaire; PHQ-9: the nine-item depression

scale of the patient health questionnaire; PHQ-15: the 15-item somatic symptom scale of the patient health questionnaire; QoL: quality of life; SF-12 MCS: mental composite score of the 12-item short-form health survey; SF-12 PCS: physical composite score of the SF-12; SOC: sense of coherence; SOC-9: the nine-item sense of coherence scale; TCM: Traditional Chinese Medicine; WI-7: the seven-item Whiteley Index.

Authors' contributions
XNN contributed to the primary statistical analysis, data interpretation, and drafting of the manuscript. WJ contributed the conception of this manuscript and was responsible for it. FK and RS were responsible for the design of this study, coordination of the work of study centers, and review of this manuscript. RL contributed to the statistical analysis and data interpretation. HX, LT, JJ, ZLM, TGQ, ZXD, and ZL were responsible for different departments and study centers, as well as for the review of this manuscript. All authors read and approved the final manuscript.

Author details
[1] Department of Psychological Medicine, Peking Union Medical College Hospital, Chinese Academy of Medical Sciences & Peking Union Medical College, Beijing 100730, People's Republic of China. [2] Department of Psychosomatic Medicine and Psychotherapy, University Medical Centre Freiburg, Freiburg, Germany. [3] Institute of Psychology, University of Freiburg, Freiburg, Germany. [4] Department of Gastroenterology, Peking Union Medical College Hospital, Chinese Academy of Medical Sciences & Peking Union Medical College, Beijing, China. [5] Department of Traditional Chinese Medicine, Peking Union Medical College Hospital, Chinese Academy of Medical Sciences & Peking Union Medical College, Beijing, China. [6] Department of Psychosomatic Medicine, Dongfang Hospital, School of Medicine, Tongji University, Shanghai, China. [7] Mental Health Centre, West China Hospital, Sichuan University, Chengdu, Sichuan, China. [8] Department of General Internal Medicine and Psychosomatics, University Hospital Heidelberg, Heidelberg, Germany.

Acknowledgements
We are very grateful to our research assistants in Shanghai (Nan Shen from Dong Fang Hospital, Heng Wu from Tongji University, Weijun Chen from the Shanghai Mental Health Centre), Beijing (Xiayuan Sun from Peking Union Medical College Hospital), Chengdu (Ling Zhang from West China Hospital), and Kunming (Ruixiang Li from Red Cross Hospital of Yunnan Province). Furthermore, we extend our sincere thanks to the German team from the University Medical Centre Freiburg that worked on this study: Wentian Li and Eva März for their work on translation; Elvira Bozkaya for her work on data management; and Emily Engbers, Anika Dold and Ma Lin for their work as data entry assistants. The cooperation of the participating patients is also gratefully acknowledged.

Competing interests
The authors declare that they have no competing interests.

Consent for publication
Not applicable.

Funding
This study was supported by the Centre for Sino-German Research Promotion [Grant Number GZ 690], the Capital Development Fund for Medical Research [Grant Number 2009-3003], and the Mental Health Capacity Building Project by the National Health and Family Planning Commission [Grant Number IHECC2013 MHCB]. All of the authors are independent from the funders. The funders of this study had no role in study design, data collection, data analysis, data interpretation, or writing of the manuscript.

References
1. Hanel G, Henningsen P, Herzog W, Sauer N, Schaefert R, Szecsenyi J, Lowe B. Depression, anxiety, and somatoform disorders: vague or distinct categories in primary care? Results from a large cross-sectional study. J Psychosom Res. 2009;67(3):189–97.
2. Hedman E, Lekander M, Ljotsson B, Lindefors N, Ruck C, Andersson G, Andersson E. Optimal cut-off points on the health anxiety inventory, illness attitude scales and whiteley index to identify severe health anxiety. PLoS ONE. 2015;10(4):e0123412.
3. Roca M, Gili M, Garcia-Garcia M, Salva J, Vives M, Garcia Campayo J, Comas A. Prevalence and comorbidity of common mental disorders in primary care. J Affect Disord. 2009;119(1–3):52–8.
4. Schaefert R, Honer C, Salm F, Wirsching M, Leonhart R, Yang J, Wei J, Lu W, Larisch A, Fritzsche K. Psychological and behavioral variables associated with the somatic symptom severity of general hospital outpatients in China. Gen Hosp Psychiatry. 2013;35(3):297–303.
5. Toft T, Fink P, Oernboel E, Christensen K, Frostholm L, Olesen F. Mental disorders in primary care: prevalence and co-morbidity among disorders. results from the functional illness in primary care (FIP) study. Psychol Med. 2005;35(8):1175–84.
6. Kessler RC, Berglund P, Demler O, Jin R, Merikangas KR, Walters EE. Lifetime prevalence and age-of-onset distributions of DSM-IV disorders in the National Comorbidity Survey Replication. Arch Gen Psychiatry. 2005;62(6):593–602.
7. Wittchen HU, Jacobi F, Rehm J, Gustavsson A, Svensson M, Jonsson B, Olesen J, Allgulander C, Alonso J, Faravelli C, et al. The size and burden of mental disorders and other disorders of the brain in Europe 2010. Eur Neuropsychopharmacol J Eur College Neuropsychopharmacol. 2011;21(9):655–79.
8. Henningsen P, Zimmermann T, Sattel H. Medically unexplained physical symptoms, anxiety, and depression: a meta-analytic review. Psychosom Med. 2003;65(4):528–33.
9. Kroenke K, Spitzer RL, Williams JB, Linzer M, Hahn SR, deGruy FV, Brody D 3rd. Physical symptoms in primary care. Predictors of psychiatric disorders and functional impairment. Arch Fam Med. 1994;3(9):774–9.
10. Lowe B, Spitzer RL, Williams JB, Mussell M, Schellberg D, Kroenke K. Depression, anxiety and somatization in primary care: syndrome overlap and functional impairment. Gen Hosp Psychiatry. 2008;30(3):191–9.
11. de Waal MW, Arnold IA, Eekhof JA, van Hemert AM. Somatoform disorders in general practice: prevalence, functional impairment and comorbidity with anxiety and depressive disorders. Br J Psychiatry J Mental Sci. 2004;184:470–6.
12. Li S, Shen Y, Zhang W, et al. Epidemiological investigation on mental disorders in 7 areas of China. Chin J Psychiatry. 1998;31:69–71.
13. Hsu LK, Folstein MF. Somatoform disorders in Caucasian and Chinese Americans. J Nerv Ment Dis. 1997;185(6):382–7.
14. Parker G, Cheah YC, Roy K. Do the Chinese somatize depression? A cross-cultural study. Soc Psychiatry Psychiatr Epidemiol. 2001;36(6):287–93.
15. Guo WJ, Tsang A, Li T, Lee S. Psychiatric epidemiological surveys in China 1960–2010: how real is the increase of mental disorders? Curr Opin Psychiatry. 2011;24(4):324–30.
16. Phillips MR, Zhang J, Shi Q, Song Z, Ding Z, Pang S, Li X, Zhang Y, Wang Z. Prevalence, treatment, and associated disability of mental disorders in four provinces in China during 2001–05: an epidemiological survey. Lancet. 2009;373(9680):2041–53.
17. Lee S, Leung CM, Kwok KP, Lam Ng K. A community-based study of the relationship between somatic and psychological distress in Hong Kong. Trans Psychiatry. 2015;52(5):594–615.
18. Lancet T. Violence against doctors: why China? Why now? What next? Lancet. 2014;383(9922):1013.
19. Wu LX, Qi L, Li Y. Challenges faced by young Chinese doctors. Lancet. 2016;387(10028):1617.
20. Dhaliwal SK, Hunt RH. Doctor-patient interaction for irritable bowel syndrome in primary care: a systematic perspective. Eur J Gastroenterol Hepatol. 2004;16(11):1161–6.
21. Deale A, Wessely S. Patients' perceptions of medical care in chronic fatigue syndrome. Soc Sci Med 1982. 2001;52(12):1859–64.
22. Hahn SR. Physical symptoms and physician-experienced difficulty in the physician-patient relationship. Ann Intern Med. 2001;134(9 Pt 2):897–904.
23. Hahn SR, Kroenke K, Spitzer RL, Brody D, Williams JB, Linzer M, deGruy FV. The difficult patient: prevalence, psychopathology, and functional impairment. J Gen Intern Med. 1996;11(1):1–8.
24. Dempster M, Howell D, McCorry NK. Illness perceptions and coping in physical health conditions: A meta-analysis. J Psychosomatic Res. 2015;79:506–13.
25. Jones CJ, Smith HE, Llewellyn CD. A systematic review of the effectiveness of interventions using the Common Sense Self-Regulatory Model to improve adherence behaviours. J Health Psychol. 2015;21:2709–24.

26. Hudson JL, Bundy C, Coventry PA, Dickens C. Exploring the relationship between cognitive illness representations and poor emotional health and their combined association with diabetes self-care. A systematic review with meta-analysis. J Psychosom Res. 2014;76(4):265–74.

27. Hiller W, Rief W, Fichter MM. Dimensional and categorical approaches to hypochondriasis. Psychol Med. 2002;32(4):707–18.

28. Lee S, Ng KL, Ma YL, Tsang A, Kwok KP. A general population study of the Chinese Whiteley-7 index in Hong Kong. J Psychosom Res. 2011;71(6):387–91.

29. Antonovsky A. Health, stress and coping. San Francisco: Jossey-Bass; 1979.

30. Huang L, Lou X, Wang A. The association between post-stroke depression and sense of coherence and social support. Chin J Gerontol. 2016;36(18):4614–6.

31. Chen J, Wu J, Liu X. Impact of sense of coherence on coping style in patients with AIDS. Chin J Modern Nurs. 2016;22(10):1436–8.

32. Zhang Y, Fritzsche K, Leonhart R, Zhao X, Zhang L, Wei J, Yang J, Wirsching M, Nater-Mewes R, Larisch A, et al. Dysfunctional illness perception and illness behaviour associated with high somatic symptom severity and low quality of life in general hospital outpatients in China. J Psychosom Res. 2014;77(3):187–95.

33. Kroenke K, Spitzer RL, Williams JB. The PHQ-15: validity of a new measure for evaluating the severity of somatic symptoms. Psychosom Med. 2002;64(2):258–66.

34. Lee S, Ma YL, Tsang A. Psychometric properties of the Chinese 15-item patient health questionnaire in the general population of Hong Kong. J Psychosom Res. 2011;71(2):69–73.

35. Qian J, Ren Z, Yu D, He X, Li C. patient health questionnaire Patient Health Questionnaire-15(PHQ-15) reliability validity detection rate psychometrics. Chin Mental Health J. 2014;28(3):173–8.

36. Zhang L, Fritzsche K, Liu Y, Wang J, Huang M, Wang Y, Chen L, Luo S, Yu J, Dong Z, et al. Validation of the Chinese version of the PHQ-15 in a tertiary hospital. BMC psychiatry. 2016;16:89.

37. Korber S, Frieser D, Steinbrecher N, Hiller W. Classification characteristics of the Patient Health Questionnaire-15 for screening somatoform disorders in a primary care setting. J Psychosom Res. 2011;71(3):142–7.

38. Xiong N, Fritzsche K, Wei J, Hong X, Leonhart R, Zhao X, Zhang L, Zhu L, Tian G, Nolte S, et al. Validation of patient health questionnaire (PHQ) for major depression in Chinese outpatients with multiple somatic symptoms: a multicenter cross-sectional study. J Affect Disord. 2015;174:636–43.

39. He R, Qin X, Ai L, Li Y, Wang W, Jin Q, Liu L, Dong G. Prevalence of anxiety disorders of outpatients in internal medicine departments of general hospitals at different level. Clin J Public Health. 2008;24(6):702–4.

40. Conradt M, Cavanagh M, Franklin J, Rief W. Dimensionality of the Whiteley Index: assessment of hypochondriasis in an Australian sample of primary care patients. J Psychosom Res. 2006;60(2):137–43.

41. Fink P, Ewald H, Jensen J, Sørensen L, Engberg M, Holm M, Munk-Jørgensen P. Screening for somatization and hypochondriasis in primary care and neurological in-patients: a seven-item scale for hypochondriasis and somatization. J Psychosom Res. 1999;46(3):261–73.

42. Flannery RB Jr, Perry JC, Penk WE, Flannery GJ. Validating Antonovsky's Sense of Coherence Scale. J Clin Psychol. 1994;50(4):575–7.

43. Schumacher J, Wilz G, Gunzelmann T, Brähler E. Antonovsky's sense of coherence scale—its validation in a population based sample and the development of a new short scale. Psychother Psychosom Med Psychol. 2000;50:472–82.

44. Li W, Leonhart R, Schaefert R, Zhao X, Zhang L, Wei J, Yang J, Wirsching M, Larisch A, Fritzsche K. Sense of coherence contributes to physical and mental health in general hospital patients in China. Psychol Health Med. 2015;20(5):614–22.

45. Van der Feltz-Cornelis CM, Van Oppen P, Van Marwijk HW, De Beurs E, Van Dyck R. A patient-doctor relationship questionnaire (PDRQ-9) in primary care: development and psychometric evaluation. Gen Hosp Psychiatry. 2004;26(2):115–20.

46. Ware J Jr, Kosinski M, Keller SD. A 12-Item short-form health survey: construction of scales and preliminary tests of reliability and validity. Med Care. 1996;34(3):220–33.

47. Lam CL, Tse EY, Gandek B. Is the standard SF-12 health survey valid and equivalent for a Chinese population? Qual Life Res Int J Qual Life Aspects Treat Care Rehab. 2005;14(2):539–47.

48. Hambleton RK, Merenda PF, Spielberger CD. Adapting educational and psychological tests for cross-cultural assessment. Mahwah: Lawrence Erlbaum Associates; 2005.

49. Pocock SJ, Assmann SE, Enos LE, Kasten LE. Subgroup analysis, covariate adjustment and baseline comparisons in clinical trial reporting: current practice and problems. Stat Med. 2002;21(19):2917–30.

50. Bartels PH, Bartels HG. Discriminant analysis. Anal Quant Cytol Histol. 2009;31(5):247–54.

51. Wei J, Zhang L, Zhao X, Fritzsche K. Current trends of psychosomatic medicine in China. Psychother Psychosom. 2016;85(6):388–90.

52. Eriksson M, Lindstrom B. Antonovsky's sense of coherence scale and the relation with health: a systematic review. J Epidemiol Community Health. 2006;60(5):376–81.

53. Ryder AG, Chentsova-Dutton YE. Depression in cultural context: "Chinese somatization," revisited. Psychiatric Clin N Am. 2012;35(1):15–36.

54. Wu H, Zhao X, Fritzsche K, Leonhart R, Schaefert R, Sun X, Larisch A. Quality of doctor-patient relationship in patients with high somatic symptom severity in China. Complement Ther Med. 2015;23(1):23–31.

3

Knowledge of and attitudes towards electroconvulsive therapy (ECT) among psychiatrists and family physicians in Saudi Arabia

Ahmad N. AlHadi[1,2*], Fahad M. AlShahrani[3,4], Ali A. Alshaqrawi[5], Mohanned A. Sharefi[6] and Saud M. Almousa[7]

Abstract

Objectives: To assess the knowledge of and attitudes towards ECT among psychiatrists and family physicians in Saudi Arabia.

Methods: The study is quantitative observational cross-sectional with a convenient sample that included psychiatrists and family physicians (including residents) in Saudi Arabia.

Results: Of the 434 questionnaires emailed, a total of 126 returned completed questionnaires (29% response rate). The mean age of respondents was 35 years old. Psychiatrists accounted for 68.3%. The majority were Saudis (95.2%) and male (70.6%). Around half were consultants and about two-thirds (62.7%) had worked in a facility that used ECT. Psychiatrists showed better knowledge than family physicians in their answers, with a mean total knowledge scoring of 8.12 (±1.25) out of 10 and 6.15 (±1.25), respectively (P < 0.0001). Among psychiatrists, 87% thought that ECT required general anesthesia, while 35% of family physicians believed so (P < 0.0001). Other items of ECT knowledge are discussed. Psychiatrists displayed a better attitude towards ECT than family physicians in all answers, with a mean score of 9.54 (±1.16) and 7.85 (±2.39), respectively (P < 0.0001).

Conclusions: Psychiatrists scored better than family physicians in both knowledge and attitude regarding ECT.

Keywords: Electroconvulsive therapy, ECT, Psychiatrist, Family physician, Knowledge, Attitude, Saudi Arabia

Background

Electroconvulsive therapy (ECT) is a therapeutic method used in the psychiatric field, first established in the 1930s [1]. It was proven then that ECT could be a life-saving modality, decreasing suicidal ideations and suicide attempts in severe cases of depression [2]. Some studies in Poland and Slovakia revealed that ECT is primarily indicated for affective disorders like depression [3], while schizophrenia was the main indication for ECT in eastern Europe and Asia [4]. A recent study found that ECT is used more often than medications in severe cases

*Correspondence: alhadi@ksu.edu.sa
[1] Department of Psychiatry, College of Medicine, King Saud University, King Saud University Medical City, PO Box 242069, Riyadh 11322, Saudi Arabia
Full list of author information is available at the end of the article

of depression [5]. Several studies did not find any serious side effects of ECT such as epilepsy, brain damage, and pain [6, 7]. The occurrence of permanent memory loss with ECT is uncommon [8]. Even if memory loss occurs, it usually spares emotional and personal memories [9].

Although ECT was found to be safe and effective [7], usage has declined by 80% among Hungarian psychiatrists in the past few years [10]. Also, half of Chuvash Republic psychiatrists believe that ECT is dangerous and it should be used as a last modality of treatment [4]. Additionally, only one-third of psychiatrists in Greece and Hungary would accept ECT as a treatment for themselves if they needed it [9, 10], while Romanian psychiatrists showed a more receptive attitude towards receiving ECT (47.5%) [11]. One of the reasons behind decreased use of ECT is poor knowledge [12, 13]. However, a

Romanian paper found no correlation between knowledge and attitude among psychiatrists [11]. On the other hand, 86.3% of Indian psychiatrists preferred that ECT be available in general psychiatric clinics [14] and most Nigerian psychiatrists recommend using ECT when it suits their patients [12].

Non-psychiatric physicians have a more negative attitude towards ECT. Also, it was found that only 22% of non-psychiatric physicians would prefer ECT over pharmacological medications, even though they all knew that ECT would be more effective than medications. In addition, the same study showed that those non-psychiatric physicians who had not completed specialty training (i.e., general practitioners and trainees) had a more positive attitude towards ECT. Nevertheless, all still held negative attitudes [9]. Furthermore, in Nigeria, almost three-quarters of psychiatric nurses believed that ECT was helpful for most psychiatric patients [15]. A recent study found that neurologists and family practitioners needed to have more knowledge of ECT [7].

Sources of knowledge can be of a great effect on the attitude towards ECT. Media was found to be the primary source of ECT knowledge for medical and nursing students [7, 16], which usually has negative image influence on the attitude [7, 16, 17]. Poor ECT education in medical schools' curricula may cause defect in physicians' attitude [4]. However, clinical practice and acquiring more knowledge of ECT promote a positive attitude towards its usage [16, 18]. A study conducted with medical students in three countries (Iraq, Egypt and United Kingdom) found that the attitudes towards ECT were affected by socio-cultural factors and the modalities of education [1], while some studies revealed no socio-cultural effect on the attitude [7]. It has been observed that in many countries, there is a demand for improving education and training for ECT among students, non-psychiatric physicians, and psychiatrists themselves [9, 10].

This study aims to assess the knowledge of and attitude towards ECT among psychiatrists and family physicians in Saudi Arabia.

Methods

The study is quantitative observational cross-sectional.

Participants

We used a convenient sampling method to include all the psychiatrists and family physicians (including residents) in Saudi Arabia who we can reach. We were able to obtain their emails or phone numbers from the Saudi Commission for Health Specialties, hospital departments, university departments, and through colleagues. The three inclusion criteria were as follows: a psychiatrist

or a family physician (including residents in training); and able to read and understand English language; and have a history of practicing medicine in Saudi Arabia.

Questionnaire

An electronic survey was emailed and sent through WhatsApp (a messaging social media application). We used a scale that has been used in previous study, so no pilot study was done. We got the permission from the author [10].

The questionnaire consists of three sections: (1) demographic data and few questions about ECT experience; (2) knowledge of ECT (10 items with total score of 10); and (3) attitudes towards ECT (11 items with total score of 11). We decided to remove one item in the knowledge subscale which was "the efficacy of the convulsive treatment has been discovered by a Hungarian psychiatrist." We think that this item is not necessary for Saudi psychiatrists or family physicians to know. Also, we changed "Hungary" to "Saudi Arabia" in some items to be more appropriate.

Data analysis

Data were analyzed by the Statistical Package for Social Sciences (SPSS) [19] (Armonk, NY, USA), version 21.0. Descriptive statistical data are presented by mean values, standard deviations, and percentages. T tests, Chi square, and Analysis of variance (ANOVA) were used to compare subgroups. Additionally, the relationship between different variables was assessed by Pearson's correlation. Statistical significance was set at 0.05.

Results
Study subjects

An online survey was sent to 435 psychiatrists and family physicians in Saudi Arabia. Completed questionnaires were returned by 126 (29% response rate). Psychiatrists comprised 68.3% ($n = 86$) of respondents; 31.7% ($n = 40$) were family physicians and general practitioners (GPs). The mean age of psychiatrists and family physicians was 34.45 (SD = 7.16) and 35.20 (SD = 7.01), respectively. The majority were male (70.6%), Saudis (95.2%), and then working in the Kingdom of Saudi Arabia (92.1%). Consultants accounted for around half of the respondents (46.8%), while 21.4% were specialists and 31.7% were residents. Most of the respondents worked in general hospitals (32.5%) followed by university hospitals (23.8%), then psychiatric hospitals (15.9%), while primary care centers accounted for only 11.9%. In addition, 15.1% worked in more than one setting. Around 44.4% of responders rated themselves as having medium knowledge of ECT, 34.1% minimal knowledge, and 21.4% a high level of knowledge. Finally, 62.7% have worked in an ECT-utilizing facility. Around 80% of psychiatrists had referred patients for ECT and would consent to receive it themselves if needed. However, among family physicians, only 5% had referred patients for ECT, and 57.5% would agree to receive it themselves ($P \leq 0.001$). Demographic data are shown in Table 1.

Knowledge

Regarding questions concerning ECT knowledge, about 60% of psychiatrists answered all questions (10 questions) correctly except for one, which concerned whether long seizure duration resulted in more effective treatment. Among family physicians, 60% answered only five

Table 1 Demographics and personal data, ECT preferences, and experience

Item	Mean or N (SD or %)			P value
	Psychiatrists N = 86 (68%)	Family physicians N = 40 (32%)	All N = 126 (100%)	
Age (mean, SD)	34.45 (7.16)	35.20 (7.01)	34.69 (7.09)	0.582
Gender				
Male	62 (72.1%)	27 (30.3%)	89 (70.6%)	0.598
Female	24 (27.9%)	13 (35.1%)	37 (29.4%)	
Education				
Resident	31 (36%)	9 (22.5%)	40 (31.8%)	0.217
Specialist (registrar)	19 (22%)	8 (20%)	27 (21.4%)	
Consultant	36 (42%)	23 (57.5%)	59 (46.8)	
Saudi	80 (93%)	40 (100%)	120 (95.2%)	0.087
Non-Saudi	6 (7%)	0 (0.0%)	6 (4.8%)	
Current work country				
Inside KSA	76 (88.4%)	40 (100%)	116 (92.1%)	0.025
Outside KSA	10 (11.6%)	0 (0.0%)	10 (7.9%)	
Region				
Riyadh	60 (70%)	24 (60%)	84 (66.7%)	0.279
Outside Riyadh	26 (30%)	16 (40%)	42 (33.3%)	
Place of work				
University	23 (27%)	7 (17.5%)	30 (24%)	0.0001
General hospital	31 (36.5%)	16 (40%)	37 (29.6%)	
Psychiatric hospital	31 (36.5%)	0 (0%)	31 (24.8%)	
Primary care center	0 (0.0%)	17 (42.5%)	17 (13.6%)	
My knowledge about ECT				
Minimal	13 (15%)	30 (75%)	43 (34.1%)	0.0001
Medium	48 (56%)	8 (20%)	56 (44.5%)	
High level	25 (29%)	2 (5%)	27 (21.4%)	
Have you ever worked in an ECT-utilizing department?				
Yes	73 (85%)	6 (15%)	79 (62.7%)	0.0001
No	13 (15%)	34 (85%)	47 (37.3%)	
Have you ever referred patients to ECT?				
Yes	66 (76.7%)	2 (5%)	68 (54%)	0.0001
No	20 (23.3%)	38 (95%)	58 (46%)	
Is there any ECT-treated person in your family or among your acquaintances?				
Yes	6 (7%)	2 (5%)	8 (6.3%)	0.67
No	80 (93%)	38 (95%)	118 (93.7%)	
Do you have a psychiatric illness in your family or in your acquaintances?				
Yes	35 (40.7%)	12 (30%)	47 (37.3%)	0.25
No	51 (59.3%)	28 (70%)	79 (62.7%)	
I would consent to receive ECT in case I was in a psychotic depressive condition				
Yes	72 (83.7%)	23 (57.5%)	95 (75.4%)	0.001
No	14 (16.3%)	17 (42.5%)	31 (24.6%)	

questions correctly out of 10 questions. Psychiatrists displayed better knowledge than family physicians in response to most questions, with a Total Knowledge Score on 10 questions of 8.12 ($\pm$1.25) and 6.15 ($\pm$1.25), respectively ($P < 0.0001$). Among psychiatrists, 87.2% thought that ECT required general anesthesia (GA) and 86% agreed that muscle relaxation is mandatory to do ECT. However, family physicians accounted for 35 and 70% on the previous two questions, respectively. Moreover, 91.9% of psychiatrists knew the number of recommended ECT weekly sessions, while only about 50% of family physicians did ($P < 0.0001$). Furthermore, about half of the family physicians agreed that ECT relieves depression faster than drugs and that it is contraindicated in patients with a history of MI, although psychiatrists scored better on both questions (74.4 and 94.2%, respectively). As for using ECT with patients aged 65 years, 88.4% of psychiatrists but only 35% of family physicians considered it acceptable ($P < 0.0001$). On the other hand, the only item family physicians answered correctly more frequently higher psychiatrists was, "The longer the seizure duration, the more effective the treatment" 87.5 versus 47.7% ($P < 0.0001$). Answers to all the items on the knowledge subscale showed a statistical significance difference between psychiatrists and family physicians except numbers 2 and 3 (Table 2).

Attitude

Psychiatrists showed a more positive attitude than family physicians in all questions, except for item numbers 2, 3, 4, and 7, with scores of 9.54 ($\pm$1.16) and 7.85 ($\pm$2.39) out of 11, respectively ($P < 0.0001$), as shown in Table 3. None of the responders agreed that ECT is used as a

punishment. Almost all psychiatrists (96.5%) and almost three-quarters (72.5%) of family physicians believed that ECT does not cause death or permanent brain damage ($P < 0.0001$). Also, roughly 95% of psychiatrists and 80% of family physicians disagreed with the statements that ECT should be illegal and is abused by psychiatrists. However, more than half of family physicians thought that ECT is only used as a final resort and among minority populations, while roughly 30% of psychiatrists agreed with that statement. Responses to the statement "ECT is used more often for treating the poor people" showed statistical insignificance difference.

Knowledge and attitude
There was positive correlation between the mean of total knowledge score and the mean of total attitude score and it was statistically significant ($r = 0.375, P < 0.0001$).

Discussion
This study assessed knowledge of and attitudes towards ECT among psychiatrists and family physicians in Saudi Arabia. Our results demonstrate that psychiatrists had better knowledge of ECT than family physicians, with the exception of one question concerning the duration of seizure. This issue is controversial. It was previously thought that "The longer the seizure duration, the more effective the treatment" is true but recent studies showed no relationship [20, 21]. Also, this difference might be explained by a better understanding of brain physiology among family physicians. Both groups in this study agreed that ECT is neither dangerous nor does it cause death. However, a recent study showed that only half of surveyed Russian psychiatrists believe that ECT is not dangerous

Table 2 Differences between psychiatrists and family physicians in knowledge scale

Knowledge scale	Correct answer (better knowledge)			P value
	Psychiatrists N = (86)	Family physicians N = (40)	All N = (126)	
ECT is used more often in Saudi Arabia than in the USA (F)	84 (97.7%)	35 (87.5%)	119 (94.4%)	0.020
ECT has been used for the first time in the 1930s (T)	54 (62.8%)	30 (75.0%)	84 (66.7%)	0.176
The anesthetic level during ECT should be as deep as possible (F)	70 (81.4%)	29 (72.5%)	99 (78.6%)	0.257
ECT is more effective, and helps to relieve depression faster than drugs do (T)	81 (94.2%)	22 (55.0%)	103 (81.7%)	0.0001
ECT is contraindicated in patients with prior history of myocardial infarction (F)	64 (74.4%)	21 (52.5%)	85 (67.5%)	0.015
In Saudi Arabia ECT can be administered only under general anesthesia (T)	75 (87.2%)	14 (35.0%)	89 (70.6%)	0.0001
ECT can be done in Saudi Arabia without muscle relaxation (F)	74 (86.0%)	28 (70.0%)	102 (81.0%)	0.033
ECT can be used over the age of 65 (T)	76 (88.4%)	14 (35.0%)	90 (71.4%)	0.0001
The longer the seizure duration, the more effective the treatment (F)	41 (47.7%)	35 (87.5%)	76 (60.3%)	0.0001
Recommended weekly frequency of the sessions are two or three (T)	79 (91.9%)	18 (45.0%)	97 (77.0%)	0.0001
Total knowledge score: mean (SD)	8.12 (1.25)	6.15 (1.25)	7.49 (1.55)	0.0001

Table 3 Differences between psychiatrists and family physicians in Attitude scale

Attitudes scale	Correct answer (positive attitude)			P value
	Psychiatrists N = 86	Family physicians N = 40	All N = 126	
Psychiatrists often abuse ECT	81 (94.2%)	32 (80.0%)	113 (89.7%)	0.015
ECT is used to control violent patients	64 (74.4%)	29 (72.5%)	93 (73.8%)	0.820
ECT is used as a punishment	86 (100%)	40 (100%)	126 (100%)	None
ECT can cause pain	55 (64.0%)	21 (52.5%)	76 (60.35%)	0.221
ECT is dangerous and may cause death	83 (96.5%)	29 (72.5%)	112 (88.9%)	0.0001
ECT should only be used as a final resort	61 (70.9%)	16 (40.0%)	77 (61.1%)	0.001
ECT is used more often for treating the poor people	81 (94.2%)	35 (87.5%)	116 (92.1%)	0.196
ECT is used more often in minority populations	59 (68.6%)	19 (47.5%)	78 (61.9%)	0.023
ECT is an outdated, obsolete procedure	82 (95.3%)	31 (77.5%)	113 (89.7%)	0.002
ECT can cause permanent brain damage	83 (96.5%)	29 (72.5%)	112 (88.9%)	0.0001
ECT should be illegal to perform	85 (98.8%)	33 (82.5%)	118 (93.7%)	0.0001
Total attitude score	9.54 (1.16)	7.85 (2.39)	9.00 (1.82)	0.0001

[4]. We believe that the improvement in the education in the medical colleges in KSA has influenced the outcome. More than half of family physicians knew that ECT relieves depression faster than drugs do. Nevertheless, around three-quarters of non-psychiatric physicians in a Greek study chose medications over ECT, despite their knowledge [9]. The explanation might be that family physicians encounter more cases and they interact more often with psychiatric physicians compared to non-psychiatric physicians (surgical and non-surgical physicians) in Greece. However, psychiatrists scored better on both questions (94.2 and 74.4%, respectively). Moreover, 91.9% of psychiatrists knew the correct number of recommended ECT weekly sessions compared to around 50% of family physicians. As the psychiatrists have a chance to practice ECT, this influenced their knowledge.

Psychiatrists showed a better attitude than family physicians in all attitudes-related questions. These findings were similar to those of a study conducted in Greece [9]. This might be explained by psychiatrists utilize ECT more often and aware of its outcome than family physicians. Similar explanation was found on other studies in British Columbia and Australia [16, 18]. In this study, 83% of psychiatrists are willing to receive ECT when indicated, which shows higher attitude compared to Greek, Hungarian, and Romanian psychiatrists [9–11]. Based on these studies and the current study, having more training and experience may improve attitude. We may link this progress to poor education in the past among medical students, non-psychiatric physicians, and even psychiatrists [4, 9, 10]. One of the reasons that a small percentage of psychiatrists were unwilling to receive ECT in the past was fear of being embarrassed if their colleagues saw experiencing incontinence during the ECT session.

Psychiatrists might also refuse ECT because they refused to believe they are ill [9] (Tables 4, 5).

Sources of knowledge can greatly influence the attitude towards ECT. Media and poor medical school curricula have a negative impact on the attitude towards and knowledge of ECT [7, 16, 17]. The media, especially in movies, represent ECT in a wrong way, depicting it as torture that destroys memories. A short psychiatry rotation and inadequate clinical exposure contribute to poor knowledge and attitude [1]. This may lead to poor knowledge among future psychiatrists as this previously affected the psychiatrists in Texas and Nigeria [12, 13]. Even though a study showed no link between knowledge and attitude [11], we believe that knowledge of ECT plays a major role. In this study, we noticed that the psychiatrists group had a higher knowledge score compared than the other group, which may reflect on their high attitude score also. This is supported by the significant positive correlation between knowledge and attitude in this study. Furthermore, another possible factor is the socio-cultural environment, which has a great effect on this society. This was observed in another study in three other countries [1]. Yet another paper was done in Turkey on medical students, psychology students, and lay people found no significance [7]. In our study, the questionnaire that we adapted did not have the option of "I do not know," which may have affected the participants' response accuracy.

Conclusion
We concluded that psychiatrists have better knowledge and attitude towards ECT than Family Physicians. From our observation, there is a correlated relation between the knowledge and attitude.

Table 4 Total knowledge score

Item	Psychiatrists (mean)	P value	Family physicians (mean)	P value	All	P value
Age	r = 0.140	0.203	r = −0.220	0.173	r = −0.007	0.936
Gender						
Male	8.18	0.469	6.22	0.605	7.58	0.302
Female	7.96		6.00		7.27	
Education						
Resident	7.87	0.398	6.00	0.497	7.45	0.551
Specialist (registrar)	8.26		6.63		7.78	
Consultant	8.25		6.04		7.39	
Saudi	8.06	0.146	6.15	No comparison	7.43	
Non-Saudi	8.83		0.0[a]		8.83	0.029
Current work country						
Inside KSA	8.05	0.195	6.15	No comparison	7.40	0.018
Outside KSA	8.60		0.0[a]		8.60	
Region						
Riyadh	8.03	0.353	6.38	0.167	7.56	0.491
Outside Riyadh	8.31		5.81		7.36	
Place of work						
University	8.13	0.955	6.29	0.915	7.70	0.0001
General hospital	8.16		6.19		7.49	
Psychiatric hospital	8.07		0.0[a]		8.07	
Primary care center	0.0[a]		6.06		6.06	
My knowledge about ECT						
Minimal	7.85	0.360	6.00	0.226	6.56	0.0001
Medium	8.04		6.38		7.80	
High level	8.40		7.50		8.33	
Have you ever worked in an ECT-utilizing department?						
Yes	8.21	0.117	5.67	0.311	8.01	0.0001
No	7.62		6.24		6.62	
Is there any ECT-treated person in your family or among your acquaintances?						
Yes	8.67	0.266	5.50	0.458	7.88	0.472
No	8.08		6.18		7.47	
Do you have a psychiatric illness in your family or in your acquaintances?						
Yes	8.26	0.390	6.08	0.829	7.70	0.242
No	8.02		6.18		7.37	
I would consent to receive ECT in case I was in a psychotic depressive condition						
Yes	8.19	0.190	6.35	0.250	7.75	0.001
No	7.71		5.88		6.71	

[a] Not included in the analysis

Table 5 Total attitude score

Item	Psychiatrists (mean)	P value	Family physicians (mean)	P value	All	P value
Age	$r = 0.190$	0.081	$r = 0.080$	0.625	$r = 0.094$	0.298
Gender						
Male	9.65	0.156	7.70	0.584	9.06	0.593
Female	9.25		8.15		8.87	
Education						
Resident	9.29	0.310	7.56	0.917	8.90	0.913
Specialist (registrar)	9.58		7.88		9.07	
Consultant	9.72		7.96		9.03	
Saudi	9.56	0.421	7.85	No comparison	8.99	0.819
Non-Saudi	9.17		0.0[a]		9.17	
Current work country						
Inside KSA	9.47	0.092	7.85	No comparison	8.91	0.070
Outside KSA	10.00		0.0[a]		10.00	
Region						
Riyadh	9.60	0.430	8.13	0.380	9.18	0.120
Outside Riyadh	9.39		7.44		8.64	
Place of work						
University	9.78	0.412	8.00	0.161	9.37	0.198
General hospital	9.55		7.00		8.68	
Psychiatric hospital	9.36		0.0[a]		9.36	
Primary care center	0.0[a]		8.59		8.59	
My knowledge about ECT						
Minimal	8.92	0.116	7.57	0.216	7.98	0.0001
Medium	9.65		8.25		9.45	
High level	9.64		10.50		9.70	
Have you ever worked in an ECT-utilizing department?						
Yes	9.70	0.001	9.00	0.205	9.65	0.0001
No	8.62		7.65		7.92	
Is there any ECT-treated person in your family or among your acquaintances?						
Yes	10.00	0.123	6.50	0.420	9.13	0.842
No	9.50		7.92		8.99	
Do you have a psychiatric illness in your family or in your acquaintances?						
Yes	9.77	0.116	7.17	0.242	9.11	0.615
No	9.37		8.14		8.94	
I would consent to receive ECT in case I was in a psychotic depressive condition						
Yes	9.60	0.259	7.78	0.839	9.16	0.146
No	9.21		7.94		8.52	

[a] Not included in the analysis

Limitations

We recommend including the option "I do not know" in the answers to improve the accuracy of participants' responses.

Abbreviations

ECT: electroconvulsive therapy; GA: general anesthesia; GPs: general practitioners; ANOVA: analysis of variance; KSA: Kingdom of Saudi Arabia.

Authors' contributions

ANA was the principal investigator, participated in the study design, manuscript writing, data collecting, and analysis. FMA, AAA, MAS, SMA participated in the study design, data collection, and writing the manuscript. All authors read and approved the final manuscript.

Author details

[1] Department of Psychiatry, College of Medicine, King Saud University, King Saud University Medical City, PO Box 242069, Riyadh 11322, Saudi Arabia. [2] SABIC Psychological Health Research & Applications Chair (SPHRAC), College of Medicine, King Saud University, King Saud University Medical City, PO Box 242069, Riyadh 11322, Saudi Arabia. [3] Family Medicine Department, King Abdulaziz Medical City, National Guard, Riyadh, Saudi Arabia. [4] College of Medicine, King Saud bin Abdulaziz University for Health Sciences, Riyadh, Saudi Arabia. [5] Department of Psychiatry, King Saud University Medical City, Riyadh, Saudi Arabia. [6] Department of Emergency Medicine, Prince Sultan Military Medical City, Riyadh, Saudi Arabia. [7] Department of Internal Medicine, King Fahad Medical City, Riyadh, Saudi Arabia.

Acknowledgements

We thank all the psychiatrists and family physicians who participated in this study. Also, we thank Dr. Imad Yaseen for helping us in data analysis.

Competing interests

The authors declare that they have no competing interests.

Consent for publication

The authors provide consent for publication.

Funding

This research was funded by the SABIC Psychological Health Research and Applications Chair, Department of Psychiatry, College of Medicine, Deanship of Post Graduate Teaching, King Saud University.

References

1. Abbas M, Mashrai N, Mohanna M. Knowledge of and attitudes toward electroconvulsive therapy of medical students in the United kingdom, Egypt, and Iraq: a transcultural perspective. J ECT. 2007;23:260–4.
2. Spiric Z, Stojanovic Z, Samardzic R, Milovanović S, Gazdag G, Marić NP. Electroconvulsive therapy practice in Serbia today. Psychiatr Danub. 2014;26:66–9.
3. Olekseev A, Ungvari GS, Gazdag G. Electroconvulsive therapy practice in Ukraine. J ECT. 2014;30:216–9.
4. Golenkov A, Ungvari GS, Gazdag G. ECT practice and psychiatrists' attitudes towards ECT in the Chuvash Republic of the Russian Federation. Eur Psychiatry. 2010;25:126–8.
5. Kellner CH, Kaicher DC, Banerjee H, Knapp RG, Shapiro RJ, Briggs MC, et al. Depression severity in electroconvulsive therapy (ECT) versus pharmacotherapy trials. J ECT. 2015;31:31–3.
6. Ray AK. Does electroconvulsive therapy cause epilepsy? J ECT. 2013;29:201–5.
7. Aki OE, Ak S, Sonmez YE, Demir B. Knowledge of and attitudes toward electroconvulsive therapy among medical students, psychology students, and the general public. J ECT. 2013;29:45–50.
8. Berg JE. Electroconvulsive treatment—more than electricity? An odyssey of facilities. J ECT. 2009;25:250–5.
9. Alevizos B, Zervas IM, Hatzimanolis J, Alevizos E. Attitudes of Greek nonpsychiatrist physicians toward electroconvulsive therapy. J ECT. 2005;21:194–5.
10. Gazdag G, Kocsis N, Tolna J, Lipcsey A. Attitudes towards electroconvulsive therapy among Hungarian psychiatrists. J ECT. 2004;20:204–7.
11. Gazdag G, Zsargó E, Kerti KM, Grecu IG. Attitudes toward electroconvulsive therapy in romanian psychiatrists. J ECT. 2011;27:e55–6.
12. James BO, Inogbo CF. Implementing modified electroconvulsive therapy in Nigeria: current status and psychiatrists' attitudes. J ECT. 2013;29:e25–6.
13. Finch JM, Sobin PB, Carmody TJ, DeWitt AP, Shiwach RS. A survey of psychiatrists' attitudes toward electroconvulsive therapy. Psychiatr Serv. 1999;50:264–5.
14. Agarwal AK, Andrade C. Indian psychiatrists' attitudes towards electroconvulsive therapy. Indian J Psychiatry. 1997;39:54–60.
15. James BO, Lawani AO, Omoaregba JO, Isa EW. Electroconvulsive therapy: a comparison of knowledge and attitudes of student nurses and staff mental health nurses at a psychiatric hospital in Nigeria. J Psychiatr Ment Health Nurs. 2010;17:141–6.
16. Oldewening K, Lange RT, Willan S, Strangway C, Kang N, Iverson GL. Effects of an education training program on attitudes to electroconvulsive therapy. J ECT. 2007;23:82–8.
17. Walter G, McDonald A, Rey JM, Rosen A. Medical student knowledge and attitudes regarding ECT prior to and after viewing ECT scenes from movies. J ECT. 2002;18:43–6.
18. Andrews M, Hasking P. Effect of two educational interventions on knowledge and attitudes towards electroconvulsive therapy. J ECT. 2004;20:230–6.
19. IBM. IBM SPSS statistics for windows. Armonk: IBM Corporation; 2011.
20. Maletzky BM. Seizure duration and clinical effect in electroconvulsive therapy. Compr Psychiatry. 1978;19:541–50.
21. American Psychiatric Association. The practice of electroconvulsive therapy: recommendations for treatment, training, and privileging. A task force report of the American Psychiatric Association. 2nd ed. Washington, DC: American Psychiatric Publishing; 2001.

4

Leveling and abuse among patients with bipolar disorder at psychiatric outpatient departments in Ethiopia

Habte Belete*

Abstract

Introduction: The World Health Organization (WHO) clearly states the importance of psychological well-being in the definition of health as "a state of complete physical, mental and social well-being and not merely the absence of disease or infirmity". However, in the community, the lives of people with bipolar disorders are often harsh and abusive. Till now, the rate and related information concerning verbal or physical abuse among patients with bipolar disorder at psychiatric outpatient clinics have not been well addressed in Ethiopian settings.

Methods: Data were collected by interviewing 411 systematically selected participants at outpatient department of Amanuel Mental Specialized Hospital. For analysis, logistic regression and adjusted odds ratios (AOR) with 95% confidence intervals (CI) were used, and $P < 0.05$ was considered statistically significant.

Results: The prevalence of abuse (verbal/physical) was 37.7%. Having two or more episodes [AOR 1.70, 95% CI (1.06, 2.74)], a history of aggression [AOR 3.06, 95% CI (1.63, 5.75)] and comorbid illness [AOR 2.21, 95% CI (1.25, 3.90)] were significantly associated.

Conclusion: The prevalence of reported abuse is high among patients with bipolar disorder, and it is important to remember the rights of patients during treatment.

Keywords: Abuse, Physical, Verbal, Bipolar, Ethiopia

Introduction

Bipolar disorder is a chronic and severe mental disorder that affects the adult population worldwide. Bipolar disorder causes substantial psychosocial morbidity that affects the patient's marriage, social contacts, occupation, communication and other aspects of life. Even if the behavior of patients with bipolar disorder is somewhat challenging to caregivers [1–3], the responses of families or caregivers to this pathological behavior should not be inhuman. The challenge to caregivers or families is not only the abnormal behavior, but also the cost of their treatment. Individuals with bipolar disorder have high rates of psychiatric and medical comorbidity, which contribute to increased utilization of healthcare resources

[4]. WHO clearly states the importance of psychological well-being in the definition of health as "a state of complete physical, mental and social well-being and not merely the absence of disease or infirmity" [5]. However, in the community the lives of people with bipolar disorders are often harsh and abusive [6]. The rate of mood disorder occurrence reaches up to 52% even among healthy individuals who have suffered from abuse or violence in their lifetimes [7]. Patients with bipolar disorder attempt suicide at a rate of at least 25 to 50% [8], and most of them complete their death wish. Psychosocial factors such as abuse have an association with suicidal attempts [9]. The problem of reported abuse (physical and verbal) in individuals with severe mental illness has received relatively little attention, even though several studies suggest an extremely high prevalence of victimization in this population.

*Correspondence: habte.belete@gmail.com
Psychiatry Department, College of Medicine and Health Science, Bahir Dar University, P.O. Box: 79, Bahir Dar, Ethiopia

There is a high prevalence of victimization by abuse (mainly physical abuse) among patients with bipolar disorders and other severe mental illnesses. Studies have revealed that physical or emotional abuse can take place because of the presence of psychosocial factors, demographic factors and living circumstances, and substance abuse [10–12].

Many studies find that patients with bipolar disorder, especially women, suffer a high rate of physical and emotional abuse [13, 14], as do homeless patients with episodically severe mental illness [15].

Unfavorable childhood experiences and stressful life events significantly predict recurrence [16]. Unfavorable experiences contribute to worsening mental and physical health and lead to poor outcomes among adults with severe mood disorders [17]. Most patients with bipolar disorder who had unfavorable life events such as physical abuse are prone to rapid cycling, suicidal behavior, early onset and higher comorbidity for other psychiatric and cognitive disorders [18, 19].

Severe emotional abuse among patients with bipolar disorder is associated with lifetime substance misuse comorbidity and rapid cycling. A history of childhood abuse among patients with bipolar disorder has an association with lifetime suicidal attempts. Multiple forms of abuse show a graded increase in the risk of suicidal attempts, rapid cycling and poor prognosis among patients with bipolar disorder [20]. Patients' exposure to abuse at an early age is associated with poor response to treatment, risk of hospitalization and an increase in residential treatments [21]. A history of abuse is common among patients with bipolar disorders [22–24]. Current reported abuse and psychosocial stressors lead to worsening morbidity [25] and increases mortality from suicide. Stressful life events carry a risk of suicidal behaviors among patients with bipolar disorders [26, 27]. In general, bipolar disorder affects the patient and families. Therefore, describing the challenge to patients and social systems is important to improve health care and to provide good mental health care in low income countries.

The prevalence of physical abuse among patients with psychiatric illnesses, including bipolar disorder, is reported to be high in studies from western countries. For instance, an American study stated that 62.8% of the participants reported physical abuse from their partners, and 45.8% of the participants reported abuse from their own family members [28]. The prevalence of physical abuse was 27.3% among patients with bipolar disorder and schizophrenia. The prevalence of adulthood physical abuse was higher among patients with major psychiatric disorders (bipolar disorders and schizophrenia) compared to patients with medical illnesses [29]. Among patients with mood disorders, the reported abuse was 35%, including various types of abuse, but 75% reported physical abuse [30].

While the western literature describes the issue of abuse among patients with bipolar disorder well, there are still few data concerning abuse among patients with bipolar disorder in Ethiopia. The nationwide prevalence of bipolar disorder is not well reported in Ethiopia. Mental health services are quiet poor, and there is only one mental hospital (Amanuel Mental Specialized Hospital) for the country. Most rural communities choose cultural, traditional and religious healing methods in Ethiopia. However, many cultural treatments for mental illness are prone to physical or verbal abuse such as insults and restraints. Therefore, the aim of this study was to determine the magnitude of abuse among patients with bipolar disorder at psychiatric outpatient clinics in Ethiopia.

Methods
Study setting
A cross-sectional survey was conducted at the outpatient department of Amanuel Mental Specialized Hospital in Addis Ababa, Ethiopia. It has 15 outpatient departments; 8 of them serve approximately 11,500 bipolar patients yearly. The hospital has 300 beds for adult psychiatry inpatients and emergency, forensic and addiction services. While there are psychiatric clinics in many different general and specialized hospitals in Ethiopia, Amanuel Mental Specialized Hospital is the only mental hospital in Ethiopia that hosts many referral cases from throughout the country. The number of follow-up patients with bipolar disorder in this hospital seems unusual. However, the hospital is the only mental hospital in Ethiopia that hosts many patients with relapse and chronic illness from all parts of the country.

Participants
The source population was participants who had been clinically diagnosed (according to the Diagnostic and Statistical Manual of Mental Disorders, 5th edition) with bipolar disorder (any type of bipolar disorder) by psychiatrists and mental health professional specialists (who have master's degrees in mental health). The patients had bipolar disorder and had been regularly followed up at Amanuel Mental Specialized Hospital, which sees a yearly average of 11,500 patients. The number of patients was estimated by taking the annual average patient follow-up by year at Amanuel Mental Specialized Hospital. The hospital uses the Diagnostic and Statistical Manual of Mental Disorders, 5th edition, to diagnose mental disorders including bipolar disorder. Those participants who presented to the outpatient departments during the study period and met the inclusion criteria comprised the study

population. The study participants were aged 18 years and above; those who were seriously ill (emotionally disturbed and unable to maintain normal conversation) and incapable of communication were excluded.

From the total 423 potential participants, 411 completed the interview, but 5 declined, 4 were unable to complete the form, and 3 were excluded for not meeting the criteria. A systematic random sampling technique was used to select participants by using the sampling fraction of 2 of 958 patients with bipolar disorder (who visit the hospital each month on average). Data were collected by well-trained, degree-holding psychiatric nurses by interviewing patients using a questionnaire translated into the local language, Amharic, which is the national working language of Ethiopia. The Ethical Review Board of the University of Gondar and Amanuel Mental Specialized Hospital approved the study, and written consent was taken from the participants. Confidentiality was maintained throughout the process by anonymous questionnaires and omitting personal identification.

Instrument

The reported physical or verbal abuse was assessed by questioning the patients and relatives and reviewing their medical records for whether or not the patients had suffered abuse (physically/verbally) from their caregivers or family members since their morbidity. The questionnaire was developed for this study. It considers physical abuse to have occurred if any of the following happened to the patients: hitting, slapping, pushing or throwing any material to harm the patient. For verbal abuse, any of the following were considered: shouting, insulting, criticizing and undermining the patient's role in the family, also by the caregiver, after the patient had been diagnosed with bipolar disorder. This tool had internal consistency (Cronbach's alpha) of 76% and was understood during the pretest. Socioeconomic status (wealth) of the study participants was assessed by using principal component analysis in which eigenvalues greater than 1 were used as extractions, and the factors to extract were fixed at five (from the lowest to highest). Participants' educational status was classified as educated or not based on whether they were receiving formal education.

Medication adherence was assessed by a standard tool, the Morisky Medication Adherence Scale 8-item tool, and levels were set as poor adherence (0–6), moderate (≥6 and <8) and good (8) on the 8-item Morsiky Medication Adherence Scale [31]. Social support was assessed using the Oslo-3 Social Support Scale, with categories of strong (12–14), moderate (9–11) and poor social support (3–8) [32]. Perceived stress was assessed by the Global Perceived Stress Scale 10-item tool, and its health concern stress level was categorized into scores of 0–11

(low), 12–15 (moderate) and 16 and above (high) [33]. Current substance use (smoking, alcohol and khat) was assessed by adopting the alcohol, smoking and substance involvement screening test [34]. Other clinical variables such as duration of the illness, age of illness onset and history of aggression were assessed by reviewing the patients' chart and self-report.

Analysis

Data were entered into Epi Data version 3.1 and analyzed using the Statistical Package for Social Sciences, version 20. Descriptive statistics were analyzed, and multivariate and binary logistic regression analysis was used to select the predictors associated with abuse. Association was determined using odds ratios by taking 95% confidence intervals, and $P < 0.05$ was considered statistically significant.

Results

The study included a total of 411 respondents with bipolar disorder, and 236 (57.4%) were females. The mean age of participant was 34.35 years (Standard Deviation: 34.35 ± 11.13 years), and most of the participants 142 (35.4%) were of Amharic ethnicity (Table 1).

Of the total participants, 139 (33.8%), 84 (20.4%) and 69 (16.8%) had anxiety symptoms, guilty feelings and grandiosity during the study period, respectively. Among total participants, 52.8% had >5 years morbidity (Table 2).

Magnitude of abuse

The magnitude of reported abuse (physical or verbal) was 37.7%. This happened after patients' diagnosis with bipolar disorder. Concerning the type of abuse, of the total participants, 104 (25.3%) reported physical abuse. For verbal abuse, 134 (32.6%) reported insults, 129 (31.4%) were criticized, 42 (10.2%) were sent away at mealtime, 138 (33.6%) were shouted at by their family members, and 53 (12.9%) were restricted from their role in the family. All patients who reported abuse also reported verbal abuses at least once during their morbidity.

Of the total patients who reported abuse, 84 (54.2%) were females; 121 (78.1%) had more than one episode, and 63 (40.6%) had poor social support. Patients who reported abuse perceived that their life was full of stress; 78 (50.3%) were scored as having high perceived stress, and 123 (79.4%) used some of these substances (alcohol, tobacco and khat).

Multivariate analysis

After multivariate analysis of abuse in relation to all explanatory variables, a history of aggressive behavior, having two or more episodes of bipolar disorder and

Table 1 Demographic predictors related to abuse in bipolar patients

Characteristics	Abuse		Overall	Chi-square (X^2) (P value)
	Yes	No		
Sex				
Male	71 (45.8%)	104 (40.6%)	175 (42.6%)	1.06 (0.30)
Female	84 (54.2%)	152 (59.4%)	236 (57.4%)	
Residency				
Urban	117 (75.5%)	177 (69.1%)	294 (71.5%)	1.91 (0.17)
Rural	38 (24.5%)	79 (30.9%)	117 (28.5%)	
Education				
No formal education	17 (11%)	52 (20.3%)	69 (16.8%)	6.04 (0.01)
Educated	138 (89%)	204 (79.7%)	342 (83.2%)	
Religion				
Christian	115 (74.2%)	196 (76.6%)	311 (75.7%)	0.29 (0.56)
Muslim	40 (25.8%)	60 (23.4%)	100 (24.3%)	
Marital status				
Currently married	58 (37.4%)	122 (47.7%)	180 (43.8%)	4.11 (0.04)
Not married	97 (62.6%)	134 (52.3%)	231 (56.2%)	
Job				
Has job	111 (71.6%)	188 (73.4%)	299 (72.7%)	0.16 (0.45)
No job	44 (28.4%)	68 (26.6%)	112 (27.3%)	
Ethnicity				
Amahara	60 (38.7%)	82 (32%)	142 (34.55%)	3.6 (0.46)
Oromo	48 (31%)	87 (34%)	135 (32.85%)	
Gurage	32 (20.6%)	50 (19.5%)	82 (20%)	
Tigray	6 (3.9%)	18 (7%)	24 (5.8%)	
Others[a]	9 (5.8%)	19 (7.5%)	28 (6.8%)	
Wealth				
Lowest	35 (22.6%)	48 (18.8%)	83 (20.2%)	2.33 (0.67)
Second	34 (21.9%)	54 (21.1%)	88 (21.4%)	
Middle	27 (17.4%)	51 (19.9%)	78 (19%)	
Fourth	35 (22.6%)	52 (20.3%)	87 (21.2%)	
Highest	24 (15.5%)	51 (19.9%)	75 (18.2%)	

[a] Wolaita, Sidama, Gamo

having a comorbid illness were found to be more statistically significant than other variables (Table 3).

Discussion

Patients' lives often change after being diagnosed as mentally ill, and the behavior of patients with bipolar disorder is mostly realted to their illness. Therefore, the response from the environment affects the psychopathology. Inappropriate handling of this behavior and abuse of the patients can occur.

The prevalence of abuse (physical or verbal) is higher in this study compared to studies from New Zealand (27.3%) [29], but lower than the 62.8% reported in the USA [28] and 75% in [30]. Factors such as methodological differences and the clinical and medico-legal factors in each

country might be responsible for this inconsistency. There is no universal agreement on how to handle the behavior of patients with mental illness, and the treatment guidelines, laws and ethical issues of each country lead to the discrepancy in the reported abuse among studies.

In the logistic regression analysis, participants who had two or more episodes of bipolar disorder had increased chances of reported abuse—almost two times more than for those who had only one episode [AOR 1.70 95% CI (1.06, 2.74)]. This may be due to the re-occurrence of affective or psychotic symptoms disturbing the family or caregivers, and the counter-response may lead the families or caregivers to mishandle the patients [35]. The episodic nature of the illness itself exposes patients with bipolar disorder to various psychosocial disadvantages

Table 2 Psychosocial and clinical factors related to abuse among patients with bipolar disorder

Characteristics	Abuse		Overall	Chi-square (X^2) (P value)
	Yes	No		
Duration of illness				
Less than a year	5 (3.2%)	15 (5.9%)	20 (4.9%)	5.06 (0.06)
1–5 years	57 (36.8%)	117 (45.7%)	174 (42.3%)	
>5 years	93 (60%)	124 (48.4%)	217 (52.8%)	
Age at onset of illness				
Before 18 years old	30 (19.4%)	38 (14.8%)	68 (16.5%)	6.74 (0.034)
Between 18 and 24 years	69 (44.5%)	92 (36%)	161 (39.2%)	
After 24 years	56 (36.1%)	126 (49.2%)	182 (44.3%)	
History of aggression				
Yes	141 (91%)	191 (74.6%)	332 (80.8%)	16.64 (0.00005)
No	14 (9%)	65 (25.4%)	79 (19.2%)	
Medication adherence				
Poor	51 (32.9%)	66 (25.8%)	117 (28.4%)	2.75 (0.25)
Moderate	57 (36.8%)	111 (43.4%)	168 (40.9%)	
Good	47 (30.3%)	79 (30.8%)	126 (30.7%)	
Perceived stress				
Low	43 (27.7%)	75 (29.3%)	118 (28.7%)	0.48 (0.78)
Moderate	34 (22%)	49 (19.1%)	83 (20.2%)	
High	78 (50.3%)	132 (51.6%)	210 (51.1%)	
Comorbid illness				
Yes	35 (22.6%)	27 (10.5%)	62 (15.1%)	10.91 (0.001)
No	120 (77.4%)	229 (89.5%)	349 (84.9%)	
Social support				
Poor	63 (40.6%)	79 (30.9%)	142 (34.5%)	4.15 (0.13)
Moderate	62 (40%)	122 (47.6%)	184 (44.8%)	
Strong	30 (19.4%)	55 (21.5%)	85 (20.7%)	
Khat chewing				
Yes	33 (21.3%)	34 (13.3%)	67 (16.3%)	4.54 (0.03)
No	122 (78.7%)	222 (86.7%)	344 (83.7%)	
Tobacco use				
Yes	38 (24.5%)	39 (15.2%)	77 (18.7%)	5.46 (0.02)
No	117 (75.5%)	217 (84.8%)	334 (81.3%)	
Alcohol use				
Yes	52 (33.5%)	61 (23.8%)	113 (27.5%)	4.58 (0.03)
No	103 (66.5%)	195 (76.2%)	298 (72.5%)	

such as unemployment, poor social relationships and high costs for their treatment [4]. This psychosocial disadvantage may cause conflicts in the patient's environment that invite abuse. Frequent episodes of illness create various challenges for the patients, including exposing them to abuse [36]. Recurrences of the psychopathology always result in difficult behaviors that distress the caregivers, leading them to be aggressive toward the patients.

Patients' previous history of aggressive behavior was one contributing factor for reporting abuse, and the odds of reporting abuse were three times larger for those with a reported history of aggressive behavior than for those without [AOR 3.06, 95% CI (1.63, 5.75)]. This had a bidirectional association with aggression and abuse in which most patients who reported abuse had a history of aggression, especially auto-aggression or suicidal attempts [20]. Family- or caregiver-related reports of abuse or mistreatment may be the primary risk factor for aggression in patients with bipolar disorder [37]. This association might be due to the relationship between aggressive behavior and the management of this behavior in the community and health care settings [38].

Comorbid medical and psychiatric illness is common in patients with bipolar disorder, having various

Table 3 Factors related to abuse in bipolar patients

Explanatory variables	Abuse (physical/verbal)		(Crude odds ratio) (95% CI)	Adjusted odds ratio (AOR) 95% CI
	Yes	No		
Marital status				
Not married	97	134	1.52 (1.01, 2.29)*	1.32 (0.86, 2.02)α
Married	58	122	1.00	1.00
Number of episodes				
One episode	34	85	1.00	1.00
Two or more episodes	121	171	1.77 (1.12, 2.81)*	1.70 (1.06, 2.74)**
History of aggression				
Yes	141	191	3.43 (1.85, 6.35)*	3.06 (1.63, 5.75)**
No	14	65	1.00	1.00
Education				
No formal education	17	52	2.07 (1.15, 3.73)*	1.73 (0.93, 3.19)α
Educated	138	204	1.00	1.00
Comorbid illness				
Yes	35	27	2.47 (1.43, 4.28)*	2.21 (1.25, 3.90)**
No	120	229	1.00	1.00
Alcohol drinking				
Yes	52	61	1.61 (1.04, 2.51)*	1.28 (0.80, 2.05)α
No	103	195	1.00	1.00

* $P < 0.05$)

** Significantly associated at $P < 0.05$), 1.00 (reference), α (not significantly associated)

impacts on patients' lives. According to this finding, the reported abuse was more than two times greater for patients who had comorbid illness than for those who did not [AOR 2.21, 95% CI (1.25, 3.90)]. This was in line with previous studies finding that illness comorbidities increase the reported abuse [28], and the reported abuse is high among patients with bipolar disorder and comorbid illness [36]. Some disorders can cause behavioral disturbances and may lead patients to develop irritable and aggressive behavior. This may cause different types of responses in the family that lead to patient abuse.

In general, patients who report abuse are not treated in accordance with human rights. The United Nations announced that all persons with a mental illness should be treated with humanity and respect for the inherent dignity of the human person [39]. However, the reported abuse in patients with mental illness has increased in recent studies, including this finding. Therefore, the rights of patients should be considered during their illness.

Conclusion
Reports of abuse are common in patients with bipolar disorder at psychiatric outpatient clinics in Ethiopia, and this needs public health attention as well as ethical considerations. A history of past aggression, the number of

episodes and comorbid illness were found to be significantly associated with abuse.

Limitations
This was a cross-sectional survey that cannot show the temporal cause-effect association of factors and abuse. This report cannot be generalized for all patients with bipolar disorder in Ethiopia since the study was only carried out in one mental hospital. The tool for assessing abuse is new, and its sensitivity and specificity have been not well reported. All these standardized tools have not been validated in our culture.

Abbreviations
AOR: adjusted odds ratio; CI: confidence interval; WHO: World Health Organization.

Acknowledgements
I acknowledge the study participants and staffs of Amanuel Mental Specialized Hospital for their cooperation.

Competing interests
The author declares that he has no competing interests.

Appendix
Physical and verbal abuse scale
Instruction

- Please encircle "yes" or "no" for each item based on the patient's experience in relation to his/her family members or caregivers since the onset of the illness.

  1. Physical abuse (any of the following)
     1.1 Hitting
     1.2 Slapping
     1.3 Pushing
     1.4 Throwing any material to harm the patient

  2. Verbal abuse (any of the following)
     2.1 Shouting
     2.2 Insulting
     2.3 Criticizing
     2.4 Undermining patient's role

Scoring

- If the patients answer "one yes" for any of the items, this is considered an experience of reported abuse for each type.
- The internal consistency (Cronbach's alpha) is 76%.

Received: 4 April 2017   Accepted: 29 June 2017
Published online: 11 July 2017

References

1. Yesavage JA. Bipolar illness: correlates of dangerous inpatient behaviour. Br J Psychiatry. 1983;143(6):554–7.
2. Feldmann TB. Bipolar disorder and violence. Psychiatr Q. 2001;72(2):119–29.
3. Volavka J. Violence in schizophrenia and bipolar disorder. Psychiatr Danub. 2013;25(1):24–33.
4. Sajatovic M. Bipolar disorder: disease burden. Am J Manag Care. 2005;11(3 Suppl):S80–4.
5. World Health Organization. Investing in mental health; 2003.
6. Freeman M, Pathare S. WHO resource book on mental health, human rights and legislation: World Health Organization; 2005.
7. Braaf DR, Meyering IB. Issues paper. 25 may 2013.
8. Jamison KR. Suicide and bipolar disorder. J Clin Psychiatry. 2000;61(suppl 9):47–51
9. McGrady A, Lynch D, Rapport D. Psychosocial factors and comorbidity associated with suicide attempts: findings in patients with bipolar disorder. Psychopathology. 2017;50(2):171–4.
10. Goodman LA, Salyers MP, Mueser KT, Rosenberg SD, Swartz M, Essock SM, et al. Recent victimization in women and men with severe mental illness: prevalence and correlates. J Trauma Stress. 2001;14(4):615–32.
11. Savitz JB, Van Der Merwe L, Stein DJ, Solms M, Ramesar RS. Neuropsychological task performance in bipolar spectrum illness: genetics, alcohol abuse, medication and childhood trauma. Bipolar Disord. 2008;10(4):479–94.
12. Hiday VA. Outpatient commitment: the state of empirical research on its outcomes. Psychol Public Policy Law. 2003;9(1–2):8.
13. Howard LM, Trevillion K, Khalifeh H, Woodall A, Agnew-Davies R, Feder G. Domestic violence and severe psychiatric disorders: prevalence and interventions. Psychol Med. 2010;40(06):881–93.
14. Meade CS, McDonald LJ, Graff FS, Fitzmaurice GM, Griffin ML, Weiss RD. A prospective study examining the effects of gender and sexual/physical abuse on mood outcomes in patients with co-occurring bipolar I and substance use disorders. Bipolar Disord. 2009;11(4):425–33.
15. Goodman LA, Dutton MA, Harris M. Episodically homeless women with serious mental illness: prevalence of physical and sexual assault. Am J Orthopsychiatry. 1995;65(4):468–78.
16. Dienes KA, Hammen C, Henry RM, Cohen AN, Daley SE. The stress sensitization hypothesis: understanding the course of bipolar disorder. J Affect Disord. 2006;95(1):43–9.
17. Lu W, Mueser KT, Rosenberg SD, Jankowski MK. Correlates of adverse childhood experiences among adults with severe mood disorders. Psychiatr Serv. 2008;59(9):1018–26.
18. Post RM, Leverich GS, Xing G, Weiss SR. Developmental vulnerabilities to the onset and course of bipolar disorder. Dev Psychopathol. 2001;13(03):581–98.
19. McIntyre RS, Soczynska JK, Mancini D, Lam C, Woldeyohannes HO, Moon S, et al. The relationship between childhood abuse and suicidality in adult bipolar disorder. Violence Vict. 2008;23(3):361–72.
20. Garno JL, Goldberg JF, Ramirez PM, Ritzler BA. Impact of childhood abuse on the clinical course of bipolar disorder. Br J Psychiatry. 2005;186(2):121–5.
21. Marchand WR, Wirth BL, Simon MC. Adverse life events and pediatric bipolar disorder in a community mental health setting. Commun Ment Health J. 2005;41(1):67–75.
22. Hyun M, Friedman SD, Dunner DL. Relationship of childhood physical and sexual abuse to adult bipolar disorder. Bipolar Disord. 2000;2(2):131–5.
23. Jaworska-Andryszewska P, Rybakowski J. Negative experiences in childhood and the development and course of bipolar disorder. Psychiatr Pol. 2016;50(5):989–1000.
24. Palmier-Claus J, Berry K, Bucci S, Mansell W, Varese F. Relationship between childhood adversity and bipolar affective disorder: systematic review and meta-analysis. Br J Psychiatry. 2016. doi:10.1192/bjp.bp.115.179655.
25. Post R, Leverich G. The role of psychosocial stress in the onset and progression of bipolar disorder and its comorbidities: the need for earlier and alternative modes of therapeutic intervention. Dev Psychopathol. 2006;18(04):1181–211.
26. Leverich GS, Altshuler LL, Frye MA, Suppes T, Keck PE Jr, McElroy SL, et al. Factors associated with suicide attempts in 648 patients with bipolar disorder in the Stanley Foundation Bipolar Network. J Clin Psychiatry. 2003;64(5):506–15.
27. McIntyre RS, Muzina DJ, Kemp DE, Blank D, Woldeyohannes HO, Lofchy J, et al. Bipolar disorder and suicide: research synthesis and clinical translation. Curr Psychiatry Rep. 2008;10(1):66–72.
28. DeGiralomo J. Physical aggression against psychiatric inpatients by family members and partners. Psychiatr Serv. 1996;47:531–3.
29. Coverdale JH, Turbott SH. Sexual and physical abuse of chronically ill psychiatric outpatients compared with a matched sample of medical outpatients. J Nerv Ment Dis. 2000;188(7):440–5.
30. Parsaik AK, Abdelgawad N, Chotalia JK, Lane SD, Pigott TA. Early-life trauma in hospitalized patients with mood disorders and its association with clinical outcomes. J Psychiatr Pract. 2017;23(1):36–43.
31. Morisky DE, Ang A, Krousel-Wood M, Ward HJ. Predictive validity of a medication adherence measure in an outpatient setting. J Clin Hypertens. 2008;10(5):348–54.
32. Bøen H. Characteristics of senior centre users–and the impact of a group programme on social support and late-life depression. 2012.
33. Cohen S, Kamarck T, Mermelstein R. A global measure of perceived stress. J Health Soc Behav. 1983;24:385–96.
34. Humeniuk R, Ali R, Babor TF, Farrell M, Formigoni ML, Jittiwutikarn J, et al. Validation of the alcohol, smoking and substance involvement screening test (ASSIST). Addiction. 2008;103(6):1039–47.
35. Ballester J, Goldstein T, Goldstein B, Obreja M, Axelson D, Monk K, et al. Is bipolar disorder specifically associated with aggression? Bipolar Disord. 2012;14(3):283–90.
36. Post RM, Altshuler LL, Kupka R, McElroy SL, Frye MA, Rowe M, et al. Verbal abuse, like physical and sexual abuse, in childhood is associated with an

earlier onset and more difficult course of bipolar disorder. Bipolar Disord. 2015;17(3):323–30.

37. Barlow K, Grenyer B, Ilkiw-Lavalle O. Prevalence and precipitants of aggression in psychiatric inpatient units. Aust N Z J Psychiatry. 2000;34(6):967–74.

38. Guzman-Parra J, Guzik J, Garcia-Sanchez JA, Pino-Benitez I, Aguilera-Serrano C, Mayoral-Cleries F. Characteristics of psychiatric hospitalizations with multiple mechanical restraint episodes versus hospitalization with a single mechanical restraint episode. Psychiatry Res. 2016;244:210–3.

39. United Nations General Assembly: Resolution 46/119: The protection of persons with mental illness and the improvement of mental health care. http://www.un.org/documents/ga/res/46/ a46r119.htm. Accessed 12 Aug 2008.

5

An arabic translation, reliability, and validation of Patient Health Questionnaire in a Saudi sample

Ahmad N. AlHadi[1,5*], Deemah A. AlAteeq[1,5], Eman Al-Sharif[2], Hamdah M. Bawazeer[2], Hasan Alanazi[2], Abdulaziz T. AlShomrani[3,5], Raafat M. Shuqdar[4,5] and Reem AlOwaybil[5]

Abstract

Background: Psychological disorders including depression and anxiety are not rare in primary care clinics. The Patient Health Questionnaire (PHQ) is a clinical diagnostic tool that is widely utilized by primary health care physicians worldwide because it provides a practical in-clinic tool to screen for psychological disorders. This study evaluated the validity of the Arabic version of the PHQ in all six modules including depression, anxiety, somatic, panic, eating, and alcohol abuse disorders.

Methods: This is a quantitative observational cross-sectional study that was conducted by administrating the translated Arabic version of PHQ to a sample of King Saud University students in Riyadh, Saudi Arabia.

Results: The sample was 731 university students who participated in this study including 376 (51.6%) females and 354 (48.4%) males with a mean age of 21.30 years. Eight mental health experts carried out the face validation process of the PHQ Arabic version. The internal consistency reliability was measured using Cronbach's alpha for the PHQ9, GAD7, PHQ15, and panic disorder modules. The results were 0.857, 0.763, 0.826, and 0.696, respectively. In comparison, the eating disorders and alcohol abuse modules demonstrated poor internal consistency due to small number of participants in these modules.

Conclusion: This study demonstrates that the Arabic version of the PHQ is a valid and reliable tool to screen for depression, anxiety, somatic, and panic disorders in a Saudi sample.

Keywords: Patient Health Questionnaire, PHQ, Arabic, Saudi Arabia, Validation

Background

Psychological disorders are relatively common in the community and in primary care patients. A recent study of three large primary care clinics in Riyadh, Saudi Arabia reported that nearly half of the patients expressed depressive symptoms [1]. Also, Al-Khathami and Ogbeide found that nearly one-third of the primary health clinic patients at Alkharj, Saudi Arabia demonstrated a high prevalence of psychological disorders [2]. Becker studied a primary care clinic in Riyadh, Saudi Arabia and showed that primary care physicians had poor diagnostic skills and could not accurately detect depression or somatization [3].

Many reliable self-report screening psychological instruments are available to help physicians in detecting psychological symptoms and improving their abilities to diagnose mental illness. Self-report questionnaires can provide an accurate diagnosis that is equally valid when compared to the structured interviews [4]. Thus, there is a widespread need to provide clinical instruments that can improve the diagnosis of psychological disorders at primary care clinics in Saudi Arabia.

The Patient Health Questionnaire (PHQ) is one of the most widely used clinical diagnostic instruments in primary care settings. It is valid and reliable in detecting

*Correspondence: alhadi@ksu.edu.sa
5 SABIC Psychological Health Research & Applications Chair (SPHRAC), College of Medicine, King Saud University, PO Box 242069, Riyadh 11322, Saudi Arabia
Full list of author information is available at the end of the article

psychological disorders. It is a self-administrated instrument that was developed in 1999 as an improved version of the original Primary Care Evaluation of Mental Disorders (PRIME-MD). It has good utility and acceptable validity compared to the original questionnaire. It measures six disorders: depression, generalized anxiety, panic, somatization, eating, and alcohol abuse disorders [4]. In the last two decades, studies have shown that the PHQ is efficient, reliable, and highly acceptable for diagnosing depression, anxiety, and somatic disorders. Löwe et al. compared the PHQ with The Hospital Anxiety and Depression Scale (HADS) and the WHO Well-being (WBI-5), tools designed for screening depression and anxiety. The PHQ had better diagnostic accuracy compared to the two well-established instruments [5]. This study used the international classification of diseases ICD-10 diagnosis criteria for depression. Conversely, the original PHQ study used the Diagnostic and Statistical Manual of Mental Disorders revised third edition and the fourth edition (DSM-III-R and DSM-IV) as criteria [4]. There is no big difference in diagnostic criteria for depression and anxiety disorders in ICD-10 and DSM-IV. Thus, it appears that the PHQ demonstrates reliable diagnostic accuracy of mental disorders whether the diagnostic criteria were based on the ICD-10 or the DSM-IV.

The PHQ has been adapted into many languages as a valuable diagnostic instrument because it exhibits high cultural sensitivity among different cultures and ethnic groups. For instance, the PHQ-9—the depression module—is a good instrument to evaluate depression cases among diverse ethnic groups in the United States such as African Americans, Chinese Americans, and Latinos [6]. Accordingly, many international adaptations of the instrument have shown that it is valid and reliable instrument. Karekla et al. examined the validity of the PHQ for a Greek population and concluded that it demonstrated good validity and reliability. Other studies also supported these findings [7]. Liu et al. [8] reported that the Chinese version of the (PHQ-9) and its subscales are valid and can accurately detect major depression in Taiwan. Furthermore, a study showed that the Patient Health Questionnaire—Somatic, Anxiety, and Depressive symptoms (PHQ-SAD), is valid and reliable for a Turkish population [9]. Many other countries and cultures adapted PHQ9 as a diagnostic and screening tool including Nepal, Nigeria, Greece, Sri Lanka, Thailand, and China [7, 10–14]. The PHQ-9 is also adapted in many medical diagnoses like AIDS, coronary artery diseases, migraine, morbid obesity, and stroke [15–19].

The PHQ was first adapted into Arabic in 2002 by a study that examined its validity in terms of detecting depression, anxiety, and somatization in primary care. The study used the Structured Clinical Interview (SCID-R) as the standard criterion and reported that the PHQ is valid in a Saudi population for diagnosing depression and somatization but not anxiety [3, 20]. However, the study did not illustrate the causes of the low sensitivity of the PHQ anxiety module. Nevertheless, its sensitivity could be improved by lowering the threshold to "several days" instead of "more than half of the days" [20]. To the best of our knowledge, no other study has shown the validity of the PHQ and its anxiety module for a Saudi population.

Other studies used the PHQ-9 to examine depression prevalence in primary care clinics. Abdelwahid and Al-shahrani reported that the prevalence of depression was 12% among patients of Family Medicine in Southeastern Saudi Arabia by using the (PHQ-9) as a detecting instrument [21]. A cross-sectional study surveyed four primary care clinics in Alkhobar, Saudi Arabia and reported that the prevalence of depression among the primary care patients was 16% by using the PHQ-9 [22]. Finally, Al-Qadhi et al. investigated the prevalence of depression in primary care clinics and reported high prevalence. They also compared the PHQ-9 and the ultra-brief version PHQ-2 and stated that the two versions are equally valid for screening depression [1]. It was evident in various studies that university students had prevalent and persistent mental health problems. In all these studies, the Arabic (Tunisian version) PHQ9 translation was used. There are no other Arabic translations available in the PHQ website other than PHQ9 and GAD7.

Until recently there was no study examining the validity of the entire PHQ with all modules in an Arabic speakers population. This study examines the validity of the PHQ in screening for depression, anxiety, somatic, panic, eating, and alcohol abuse disorders in a population of university students.

Methods
This is a quantitative observational cross-sectional study.

Subjects and procedure
We recruited university students from King Saud University in Riyadh, Saudi Arabia. The sample was collected through convenience sampling. We included students agreeing to participate in the study and able to read and understand Arabic. Almost all participants are Saudi and all of them are fluent in Arabic and English languages. We offered questionnaire to all university students in the medical college through representatives in each class. Data were collected from January to May 2015.

Sample size calculation

$$n = \left(Z_{a/2}\right)^2 s^2 / d^2$$

s standard deviation = 4.91 of PHQ-9 from previous study [1]; d the accuracy of estimate, we chose 1 difference score in the total score of PHQ-9 score; $Z_{a/2}$ a normal deviate reflects the type I error which = 1.96 for 95% confidence level; Sample size = $(1.96)^2 * (4.91)^2/(1)^2 = 3.84 * 24.11/1 = 92.58-93$ participants; So the required sample for power analysis is 93 participants.

Measures

We used a paper and pen questionnaire. The questionnaire included demographic data and formal (not dialect) Arabic translation of the whole PHQ. PHQ consists of six modules. Depression (PHQ9-9 items), generalized anxiety (GAD7-7 items), and somatization (PHQ15-15 items) modules have items with Likert scales. Panic (15 items), eating (8 items), and alcohol abuse (5 items) modules are all Yes/No answers. The Arabic version is exactly the same structure of the original English scale. We followed the guidelines of Sousa et al. in translation, adaptation, and validation of PHQ [23]: Step 1: forward translation—translation of the PHQ into the Arabic language by two independent translators. Step 2: synthesis I—comparison of the two translated versions of the PHQ and the development of an initial translated version. Step 3: blind back-translation of the preliminary initial translated version of the PHQ from Arabic to English. Step 4: synthesis II—comparison of the two back-translated versions of the PHQ. Step 5: pilot testing of the pre-final version of the instrument in Arabic. We also did face validity by sending the pre-final version to eight referees from mental health experts.

Ethical

The PHQ measures are in the public domain. No permission was required to reproduce, translate, display, or distribute. IRB approval from King Saud University was granted before data collection was begun.

Data analysis

Data were analyzed using the Statistical Package for Social Sciences (SPSS) [24] (Armonk, NY, USA) version 21.0. Descriptive statistical data are presented by mean values, standard deviations, and percentages for the sociodemographic variables. Pearson's correlation was used to assess the relationship between different variables. We used Cronbach's alpha coefficients, corrected item-total correlation and inter-item correlation matrix analysis to assess the internal consistency reliability. A Cronbach's alpha of ≥ 0.7 and item-total correlation of >0.2 were considered statistically acceptable [25]. Only statistically significant differences at $p < 0.05$ were reported.

Results

We recruited 731 university students out of 1400 students with response rate of 52%. Almost half of them were female 376 (51.6%) with a mean age of 21.30 (SD = 1.46) years. Almost all the participants were single. Table 1 shows the demographic characteristics of the sample.

Translation process

It took approximately 2 months to finalize the process. We hired independent certified translators who are not familiar with the questionnaire. The authors of this study were the focus group that made the synthesis. All are fluent in both Arabic and English languages—some of them are mental health experts and some of them were medical students.

Validity analysis

Face validity was carried out by a group of eight experts in mental health (psychiatrists and psychologists) fluent in Arabic and English. The final draft of the Arabic version with the original English scale and was sent via email. They completed a form stating whether they agree with the translation of each item or not and provided comments or alternative translations. They agreed on approximately 98% of the translation with few comments and suggestions. The authors reviewed all feedback

Table 1 Demographic characteristics

Demographic characteristics	Study sample = n (%) = 731 (100%)
Gender	
Male	354 (48.4%)
Female	376 (51.6%)
Age	
Mean (SD)	21.30 (1.46)
Social status	
Married	14 (1.9%)
Single	717 (98.1%)
Medical diagnoses	65 (8.9%)
Diabetes mellitus	8 (1.1%)
Hypothyroidism	3 (0.4%)
Asthma	21 (2.9%)
Irritable bowel syndrome	4 (0.5%)
Others	28 (3.8%)
Psychiatric diagnoses	19 (2.6%)
Depression	7 (1.0%)
Generalized anxiety disorder	1 (0.1%)
Obsessive compulsive disorder	6 (0.8%)
Social anxiety disorder	1 (0.1%)
More than one	4 (0.5%)

All are self-reported

points and included them in the final version of the Arabic translation.

Reliability and item analysis
PHQ-9
Table 2 shows the mean scores and standard deviation for all PHQ-9 items. The most frequently endorsed item was "Feeling tired." Suicidal ideation was the item that was endorsed the least. Cronbach's alpha was 0.857. All items, if deleted, would decrease the total scale of Cronbach's alpha except item 9 (suicidal ideation). All items correlated with the total scale to a good degree (lowest $r = 0.378$). Inter-item correlations range between 0.177 and 0.648 as shown in Table 3.

GAD-7
Table 4 shows the mean scores and standard deviation for all GAD7 items. The most frequently endorsed item

was "Feeling nervous, anxious, on edge, or worrying a lot about different things." "Feeling restless so that it is hard to sit still" was the item that was endorsed the least. Cronbach's alpha was 0.763. All items, if deleted, would decrease the total scale of Cronbach's alpha. All items correlated with the total scale to a good degree (lowest $r = 0.410$). Inter-item correlations range between 0.204 and 0.426 as shown in Table 5.

PHQ-15
We calculated it as instructed in PHQ instruction manual [26] by assigning scores of 0, 1, and 2 to the response categories of (not at all, bothered a little, and bothered a lot) for the 13 somatic symptoms of the PHQ (items 1a-1 m). Also, 2 items from the PHQ-9 were added (sleep and energy) and scored 0 (not at all), 1 (several days) or 2 (more than half the days or nearly every day). Table 6 shows the mean scores and standard deviation for all

Table 2 Item statistics for PHQ-9 (major depression disorder)

PHQ-9 items	Mean	Std. deviation	Corrected item-total correlation	Cronbach's alpha if item deleted	Change in Cronbach's alpha if item deleted
Little interest or pleasure in doing things	1.08	0.843	0.654	0.835	−0.022
Feeling down, depressed, or hopeless	0.98	0.853	0.698	0.831	−0.026
Trouble falling or staying asleep, or sleeping too	1.27	1.042	0.558	0.846	−0.011
Feeling tired or having little energy	1.33	0.953	0.674	0.832	−0.025
Poor appetite or overeating	0.99	1.014	0.577	0.843	−0.022
Feeling bad about yourself—or that you are a failure or have let yourself or family down	0.77	0.951	0.626	0.838	−0.009
Trouble concentrating on things, such as reading the newspaper or watching TV	0.67	0.864	0.534	0.847	−0.010
Moving or speaking so slowly that other people could have or the opposite?	0.45	0.789	0.548	0.845	−0.012
Thoughts that you would be better off dead or of hurting	0.16	0.543	0.378	0.859	0.002
Total	7.71	5.433	0.400	0.857	0.000

Table 3 Inter-item correlation matrix for PHQ-9 (major depression disorder)

PHQ-9 items	Item 1	Item 2	Item 3	Item 4	Item 5	Item 6	Item 7	Item 8	Item 9
Little interest or pleasure in doing things	1.000	–	–	–	–	–	–	–	–
Feeling down, depressed, or hopeless	0.648	1.000	–	–	–	–	–	–	–
Trouble falling or staying asleep, or sleeping too	0.431	0.439	1.000	–	–	–	–	–	–
Feeling tired or having little energy	0.553	0.507	0.583	1.000	–	–	–	–	–
Poor appetite or overeating	0.397	0.454	0.410	0.468	1.000	–	–	–	–
Feeling bad about yourself or that you are a failure or have let yourself or family down	0.485	0.578	0.356	0.444	0.445	1.000	–	–	–
Trouble concentrating on things, such as reading the newspaper or watching TV	0.377	0.376	0.345	0.417	0.368	0.398	1.000	–	–
Moving or speaking so slowly that other people could have or the opposite?	0.389	0.421	0.290	0.388	0.383	0.403	0.462	1.000	–
Thoughts that you would be better off dead or of hurting	0.265	0.370	0.177	0.236	0.223	0.347	0.219	0.348	1.000

Table 4 Item statistics GAD-7 generalized anxiety disorder

GAD-7 items	Mean	Std. deviation	Corrected item-total correlation	Cronbach's alpha if item deleted	Change in Cronbach's alpha if item deleted
Feeling nervous, anxious, on edge, or worrying a lot about different things	1.31	0.486	0.423	0.747	−0.016
Feeling restless so that it is hard to sit still	0.49	0.646	0.483	0.733	−0.030
Getting tired very easily	0.91	0.720	0.595	0.707	−0.056
Muscle tension, aches, or soreness	0.55	0.674	0.441	0.742	−0.021
Trouble falling asleep or staying asleep	0.92	0.743	0.410	0.751	−0.012
Trouble concentrating on things, such as reading a book or watching TV	0.71	0.714	0.529	0.723	−0.040
Becoming easily annoyed or irritable	1.06	0.662	0.505	0.729	−0.034
Total	5.95	3.004	0.317	0.763	0.000

PHQ-15 items. The most frequently endorsed item was "Feeling tired or low energy." "Pain or problems during sexual intercourse" was the item that was endorsed the least. Cronbach's alpha was 0.826. All items, if deleted, would decrease the total scale Cronbach's alpha with the exception of "Pain or problems during sexual intercourse." All items correlated with the total scale to a good degree (lowest $r = 0.207$) except item 5 "Pain or problems during sexual intercourse" with $r = 0.032$. Inter-item correlations range between −0.040 and 0.588 as shown in Table 7.

Other scales

Panic disorder, eating disorders, and alcohol abuse sections were all Yes/No answers. It is different than PHQ-9, GAD-7, and PHQ-15, which are Likert scale answers.

The panic disorder scale consists of 15 items. It started with a single question "In the last 4 weeks, have you had an anxiety attack suddenly feeling fear or panic?" If the subject answered "No" then there was no need to complete the rest of the items. The next 3 items asked about attack details, and the next 11 items focused on the physical symptoms during attacks. It measures the diagnosis not the severity. Cronbach's alpha was 0.696. All items, if deleted, would decrease the total scale of Cronbach's

alpha except "Have you had an anxiety attack—suddenly fear or panic?", "Has this ever happened before?" and "Did you tremble or shake?" they will increase alpha to 0.700, 0.709, and 0.707, respectively.

Bulimia nervosa and binge eating disorder have 8 items. Cronbach's alpha was 0.110. Again, it measures the diagnosis not the severity. This scale started with 2 items. If any were answered with a "Yes" then the participant needs to proceed; otherwise, he stops.

The alcohol abuse scale consisted of 5 items. Cronbach's alpha was 0.280. This scale starts with a question: "Do you ever drink alcohol (including beer or wine)?" If participant checks "NO" then he needs to stop and not answer the remaining 5 items.

Discussion

This study evaluated the validity and reliability of the PHQ in a sample of university students. The PHQ is very helpful tool for diagnosis and also for severity measures for many psychiatric disorders. Some studies already used the PHQ-9, GAD-7, and PHQ-15 in Saudi Arabia. Most of them used a straightforward translation method or the Tunisian Arabic version of the PHQ-9 in PHQ screeners website [22].

Table 5 Inter-item correlation matrix GAD-7 generalized anxiety disorder

GAD-7 items	Item 1	Item 2	Item 3	Item 4	Item 5	Item 6	Item 7
Feeling nervous, anxious, on edge, or worrying a lot about different things	1.000	–	–	–	–	–	–
Feeling restless so that it is hard to sit still	0.314	1.000	–	–	–	–	–
Getting tired very easily	0.336	0.369	1.000	–	–	–	–
Muscle tension, aches, or soreness	0.204	0.288	0.426	1.000	–	–	–
Trouble falling asleep or staying asleep	0.224	0.236	0.352	0.240	1.000	–	–
Trouble concentrating on things, such as reading a book or watching TV	0.284	0.383	0.389	0.297	0.319	1.000	–
Becoming easily annoyed or irritable	0.332	0.324	0.410	0.277	0.260	0.384	1.000

Table 6 Item statistics for PHQ-15 (Somatization Disorder Scale)

PHQ-15 items	Mean	Std. deviation	Corrected item-total correlation	Cronbach's alpha if item deleted	Change in Cronbach's alpha if item deleted
Stomach pain	0.73	0.692	0.515	0.811	−0.015
Back pain	0.75	0.731	0.454	0.815	−0.011
Pain in your arms, legs, or joints (knees, hips, etc.)	0.69	0.717	0.498	0.812	−0.014
Menstrual cramps or other problems with your	0.57	0.761	0.460	0.815	−0.011
Pain or problems during sexual intercourse	0.00	0.053	0.032	0.830	0.004
Headaches	0.91	0.707	0.417	0.818	−0.008
Chest pain	0.28	0.513	0.353	0.821	−0.005
Dizziness	0.49	0.630	0.502	0.812	−0.014
Fainting spells	0.05	0.257	0.207	0.827	0.001
Feeling your heart pound or race	0.60	0.684	0.525	0.811	−0.015
Shortness of breath	0.40	0.600	0.499	0.813	−0.013
Constipation, loose bowels, or diarrhea	0.73	0.737	0.514	0.811	−0.015
Nausea, gas, or indigestion	0.80	0.767	0.580	0.806	−0.020
Trouble falling or staying asleep, or sleeping too	1.11	0.819	0.398	0.821	−0.005
Feeling tired or having little energy	1.17	0.734	0.509	0.811	−0.015
Total	9.28	5.331	0.224	0.826	0.000

The PHQ-9 showed good internal consistency with Cronbach's alpha of 0.857. Usually, self-reported scales are considered to have good reliability if Cronbach's alpha ranges between 0.70 and 0.95 [25]. This is consistent with the results of PHQ in the US where the alpha coefficient ranged from 0.79 to 0.89 [6, 27]. It also agrees with a Nigerian study that showed the alpha PHQ9 to be 0.85 [11]. The suicidal ideation item is the only item that if deleted will increase the reliability by 0.002. This small increment does not motivate removing the item. However, there is another version of PHQ-9 without this item. It is called PHQ-8 and is used mainly in non-depression research studies [26]. All other items correlated to the total scale nicely. Ideally, the average inter-item correlation for a set of items is better between 0.20 and 0.40 [28].

The GAD-7 reliability is acceptable with Cronbach's alpha of 0.763, and all the items are nicely correlated with the total scale and also to each other. The PHQ-SADS includes PHQ-9, GAD-7, and PHQ-15 measures plus panic measure from the original PHQ. However, GAD7 in PHQ is not the same as in PHQ-SADS in many points. First, only 3 items are the same in both versions of GAD7. Second, answers in GAD7 of the PHQ include 3 options "Not at all, several days, and more than half the days" where "nearly every day" is added in GAD-7 of PHQ-SADS. Third, duration of symptoms is 4 weeks in GAD-7 of PHQ, while it is 2 weeks in GAD-7 of PHQ-SADS. We used GAD7 of the PHQ and found it to be reliable. We do not know which version of GAD7 was used in Becker et al. which found that the anxiety scale is not valid in

Arabic (Saudi Arabia) [20]. We tried to get this information or to get the Arabic version that was used but we were unable because of no response from the authors.

The PHQ-15 somatization scale showed good internal consistency with Cronbach's alpha with 0.826. A Greek study found PHQ-15 Cronbach's alpha to be 0.73 for women and 0.71 for men [29]. In a Swedish sample, the alpha coefficients of the PHQ-15 ranged from 0.75 to 0.85 between study groups [30]. Becker et al. found sensitivity and specificity for Arabic somatization scale 0.65 and 0.96, respectively [20]. All PHQ-15 items are nicely correlated with the total scale with the exception of item 5 "Pain or problems during sexual intercourse." This item showed poor correlation with other items in inter-item correlations. The inter-item correlations of the PHQ-15 showed 5 negative scores out of 15 scores—none of these were >0.2. This could be because almost all participants were single (98.1%). Only 10 of the participants answered this question, and the rest of participants left it blank. Eight chose "not at all," and only two chose "bothered a little." To correctly test this item, it is better to select a cohort with more married participants.

Other scales

Panic disorder scale showed acceptable internal consistency with alpha = 0.696. This confirms a Greek study that found alpha = 0.73 [7]. We believe that the items—that if they are deleted may increase the reliability—are worth to stay in the scale. First, the increase is not that much (a 0.013 maximum). Second, they are crucial—especially

Table 7 Inter-item correlation matrix for PHQ-15 (Somatization Disorder Scale)

PHQ-15 items	Item 1	Item 2	Item 3	Item 4	Item 5	Item 6	Item 7	Item 8	Item 9	Item 10	Item 11	Item 12	Item 13	Item 14	Item 15
Stomach pain	1.000	–	–	–	–	–	–	–	–	–	–	–	–	–	–
Back pain	0.346	1.000	–	–	–	–	–	–	–	–	–	–	–	–	–
Pain in your arms, legs, or joints (knees, hips, etc.)	0.288	0.458	1.000	–	–	–	–	–	–	–	–	–	–	–	–
Menstrual cramps or other problems with your periods	0.328	0.255	0.277	1.000	–	–	–	–	–	–	–	–	–	–	–
Pain or problems during sexual intercourse	0.021	0.019	0.060	0.101	1.000	–	–	–	–	–	–	–	–	–	–
Headaches	0.222	0.199	0.253	0.289	−0.031	1.000	–	–	–	–	–	–	–	–	–
Chest pain	0.198	0.221	0.223	0.117	−0.029	0.181	1.000	–	–	–	–	–	–	–	–
Dizziness	0.245	0.307	0.321	0.273	0.001	0.323	0.214	1.000	–	–	–	–	–	–	–
Fainting spells	0.099	0.135	0.130	0.098	−0.011	0.051	0.191	0.172	1.000	–	–	–	–	–	–
Feeling your heart pound or race	0.272	0.222	0.293	0.249	−0.008	0.294	0.289	0.369	0.183	1.000	–	–	–	–	–
Shortness of breath	0.241	0.262	0.273	0.230	0.054	0.255	0.346	0.354	0.205	0.484	1.000	–	–	–	–
Constipation, loose bowels, or diarrhea	0.424	0.221	0.262	0.310	0.020	0.219	0.199	0.234	0.154	0.314	0.260	1.000	–	–	–
Nausea, gas, or indigestion	0.505	0.264	0.351	0.351	0.049	0.234	0.221	0.300	0.120	0.327	0.315	0.588	1.000	–	–
Trouble falling or staying asleep, or sleeping too	0.226	0.182	0.206	0.198	−0.040	0.236	0.141	0.224	−0.009	0.256	0.201	0.203	0.229	1.000	–
Feeling tired or having little energy	0.248	0.248	0.257	0.304	0.024	0.257	0.155	0.325	0.094	0.308	0.277	0.289	0.295	0.525	1.000

the first one, which is the gate for the scale. Also, the second item focuses on attack recurrence, which is a criterion for panic disorder diagnosis. The least important item is shaking and tremor although it is among common physical symptoms in the panic attack.

Unfortunately, eating disorders and alcohol abuse modules have low internal consistency scores. This can be explained by the small number who answered these modules and small number of items. The Cronbach alpha depends on the sample size and on the items number in the scale. Small item numbers (<10) have Cronbach alpha values that are usually very small [28]. Eating disorder modules have only 8 items and were answered by only 41 participants (5.6%). This is not consistent with other studies. For example, the Greek study found that Cronbach's alpha for an eating disorder module is 0.70 [7].

The alcohol abuse scale showed low reliability. Alcohol drinking is prohibited and illegal in Saudi Arabia. This low reliability score could be due to the low participation rate in this section. It has only 5 items, and only 6 participants (<1%) answered the scale. All were male. Although no females answered the scale, the last item in the scale stated "Driving under the influence," and this cannot be measured in Saudi women because it is illegal for females to drive in Saudi Arabia.

Conclusion
The PHQ Scale is a widely used tool with many translations worldwide. The Arabic version of the PHQ is a valid and reliable measure to screen depression, anxiety, somatic, and panic disorders in a Saudi sample. Eating disorders and alcohol abuse modules need to be administered on different samples to have more participation. We hope our study will encourage researchers and practitioners to conduct more studies in Saudi Arabia regarding mental health disorders.

Limitations
Our study has several limitations. First, the study was conducted among university students; therefore, it cannot be generalized. Second, it would be better if the reliability was examined through test–retest and not limited to the internal consistency tests. Third, we did not do convergent validity by comparing the scale to another gold standard. Fourth, there were few participants in the eating disorder and alcohol abuse modules.

Clinical implications
The application of validated and reliable Arabic PHQ will have a better impact in the recognition and detection of various mental health disorders that are under-diagnosed.

Abbreviations
ANOVA: analysis of variance; DSM: Diagnostic and Statistical Manual of Mental Disorders; GAD7: PHQ—generalized anxiety disorder items; HADS: Hospital Anxiety and Depression Scale; ICD: international classification of diseases; PHQ-SAD: Patient Health Questionnaire—Somatic, Anxiety, and Depressive symptoms; PHQ: Patient Health Questionnaire; PHQ15: PHQ—somatization disorder items; PHQ9: PHQ—major depressive disorder items; PRIME-MD: Primary Care Evaluation of Mental Disorders; SCID-R: Structured Clinical Interview; WBI-5: WHO Well-being Inventory.

Authors' contributions
ANA was the principal investigator, participated in the study design, manuscript writing and data collecting and analysis. DAA, EA, HMB, HA, ATA, RMS, RA participated in the study design, data collection, and writing the manuscript. All authors read and approved the final manuscript.

Author details
[1] Department of Psychiatry, College of Medicine, King Saud University, Riyadh, Saudi Arabia. [2] College of Medicine, King Saud University, Riyadh, Saudi Arabia. [3] College of Medicine, Al Imam Mohammad Ibn Saud Islamic University, Riyadh, Saudi Arabia. [4] College of Medicine, Taibah University, Madinah, Saudi Arabia. [5] SABIC Psychological Health Research & Applications Chair (SPHRAC), College of Medicine, King Saud University, PO Box 242069, Riyadh 11322, Saudi Arabia.

Acknowledgements
We would like to thank all people who shared in this study especially the students, the translators, and mental health experts who reviewed the translation. Also we thank Mohammed K. Al-Anazi, Abdulrahman S. AlBakheet, and Khulood K. AlRaddadi for helping us in collecting the data. This research was full financially supported by SABIC Psychological Health Research and Applications Chair, Department of Psychiatry, College of Medicine, Deanship of Post Graduate teaching, King Saud University.

Competing interests
The authors declare that they have no competing interests.

Funding
This research was funded by the SABIC Psychological Health Research and Applications Chair, Department of Psychiatry, College of Medicine, Deanship of Post Graduate Teaching, King Saud University.

References
1. Al-Qadhi W, Ur Rahman S, Ferwana MS, Abdulmajeed IA. Adult depression screening in Saudi primary care: prevalence, instrument and cost. BMC Psychiatry. 2014;14(1):190. doi:10.1186/1471-244X-14-190.
2. Al-Khathami AD, Ogbeide DO. Prevalence of mental illness among Saudi adult primary-care patients in Central Saudi Arabia. Saudi Med J. 2002;23(6):721–4. doi:10.15537/4102.
3. Becker SM. Detection of somatization and depression in primary care in Saudi Arabia. Soc Psychiatry Psychiatr Epidemiol. 2004;39(12):962–6. doi:10.1007/s00127-004-0835-4.
4. Spitzer RL, Kroenke K, Williams JB. Validation and utility of a self-report version of PRIME-MD: the PHQ primary care study. Primary Care Evaluation of Mental Disorders. Patient Health Questionnaire. JAMA. 1999;282(18):1737–44. doi:10.1001/jama.282.18.1737.
5. Löwe B, Gräfe K, Zipfel S, Witte S, Loerch B, Herzog W. Diagnosing ICD-10 depressive episodes: superior criterion validity of the Patient Health Questionnaire. Psychother Psychosom. 2004;73(6):386–90. doi:10.1159/000080393.
6. Huang FY, Chung H, Kroenke K, Delucchi KL, Spitzer RL. Using the Patient Health Questionnaire-9 to measure depression among racially and ethnically diverse primary care patients. J Gen Intern Med. 2006;21(6):547–52. doi:10.1111/j.1525-1497.2006.00409.x.

7.   Karekla M, Pilipenko N, Feldman J. Patient health questionnaire: Greek language validation and subscale factor structure. Compr Psychiatry. 2012;53(8):1217–26. doi:10.1016/j.comppsych.2012.05.008.

8.   Liu S-I, Yeh Z-T, Huang H-C, et al. Validation of Patient Health Questionnaire for depression screening among primary care patients in Taiwan. Compr Psychiatry. 2011;52(1):96–101. doi:10.1016/j.comppsych.2010.04.013.

9.   Yazici Güleç M, Güleç H, Simşek G, Turhan M, Aydin Sünbül E. Psychometric properties of the Turkish version of the Patient Health Questionnaire—Somatic, Anxiety, and Depressive symptoms. Compr Psychiatry. 2012;53(5):623–9. doi:10.1016/j.comppsych.2011.08.002.

10. Kohrt BA, Luitel NP, Acharya P, Jordans MJD. Detection of depression in low resource settings: validation of the Patient Health Questionnaire (PHQ-9) and cultural concepts of distress in Nepal. BMC Psychiatry. 2016;16(1):58. doi:10.1186/s12888-016-0768-y.

11. Adewuya AO, Ola BA, Afolabi OO. Validity of the patient health questionnaire (PHQ-9) as a screening tool for depression amongst Nigerian university students. J Affect Disord. 2006;96(1–2):89–93. doi:10.1016/j.jad.2006.05.021.

12. Hanwella R, Ekanayake S, De Silva VA. The validity and reliability of the sinhala translation of the patient health questionnaire (PHQ-9) and PHQ-2 screener. Depress Res Treat. 2014. doi:10.1155/2014/768978.

13. Wang W, Bian Q, Zhao Y, et al. Reliability and validity of the Chinese version of the Patient Health Questionnaire (PHQ-9) in the general population. Gen Hosp Psychiatry. 2014;36(5):539–44. doi:10.1016/j.genhosppsych.2014.05.021.

14. Lotrakul M, Sumrithe S, Saipanish R. Reliability and validity of the Thai version of the PHQ-9. BMC Psychiatry. 2008;8:46. doi:10.1186/1471-244X-8-46.

15. Monahan PO, Shacham E, Reece M, et al. Validity/reliability of PHQ-9 and PHQ-2 depression scales among adults living with HIV/AIDS in Western Kenya. J Gen Intern Med. 2009;24(2):189–97. doi:10.1007/s11606-008-0846-z.

16. Thombs BD, Ziegelstein RC, Whooley MA. Optimizing detection of major depression among patients with coronary artery disease using the patient health questionnaire: data from the heart and soul study. J Gen Intern Med. 2008;23(12):2014–7. doi:10.1007/s11606-008-0802-y.

17. Seo J-G, Park S-P. Validation of the Patient Health Questionnaire-9 (PHQ-9) and PHQ-2 in patients with migraine. J Headache Pain. 2015;16:65. doi:10.1186/s10194-015-0552-2

18. Cassin S, Sockalingam S, Hawa R, et al. Psychometric properties of the patient health questionnaire (PHQ-9) as a depression screening tool for bariatric surgery candidates. Psychosomatics. 2013;54(4):352–8. doi:10.1016/j.psym.2012.08.010.

19. de Man-van Ginkel JM, Gooskens F, Schepers VPM, Schuurmans MJ, Lindeman E, Hafsteinsdóttir TB. Screening for poststroke depression using the Patient Health Questionnaire. Nurs Res. 2012;61(5):333–41. doi:10.1097/NNR.0b013e31825d9e9e.

20. Becker S, Al Zaid K, Al Faris E. Screening for somatization and depression in Saudi Arabia: a validation study of the PHQ in primary care. Int J Psychiatry Med. 2002;32(3):271–83.

21. Abdelwahid HA, Al-shahrani SI. Screening of depression among patients in Family Medicine. Saudi Med J. 2011;32(9):948–52.

22. Aldabal B, Koura M, Alsowielem L. Magnitude of depression problem among primary care consumers in Saudi Arabia. Koura MR, ed. Int J Med Sci Public Heal. 2014;4(2):205–10. doi:10.5455/ijmsph.2015.2010201439.

23. Sousa VD, Rojjanasrirat W. Translation, adaptation and validation of instruments or scales for use in cross-cultural health care research: a clear and user-friendly guideline. J Eval Clin Pract. 2011;17(2):268–74. doi:10.1111/j.1365-2753.2010.01434.x.

24. IBM SPSS Inc. SPSS Statistics for Windows. 2012;Version 21.

25. Tavakol M, Dennick R. Making sense of Cronbach's alpha. Int J Med Educ. 2011;2:53–5. doi:10.5116/ijme.4dfb.8dfd.

26. Patient Health Questionnaire (PHQ) Screeners Instruction Manual. https://phqscreeners.pfizer.edrupalgardens.com/sites/g/files/g10016261/f/201412/instructions.pdf. Accessed 27 July 2016.

27. Lee PW, Schulberg HC, Raue PJ, Kroenke K. Concordance between the PHQ-9 and the HSCL-20 in depressed primary care patients. J Affect Disord. 2007;99(1–3):139–45. doi:10.1016/j.jad.2006.09.002.

28. Pallant J. SPSS survival manual: a step by step guide to data analysis using the SPSS program. 4th ed. Maidenhead: Open University Press; 2010.

29. Hyphantis T, Kroenke K, Papatheodorou E, et al. Validity of the Greek version of the PHQ 15-item Somatic Symptom Severity Scale in patients with chronic medical conditions and correlations with emergency department use and illness perceptions. Compr Psychiatry. 2014;55(8):1950–9. doi:10.1016/j.comppsych.2014.08.042.

30. Nordin S, Palmquist E, Nordin M. Psychometric evaluation and normative data for a Swedish version of the Patient Health Questionnaire 15-Item Somatic Symptom Severity Scale. Scand J Psychol. 2013;54(2):112–7.

6

Validation of the Italian version of the dissociative experience scale for adolescents and young adults

Concetta De Pasquale[1]*, Federica Sciacca[2] and Zira Hichy[3]

Abstract

Background: The Dissociative Experience Scale for adolescent (A-DES), a 30-item, multidimensional, self-administered questionnaire, was validated using a large sample of American young people sample. We reported the linguistic validation process and the metric validity of the Italian version of A-DES in the Italy.

Methods: A set of questionnaires was provided to a total of 633 participants from March 2015 to April 2016. The participants consisted of 282 boys and 351 girls, and their average age was between 18 and 24 years old. The translation process consisted of two consecutive steps: forward–backward translation and acceptability testing. The psychometric testing was applied to Italian students who were recruited from the Italian Public Schools and Universities in Sicily. Informed consent was obtained from all participants at the research. All individuals completed the A-DES. Reliability and validity were tested.

Results: The translated version was validated on a total of 633 Italian students. The reliability of A-DES total is .926. It is composed by 4 subscales: Dissociative amnesia, Absorption and imaginative involvement, Depersonalization and derealization, and Passive influence. The reliability of each subscale is: .756 for dissociative amnesia, .659 for absorption and imaginative involvement, .850 for depersonalization and derealization, and .743 for passive influence.

Conclusions: The Italian version of the A-DES constitutes a useful instrument to measure dissociative experience in adolescents and young adults in Italy.

Keywords: A-DES, Adolescents, Young adults, Dissociative experience, Validation, Scale, Questionnaire

Background

Dissociation can be defined as a lack of integration of thoughts, feeling, and experiences into the normal stream of consciousness [1]. Putman has identified four categories of dissociation including memory dysfunction, disturbances in identity, passive influence, and absorption [2]. Dissociative memory dysfunctions are a form of amnesia for events, intrusive memories or flashbacks. They include phenomena such as the inability to understand if a memory is an actual event or information obtained by hearing, thinking, or reading about the event. Disturbances in identity include feelings of being more than one person (dissociative identity), distortions in the perceptions of one's own body (depersonalization), and the inability to remember important personal information (dissociative amnesia). Passive influence involves a feeling that one's behaviors are caused by a force from within. Absorption refers to a very intense focusing of attention [3]. Dissociative experiences can happen to everyone, but in adolescent populations, they are more common in adolescents populations than in adults population [4]. In recent decades, the progress of technology and internet has come to develop some "side effects". Zanon et al. showed a possible correlation between the use of the internet, the dissociative experience and the presence of specific personality traits [5], while Craparo correlated internet addiction with alexithymia and dissociative experience [6].

*Correspondence: depasqua@unict.it
[1] Department of Medical Surgeon Science and Applied Technology. GF Ingrassia, University of Catania, Catania, Italy
Full list of author information is available at the end of the article

We report the linguistic validation process and the metric validity of the Italian version of the A-DES in the Italy.

Methods
Sample
Participants were randomly selected from Italian Public High Schools and University in Sicily. Participants in the High Schools were selected after the informed consent granted by the head teacher, and the questionnaires were administered during regular classes. Participants from University were contacted in various study rooms. Informed consent was obtained from all participants at the research.

General characteristics
The following parameters were collected from the students: gender, age, school or university, main use of smartphones.

Dissociative experience scale
The A-DES is a well-validated specific questionnaire for adolescents with dissociative symptoms in USA [1] that includes 30 questions describing memory dysfunctions, disturbances in identity, passive influence, and absorption [2]. Each item presents a statement in the first person form (e.g., "My body feels as if it doesn't belong to me"). Under each of these statements, subjects mark the frequency of these experiences on a scale from 0 to 10 with 0 labeled "never" and 10 labeled "always". The Total of A-DES scores are equal to the mean of all item scores. Subscale scores can also be calculated in four areas: dissociative amnesia (items 2, 5, 8, 12, 15, 22 and 27), absorption and imaginative involvement (items 1, 7, 10, 18, 24 and 28), depersonalization and derealization (items 3, 6, 9, 11, 13, 17, 20, 21, 25, 26, 29, and 30), and passive influence (items 4, 14, 6, 9 and 23) [1].

General organization
The development and linguistic validation of a questionnaire is based on two main steps. They were organized as follows: 1. the translation and the cultural adaptation process 2. The psychometric testing. The two steps were planned under the coordination of a team that included the Italian Researcher, Psychologist and Psychiatrist to of the University of Catania.

Translation and cultural adaptation process
The developers provided a conceptual definition of the original items to clarify the notions investigated in each item of the original American questionnaire. The original version of the scale was drawn by five American

psychologist of "The University of Arkansas" [1]. The translation and the cultural adaptation processes were organized into steps. Forward translation of the SAS-SV from English into Italian was performed by two native Italian speakers who were also fluent in English. Any differences between the 2 translated versions were discussed by the translators. An agreed upon (?) forward-translated version of the A-DES was produced. The misinterpretation and acceptability were checked. Some terms were reworded and a new version was produced.

Psychometric testing
The latest version was validated in a larger sample of Italian students to test the psychometric properties and to check the reliability.

Statistical analyses
A confirmatory factor analysis was performed using the SPSS 22 software (Statistical Package for Social Science).

The reliability of instruments were calculated using Cronbach's alpha.

Results
Sample characteristics
The study sample included 633 ($M = 317.25$, $SD = 183.16$) Italian student recruited from Public Schools and Universities and selected from March 2015 to April 2016. The participants consisted of 282 boys and 351 girls, aged between 13 and 24 years old ($M = 18.24$, $SD = 3.05$). Table 1 reports the distribution of the socio-demographic variables of the sample.

Item analysis and reliability
Table 2 shows item analysis of four factor of Dissociative Experience Scale for Adolescent for Italian samples. Regarding internal consistency all the item-total correlations appeared adequate, and there were no changes in the value of alpha excluding item. Finally In the end all alpha coefficients (Dissociative Amnesia = .76, Absorption and imaginative involvement = .66; Depersonalization and derealization = .85; Passive influence = .74) and the split-half correlation (Dissociative Amnesia = .63, Absorption and imaginative involvement = .48; Depersonalization and derealization = .67; Passive influence = .57) were adequate.

Factor structure
Because the relationship between observed variables and their underlying latent constructs was already confirmed in previous study [1], in this study we performed a confirmatory factor analysis [7] to verify if the same relationships can be find in our sample. To verify the adequacy

Table 1 Distribution of the socio-demographic variables of the sample

Variables	N	(N=633) %	Mean
Age	633		18.24
Sex			
Males	282	44.5	
Females	351	55.5	
School/University			
Art school	1	.2	
Catering collage	93	13.6	
Archaeology faculty	1	.2	
Architecture faculty	10	1.6	
Economic faculty	3	.5	
Pharmacy faculty	1	.2	
Jurisprudence faculty	7	1.1	
Engineering faculty	21	3.3	
Medical faculty	3	.5	
Psychology faculty	146	23.1	
Education faculty	111	17.5	
Secondary school specializing in scientific subjects	200	31.6	
Tourism faculty	2	.3	
Physical education	4	.6	
Natural science	1	.2	
Social science	4	.6	
Tourism high school	25	4.0	

N sample number, % percentage

Table 2 Item analysis of four factor of dissociative experience scale for adolescent for Italian samples

	M	SD	Item-total correlation	Alpha if item deleted	Factorloading
Dissociative amnesia					
2	1.32	2.178	.433	.925	.48
5	2.60	2.946	.538	.923	.57
8	1.29	2.370	.619	.922	.68
12	2.74	2.688	.408	.925	.41
15	1.18	2.347	.522	.923	.57
22	1.10	2.248	.573	.923	.63
27	2.29	3.070	.599	.922	.61
Absorptionand imaginative involvement					
1	2.85	2.549	.280	.927	.32
7	2.60	2.579	.85	.924	.51
10	4.54	3.027	.347	.926	.34
18	2.52	2.862	.570	.923	.66
24	1.40	2.402	.592	.923	.69
28	1.07	2.175	.529	.923	.54
Depersonalization andderealization					
3	2.49	2.579	.449	.924	.45
6	1.11	2.127	.637	.922	.63
9	1.85	2.636	.415	.925	.42
11	2.64	3.124	.501	.924	.49
13	.82	2.030	.563	.923	.66
17	3.97	3.224	.321	.927	.35
20	2.35	2.951	.604	.922	.63
21	1.61	2.611	.595	.922	.67
25	1.30	2.504	.608	.922	.70
26	1.94	2.797	.625	.922	.68
29	1.21	2.520	.566	.923	.64
30	.75	1.995	.642	.922	.75
Passive influence					
4	3.27	2.794	.472	.924	.49
14	2.12	2.809	.568	.923	.58
16	1.47	2.302	.581	.923	.63
19	2.78	3.000	.588	.922	.64
23	1.41	2.450	.661	.922	.72

M mean, SD standard deviation

of the models we used the χ^2: a solution fits well the data well when χ^2 is non-significant ($p > .05$). Given that this statistic is sensitive to sample size, the two-index strategy [8] proposing combined use of comparative fit index [9] and standardized root mean square residual [10] was applied. The model fits the data well if CFI is greater than or equal to .95 and SRMR is smaller than or equal to .08. Goodness of fit indexes are: $\chi^2(399) = 2132.88$, $p < .001$, CFI = .96, SRMR = .067; as you can see, although the χ^2 is significant, SRMR and CFI meet completely the criteria. Moreover, all factor loadings were significant, $p < .001$ (Table 2).

We also tested a second order factor structure whit one superordinate factor [7]. Goodness of fi indexes are: $\chi^2(401) = 2163.40$, $p < .001$, CFI = .96, SRMR = .067; also in this case, although the χ^2 is significant, SRMR and CFI meet completely the criteria. Moreover, all factor loadings were significant, $p < .001$ (Table 3). Finally, all inter-factor correlations were significant ($p < .001$) and reliability coefficient were high (alpha = .93; split-half correlation = .76).

Discussion

The scale possessed a good internal consistency, all factors show good saturation. The DES in Italian version is valid. This scale is useful for detecting the dissociative experience and various events such as amnesia, depersonalization, passive influence and absorption.

It can be used to implement prevention projects in the screening.

The scale can be used both as a single factor, both with the four separate factors (Dissociative Amnesia,

Table 3 Factor structure of DES

		M	SD	Factorloading	Correlation			
					1	2	3	4
1	Amnesia	1.7883	1.63723	.96				
2	Absorption	2.4953	1.58881	.94	.721			
3	Depersonalization	1.8372	1.60949	.91	.734	.664		
4	Influence	2.2079	1.88347	.98	.716	.653	.753	
DES_Tot		2.0192	1.47459					

M mean, *SD* standard deviation

Absorption and imaginative involvement, Depersonalization and derealization, and Passive influence).

We reporte in Additional file 1 Italian version of the dissociative experience scale for Adolescent.

Conclusion

New technologies related to social communication have made problematic the quality of existence. The Teenagers now spends more and more time in front of the smartphone and the Internet, mainly to communicate with others through messages, social networks, calls, finding in them a more accessible means of communication more accessible, easy, free from anxiety and fear, a defense from on the other. It brings more and more to escape from the real relationship.

Literature shows they are absent for other dissociative disorders such as significant "dissociative trance from display screen" shown in the study of Caretti and coworkers [11].

Directly proportional to the degree of reliance on smartphones is the presence of mild dissociative symptoms related to the size of the " absorption and imaginative assimilation", the tendency to engage his their mind in situations of altered and highly focused attention [12].

The aim of this study was to test the validity of the Dissociative Experience scale in Italian to analyze dissociative experience in Italian adolescents who use technological communication instruments.

At present there is insufficient evidence-based literature to establish diagnostic criteria and clinical symptoms needed to identify repetitive patterns of behavior and excessive, comparable to those produced by "Disorders related to substances and disorders Addiction" [13]. The use of this instrument can be an added value for a useful comparison on important issues that limit the educational process and human planning, preventing him from seizing the opportunities necessary for it to achieve maturation and personality development in all his physical and psychic potential, intellectual and moral.

Authors' contributions

CD conceived of the study, and participated in its design and coordination and helped to draft the manuscript. FS participated in the design of the study and helped to draft the manuscript. ZH performed the statistical analysis of the study. All authors read and approved the final manuscript.

Author details

[1] Department of Medical Surgeon Science and Applied Technology. GF Ingrassia, University of Catania, Catania, Italy. [2] Department of Education Science, University of Catania, Via Teatro Greco, 84, Catania, Italy. [3] Department of Education of Education Science, University of Catania, Via Teatro Greco, 84, Catania, Italy.

Acknowledgements

Not applicable.

Competing interests

The authors declare that they have no competing interests.

Consent for publication

The material was collected anonymously after obtaining the consent of the student, if of legal age, the parents, for underage students, and the school administrator.

References

1. Bernestein EM, Putman FW. Development, reliability, and validation of a dissociative scale. J Nerv Ment Dis. 1986;174:727–34.
2. Putman FW. Dissociative disorders in children and adolescent. In: Lynn SJ, Rhue JW, editors. Dissociation: clinical and theoretical perspectives. New York: Guilford Press; 1994. p. 175–89.
3. Smith SR, Carlson EB. Reliability and validity of the adolescent dissociative experiences scale. Dissociation. 1997;9(2):125–9.
4. Putman FW. Dissociative disorders in children and adolescent: a developmental perspective. Psychiatr Clin North Am. 1991;14:519–31.
5. Zanon I, Bertin I, Fabbri Bombi A. Trance dissociativa e internet dipendenza: studio su un campione di utenti della rete. Official J Ital Soc Psychopathol, Pacini editore medicina. 2002;8(4).
6. Craparo G. Internet addiction, dissociation and alexithymia. Proced Soc Behav Sci. 2011;30(2011):1051–6.
7. Jöreskog KG, Sörbom D. LISREL 8 user's reference guide. Chicago: Scientific Software International; 1996.
8. Hu L, Bentler PM. Cutoff criteria for fit indexes in covariance structure analysis: conventional criteria versus new alternatives. Struct Equ Model. 1999;6:1–55. doi:10.1080/10705319909540110.
9. Bentler PM. Comparative fit indexes in structural models. Psychol Bull. 1990;107:238–46. doi:10.1037/0033-2909.107.2.238.

10. Bentler PM. EQS structural equations program manual. Encino: Multivariate Software; 1995.
11. Caretti V. Psicodinamica della trance dissociativa da videoterminale. In: Cantelmi T, Del Miglio C, Talli M, D'Andrea A, editors. La mente in Internet. Psicopatologia delle condotte on-line. Padova: Piccin; 2000.
12. Tellegen A, Atkinson G. Openness to absorbing and self-altering experiences ("absorption"), a trait related to hypnotic susceptibility. J Abnorm Psychol. 1974;83(3):268.
13. American Psychiatric Association. Diagnostic and statistical manual of mental disorders (DSM-5®). Arlington: American Psychiatric Publishing; 2013.

7

Mental, neurologic, and substance use (MNS) disorders among street homeless people in Ethiopia

Getinet Ayano*, Dawit Assefa, Kibrom Haile, Asrat Chaka, Haddish Solomon, Petros Hagos, Zegeye Yohannis, Kelemua Haile, Lulu Bekana, Melkamu Agidew, Seife Demise, Belachew Tsegaye and Melat Solomon

Abstract

Background: About 25–60% of the homeless population is reported to have some form of mental disorder. To our knowledge, there are no studies aimed at the screening, diagnosis, treatment, care, rehabilitation, and support of homeless people with mental, neurologic, and substance use (MNS) disorders in general in Ethiopia. This is the first study of its kind in Africa which was aimed at screening, diagnosis, care, treatment, rehabilitation, and support of homeless individuals with possible MNS disorder.

Methods: Community-based survey was conducted from January to March 2015. Homeless people who had overt and observable psychopathology and positive for screening instruments (SRQ20, ASSIST, and PSQ) were involved in the survey and further assessed for possible diagnosis by structured clinical interview for DSM-IV diagnoses and international diagnostic criteria for seizure disorders for possible involvement in care, treatment, rehabilitation services, support, and training. The Statistical Program for Social Science (SPSS version 20) was used for data entry, clearance, and analyses.

Results: A total of 456 homeless people were involved in the survey. Majority of the participants were male ($n = 402$; 88.16%). Most of the homeless participants had migrated into Addis Ababa from elsewhere in Ethiopia and Eritrea (62.50%). Mental, neurologic, and substance use disorders resulted to be common problems in the study participants (92.11%; $n = 420$). Most of the participants with mental, neurologic, and substance use disorders (85.29%; $n = 354$) had psychotic disorders. Most of those with psychosis had schizophrenia (77.40%; $n = 274$). Almost all of the participants had a history of substance use (93.20%; $n = 425$) and about one in ten individuals had substance use disorders (10.54%; $n = 48$). Most of the participants with substance use disorder had comorbid other mental and neurologic disorders (83.33%; $n = 40$).

Conclusion and recommendation: Mental, neurologic, and substance use disorders are common (92.11%) among street homeless people in Ethiopia. The development of centers for care, treatment, rehabilitation, and support of homeless people with mental, neurologic, and substance use disorders is warranted. In addition, it is necessary to improve the accessibility of mental health services and promote better integration between mental and primary health care services, as a means to offer a better general care and to possibly prevent homelessness among mentally ill.

Background

Homelessness problem is most often caused by multiple and interrelated individual structural depreciation.

It leads to maladjustment and creates problems related to issues of social, economic, health, and starvation [1]. Homelessness is defined in various ways; in this study, homelessness indicates only those sleeping in designated shelters or public spaces. Broadly the term can include people living in marginal accommodation, as well as

*Correspondence: ayanogetinet@yahoo.com
Research and Training Department, Amanuel Mental Specialized Hospital, PO box: 1971, Addis Ababa, Ethiopia

roofless people. Some studies include the former, while in others the definition includes only those sleeping in designated shelters or public spaces. The features of a definition of homelessness that are useful in any locality, however, are the lack of appropriate housing and the social marginalization of the individual [2, 3].

Majority of those people sleeping in designated shelters or public spaces have nationalities of the country of residence but some of them may be immigrants or nationality of other countries. The population of homeless persons is very diverse: it includes representatives from all ethnic groups, the young and the old, women and men, single persons and families, people from both urban and rural environments, and people with physical and/or mental problems [4, 5]. Most of the homeless individuals are between 31 and 50 years of age, are unmarried, and are unemployed [6–10].

Homeless people are more likely than the general population to have mental, neurologic, and substance use disorders. Evidence from different countries indicated that most of the homeless people suffer from mental illnesses such as depression, schizophrenia, substance abuse, psychotic disorders, and personality disorders. The prevalence of these disorders among homeless populations varies from country to country, and the precise cultural, national, psychosocial, and neurobiological determinants of these differences remain unclear. However, trends in mental disorders, homelessness, drug abuse, and crime suggest that Western industrial societies are becoming increasingly harmful to psychological and social well-being [11, 12].

According to different studies, 25–50% of the homeless population is reported to have some form of mental disorder [13–15] in high-income countries. This rises to about 60% among those who are street homeless. Severe mental disorders (SMD) and addictive or substance use disorders are the most common conditions among homeless individuals. In a meta-analysis of 29 studies conducted from 1979 to 2005, alcohol and drug dependence are the most common problems in homeless people with a pooled prevalence estimate of 38 and 24%, respectively, followed by psychosis with the pooled prevalence estimate of 13% [16]. Other studies indicated that 20–25% of the homeless population in the United States suffers from some form of severe mental illness. In comparison, only 6% of Americans are severely mentally ill [17]. In addition, in United States, mental illness was the third largest cause of homelessness [17].

As compared to general populations, homeless persons suffer from a high prevalence of physical disease, mental illness, and substance abuse [18–28]. Homelessness is associated with an increased risk of infections such as tuberculosis and human immunodeficiency virus (HIV) disease [29–34]. Among the homeless, access to health care is often suboptimal [35–39]. Homeless persons also experience severe poverty and often come from disadvantaged minority communities, factors that are independently associated with poor health [40–45].

Evidences from different studies have shown that the presence of mental disorders homeless people increases likelihood that the person spends longer periods as homeless [46], increased risk of mortality from general medical causes, suicide [47–49] and drug-related causes [50] and also increases vulnerability of the homeless person, including violent victimization [51] and criminality [52–54].

Evidence from studies in China [55], Nigeria [56], and Ethiopia [57] in people with schizophrenia revealed prevalence estimates of homelessness, i.e., 7.8, 4, and 7%, respectively. To our knowledge, there are no studies aimed at the screening, diagnosis, treatment, care, rehabilitation, and support of homeless people with mental, neurologic, and substance use (MNS) disorders in general in Ethiopia. This is the first study of its kind in Ethiopia, probably in Africa which aimed at screening, diagnosis, care, treatment, rehabilitation, and support of homeless individuals with possible MNS disorder. Furthermore, this study was aimed at creating continued rehabilitation, training, and other support for homeless people with MNS disorder in Ethiopia.

Methods

Study setting and design

Community-based survey was conducted from January to March 2015, at Addis Ababa, Ethiopia. Addis Ababa is the capital and largest city of Ethiopia. It has a population of 3,384,569 according to the 2015 population census, with annual growth rate of 3.8%. This number has been increased from the originally published 2,738,248 figure and appears to be still largely underestimated [58, 59]. As a chartered city, Addis Ababa has the status of both a city and a state. It is where the African Union is and its predecessor the OAU was based. It also hosts the headquarters of the United Nations Economic Commission for Africa (ECA) and numerous other continental and international organizations. Addis Ababa is therefore often referred to as "the political capital of Africa" due to its historical, diplomatic, and political significance for the continent [60]. In Ethiopia, particularly in major cities, homelessness is a manifest problem. In Addis Ababa, for example, the city administration estimates the number of homeless individuals to be around 50,000. A total of 456 homeless individuals were participated in the survey.

Study population

A total of 456 homeless people (homelessness) equated with street homelessness (rooflessness) were included in the survey. All homeless people are included from Addis Ababa, Ethiopia.

Sampling procedures
Study participants were included using multistage cluster sampling technique. We randomly selected 30 wards (kebeles) from a total of 98 in Addis Ababa, and everyone within the chosen wards (kebeles) who fulfilled the inclusion criteria was sampled.

Inclusion and exclusion criteria
Homeless people who had overt and observable psychopathology and positive for screening instruments (SRQ20, ASSIST and PSQ) were involved in the survey and further assessed for possible diagnosis by structured clinical interview for DSM-IV diagnoses and international diagnostic criteria for seizure disorders for possible involvement for care, treatment, rehabilitation service, support, and trainings.

Data collection, processing, and analyses
Data were collected by trained psychiatry professionals. The SRQ20, ASSIST, and PSQ were used for screening for possible problems, and Structured Clinical Interview of DSM-IV (SCID) was administered by psychiatry professionals and used to assess mental, neurologic, and substance use disorders. The Statistical Program for Social Science (SPSS version 20) was used for data entry, clearance, and analyses. Sociodemographic and clinical factors (diagnosis, history of alcohol, cannabis, nicotine, and khat abuse or dependence) were analyzed and reported using words, tables, and charts.

Ethical consideration
The survey was led by Amanuel Mental Specialized Hospital and was collaborative work with the Federal Ministry of Health of Ethiopia and Addis Ababa Health Bureau. Ethical approval was obtained from Amanuel Mental Specialized Hospital and Addis Ababa Health bureau Research Ethics Committee (REC). Written informed consent was obtained from each study participant and they were informed about their rights to interrupt the interview at any time. Confidentiality was maintained at all levels of the survey. The survey or research team facilitated admission, in collaboration with the district administration and Amanuel Mental Specialized Hospital, for those who had possible mental, neurologic, and substance use disorders and considered at immediate risk, including admission to a rehabilitation unit. All homeless people with possible mental, neurologic, and substance use disorders were evaluated by a specialist for diagnosis and further management and most of them were treated in inpatient unit at primary-,

secondary-, and tertiary-level health institutions for 3–6 months.

Results
Sociodemographic characteristics of participants
A total of 456 homeless people were involved in the survey. Majority of the participants were male ($n = 402$; 88.16%). Most of the homeless participants had migrated into Addis Ababa from elsewhere in Ethiopia and Eritrea (62.50%). Most homeless participants were chronically homeless, with over three-fourths (79.61%) having been homeless for 2 years or longer; only 20.39% of participants were homeless for less than 2 years (Table 1).

Magnitude and types of specific disorders among homeless people with mental, neurologic, and substance use disorders
In general, a majority of the participants included in the survey had some form of MNS disorder (92.11%; $n = 420$), and more than three-fourths of cases (85.29%; $n = 354$) were psychotic disorders. Most of those with psychosis had schizophrenia (77.40%; $n = 274$). Almost all of the participants had a history of substance use (93.20%; $n = 425$) and about one in ten individuals had substance use disorders (10.54%; $n = 48$). Most of the substance use disorder was comorbid with other mental and neurologic disorders (83.33%; $n = 40$) (Table 2).

Table 1 Sociodemographic characteristics of homeless people ($n = 456$), Addis Ababa, Ethiopia, 2015

Variable	Frequency	%
Gender		
Female	54	11.84
Male	402	88.16
Regions (place of birth/residence before homelessness)		
Addis Ababa	171	37.50
Oromia	79	17.32
Amhara	83	18.20
South Ethiopia	64	14.04
Tigray	10	2.20
Diredawa	6	1.32
Harar	8	1.76
Somali	2	0.44
Eritrea	8	1.76
Others	25	5.46
Duration of homelessness		
< 6 months	27	5.92
6–12 months	30	6.58
1–2 years	36	7.89
2–5 years	112	24.56
> 5 years	251	55.05

Table 2 Prevalence of mental, neurologic, and substance use disorders among homeless participant, Addis Ababa, Ethiopia ($n = 456$) Addis Ababa, Ethiopia, 2015

Type of mental disorders	Frequency	%
Schizophrenia	274	60.09
Psychotic disorders NOS	45	9.87
Major depressive disorders with psychotic features	23	5.04
Substance-induced psychotic disorders	31	6.79
Major depressive disorders	21	4.61
Brief psychotic disorders	4	0.88
General anxiety disorders	4	0.88
Catatonia (unspecified)	1	0.21
Substance use history	425	93.20
Substance use disorders	48	10.53
Epilepsy	8	1.75
Comorbid mental and substance use disorders	40	83.33
No illness	36	7.89
Overall mental neurologic and substance use disorders	420	92.11

Discussion

The current survey revealed that a significant portion of homeless study participants had mental, neurologic, and substance use disorders and the high burden of mental, neurologic, and substance use disorders among street homeless in Ethiopia. To our knowledge, there are no studies aimed at screening, diagnosis, treatment care, rehabilitation, and establishment of continued support and networks for homeless people with MNS disorder in general in Ethiopia.

This study revealed that the homeless people have very diverse sociodemographic characteristics in Ethiopia; this was comparable to that seen in homeless people in high-income country settings [4, 5]. In this survey majority, the participants had some form of MNS disorder (92.11%; $n = 420$), and more than three-fourths of cases (85.29%; $n = 354$) had psychotic disorders. Most of those with psychosis had schizophrenia (77.40%; $n = 274$). These findings were higher than the findings of Brazil (49%) [61] and other high-income countries (60%) [13]. The possible reason for the higher rate of mental disorder in our survey may be because in our study those who had overt and observable psychopathology and positive by screening instruments were involved, who are known to have higher rates of mental, neurologic, and substance use disorders.

The findings of the current study revealed that most of those homeless people with psychosis had schizophrenia (77.40%; $n = 274$). This finding was higher than the study done in high-income countries which revealed 20–25% of the homeless population in the United States suffers from

some form of severe mental illness including schizophrenia [17]. The possible reason for the higher rate of schizophrenia in our survey may be because in our study those who had overt and observable psychopathology and positive by screening instruments were involved, who are known to have higher rates of mental, neurologic, and substance use disorders.

In addition, we found that one in ten individuals had substance use disorders (10.54%; $n = 48$). These results are lower than a report from a meta-analysis of 29 studies conducted from 1979 to 2005, which revealed pooled prevalence estimate alcohol and drug dependence, i.e, 38 and 24%, respectively, among homeless individuals [16]. The possible reason for this difference might be due to the instrument they used, socioeconomic and cultural difference, and the sample included in the study.

Limitation of the study

In our study, those who had overt and observable psychopathology and positive by screening instruments were involved, who are known to have higher rates of mental, neurologic and substance use disorders.

Conclusion and recommendations

Mental, neurologic, and substance use disorders resulted to be common problems in the study participants (92.11%; $n = 420$). Most of the participants with mental, neurologic, and substance use disorders (85.29%; $n = 354$) had psychotic disorders. Most of those with psychosis had schizophrenia (77.40%; $n = 274$). Almost all of the participants had a history of substance use (93.20%; $n = 425$) and about one in ten individuals had substance use disorders (10.54%; $n = 48$). In the current study, it was found that comorbid substance use disorder with other mental and neurologic disorders was a more frequent phenomenon among homeless people and that majority of those who have mental and neurologic disorders have co-occurring substance use disorders as compared to those who have no mental and neurologic disorders. Our findings indicate that attention needs to be given to screen and assess mental, neurologic, and substance use disorders in homeless people. The development of centers for care, treatment, rehabilitation, and support of homeless people with mental, neurologic, and substance use disorders is warranted. In addition, it is necessary to improve the accessibility of mental health services and promote better integration between mental and primary health care services, as a means to offer a better general care and to possibly prevent homelessness among mentally ill.

Authors' contributions
GA conceived the study and was involved in the study design, reviewed the article, analysis, report writing, and drafted the manuscript, DA, KH, AC, ZY, HS,

MA, BT, KH, MS, SD, and LB were involved in the study design and analysis and drafted the manuscript. All authors read and approved the final manuscript.

Acknowledgements
The authors acknowledge the Federal Ministry of Health, Ethiopia for funding the study. The authors appreciate the study participants for their cooperation in providing the necessary information.

Competing interests
The authors declare that they have no competing interests.

Consent for publication
Not applicable

Funding
This research work is funded by the Federal Ministry of Health of Ethiopia.

References

1. Kuhn R, Culhane DP. Applying cluster analysis to test a typology of homelessness by pattern of shelter utilization: Results from the analysis of administrative data. American Journal of community psychology. 1998;26(2):207–32.
2. Scott J. Homelessness and mental illness. Br J Psychiatry. 1993;162:314–24.
3. Arce AA, Vergare MJ. Identifying and characterizing the mentally ill among the homeless. In: Lamb HR, editor. The homeless mentally ill: a task force report of the American Psychiatric Association. Washington: American Psychiatric Association; 1984. p. 75–89.
4. Burt MR. Over the edge: the growth of homelessness in the 1980s. New York: Russell Sage Foundation; 1992.
5. Robertson MJ, Greenblatt M. Homelessness: a national perspective. New York: Plenum Press; 1992.
6. Brandt P, Munk-Jorgensen P. Homeless in Denmark. In: Bughra D, editor. Homelessness and mental health. Cambridge: Cambridge University Press; 1996. p. 189–96.
7. Fernandez J. Homelessness: an Irish perspective. In: Bughra D, editor. Homelessness and mental health. Cambridge: Cambridge University Press; 1996. p. 209–29.
8. Koegel P, Burnam MA, Baumohl J. The causes of homelessness. In: Baumohl J, editor. Homeless in America. New York: Oryx Press; 1996.
9. O'Flaherty B. Making room: the economics of homelessness. Cambridge: Harvard University Press; 1996.
10. Rossler W, Salize HJ. Continental European experience: Germany. In: Bughra D, editor. Homelessness and mental health. Cambridge: Cambridge University Press; 1996. p. 197–208.
11. Eckersley R. Failing a generation: the impact of culture on the health and well-being of youth. J Paediatr Child Health. 1993;29(Suppl. 1):16–9.
12. Fazel S, Khosla V, Doll H, Geddes J. The prevalence of mental disorders among the homeless in western countries: systematic review and meta-regression analysis. PLoS Med. 2008;5(12):e225. https://doi.org/10.1371/journal.pmed.0050225.
13. Scott J. Homelessness and mental illness. Br J Psychiatry. 1993;162:314–24.
14. Breakey WR, Fischer PJ, Kramer M. Health and mental health problems of homeless men and women living in Baltimore. JAMA. 1989;262:1352–7.
15. Gelberg L, Linn LS. Demographic differences in health status of homeless adults. J Gen Intern Med. 1992;7:601–8.
16. Koegel P, Burnam MA. Alcoholism among homeless adults in the inner-city of Los Angeles. Arch Gen Psychiatry. 1988;45:1011–8.
17. Substance Abuse and Mental Health Services Administration, Center for Mental Health Services. Homelessness. http://mentalhealth.samhsa.gov/cmhs/Homelessness/. Accessed Jun 11, 2009
18. Breakey WR, Rischer PJ, Kramer M, et al. Health and mental health problems of homeless men and women in Baltimore. JAMA. 1989;262:1352–7.
19. Bassuk EL, Rubin L, Lauriat A. Is homelessness a mental health problem? Am J Psychiatry. 1984;141:1546–50.
20. Koegel P, Burnam A, Farr RK. The prevalence of specific psychiatric disorders among homeless individuals in the inner city of Los Angeles. Arch Gen Psychiatry. 1988;45:1085–92.
21. Koegel P, Burnam MA. Alcoholism among homeless adults in the inner city of Los Angeles. Arch Gen Psychiatry. 1988;45:1011–8.
22. Susser E, Struening EL, Conomver S. Psychiatric problems in homeless men. Arch Gen Psychiatry. 1989;46:845–50.
23. Gelberg L, Linn LS, Usatine RP, Smith MH. Health, homelessness, and poverty: a study of clinic users. Arch Intern Med. 1990;150:2325–30.
24. Ferenchick GS. Medical problems of homeless and nonhomeless persons attending an inner-city health clinic. Am J Med Sci. 1991;301:379–82.
25. Fischer PJ, Breakey WR. The epidemiology of alcohol, drug, and mental disorders among homeless persons. Am Psychol. 1991;46:1115–28.
26. Centers for Disease Control (CDC). Characteristics and risk behaviors of homeless black men seeking services from the community homeless assistance plan—Dade County, Florida, August 1991. MMWR. 1991;40:865–8.
27. Gelberg L, Linn LS. Demographic differences in health status of homeless adults. J Gen Intern Med. 1992;7:601–8.
28. Gelberg L, Leake BD. Substance use among impoverished medical patients: the effect of housing status and other factors. Med Care. 1993;31:757–66.
29. Brudney K, Dobkin J. Resurgent tuberculosis in New York City. Am Rev Respir Dis. 1991;144:745–9.
30. Concato J, Rom WN. Endemic tuberculosis among homeless men in New York City. Arch Intern Med. 1994;154:2069–73.
31. Barnes PF, El-Hajj H, Preston-Martin S, et al. Transmission of tuberculosis among the urban homeless. JAMA. 1996;275:305–7.
32. Torres RA, Mani S, Altholz J, Brickner PW. Human immunodeficiency virus infection among homeless men in a New York City shelter. Arch Intern Med. 1990;150:2030–5.
33. Allen DM, Lehman JS, Green TA, et al. HIV infection among homeless adults and runaway youth, United States, 1989–1992. AIDS. 1994;8:1593–8.
34. Zolopa AR, Hahn JA, Gorter R, et al. HIV and tuberculosis infection in San Francisco's homeless adults. JAMA. 1994;272:455–61.
35. Elvy A. Access to care. In: Brickner PW, Scharer LK, Conanan B, et al., editors. Health care of homeless people. New York: Springer Publishing Co; 1985. p. 223–31.
36. Brickner PW, Scanlan BC, Conanan B, et al. Homeless persons and health care. Ann Intern Med. 1986;104:405–9.
37. Robertson MJ, Cousineau MR. Health status and access to health services among the urban homeless. Am J Public Health. 1986;76:561–3.
38. Stark LR. Barriers to health care for homeless people. In: Jahiel RI, editor. Homelessness: a prevention oriented approach. Baltimore: Johns Hopkins University Press; 1992. p. 151–64.
39. Gelberg L, Gallagher TC, Andersen RM. KoegelP. Competing priorities as a barrier to medical care among homeless adults in Los Angeles. Am J Public Health. 1997;87:217–20.
40. Fein O. The influence of social class on health status. J Gen Intern Med. 1995;10:577–86.
41. Bucher HC, Ragland DR. Socioeconomic indicators and mortality from coronary heart disease and cancer. Am J Public Health. 1995;85:1231–6.
42. McDonough P, Duncan GJ, Williams D, House J. Income dynamics and adult mortality in the United States, 1972 through 1989. Am J Public Health. 1997;87:1476–83.
43. Lantz PM, House JS, Lepkowski JM, et al. Socioeconomic factors, health behaviors, and mortality. JAMA. 1998;279:1703–8.
44. Geronimus AT, Bound J, Waidmann TA, et al. Excess mortality among blacks and whites in the United States. N Engl J Med. 1996;335:1552–8.
45. Singh GK, Yu SM. Trends and differentials in adolescent and young adult mortality in the United States, 1950 through 1993. American Journal of Public Health. 1996;86(4):560–4.
46. Morse G, Shields NM, Hanneke CR, McCall GJ, Calsyn RJ, Nelson B. St. Louis' homeless: mental health needs, services, and policy implications. Psychosoc Rehabil J. 1986;9:39–50.

47. Babidge NC, Buhrich N, Butler T. Mortality among homeless people with schizophrenia in Sydney, Australia: a 10 year follow-up. Acta Psychiatr Scand. 2001;103:105–10.

48. Hwang SW. Mortality among men using homeless shelters in Toronto, Ontario. JAMA. 2000;283:2152–7.

49. Prigerson HG, Desai RA, Liu-Mares W, Rosenheck RA. Suicidal ideation and suicide attempts in homeless mentally ill persons: age-specific risks of substance abuse. Soc Psychiatry Psychiatr Epidemiol. 2003;38:213–9.

50. Barrow SM, Herman DB, Cordova P, Struening EL. Mortality among homeless shelter residents in New York City. Am J Public Health. 1999;89:529–34.

51. Walsh E, Moran P, Scott C, McKenzie K, Burns T, Creed F, Tyrer P, Murray RM, Fahy T. Prevalence of violent victimisation in severe mental illness. Br J Psychiatry. 2003;183:233–8.

52. Brennan P, Mednick S, Hodgins S. Major mental disorders and criminal violence in a Danish birth cohort. Arch Gen Psychiatry. 2000;57:494–500.

53. Fazel S, Grann M. The population impact of severe mental illness on violent crime. Am J Psychiatry. 2006;163:1397–403.

54. Gelberg L, Linn LS, Leake BD. Mental health, alcohol and drug use, and criminal history among homeless adults. Am J Psychiatry. 1988;145:191–6.

55. Ran MS, Chan CLW, Chen EYH, Xiang MZ, Caine ED, Conwell Y. Homelessness among patients with schizophrenia in rural China: a 10-year cohort study. Acta Psychiatr Scand. 2006;114:118–23.

56. Gureje O, Bamidele R. Thirteen-year social outcome among Nigerian outpatients with schizophrenia. Soc Psychiatry Psychiatr Epidemiol. 1999;34:147–51.

57. Kebede D, Alem A, Shibre T, Negash A, Fekadu A, Fekadu D, Deyassa N, Jacobsson L, Kullgren G. Onset and clinical course of schizophrenia in Butajira-Ethiopia—a community-based study. Soc Psychiatry Psychiatr Epidemiol. 2003;38:625–31.

58. Central Statistical Agency of Ethiopia. "Census 2007, preliminary (pdf-file)" (PDF). Archived (PDF) from the original on 18 December 2008. Retrieved 7 Dec 2008.

59. Givental E. Addis Ababa Urbanism: Indigenous Urban Legacies and Contemporary Challenges. J Geography Geology. 2017;9(1):25.

60. "United Nations Economic Commission for Africa". UNECA. Accessed 5 May 2012.

61. Lovisi GM, Mann AH, Coutinho E, Morgado AF. Mental illness in an adult sample admitted to public hostels in the Rio de Janeiro metropolitan area. Braz Soc Psychiatry Psychiatr Epidemiol. 2003;38:496–501.

8

Neurological soft signs in Tunisian patients with first-episode psychosis and relation with cannabis use

Ahmed Mhalla[1,2*], Bochra Ben Mohamed[1,2], Christoph U. Correll[3,4,5], Badii Amamou[1,2], Anouar Mechri[1,2] and Lotfi Gaha[1,2]

Abstract

Background: Neurological soft signs (NSS) are minor non-localizing neurological abnormalities that are conceptualized as neurodevelopmental markers that mediate the biological risk for psychosis. We aimed to explore the relationship between NSS and cannabis use, an environmental risk factor of psychosis.

Methods: This was a cross-sectional study in consecutively admitted patients hospitalized for first-episode psychosis. NSS were assessed by the NSS scale (23 items exploring motor coordination, motor integrative function, sensory integration, involuntary movements or posture, quality of lateralization). Presence of NSS was defined as a NSS scale total score ≥ 9.5. Cannabis use was ascertained with the cannabis subsection in the Composite International Diagnostic Interview.

Results: Among 61 first-episode psychosis patients (mean age $= 28.9 \pm 9.4$ years; male $= 86.9\%$, antipsychotic-naïve $= 75.4\%$), the prevalence of current cannabis use was 14.8% (heavy use $= 8.2\%$, occasional use $= 6.6\%$). NSS were present in 83.6% of the sample (cannabis users $= 66.7\%$ versus cannabis non-users $= 85.5\%$, $p = 0.16$). The mean total NSS score was 15.3 ± 6.7, with a significant lower total NSS score in cannabis users (11.2 ± 5.6 versus 16.0 ± 6.7, $p = 0.048$). Differences were strongest for the "motor coordination" ($p = 0.06$) and "involuntary movements" ($p = 0.07$) sub-scores.

Conclusions: This study demonstrated a negative association between cannabis use and NSS, especially regarding motor discoordination. This finding supports the hypothesis that a strong environmental risk factor, such as cannabis, may contribute to the onset of psychosis even in the presence of lower biological and genetic vulnerability, as reflected indirectly by lower NSS scores. Nevertheless, additional studies are needed that explore this interaction further in larger samples and considering additional neurobiological and environmental risk factors.

Keywords: Schizophrenia, First episode, Cannabis, Neurological soft signs

Introduction

Neurological soft signs (NSS) are minor non-localizing neurological abnormalities determined by clinical examination [1]. NSS concern four main areas of neurological functioning: motor coordination, sensory integration, sequencing of complex motor acts, and primitive developmental reflexes [2]. NSS have been conceptualized as neurodevelopmental markers that mediate the biological propensity for the development of psychosis. This conceptualization was established on the basis of many observations showing higher rates of NSS not only among people with schizophrenia, but also among treatment-naive patients with first-episode psychosis (FEP) [3, 4], non-psychotic siblings, and subjects considered at high risk for psychosis [5–8]. The prevalence of NSS in patients with FEP has been reported to range from 20 to

*Correspondence: ahmed.mhalla@yahoo.fr
[1] Psychiatry Department, Fattouma Bourguiba Hospital, 5000 Monastir, Tunisia
Full list of author information is available at the end of the article

Neurological soft signs in Tunisian patients with first-episode psychosis and relation...

57

97%, depending on the study sample and methodology, and NSS seem to precede psychotic symptoms [3, 4, 9].

Cannabis is the most widely used illicit drug in patients with psychosis [10], and the median cannabis use disorder rates are as high as 28.6% for current and 44.4% for life-time prevalence [11]. Longitudinal studies have reported an increased likelihood for developing schizophrenia and other psychoses after cannabis use [12–17], especially when cannabis use has been moderate to severe and/or started in the early teens [14, 18–20]. The relationship between cannabis and psychosis seems fairly specific to schizophrenia, as compared to other mental disorders [21, 22]. This relationship cannot be explained by potentially confounding factors, such as premorbid disorders, other types of drug use, intoxication effects, personality traits, sociodemographic markers, or intellectual ability [22]. Accordingly, several reviews conclude that there is an increased risk for psychosis in individuals who have used cannabis, typically in the magnitude of an odds ratio of 1.5–2 [22–24]. However, there are also opposing views on cannabis as a risk factor for psychosis. Some authors propose that there is a causal relationship between cannabis use and psychosis [25, 26]. Others suggest that cannabis use only precipitates psychosis in vulnerable individuals on their pathway to the disorder [25–27]. Cannabis consumption usually precedes the onset of psychosis [28, 29]. However, most individuals do not develop psychosis after cannabis use, suggesting that risk of psychosis must be modulated by other factors. In line with this conceptualization, data from recent comprehensive studies suggest that cannabis is an environmental risk factor that interacts with genetic and biological vulnerabilities for psychosis [30, 31].

While different authors have studied the association between NSS and perinatal factors, such as obstetric complications [32–34], few studies have investigated the interaction between NSS and non-perinatal environmental factors, such as cannabis use [35–37].

The aim of this study was to explore the relationship between neurodevelopmental markers reflecting neurobiological vulnerability (NSS) and an environmental risk factor (cannabis use) in a sample of Tunisian patients with FEP. The hypothesis was that the cannabis pathway to psychosis may reflect less neurobiological vulnerability.

Patients and methods

Study design

This was a cross-sectional study conducted over a period of 14 months (from July 2012 to September 2013) in the psychiatry department of Fattouma Bourguiba Hospital in Monastir, Tunisia, in consecutively admitted patients hospitalized for FEP according to Diagnostic and

Statistical Manual of Mental Disorders (DSM-IV) criteria [38]. Patients had the diagnosis of schizophrenia, schizophreniform disorder, brief psychotic disorder, delusional disorder, substance-induced psychotic disorder, or psychotic disorder not otherwise specified. Exclusion criteria were: age >55 years old, prior hospitalization or consultation in a psychiatric unit, diagnosis of psychotic disorder due to medical condition, mental retardation, a history of major neurological disorder and unwillingness to consent to participate in the study.

Measures and assessment tools

Sociodemographic and clinical data were collected both with a pre-established questionnaire and based on medical record review. The premorbid functioning was evaluated by the Premorbid Adjustment Scale (PAS) [39, 40] based on patient interview, the duration of untreated psychosis (DUP) was estimated by interviewing the caregiver/family and the patient, the psychometric assessment was conducted by the Positive and Negative Syndrome Scale (PANSS) [41], and the Global Assessment of Functioning scale (GAF) [42] based on patient interview.

The neurological evaluations were carried-out using the neurological soft signs (NSS) scale by Krebs et al. The NSS scale explores 23 minor neurological signs that are rated from 0 to 3 and distributed in five main domains: motor coordination, motor integration, sensory integration, involuntary movements or posture, and quality of lateralization. The threshold value for this scale was fixed at 9.5 as recommended in the original version [43]. Neurological side effects of antipsychotics were evaluated by the Simpson Angus (SA) scale [44].

The PANSS and the GAF scales were administered within 72 h of the patient's hospitalization. The NSS scale and the Simpson Angus scale were completed within seven days of hospitalization.

We ascertained the use of cannabis with the cannabis subsection of the Composite International Diagnostic Interview (CIDI), included within the section of substance use. According to the CIDI, patients were considered to be cannabis users if they had taken cannabis on five or more occasions; patients were considered as "heavy cannabis users" when the frequency of cannabis use was daily or nearly every day.

Statistical analyses

All statistical analyses were performed with SPSS for Windows, Version 21.0.

The independent factor was cannabis use, which divided the study sample in two groups: in-patients with current cannabis use versus in-patients without current cannabis use. The Mann–Whitney non-parametric test, the Chi-square test, the Fisher's exact test and the Pearson correlation coefficient were used for the between-group analysis. The statistical significance was set at 5%. Additionally, for the presence/absence of NSS, defined by the threshold value of >9.5 on the NSS Scale, we performed a logistic regression with cannabis use as well as smoking, alcohol use, PANSS positive score, PANSS negative score, PANSS disorganization score, PAS total score, and Simpson Angus score as variables entered into the model. The variables included were the significant ones at the statistical threshold of 0.25. All tests were two-sided with $\alpha = 0.05$. Due to the exploratory nature of the analyses, we did not correct for multiple comparisons.

Results

Sociodemographic, clinical, therapeutic use characteristics

At the end of the study period, 71 consecutively enrolled patients met the inclusion and exclusion criteria. Of these, 10 were not recruited: 4 patients due to premature discharge against medical advice and 6 patients refused study participation. Altogether, 61 in-patients were included in this study.

The study sample contained 53 men (86.9%) and 8 women; the mean age was 28.9 ± 9.4 year-old. The majority had a low educational level or was unschooled (70.5%) and single (75.4%). Family history of mental illness was present in 24.6% of the patients; consisting mainly of psychotic disorders in first-degree relatives (Table 1). The majority of the patients (67.2%) had never taken psychotropic treatment before the hospitalization; only 24.6% had received antipsychotic treatment, most often only for a few days before hospitalization and 8.2% had received antidepressant treatment. The main diagnosis was schizophreniform disorder (42.6%), the mean DUP was 39.6 ± 63.7 weeks; and the majority of patients were treated with first-generation antipsychotics (68.8%) (Table 2).

Cannabis use

The prevalence of the current cannabis use in this population was 14.8%, with heavy use among 8.2% of the patients and occasional use among 6.6%.

Neurological soft signs (NSS)

NSS evaluation

The mean NSS score was 15.3 ± 6.7 (ranging from 4 to 32.5). The highest sub-scores were noted in the domain of motor coordination (6.1 ± 2.7) (Table 3). Using the threshold value of ≥9.5 on the NSS scale, NSS were present in 83.6% of the total patient sample.

NSS and clinical and therapeutic characteristics

Correlations were found between the NSS total scores and the Poor Premorbid Functioning ($r = 0.32$, $p = 0.04$), the PANSS total scores ($r = 0.36$, $p = 0.005$), and the negative ($r = 0.45$, $p < 0.001$) and disorganization sub-scores ($r = 0.41$, $p = 0.001$), the CGI-severity scores ($r = 0.30$, $p = 0.02$), the impairment functioning in the GAF ($r = -0.26$, $p = 0.04$) and with extrapyramidal symptoms ($r = 0.52$, $p < 0.001$) (Table 3).

NSS and cannabis use

Comparing NSS scores between patients with and without cannabis use demonstrated significantly lower total NSS scores of in patients with cannabis use: 11.2 ± 5.6 versus 16.0 ± 6.7 ($p = 0.048$) (Table 4). The linear regression model showed that this association remained significant after adjustment for two potentially confounding factors that have been associated with NSS: negative symptoms and neurological side effects of antipsychotics (Table 5).

There was also an inverse, but not significant relationship between the use of cannabis and the motor coordination and the involuntary movements sub-scores (Table 3).

Table 1 Sociodemographic characteristics

Variables	Total number of patients (n = 61)	Cannabis users (n = 9)	Cannabis non-users (n = 52)	p
Age	28.9 ± 9.4	27.4 ± 7.8	29.2 ± 10	0.81
Male sex	53 (86.9%)	9 (100%)	44 (84.6%)	0.61
Psychiatric family history	15 (24.6%)	2 (22.2%)	13 (25.0%)	0.33
University studies	18 (29.5%)	3 (33.3%)	15 (28.8%)	0.57
Marital status				
Single	46 (75.4%)	7 (77.8%)	39 (75%)	0.72
Married	11 (18%)	1 (11.1%)	10 (19.2%)	
Divorced	4 (6.6%)	1 (11.1%)	3 (5.8%)	
Currently employed	27 (44.3%)	8 (88.9%)	6 (11.5%)	0.91
Premorbid Adjustment Scale score	19.2 ± 7.9	18.7 ± 8.5	22.6 ± 7.6	0.23

Table 2 Clinical and therapeutic characteristics

Variables	Total number of patients (n = 61)	Cannabis users (n = 9)	Cannabis non-users (n = 52)	p
Psychiatric diagnosis				
Schizophrenia	20 (32.9%)	5 (55.5%)	15 (28.8%)	
Schizophreniform disorder	26 (42.6%)	1 (11.1%)	25 (48.1%)	
Brief psychotic disorder	10 (16.4%)	1 (11.1%)	9 (17.2%)	0.10
Cannabis-induced psychosis	3 (4.9%)	2 (22.2%)	1 (1.9%)	
Delusional psychosis	1 (1.6%)	0 (0%)	1 (1.9%)	
Psychotic disorder not otherwise specified	1 (1.6%)	0 (0%)	1 (1.9%)	
PANSS total score	99.5 ± 20.6	101.6 ± 20.5	99.1 ± 20.8	0.65
PANSS positive score	25.1 ± 6	27 ± 6.3	24.8 ± 6	0.43
PANSS negative score	24.3 ± 9.3	25.7 ± 9.8	24 ± 9.3	0.56
GAF score	32.4 ± 8	30 ± 5.6	33.5 ± 8.3	0.28
Duration of untreated psychosis (weeks)	39.6 ± 63.7	28.6 ± 35.2	41.5 ± 87.4	0.45
Antipsychotic treatment				
First-generationantipsychotic	25(41%)	4 (44.4%)	21 (40.4%)	
Second-generationantipsychotic	19 (31.1%)	2 (22.2%)	17 (32.7%)	0.84
Co-treatment of first- and second-generation antipsychotics	17 (27.8%)	3 (33.3%)	14 (26.9%)	
Chlorpromazine equivalent	619.8 ± 419.8 mg	914.0 ± 629.8 mg	568.8 ± 356.6 mg	0.16
Simpson Angus scale score	3.8 ± 3.2	4.3 ± 2.6	3.7 ± 3.	0.37
Duration of hospitalization (days)	29.1 ± 16.6	43.3 ± 15.5	26.7 ± 15.6	0.005

GAF Global Assessment of Functioning, *PANSS* Positive and Negative Symptom Scale

Table 3 Correlations between NSS and clinical and therapeutic characteristics

	NSS total score
PAS total score	$r = 0.32, p = 0.04$
PANSS total score	$r = 0.36, p = 0.005$
PANSS positive score	$r = -0.06, p = 0.69$
PANSS negative score	$r = 0.45, p < 0.001$
PANSS disorganization score	$r = 0.41, p = 0.001$
CGI-severity score	$r = 0.30, p = 0.02$
GAF score	$r = -0.26, p = 0.04$
SA score	$r = 0.52, p < 0.001$

NSS neurological soft signs, *PAS* Premorbid Adjustment Scale, *PANSS* Positive and Negative Syndrome Scale, *GAF* Global Assessment of Functioning, *CGI* Clinical Global Impression, *SA* Simpson Angus

There was also a significant association between heavy cannabis use and lower total NSS scores ($p = 0.048$).

Altogether, 66.7% of the patients with cannabis use exceeded the threshold value of 9.5 versus 85.5% of the non-users ($p = 0.16$). Similarly, a logistic regression analysis, with the presence of NSS as dependant variable and cannabis use, smoking, alcohol use, PANSS positive score, PANSS negative score, PANSS disorganization score, PAS total score and Simpson Angus score as covariates, did not show a significant association between presence of NSS and current cannabis use ($p = 0.12$).

Discussion

In this study, the prevalence of NSS was 83.6%, given the threshold score of 9.5 suggested by the NSS scale authors [43]. Studies that evaluated patients with first-episode psychosis reported a high prevalence of NSS, ranging from 20% for the Scottish Schizophrenia Research Group [9] to 97.1% for Browne et al. [4] (Table 6).

In this study, we examined the relationship between cannabis use and NSS in FEP patients; cannabis users had significantly fewer NSS than patients without a history of cannabis use. This findings were similar to those reported by Ruiz-Veguilla et al. [36] who studied cannabis use and NSS among 92 patients with FEP (64% males, mean age: 26.9 ± 10.1 years old). The authors found that heavy cannabis users (55% of the sample of the study) had significantly less NSS assesses with the Neurological Evaluation Scale independent of potential confounders, such as sex, age, family history of psychosis, and negative symptoms [36]. A similar association was also found by Stirling et al. [37] in a sample of 112 non-depressed FEP patients (56.2% males, mean age: 26.3 years old) with 38% of cannabis users. Other studies demonstrated a lower NSS scores for patients with chronic schizophrenia and

Table 4 Neurological soft signs scale scores in patients with and without cannabis use

Neurological soft signs scale scores: median, (interquartile range)	Total number of patients ($n = 61$)	Cannabis use		Statistic tests
		Yes ($n = 9$)	No ($n = 52$)	
Motor coordination sub-score	6.0 (4.3, 9.0)	3.5 (2.3,8.0)	6 (4.5, 9.0)	$p = 0.06$
Motor integration sub-score	3.0 (1.5, 5.3)	2.5 (1.3, 4.0)	3(1.5, 5.5)	$p = 0.51$
Sensory integration sub-score	3.5 (1.5, 4.8)	2.0 (1.0, 4.0)	3.5 (1.5, 5.4)	$p = 0.20$
Involuntary movements or posture sub-score	0 (0, 0)	0 (0, 0.3)	0.3 (0, 0.3)	$p = 0.07$
Quality of lateralization sub-score	1.0 (0, 1.0)	1 (0, 1.5)	1.0 (0, 3.0)	$p = 0.20$
Total score	13.5 (11.0, 19.5)	11.5 (6.0, 14.3)	14.5 (11.5, 20.75)	$p = 0.048$
Total score >9.5 (N, %)	51 (83.6%)	6 (66.6%)	45 (86.5%)	$p = 0.16$

Table 5 Linear regression NSS total scores, PANSS negative scores and Simpson Angus scores

	Standardized coefficient beta	CI	p value
Cannabis use	−0.315	(−9.41, −2.41)	0.001
PANSS negative score	0.402	(0.15, 0.42)	<0.001
Simpson Angus score	0.476	(0.59, 1.36)	<0.001

PANSS Positive and Negative Symptom Scale

a history of cannabis use than for those without cannabis use. For example, Bersani et al. [45] investigated NSS in 25 male cannabis-consuming and 25 male non-consuming schizophrenia patients, using the Neurological Evaluation Scale and concluded that non-consuming patients showed a higher incidence of NSS. Joyal et al. [35], in a study of 16 men with and 14 men without a dual diagnosis of drug abuse and schizophrenia, reported that drug abuse was associated to fewer frontal soft signs.

Three possible explanations are suggested for this seemingly paradoxical relationship between cannabis use and NSS in FEP. First, some cannabis components may have neuroprotective effects by inhibiting the glutamatergic excitotoxicity system [46, 47]. Second, this association could be explained by the fact that cannabis would act more directly on the onset of psychosis in genetically less vulnerable individuals [19, 48] since NSS are shown to reflect a genetic liability to psychosis. In this context, cannabis use may be the environmental factor that reveals or potentiates the vulnerability to psychosis. Accordingly, it is likely that cannabis could increase the effects of genetic risk factors for psychosis. Thus, cannabis users may follow a different pathway (with less neurobiological vulnerability factors) in developing psychotic disorders compared to patients without a history of cannabis use [36, 48]. Third, the inverse association between NSS and cannabis use could be explained by a relationship between severe NSS with other clinical characteristics that would limit a subject's personal access to cannabis [47]. In fact, most studies that examined NSS in FEP, in concordance with the results of this study, concluded that NSS were associated with more negative symptoms [2, 49, 50], disorganization symptoms [2, 49, 50] and illness severity [2]. These illness dimensions can limit the patients' social interaction abilities and diminish their motivation or ability to obtain cannabis.

This study also showed an inverse, but not significant relationship between the use of cannabis and both "motor coordination" ($p = 0.06$) and "involuntary movements"

Table 6 Prevalence of neurological soft signs in first-episode psychosis

Authors (year)	N	Study population	Instrument to assess NSS	Prevalence of NSS (%)
The Scottish Schizophrenia Research Group [9]	49	First-episode schizophrenia	NES scale	20
Flyckt et al. [59]	31	First-episode psychosis	NES scale	78
Browne et al. [4]	35	First-episode schizophrenia or schizophreniform disorder	NES scale CNE scale	97
Emsley et al. [60]	66	First-episode psychosis, schizophreniform disorder or schizoaffective disorder	NES scale	68
Ruiz-Veguilla et al. [36]	92	First-episode psychosis	NES scale	45
Our study	61	First-episode psychosis	NSS scale	84

CNE Condensed Neurological Examination, *NES* Neurological Evaluation Scale, *NSS* neurological soft signs, *NSS scale* Neurological Soft Signs scale

($p = 0.07$) sub-scores. To our knowledge, no other study explored the interaction between cannabis use and the different sub-groups of NSS in FEP patients. The available data about this topic are restricted to studies with non-psychotic populations that showed greater impairment of motor functioning in patients with cannabis use. Dervaux et al. [51] compared the impact of cannabis use on NSS among patients with cannabis dependence and healthy controls and demonstrated that higher NSS scores were associated especially with motor coordination difficulties in cannabis users. Roser et al. [52] reported impairment in motor speed after cannabis use. These results could be explained by the important role of the endocannabinoid system in the control of movements. In fact, a prominent distribution of the cannabinoid 1 (CB1) receptors in the basal ganglia has been described in patients with movements disorders [53, 54], and cannabis, when interacting with CB1 receptors, induces dopamine release and an increase in motor response [55]. Heavy cannabis consumption may also lead to deterioration in the control system balance and thereby contribute to motor inhibition [56]. The dose-dependent response of motor coordination to cannabis may be due to the involvement of GABAergic and glutamatergic systems as a target of cannabis and its psychoactive component Delta-(9)-tetrahydrocannabinol (THC) [56], or the development of sensitization and adaptive process, which leads to dopamine decrease in prefrontal regions after repeated use [57, 58]. This finding may explain the impairment of motor skills reported over non-psychotic patients.

Conversely, however, higher cannabis consumption may produce a different response, which consists of a motor stimulation instead of inhibition depending on the adaptive mechanism put in place [47]. It is possible that this stimulatory effect could explain the inverse relation between motor coordination and cannabis in this study. Additionally, we investigated in-patients without any access to cannabis at the time of investigation. Hence, acute cannabis effects would not have been influenced our results and we assessed cannabis use more as a trait marker or risk factor for FEP. The fact that we found less motor coordination in patients with cannabis use and FEP strengthens our hypothesis that cannabis use might bring out psychosis risk in those individuals with less other neurobiological risk factors, as motor dysfunction, together with low intellectual quotient, was identified as one of the two strongest biological markers for schizophrenia risk in a recent meta-analysis [15].

There are several limitations to this study. First, the study was not based on a sample size calculation; the sample size, especially of the cannabis users, is small, although it lies within the range of similar FEP studies on this topic. Second, we did not confirm absence of cannabis use by urine screening and we did not have data regarding the exact time between the NSS evaluation and last cannabis consumption. Third, in view of the need for urgent treatment, it hasn't been always possible to assess NSS before antipsychotic administration, which would have been better for NSS evaluation. Finally, we did not collect data on the amount of cannabis use.

This study demonstrated a negative association between cannabis use and NSS, especially regarding motor coordination. This finding supports the hypothesis that a strong environmental risk factor, such as cannabis, may contribute to the onset of psychosis even in the presence of lower biological and genetic vulnerability, as reflected indirectly by lower NSS scores. Nevertheless, due to the limitations of our study and its exploratory nature, this question remains open, and additional studies are needed to explore this interaction further. Such studies should have sufficiently large samples of cannabis users and non-users and consider cannabis and NSS in the context of additional neurobiological and environmental risk factors.

Conclusions

Our study demonstrated a negative association between cannabis use and NSS, especially regarding motor discoordination. This finding supports the hypothesis that a strong environmental risk factor, such as cannabis, may contribute to the onset of psychosis even in the presence of lower biological and genetic vulnerability, as reflected indirectly by lower NSS scores. Nevertheless, additional studies are needed that explore this interaction further in larger samples and considering additional neurobiological and environmental risk factors.

Abbreviations

NSS: neurological soft signs; FEP: first-episode psychosis; DSM: Diagnostic and Statistical Manual of Mental Disorders; PAS: Premorbid Adjustment Scale; DUP: duration of untreated psychosis; PANSS: Positive and Negative Syndrome Scale; GAF: Global Assessment of Functioning scale; CIDI: Composite International Diagnostic Interview; CB1: cannabinoid 1; THC: Delta-(9)-tetrahydrocannabinol.

Authors' contributions

AM, BBM have made substantial contributions to conception and design, acquisition of data, analysis and interpretation of data; have been involved in drafting the manuscript and have given final approval of the version to be published. CUC has made substantial contributions to analysis and interpretation of data; has revising the manuscript critically for important intellectual content; and has given final approval of the version to be published. BA has made substantial contributions to acquisition of data; has been involved in drafting the manuscript; and has given final approval of the version to be published. AM has made substantial contributions to conception and design, acquisition of data, analysis and interpretation of data; has been involved in drafting the manuscript; has revising the manuscript critically for important intellectual content; and has given final approval of the version to be published. LG has made substantial contributions to analysis and interpretation of data; has revising the manuscript critically for important intellectual content; and has given final approval of the version to be published. All authors read and approved the final manuscript.

Author details
[1] Psychiatry Department, Fattouma Bourguiba Hospital, 5000 Monastir, Tunisia.
[2] Faculty of Medicine of Monastir, University of Monastir, Monastir, Tunisia.
[3] Department of Psychiatry, The Zucker Hillside Hospital, Glen Oaks, NY, USA.
[4] Department of Psychiatry and Molecular Medicine, Hofstra Northwell School of Medicine, Hempstead, NY, USA. [5] Center for Psychiatric Neuroscience, Feinstein Institute for Medical Research, Manhasset, NY, USA.

Acknowledgements
Our sincere acknowledgements to Professor Christoph U. Correll for his meticulous revision and advice thoroughly motivated—as we feel it— by an innate move to boost junior colleagues. That occurs despite our professor's overloaded agenda, as we know for sure.

Competing interests
Dr. Correll has been a consultant and/or advisor to or has received honoraria from: Alkermes, Allergan, Bristol-Myers Squibb, Forum, Gerson Lehrman Group, Intra Cellular Therapies, Janssen/J&J, LB Pharma, Lundbeck, Medavante, Medscape, Neurocrine, Otsuka, Pfizer, ProPhase, Sunovion, Supernus, Takeda, and Teva. He has provided expert testimony for Bristol-Myers Squibb, Janssen, and Otsuka. He served on a Data Safety Monitoring Board for Lundbeck and Pfizer. He received grant support from Takeda. The other authors report no competing interests.

Ethical approval
The ethics committee and the thesis committee of the faculty of medicine of Monastir have approved the protocol of this study. Informed consent to participate in the study was obtained from both participants and their parent or legal guardian.

References
1. Heinrich DW, Buchanan RW. Significance and meaning of neurological signs in schizophrenia. Am J Psychiatr. 1988;145:11–8.
2. Dazzan P, Murray RM. Neurological soft signs in first-episode psychosis: asystematic review. Br J Psychiatry. 2002;43(Suppl 1):50–7.
3. Venkatasubramanian G, Latha V, Gangadahr BN, Janakiramaiah N, Subbakrishna DK, Jayakumar PN, et al. Neurological soft signs in never-treated schizophrenia. Acta Psychiatr Scand. 2003;108:144–6.
4. Browne S, Clarke M, Gervin M, Lane A, Waddington JL, Larkin C, et al. Determinants of neurological dysfunction in first episode schizophrenia. Psychol Med. 2000;30:1433–41.
5. Barkus E, Stirling J, Hopkins R, Lewis S. The presence of neurological soft signs along the psychosis proneness continuum. Schizophr Bull. 2006;32:573–7.
6. Boks MP, Liddle MP, Burgerhof JG, Knegtering R, Van den Bosch RJ. Neurological soft signs discriminating mood disorders from first episode schizophrenia. Acta Psychiatr Scand. 2004;110:29–35.
7. Keshavan MS, Sanders RD, Sweeney JA, Diwadkar VA, Goldstein G, Pettegrew JW, et al. Diagnostic specificity and neuroanatomical validity of neurological abnormalities in first-episode psychosis. Am J Psychiatry. 2003;160:1298–304.
8. Woods BT, Kinney DK, Yurgelum-Tood D. Neurological abnormalities in schizophrenic patients and their families. I: comparison of schizophrenic, bipolar and substance abuse patients and normal controls. Arch Gen Psychiatry. 1986;43:657–63.
9. The Scottish Schizophrenia Research Group. The Scottish First Episode Schizophrenia Study. I. Patient identification and categorisation. Br J Psychiatry. 1987;150:331–3.
10. Regier DA, Farmer ME, Rae DS, Locke BZ, Keith SJ, Judd LL. Comorbidity of mental disorders with alcohol and other drug abuse. Results from the epidemiologic catchment area (ECA) study. JAMA. 1990;264:2511–8.
11. Koskinen J, Lohonen J, Koponen H, Isohanni M, Miettunen J. Rate of cannabis use disorders in clinical samples of patients with schizophrenia: a meta-analysis. Schizophr Bull. 2010;361:115–30.
12. Andreasson S, Allebeck P, Engstrom A, Rydberg U. Cannabis and schizophrenia. a longitudinal study of Swedish conscripts. Lancet. 1987;2:1483–6.
13. Gage SH, Hickman M, Zammit S. Association between cannabis and psychosis: epidemiologic evidence. Biol Psychiatry. 2016;79(7):549–56.
14. Marconi A, Di Forti M, Lewis CM, Murray RM, Vassos E. Meta-analysis of the association between the level of cannabis use and risk of psychosis. Schizophr Bull. 2016;42:1262–9.
15. Matheson SL, Shepherd AM, Laurens KR, Carr VJ. A systematic meta-review grading the evidence for non-genetic risk factors and putative antecedents of schizophrenia. Schizophr Res. 2011;133:133–42.
16. Sarrazin S, Louppe F, Doukhan R, Schürhoff F. A clinical comparison of schizophrenia with and without pre-onset cannabis use disorder: a retrospective cohort study using categorical and dimensional approaches. Ann Gen Psychiatry. 2015;14:44.
17. Zammit S, Allebeck P, Andreasson S, Lundberg I, Lewis G. Self reported Cannabis use as a risk factor for schizophrenia in Swedish conscripts of 1969: historical cohort study. BMJ. 2002;325:1199.
18. Caspi A, Moffitt TE, Cannon M, Mcclay J, Murray R, Harrington H. Moderation of the effect of adolescent-onset cannabis use on adult psychosis by a functional polymorphism in the catechol-O-methyltransferase gene: longitudinal evidence of a gene × environment interaction. Biol Psychiatry. 2005;57:1117–27.
19. Di Forti M, Sallis H, Allegri F, Trotta A, Ferraro L, Stilo SA. Daily use, especially of high-potency cannabis, drives the earlier onset of psychosis in cannabis users. Schizophr Bull. 2014;40:1509–17.
20. Konings M, Henquet C, Maharajh HD, Hutchinson G, Van Os J. Early exposure to cannabis and risk for psychosis in young adolescents in Trinidad. Acta Psychiatr Scand. 2008;118:209–13.
21. Chambers RA, Krystal JH, Self DW. A neurobiological basis for substance abuse comorbidity in schizophrenia. Biol Psychiatry. 2001;50:71–83.
22. Moore TH, Zammit S, Lingford-Hughes A, Barnes TR, Jones PB, Burke M. Cannabis use and risk of psychotic or affective mental health outcomes: a systematic review. Lancet. 2007;370:319–28.
23. Arseneault L, Cannon M, Witton J, Murray RM. Causal association between cannabis and psychosis: examination of the evidence. Br J Psychiatry. 2004;184:110–7.
24. Semple DM, Mcintosh AM, Lawrie SM. Cannabis as a risk factor for psychosis: systematic review. J Psychopharmacol. 2005;19:187–94.
25. Van Winkel R, Kuepper R. Epidemiological, neurobiological, and genetic clues to the mechanisms linking cannabis use to risk for non affective psychosis. Annu Rev Clin Psychol. 2014;10:767–91.
26. Hall W. Cannabis use and psychosis. Drug Alcohol Rev. 1998;17:433–44.
27. Martin AK, Robinson G, Reutens D, Mowry B. Cannabis abuse and age at onset in schizophrenia patients with large, rare copy number variants. Schizophr Res. 2014;155(1–3):21–5.
28. Degenhardt L, Tennant C, Gilmour S, Schofield D, Nash L, Hall W. The temporal dynamics of relationships between cannabis, psychosis and depression among young adults with psychotic disorders: findings from a 10-month prospective study. Psychol Med. 2007;37:927–34.
29. Valmaggia LR, Day FL, Jones C, Bissoli S, Pugh C, Hall D. Cannabis use and transition to psychosis in people at ultra-high risk. Psychol Med. 2014;44:2503–12.
30. Di Forti M, Iyegbe C, Sallis H, Kolliakou A, Falcone MA, Paparelli A, et al. Confirmation that the AKT1 (rs2494732) genotype influences the risk of psychosis in cannabis users. Biol Psychiatry. 2012;72:811–6.
31. Van Winkel R, Genetic Risk and Outcome of Psychosis (GROUP) Investigators. Family-based analysis of genetic variation underlying psychosis-inducing effects of Cannabis: sibling analysis and proband follow-up. Arch Gen Psychiatry. 2011;68:148–57.
32. Cantor-Graae E, Ismail B, McNeil TF. Are neurological abnormalities in schizophrenic patients and their siblings the result of perinatal trauma? Acta Psychiatr Scand. 2000;101:142–7.
33. Lane A, Colgan K, Moynihan F, Burke T, Waddington JL, Larkin C, O'Callaghan E. Schizophrenia and neurological soft signs: gender differences in clinical correlates and antecedent factors. Psychiatry Res. 1996;64:105–14.
34. Peralta V, Cuesta MJ, Serrano JF. Obstetric complications and neurological abnormalities in neuroleptic-naive psychotic patients. Eur Arch Psychiatry Clin Neurosci. 2006;250:407–13.

35. Joyal CC, Hallé P, Lapierre D, Hodgins S. Drug abuse and/or dependence and better neuropsychological performance in patients with schizophrenia. Schizophr Res. 2003;63:297–9.

36. Ruiz-Veguilla M, Gurpegui M, Barrigón ML, Ferrín M, Marín E, Rubio JL, et al. Fewer neurological soft signs among first episode psychosis patients with heavy cannabis use. Schizophr Res. 2009;107:158–64.

37. Stirling J, Lewis S, Hopkins R, White C. Cannabis use prior to first onset psychosis predicts spared neurocognition at 10 year follow up. Schizophr Res. 2005;75:135–7.

38. American Psychiatric Association. Diagnostic and statistical manual of mental disorders (DSM-IV), vol. 4. Washington, DC: American Psychiatric Association; 1994.

39. Cannon-Spoor HE, Potkin SG, Wyatt RJ. Measurement of premorbid adjustment in chronic schizophrenia. Schizophr Bull. 1982;8:470–84.

40. Van Mastrigt S, Addington J. Assessment of premorbid function in first-episode schizophrenia: modifications to the Premorbid Adjustment Scale. J Psychiatry Neurosci. 2002;27(2):92–101.

41. Stanley RK, Opler LA, Lindenmayer JP. Reliability and validity of the Positive and Negative Syndrome Scale for schizophrenics. Psychiatry Res. 1987;23:99–110.

42. Startup M, Jackson MC, Bendix S. The concurrent validity of the Global Assessment of Functioning (GAF). Br J Clin Psychol. 2002;41(4):417–22.

43. Krebs MO, Gut-Fayand A, Bourdel MC, Dischamp J, Olie JP. Validation and factorial structure of a standardized neurological examination assessing neurological soft signs in schizophrenia. Schizophr Res. 2000;45:245–60.

44. Simpson GM, Angus JW. A rating scale for extrapyramidal side effects. Acta Psychiatr Scand. 1970;212:11–9.

45. Bersani G, Orlandi V, Gherardelli S, Pancheri P. Cannabis and neurological soft signs in schizophrenia: absence of relationship and influence on psychopathology. Psychopathology. 2002;35:289–95.

46. Stone JM, Morrison PD, Pilowsky LS. Glutamate and dopamine dysregulation in schizophrenia—a synthesis and selective review. J Psychopharmacol. 2007;21:440–52.

47. Ruiz-Veguilla M, Callado LF, Ferrin M. Neurological soft signs in patients with psychosis and cannabis abuse: a systematic review and meta-analysis of paradox. Curr Pharm Des. 2012;18(32):5156–64.

48. Loberg E-M, Helle S, Nygard M, Berle JO, Kroken RA, Erik Johnsen E. The cannabis pathway to non-affective psychosis may reflect less neurobiological vulnerability. Front Psychiatry. 2014;18:5–159.

49. Hui C, Wong G, Chiu C. Potential endophenotype for schizophrenia: neurological soft signs. Ann Acad Med Singap. 2009;38:408–13.

50. Mhalla A, Boussaid N, Gassab L, Mechri A, Gaha L. Minor neurological and physical anomalies in patients with first-episode psychosis. Encephale. 2013;39:149–54.

51. Dervaux A, Bourdel MC, Laqueille X, Krebs MO. Neurological soft signs in non-psychotic patients with cannabis dependence. Addict Biol. 2013;18(2):214–21.

52. Roser P, Gallinat J, Weinberg G, Juckel G, Gorynia I, Stadelmann AM. Psychomotor performance in relation to acute oral administration of Delta9-tetrahydrocannabinol and standardized cannabis extract in healthy human subjects. Eur Arch Psychiatry Clin Neurosci. 2009;259:284–92.

53. de Lopez Jesus M, Sallés J, Meana JJ, Callado LF. Characterization of CB1 cannabinoid receptor immunoreactivity in postmortem human brain homogenates. Neuroscience. 2006;140:635–43.

54. Fernández-Ruiz J. The endocannabioid system as a target for the treatment of motor dysfunction. Br J Pharmacol. 2009;156:1029–40.

55. Bossong MG, van Berckel BN, Boellaard R, et al. Δ-9-Tetrahydrocannabinol induces dopamine release in the human striatum. Neuropsychopharmacology. 2009;34:759–66.

56. Fernández-Ruiz J, Hérnandez M, Ramos JA. Cannabinoid–dopamine interaction in the pathophysiology and treatment of CNS disorders. CNS Neurosci Ther. 2010;16:72–91.

57. Van Os J, Kenis G, Rutten BP. The environment and schizophrenia. Nature. 2010;468:203–12.

58. Kuepper R, Morrison PD, Van Os J, Murray RM, Kenis G, Henquet C. Does dopamine mediate the psychosis-inducing effects of Cannabis? A review and integration of findings across disciplines. Schizophr Res. 2010;121:107–17.

59. Flyckt L, Sydow O, Bjerkenstedt L, et al. Neurological signs and psychomotor performance in patients with schizophrenia, their relatives and healthy controls. Psychiatry Res. 1999;86:113–29.

60. Emsley R, Turner HJ, Oosthuizen PP. Neurological abnormalities in first-episodeschizophrenia: temporal stability and clinical and outcome correlates. Schizophr Res. 2005;75:35–44.

9

A multilevel longitudinal study of obsessive compulsive symptoms in adolescence: male gender and emotional stability as protective factors

Vasilis Stavropoulos[1,2], Kathleen A. Moore[2], Helen Lazaratou[1]* ⓘ, Dimitris Dikeos[1] and Rapson Gomez[2]

Abstract

The severity of obsessive compulsive symptoms (OCS) is suggested to be normally distributed in the general population, and they appear to have an impact on a range of aspects of adolescent development. Importantly, there are individual differences regarding susceptibility to OCS. In the present repeated measures study, OCS were studied in relation to gender and emotional stability (as a personality trait) using a normative sample of 515 adolescents at ages 16 and 18 years. OCS were assessed with the relevant subscale of the SCL-90-R and emotional stability with the Five Factor Questionnaire. A three-level hierarchical linear model was calculated to longitudinally assess the over time variations of OCS and their over time links to gender and emotional stability, while controlling for random effects due to the nesting of the data. Experiencing OCS increased with age (between 16 and 18 years). Additionally, male gender and higher emotional stability were associated with lower OCS at 16 years and these remained stable over time. Results indicate age-related and between individual differences on reported OCS that need to be considered for prevention and intervention planning.

Keywords: Obsessive compulsive symptoms, Adolescence, Gender, Development, Emotional stability

Background

Over the past two decades, significant emphasis has been placed on understanding the etiology of obsessive compulsive symptoms (OCS) [1, 2]. OCS entail recurrent and persistent thoughts that are experienced as intrusive, but which cannot be ignored (obsessions). Individuals often engage in repetitive physical or mental acts (compulsions) aimed at reducing or removing the stress induced by the obsessions. The severity of OCS is suggested to be normally distributed in the general population and often constitutes a transient part of normal development (e.g., commonplace childhood rituals such as not walking on pavement lines) [3, 4]. However, OCS over a specific threshold may result in obsessive compulsive disorder (OCD), which is a chronic psychiatric condition, with potentially serious repercussions [5] OCD includes either obsessions or compulsions or a combination of both. It tends to compromise the quality of life and the well-being of the individual in significant ways by causing distress and interfering with everyday functioning [1, 3].

Research has advanced knowledge regarding the nature and the etiology of OCS [6]. In particular, OCS have been described as heterogeneous, varying across several different dimensions (i.e., cleaning/contamination, forbidden thoughts, symmetry/ordering-counting, hoarding/acquiring and retaining objects) [3, 7, 8]. The broader OCS dimensions (content of OCS) experienced by individuals remain relatively stable over time (i.e., propensity to experience forbidden thoughts is likely to shift from thoughts of violence to thoughts of religion, but is less likely to shift from forbidden thoughts to hoarding [1, 9]; however, the severity/intensity of OCS may vary over developmental phases [1]. For instance, obsessions

*Correspondence: elazar@med.uoa.gr
[1] National and Kapodistrian University of Athens, Vas Sofias 72, 11528 Athens, Greece
Full list of author information is available at the end of the article

related to fear and loss of others are typically higher in childhood and sexual obsessions tend to present more during adolescence [10]. Although there is consensus that levels of OCS fluctuate over developmental phases, there is a dearth of longitudinal studies that focus specifically on factors associated with particular developmental trajectories [1]. As it is considered a high-risk period for the onset of OCS and the diagnosis of OCD, explaining variations in the severity of OCS during adolescence appears particularly important [2]. Also, identifying factors that may contribute to higher OCS severity in adolescents could provide useful clinical guidelines for more effective prevention and treatment interventions.

Conceptual framework

To address these needs an integrative, multilevel approach that blends elements and concepts from the OCS literature and from the risk and resilience framework was used [4, 11, 12]. Specifically, Abramowitz et al. [4] contended that OCS may often constitute a part of normal development that may be better approached dimensionally, that is on a continuum from minimum to maximum OCS, rather than categorically (presence vs absence of OCS). In that context, pathological aspects of OCS have been defined as extreme versions of normative cognitive and emotional processes [11]. There is evidence supporting a multidimensional model of OCD/OCS, where the complex clinical presentation of OCD has been summarized through a combination of a number of consistent, temporally stable symptom dimensions. These are conceptualized on a spectrum of likely coexisting syndromes that may embrace normal obsessive–compulsive phenomena extending beyond the traditional nosological boundaries of OCD [13]. Subsequently, from an evolutionary psychology perspective, it is assumed that obsessions and compulsions derive from a mental human module that unconsciously produces risk scenarios. Within this framework, obsessions act as unintentional and ego-dystonic (e.g., not aligning with the person's ego driven choices) indirect-medium or longer term risk avoidance mechanisms, which lead to future risk avoidance behaviors (this function is different to anxiety which aims to decrease immediate and direct risks [14]. These approaches to OCS are in accord with the risk and resilience theoretical framework, in which behaviors are supported to constantly vary because of the interplay of developmental (age-related), individual and contextual risk and protective factors [11]. To better investigate the effects and the interactions of risk and protective factors across each of the levels involved (age-related changes, individual and contextual), the risk and resilience framework is best employed using multiple levels of analyses [15, 16]. Such models of analyses enable the investigation

of lifespan variations across individuals controlling for ecological-contextual effects. Accordingly, the present longitudinal study examined OCS dimensionally using a normative sample of Greek adolescents (assessed at 16 and again at 18 years of age) to determine the effects of potential risk (i.e., over time changes) and protective factors (i.e., gender and emotional stability).

Adolescence and OCS

In terms of age-related factors associated with variations in the severity of OCS, the focus in the present study was on adolescence, specifically the period between 16 and 18 years. Adolescence is a pivotal developmental stage [17]. It is a critical time for the development of OCS symptoms in general and the onset of OCD in particular [3, 18] and a time of multiple and concurrent life transitions including school, peer relationships, and family interactions [19]. These developmental turning points have been assumed to potentially trigger and/or exacerbate OCS among vulnerable individuals [6].

The period between 16 and 18 years is particularly critical for adolescents in Greece (from where the current sample was sourced). These years coincide with the first two grades of lyceum (secondary high school), during which period students become entitled to select, for the first time, the type of education they wish to pursue (academic or vocational track), as well as specific topics upon which their subsequent tertiary education entry exams are based [20]. Interestingly, this period of elevated educational accountability for Greek adolescents overlaps with a time of high prevalence of OCS [21]. Given that OCS have been suggested to have a gradual onset [3] and that prospective studies have contended that OCS severity varies over time [22] the need for longitudinal research to address this particular age range and population is compelling. In the present study, these potential age-related effects are studied in light of their interaction with gender and emotional stability.

Gender

Gender has been repeatedly examined as a factor that differentiates OCS over the life course and during adolescence in particular [23–26]. Literature referring to OCD diagnosed patients contends that gender appears to affect OCS in regard to their expression (e.g., type of symptoms experienced across genders), their age of onset and their presented comorbid disorders [23]. Specifically, considering OCS types, while males appear to present more frequently sexual, religious, doubt and checking obsessions, and repeating compulsions, females seem to be more vulnerable to fears of contamination [23]. In regard to the age of initiation of OCS, males diagnosed with OCD incline to demonstrate an earlier onset than females, a more chronic pattern of symptoms and a greater social impairment [23, 24]. In that line, considering comorbidity, OCD male patients present more frequently with social phobia, tic and substance use disorders than their female counterparts, who tend to be higher in depression, suicidal thoughts, eating and impulse-control disorders [23, 24]. These findings are complimented by some adolescent community sample studies, which revealed a significantly higher OCS prevalence for males than females [27]. However, other findings based on clinical, as well as community samples, showed that gender did not associate with either the OCS heterogeneity or differences in the OCS prevalence rates [25, 28]. At this point, it should be noted that the international literature supports that females are at higher risk for anxiety and fear related symptoms, such as OCS are classified, partially due to socialization processes that encourage a feeling of sensitivity and vulnerability, which predisposes and precipitates anxious manifestations [26]. These inconsistencies considering gender's effect on OCS and OCD between findings related to clinical and community samples, as well as studies across different age groups and national populations necessitate further examination.

Emotional stability and OCS

Research has suggested several significant associations between individual level variables and susceptibility to OCS including different forms of psychopathological symptoms and impairments in executive functioning [29, 30]. In this context, OCS have been repeatedly related to personality traits [31–36]. The link between emotional stability, as a personality trait, and OCS is emphasized here. Emotional stability describes the level that a person presents to be emotionally stable under various conditions and not prone to anxiety, depression, and/or other types of high emotional fluctuations [37].

Inclusion of emotional stability in the multilevel conceptualization of OCS was prompted by several empirical findings and observations. High emotional stability (more frequently assessed by its antithesis, neuroticism) has been identified as an individual level resource for a range of psychopathological forms [38–40]. In particular, emotional stability (low neuroticism) has been repeatedly related to lower OCS and OCD in both community and clinical, adult and adolescent samples [32–34, 41–44]. While various instruments have been used to assess each construct, such as the several scales loosely entitled Big Five [45, 46], and Eysenck's Personality Inventory [47] to assess personality traits and the Maudsley Obsessive Compulsive Inventory [48] Obsessive Compulsive Inventory [49] and the Y-BOCS [50] to assess OCD, results consistently demonstrate associations between the two.

Despite the significant body of research conducted in regard to the association between emotional stability and OCS, there is (to the best of the authors' knowledge) a dearth of studies adopting a risk and resilience approach with an emphasis on the developmental period of late adolescence. Such an approach would require a longitudinal examination of the link between emotional stability and OCS, concurrently controlling (taking into consideration) for the effects of the proximal context/environment of the individual. Addressing this gap appears to be important as emotional stability presents age-related variations that seem to be more intense during late adolescence [51]. Specifically, emotional regulation skills, which have been closely associated with emotional stability [44, 52], have been shown to vary over adolescent developmental periods with mid adolescence showing the smallest repertoire of emotion regulation strategies [53]. Furthermore, social-investment theory suggests that personality maturation, which is interwoven with a gradual increase of emotional stability scores, is largely the outcome of normative life transitions to adult roles [51]. Subsequently, the period of late adolescence examined in the present study (16–18 years) is assumed to be characterized by progressively higher emotional stability scores that could have a progressively protective effect on adolescents' vulnerability to OCS. This hypothesis is underscored by the fact that the age of onset of OCD is bimodal, with early-onset before 10 years and late-onset after the age of 17 [54]. Therefore, it can be argued that these two points in time truncate any possible correlation between age and OCS, which overlaps with a transitional period for the development of emotional stability. Interestingly, late adolescence, specifically 16–18 years of age is considered to involve high levels of change in personality traits, including emotional stability [55]; and is suggested to be a peak period for the onset of OCS [3, 18].

Similarly, emotional stability as a personality trait is expected to vary due to different contextual (i.e., classroom) effects [56]. It has been found that an individual's behaviors and personality traits are calibrated by functionality requirements, which initiate as conditional adaptations that become more permanent the longer the person is exposed to the effects of a specific context [56, 57]. Such contextual effects (i.e., classroom) on levels of emotional stability could influence its association with OCS during late adolescence and, therefore, need to be controlled/addressed by the conducted analyses (i.e., in the present study random effects due to the classroom of the participants were controlled at level 3).

The present study

This repeated measures research focuses on individual differences in OCS from 16 to 18 years in a normative sample of Greek adolescents. These differences were examined both between and within individuals, through the use of three-level hierarchical linear modeling (HLM) for analyzing nested data [20]. This process enables the investigation of intra-individual (over time changes within individuals) change along with between individual differences, controlling for random effects due to the nesting of the data (classroom of the individuals). The following research hypotheses were addressed:

H1 It is hypothesized that participants' OCS scores will increase between the ages of 16 and 18 years. This is in accordance with previous studies that support an increase of OCS during developmental phases which are marked by critical life events, such as the nationwide entry exams sat by Greek adolescents hoping to gain entry to a tertiary institution [51].

H2 Based socialization processes that increase the vulnerability of females to OCS and gender related differences revealed in community sample adolescent samples, it is envisaged that male adolescents will report lower OCS scores both at the age of 16 and prospectively [26, 27].

H3 Based on the protective role of emotional stability for OCS and OCD, it is hypothesized that more emotionally stable adolescents will report lower OCS scores over time [32–34].

Methods

Participants

This survey received approval from: (i) The Ministry of Education, (ii) The Teachers' Council, and (iii) Parents' consent. The sample was selected from the Athens metropolitan area and a specific regional area using the method of randomized stratified selection based on the latest inventory card of the Ministry of Education (2010). The ratios of high schools and students were identified: (1) between the metropolitan area and the selected regional population and (2) between academic vs vocational track high schools. Based on these quotas participants were randomly (by lottery) selected at the classroom level (for exact quotas see Table 1).

The sample consisted of 515 Greek students embedded in 33 classrooms. X^2 analysis confirmed that the sample did not significantly differ from the original population regarding area of residence and the type of school of the participants $X^2 = 1.58$, DF 1,3, $p = .66$. Parents' consent was 98% and the students' response rate was over 95%. With respect to parents' and guardians' socioeconomic profile, 80.2% were married, 6.2% of the mothers and 6.8% of the fathers were unemployed, and 77.9% of the

mothers and 64.5% of the fathers had completed education equal or above high school at time 1. The estimated maximum sampling error with a size of 515 is 4.32% ($Z = 1.96$, confidence level 95%).

Participants were assessed twice, two school years apart, and their responses matched with a unique code (Time 1: age $M = 15.68$ years, SD $= .65$, range 15.5–16.5, 53.6% females, 46.4% males; Time 2: age $M = 17.67$ years, SD $= .54$, range 16.5–17.5, 54.6% females, 45.4% males). The retention rate was high (72%) with attrition due to changes of school, and school and research drop outs. To evaluate the attrition effects, attrition was used as an independent variable (dummy coded 1 = Attrition, 0 = no attrition) at level 2 of the Hierarchical Linear Modeling-HLM analyses in order to assess whether it effected OCS scores and its associations with the other independent variables. Results confirmed that attrition did not have any significant effects on OCS symptoms and their association with emotional stability (Table 2).

Table 1 Original population and sample proportions

	Area of residence		Total
	Regional area (Korinthia)	Athens metro area	
Population			
Type of school			
Vocational track			
N	744	13,560	14,304
% of total population	.83%	15.12%	15.95%
Academic track			
N	2769	72,614	75,383
% of total population	3.09%	80.96%	84.05%
Total			
N	3513	86,174	89,687
% of total population	3.91%	96.08%	100%
Study sample			
Type of school			
Vocational track			
N	7	49	56
% of sample	1.40%	9.50%	10.90%
Academic track			
N	34	425	459
% of total sample	6.60%	82.50%	89.10%
Total			
N	41	474	515
% of total sample	8.00%	92.00%	100.00%

Population refers to the actual relevant student population of the Athens Metro Area and the Regional Area (Korinthia) in 2010 and sample to the study's sample

Instruments

Symptom Check List 90 Revised (SCL-90-R)

To assess OC, the relevant subscale of the SCL-90–R questionnaire [58] was used. This scale includes ten items and reflects symptoms typical of obsessive–compulsive disorder. The emphasis is on thoughts, impulses, and actions that are experienced as irresistible by the individual but are of an ego-dystonic or undesired nature (e.g., "Having to check and double check what you do?", "Unwanted thoughts, words, or ideas that won't leave your mind", "Having thoughts about sex that bother you a lot"). Experiences of cognitive attenuation are also included in this dimension. Adolescents reported the intensity of their symptoms on a 5-point Likert scale (0 = *not at all* to 4 = *all the time*). Scores ranged from 0 to 4, where 0 indicated minimum and 4 indicated maximum symptoms. In the present study, the internal reliability of the OCS subscale was acceptable Cronbach $\alpha = .79$. The use of the OCS subscale of the SCL-90 was preferred here due to its standardization for Greek samples and for reasons of comparability with other Greek studies [20, 59, 60].

Five Factor Questionnaire for Children (FFQ)

To assess emotional stability, the FFQ emotional stability subscale was used [61]. The questionnaire consists of five subscales: extraversion, emotional stability, conscientiousness, agreeableness, and openness to experience. Each subscale includes eight bipolar adjectives (e.g., "I am calm—I am hypersensitive") that are answered on a 5-point scale (1 = very, 2 = somewhat, 3 = neither/nor, 4 = somewhat, 5 = very) situated in between. The mean for the emotional stability subscale was calculated resulting in a range from 1 to 5, indicating the minimum and the maximum presence of the trait. The internal consistency of the emotional stability subscale in the current was Cronbach $\alpha = .71$.

Procedures

The first time point assessments were collected in the school year 2009–2010 and the second time point assessments were collected in the school year 2011–2012. The

Table 2 Assessment of the attrition effects in HLM analyses

	Fixed effects with Robust standard errors				
	b_i	SE	T	DF	P_i
Attrition	.07	.09	.76	32	.452
Emotional stability attrition*	.01	.13	.08	32	.934

Attrition refers to participants who did not complete two measurements. To evaluate the attrition effects attrition was used as an independent variable (dummy coded 1 = Attrition, 0 = not attrition) at level 2 of the HLM analyses to assess whether it effects OCS and their associations with emotional stability

process of data collection was identical between the two time points. A specially trained research team of 13 undergraduate, postgraduate, and PhD students of the Department of Psychology of the University of Athens collected the data in the participants' classrooms during the first two or the last two school hours (45 min each) of a school day, according to the permission provided by the Ministry of Education. The adolescents were motivated to participate in the study by the fact that they would not have to attend subjects taught during the time of the study and they would not be considered as absent from lessons. It should be noted that according to the Greek school regulation, students are allowed to progress to the next grade on the condition that they have not exceeded 50 school hours of unjustified absence per school year.

Statistical analyses

Multilevel modeling was used to statistically analyze a data structure where measurements at two time points (Level 1) were nested within individuals (Level 2), who were nested within classrooms (Level 3) [1]. This approach was chosen to enable the study to disentangle and examine age-related changes on OCS at Level 1 and the effect of gender and emotional stability at Level 2, while controlling for possible random effects due to the nesting-clustering of the data (participants within classrooms) at Level 3 (see Fig. 1: multilevel data structure) [2]. Subsequently, HLM 6.0.8 software was used [62]. Model testing proceeded in successive phases, such that each of the examined conditions were first studied separately, before included in the full model (Raudenbush et al. [62]): (1) Unconstraint (null) model; (2) Random ancova model (Level 1 predictor); (3) Means as outcomes model (Level 2 predictors-gender and emotional stability); (4) Random coefficient (regression slope-full model) model (Levels 1 and 2 predictors-time and gender and emotional stability). Due to the results not being statistically significantly different, only the full model will be reported here. In this context, OCS (Level-1 outcome variable) were predicted for each individual at Level 1 by time in the study. Time was centered at time 1 such that the individual intercepts referred to the initial Level of OCS (Time 1 = 0, Time 2 = 1). The individual initial Level and the individual linear change over the two assessments (slope) were predicted at Level 2 by gender (females = 0, males = 1) and emotional stability. Finally, random effects due to the clustering of the participants were controlled through random effects equations at Level 3 in regard to both the main effects of time, gender, and emotional stability, as well as the cross-level interactions between time and emotional stability and time and gender (slopes). To control for mis-specification (i.e., lack of linearity) and the distributional assumptions at each

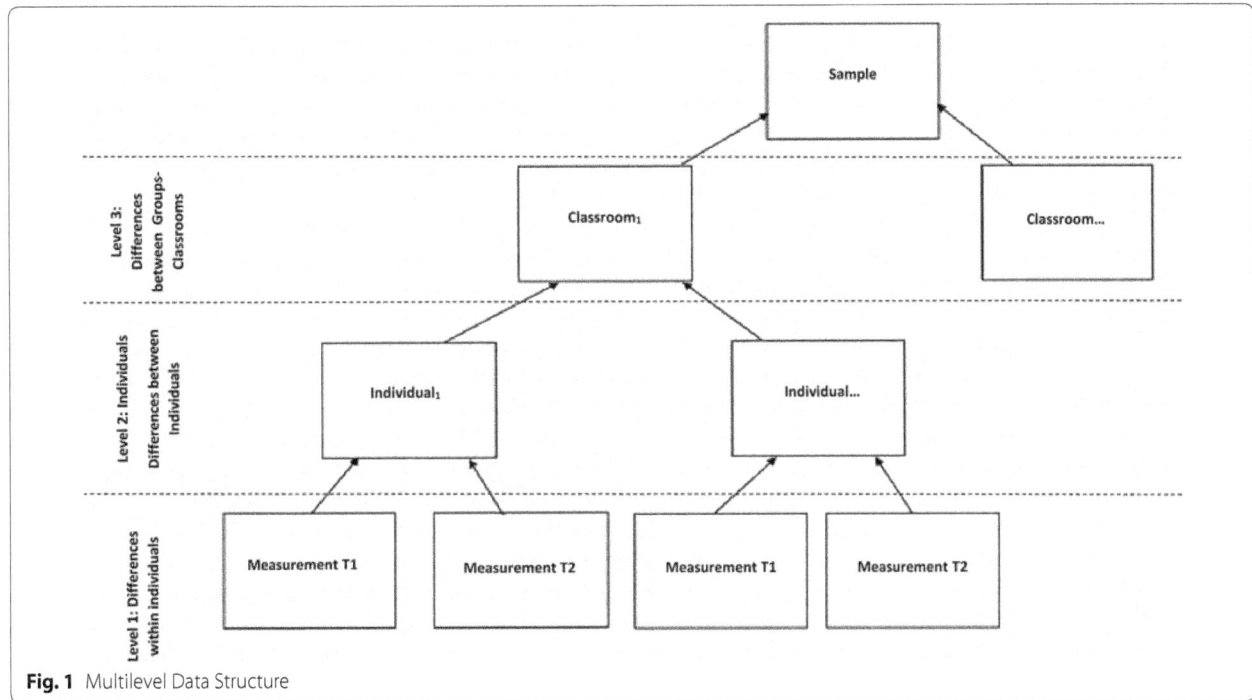

Fig. 1 Multilevel Data Structure

level (lack of normality, heteroscedasticity), HLM results accounting for robust standard errors (which are insensitive to possible violations of these assumptions) were calculated. Considering missing values, whereas they do not present a problem at Level 1 in HLM and did not occur at Level 3 (classrooms), missing values at Level 2 (individuals) were addressed. Although they were unsystematic, to avoid listwise deletion, multiple imputation was applied (five Maximum Likelihood imputations using SPSS) using all available Level 2 variables. This type of imputation was selected as it outperforms listwise deletion for parameters involving many recouped cases and results to improve standard error estimates [63]. Based on previous literature, all multilevel analyses were calculated five times and their results were averaged [64]. Prior the HLM analyses, the means, standard deviations, intercorrelations between the HLM variables were estimated (Table 3).

Results

To assure that the three levels contributed to variation in OCS scores, the level components were calculated from the unconditional model ($X^2 = 1096.49$, DF = 474, $p = .001$; $X^2 = 44.25$, DF = 32, $p = .07$). As an additional step, the intra class correlation (ICC) was calculated to determine which percentage of the variance in OCS is attributable to classroom membership (Level 3), which percentage is attributable to between individual differences (Level 2) and which to over time differences within individuals (Level 1). Results suggested that 42.32%

Table 3 Means, standard deviations, correlations

Time	Mean	S D	1	2	3
1. Emotional stability time 1	3.11	.43			
2. Emotional stability time 2	3.30	.62	− .03		
3. OCS time 1	1.17	.70	− .10*	− .02	
4. OCS time 2	1.26	.69	.04	− .31*	.04

$*p \leq .05$

(variance component = .204) of the variance in OCS is at the first Level (over time differences within individuals), 55.60% (variance component = .268) at Level 2 (the individual level) and 2.08% (variance component = .010) at Level 3 (between classrooms-controlled in the present analyses).

Therefore, HLM equations were calculated (see "Appendix"). The Level 1 intercept for the cross-sectional findings at the age of 16 years was 1.27 (this represents the estimated mean OCS score for adolescents of mean emotional stability controlling for random effects due to classroom participation). Considering how OCS change between 16 and 18 years (*hypothesis* 1), the time coefficient was $b = .15$ ($p = .001$). This indicated that the average OCS score increased to 1.42 ($1.27 + .15 = 1.42$) at the age of 18 for adolescents of mean emotional stability.

Gender was associated with OCS (*hypothesis* 2), $b = − .20$ ($p = .012$). Consequently, the average OCS score of male adolescents (0 = females, 1 = males) decreased to 1.00 ($1.27 − .20$) at the age of 16.

Considering the effect of gender over time, the coefficient was $b = -.11$ ($p = .144$) indicating that the effect of the cross-level interaction of gender with time was not significant.

Emotional stability was associated with OCS (*hypothesis* 3), $b = -.19$ ($p = .001$). Consequently, the average OCS score of adolescents who scored one point higher than the estimated mean in emotional stability decreased to 1.08 ($1.27 - .19 = 1.08$) at the age of 16. Considering the effect of emotional stability at time 1 on OCS at time 2, the coefficient was $b = .49$ ($p = .300$) indicating that the effect of the cross-level interaction of emotional stability with time was not significant (see slope on Fig. 2: Emotional stability and OCS over time).

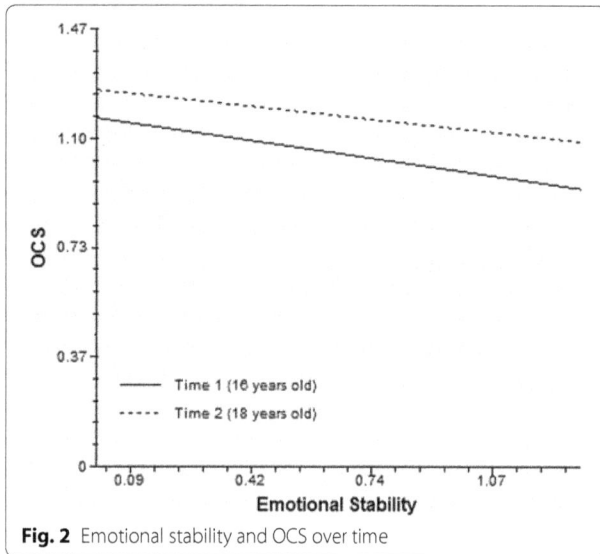

Fig. 2 Emotional stability and OCS over time

Emotional stability and OCS over time). The complete model explained 11% of the overall OCS variance resulting from 5, 5, and 1% of Levels 1, 2, 3, respectively. Analyses controlled for random effects due to other individual level random effects and classroom nesting/clustering (see "Appendix" for equations) (Table 4).

Discussion

In the present study, an integrative, multilevel approach that combined elements and concepts from the OCS literature and the risk and resilience framework was adopted to examine variations in OCS severity in a normative sample of Greek adolescents (assessed at 16 and 18 years of age). Specifically, the aim was to examine age-related change in OCS between 16 and 18 years taking into consideration the effects of emotional stability and male gender as individual level protective factors, while controlling for clustering (classroom) effects. This integrative framework was operationalized via a multilevel hierarchical linear model. The model was composed of three levels: the temporal factors (i.e., OCS over time), emotional stability, and gender as an individual level factors and controlled for random effects due to the nesting of the data (classrooms of participants). Multilevel analysis demonstrated that OCS increased between 16 and 18 years. Furthermore, male adolescents and adolescents higher in emotional stability were significantly less susceptible to OCS at the age of 16 years and these associations did not vary over time.

Age-related changes and OCS

The effect of age on OCS severity has been studied repeatedly [1, 4, 10, 11] albeit with equivocal results. In

Table 4 HLM analysis predicting adolescents' OCS scores

	Presence score									
	Fixed effects without Robust standard errors					Fixed effects with Robust standard errors				
	b_i	SE	T	DF	p_1	b_i	SE	T	DF	p_1
Cross-sectional results										
Intercept	1.27	.04	29.83	32	.001	1.27	.04	32.30	32	.001
Emotional stability	−.19	.08	−2.49	32	.004	−.19	.06	−2.94	32	.001
Gender	−.20	.06	−3.28	32	.003	−.20	.05	−4.23	32	.006
Over time results										
Intercept (time)	.15	.05	3.12	32	.004	.15	.04	4.29	32	.001
Emotional stability	.06	.09	.69	32	.494	.06	.06	1.05	32	.300
Gender	−.11	.08	−1.35	32	.187	−.11	.07	−1.50	32	.144

Table 3 summarizes the main results regarding the individual factors examined and is divided into four parts. The upper left part presents the cross-sectional findings without controlling for random effects. The lower left part presents the over time change results without controlling for random effects. The upper right part presents the cross-sectional findings after controlling for random effects at Levels 2 (individual) and 3 (Classroom). The lower right part presents the over time change results after controlling for random effects at Levels 2 (individual) and 3 (Classroom). Controlling for random effects mildly differentiated the results, and therefore, only the results after controlling for random effects were considered and reported in the text (right side of the table) our longitudinal assessment of a normative and representative sample of adolescents in Greece, the results revealed that OCS scores increased significantly between 16 and 18 years, encompassing one of the bimodal periods for onset of OCD. In another prospective study, Alvarenga et al. [5] reported a gradual increase of OCS in children aged 6–12 years which accords with the lower age peak for onset. However, in their study of adolescents diagnosed with OCD, De la Cruz et al. [1] found a tendency towards a negative relationship between OCD symptoms and age. These equivocal findings could be attributed to the different sampling methodologies (community vs clinical samples) or scales used and even the different age ranges and cultural backgrounds of the participants. However, the general consensus from past studies is that the increase of OCS and the onset of OCD occurs most often either during late adolescence, as found in the current study, or before the age of 10 [4, 18]. Indeed, Fineberg et al. [22] discussed the dearth of prospective studies which have considered the progression of OCS across developmental phases and recommended longitudinal research at these times with non-clinical populations.

The results of the present study support the results of past studies which have indicated that challenging life events exert a possible causal effect on OCS [4, 6]. In particular, Abramowitz et al. [4], Mataix-Cols et al. [65], and Stewart et al. [66] suggested that times of educational-family transitions and student exams may act as a trigger or exacerbate OCS among more vulnerable individuals. Such an event was certainly present for the current sample of students who were faced with their national university entrance examinations, which succeeded time point 2 measurement. It can be argued that students' increased pressure associated with this educational challenge could contribute to the increase in the reported OCS scores in the current sample. Given that: (a) to the best of the authors' knowledge this is the first prospective study of OCS severity in adolescents in Greece during the period between 16 and 18 years and; (b) the sample in the present study included exclusively high school students (and not late adolescents who were not attending lyceum/secondary high school), this conclusion needs to be addressed with caution.

Despite the need for more longitudinal and cross-cultural studies of typical adolescent development between 16 and 18 years, our results have direct implications for planning prevention and treatment initiatives. The need for more prevention resources and programs to be allocated to adolescents before the age of 16 years in order to prevent age-related OCS behaviors from escalating into clinical problems later in life is highlighted—especially for more vulnerable individuals.

Gender

In terms of the individual level protective factors assessed here, being a male was found to significantly reduce OCS symptoms at the age of 16 and this effect remained stable over time. This finding, at least partially, agrees with past research illustrating that gender associates with differentiations in OCS (e.g., expression/type, age of onset, comorbidity; see above) [23]. However, the present finding appears inconsistent with regard to the direction of the differences in OCS across genders. Specifically, findings based on clinical samples have indicated that males tend to experience more intense OCS, interwoven with significantly higher social impairment [23, 24]. However, it should be noted that these differences refer to clinical samples, while the present study examined a normative community sample of Greek adolescents. Therefore, one could assume that while late adolescent males tend to present lower OCS levels in general, it is likely that when they present OCS to the extent that these might exceed the diagnostic thresholds, these tend to associate with higher levels of impairment than females. This hypothesis is consistent with differences in the phenomenology of other clinical manifestations across genders and between community and clinical samples [67, 68]. A potential explanation of this finding (e.g., adolescent males lower on OCS than females) could be viewed in the context of "gender appropriateness hypothesis" [68]. This suggests that females are more vulnerable to anxiety and fear related symptoms, including OCS, due to socialization effects that may cultivate a self-perception of sensitivity and vulnerability that attracts anxious manifestations [26]. Nevertheless, inconsistencies considering gender's effect on OCS and OCD between clinical and community sample studies, various age groups and national populations are not uncommon and may indicate specific age, type of sample (clinical vs community), and national group limitations in the generalizability of the findings [23–26].

Emotional stability and OCS

Emotional stability was additionally found to reduce the severity of OCS reported by adolescents. Other studies have similarly shown that higher emotional stability (lower neuroticism) is associated with decreased susceptibility to psychopathological symptoms in general [37, 39, 40] as well as OCS and OCD in particular [32–34, 41–43] by decreasing individuals' vulnerability to pressure. In other fields of research, emotional stability has been associated with higher vulnerability to shame, psychological inflexibility, and emotional dysregulation [44] resulting in higher levels of anxiety. Lower emotional stability that increases anxiety could in turn trigger and/or reinforce OCS [8].

The current results suggest that the relationship between emotional stability and OCS does not significantly change in adolescents aged between 16 and 18 years old. This finding indicates that this association (and not emotional stability or OCS independently) is broadly stable during this specific developmental phase. In light of the significance of developmental timing, as highlighted in the risk and resilience framework [12], this finding may mean that adolescents low in emotional stability may have an earlier onset than late adolescence, and may be more vulnerable to developing OCS in subsequent times of stress. This is in line with international literature that has suggested such a gradual increase in the levels of emotional stability over developmental periods from early to late adolescence and emphasizes the need of emotional stability to be considered in the planning of OCS prevention and intervention initiatives [51]. In particular, OCS prevention and treatment programs in adolescence could include psychoeducation activities in regard to emotional stability (e.g., explaining how reacting calmly and stable to pressure may protect from the development of OCS symptoms); this would reinforce the individuals' level of OCS risk awareness and self-reflection. However, given the paucity of relevant research, it is important to interpret this suggestion with caution.

Conclusion, implications, limitations and further research

The present study illustrated the benefits of applying a longitudinal, contextualized methodology when investigating OCS in adolescence. This study's strengths entail (a) the longitudinal design, (b) a normative and representative sample, and (c) the use of multilevel analyses that enabled the combined examination of developmental risks (i.e., aging between 16 and 18 years) and individual resources (i.e., emotional stability) in regard to OCS. Subsequently, the results have implications for OCS prevention and treatment in adolescence. Specifically, prevention or treatment strategies that would increase emotional stability levels are suggested to be more beneficial when applied before the age of 16 years in reducing OCS severity. Furthermore, Greek adolescents presenting OCS may benefit more by targeted group interventions that will aim to reduce the levels of pressure between 16 and 18 years [69]. Prevention initiatives and programs should ideally embrace an element of gender differentiation (during the period between 16 and 18 years) to address the progressively higher OCS risk in females, and include psychoeducation modules referring to teacher, parents, and mental health practitioners regarding the potential OCS developmental trajectory related increase between 16 and 18 years.

Despite its strengths, this study has limitations. First, findings were based on self-report questionnaires, while the use of the OC subscale of SCL-90 as the only measure of OCS restricted the investigation of OCS in a multidimensional fashion. Although the SCL-90-OC subscale has been used in prospective OCS studies in the past [22] and has been adapted and widely applied in Greek adolescent, school and community samples [20, 70, 71], the use of more comprehensive, specific and sensitive OCS measurements should be adopted in future multilevel studies involving the school context.

Second, the use of a school sample to prospectively examine OCS raises questions considering the applicability of the findings to clinical samples. Therefore, similar longitudinal and contextualized studies are required to be replicated in clinical samples. Counterintuitively, the use of normative samples enables the dimensional investigation of OCS, which is significant for prevention purposes given their canonical distribution in the general population [4].

Finally, the sample was measured only twice and there was attrition between the two measurements. The 16–18 years old age range of participants coincides with a specific educational transition for Greek adolescents, which may narrow the applicability of the findings. Despite these factors, the study is novel in that there is a paucity of large cohort, longitudinal work in this area. Provided the statistical control of the attrition effects applied, the results contribute to the knowledge of school population differences, trait, and age-related factors affecting the experience of OCS. This study's impact could be relevant both in an applied sense, for school interventions, and also in terms of widening further avenues of research relating to the school context and psychopathology. Future multilevel OCS studies within the school context should include samples of different cultural backgrounds, and investigate more than two time points and wider age ranges.

Authors' contributions

VS contributed to hypotheses formulation, data collection, and analyses. KM contributed to the literature review and hypotheses formulation. HL contributed to the literature review. DD contributed to the data analyses. RG contributed to the structure and sequence of theoretical arguments. All authors read and approved the final manuscript.

Author details

[1] National and Kapodistrian University of Athens, Vas Sofias 72, 11528 Athens, Greece. [2] Federation University Australia, Mount Helen, Ballarat, VIC, Australia.

Acknowledgements

Not Applicable.

Competing interests

The authors of the present study do not report any competing interest.

Consent for publication
Authors confirm that this paper has not been either previously published or submitted simultaneously for publication elsewhere. Authors assign copyright or license the publication rights in the present article.

Funding
Data collection in Greece for this study has been co-financed by the European Union (European Social Fund—ESF) and Greek national funds, under the Operational Program "Education and Lifelong Learning" of the National Strategic Reference Framework (NSRF)—Research Funding Program: Heracleitus II.

Appendix

Level 1 equation:

$$Y = \Pi_0 + \Pi_1 * (\text{time}) + \varepsilon$$

Level 2 equations:

$$\Pi_0 = \beta_{00} + \beta_{01} * (\text{Emotional Stability})$$
$$+ \beta_{02} * (\text{Gender}) + \rho_0$$

$$\Pi_1 = \beta_{10} + \beta_{11} * (\text{Emotional Stability})$$
$$+ \beta_{12} * (\text{Gender}) + \rho_{01}$$

Level 3 equations:

$$\beta_{01} = \gamma_{010} + u_{01}$$

$$\beta_{01} = \gamma_{010} + u_{01}$$

$$\beta_{10} = \gamma_{100} + u_{10}$$

$$\beta_{11} = \gamma_{110} + u_{11}$$

ε, ρ and u parameters refer to controls of random effects at the three levels

Note 1: The data abides with the sample size requirements suggesting: (a) a minimum ratio of $10_{\text{clusters}}/5_{\text{participants}}$ to test for fixed effects and cross-level interactions in models with one explanatory variable at each of the levels, and: (b) a minimum requirement of 30 clusters for testing standard errors of fixed effects [15, 16].

Note 2: Conducting covariance based structural equation modeling (CBSEM) was not selected as: (a) it requires at least three or four indicators (the current study includes two time points) for every latent variable (growth) [72] and; (b) it assumes multi-normal distribution of the observed variables to ensure meaningful results-which is rarely the case in empirical research [73]. Similarly, latent growth modeling (LGM) was not chosen as it assumes that Level 1 predictors with random effects have the same distribution across all participants in each

subpopulation-while HLM allows different distributions [62]. Finally, HLM was preferred over partial least square analysis (PLS), as it estimates the effects of variables on the outcome variable at one level (i.e., individual), while at the same time taking into account the effect of variables on the outcome variable at another level (i.e., classroom) [62].

References
1. De la Cruz LF, Micali N, Roberts S, Turner C, Nakatani E, Heyman I, Mataix-Cols D. Are the symptoms of obsessive-compulsive disorder temporally stable in children/adolescents? A prospective naturalistic study. Psychiatry Res. 2013;209(2):196–201. https://doi.org/10.1016/j.psychres.2012.11.033.
2. Frydman I, Pedro E, Torres AR, Shavitt RG, Ferrão YA, Rosário MC, Fontenelle LF. Late-onset obsessive-compulsive disorder: risk factors and correlates. J Psychiatr Res. 2014;49:68–74. https://doi.org/10.1016/j.jpsychires.2013.10.021.
3. Abramowitz JS, Taylor S, McKay D. Obsessive-compulsive disorder. Lancet. 2009;374(9688):491–9. https://doi.org/10.1016/S0140-6736(09)60240-3.
4. Abramowitz JS, Fabricant LE, Taylor S, Deacon BJ, McKay D, Storch EA. The relevance of analogue studies for understanding obsessions and compulsions. Clin Psychol Rev. 2014;34(3):206–17. https://doi.org/10.1016/j.cpr.2014.01.004.
5. Alvarenga PG, Cesar RC, Leckman JF, Moriyama TS, Torres AR, Bloch MH, Miguel EC. Obsessive-compulsive symptom dimensions in a population-based, cross-sectional sample of school-aged children. J Psychiatr Res. 2015;62:108–14. https://doi.org/10.1016/j.jpsychires.2015.01.018.
6. Barton R, Heyman I. Obsessive–compulsive disorder in children and adolescents. Paediatr Child Health. 2013;23(1):18–23. https://doi.org/10.1016/j.paed.2012.10.002.
7. Bloch MH, Landeros-Weisenberger A, Rosario MC, Pittenger C, Leckman JF. Meta-analysis of the symptom structure of obsessive-compulsive disorder. FOCUS. 2015;13(2):232–43. https://doi.org/10.1176/appi.focus.130209.
8. Clark DA, Simos G. Obsessive–compulsive spectrum disorders: diagnosis, theory, and treatment. In: CBT for anxiety disorders: a practitioner book. Hoboken, New Jersey, United States: John Wiley & Sons, Ltd.; 2013. p. 25–55. https://doi.org/10.1002/9781118330043.ch2.
9. Fullana MA, Mataix-Cols D, Caspi A, Harrington H, Grisham JR, Moffitt TE, Poulton R. Obsessions and compulsions in the community: prevalence, interference, help-seeking, developmental stability, and co-occurring psychiatric conditions. Am J Psychiatry. 2009;166(3):329–36.
10. Geller DA, Biederman J, Faraone S, Agranat A, Cradock K, Hagermoser L, Coffey BJ. Developmental aspects of obsessive compulsive disorder: findings in children, adolescents, and adults. J Nerv Ment Dis. 2001;189(7):471–7.
11. Clark DA. Innovation in obsessive compulsive disorder: a commentary. J Behav Ther Exp Psychiatry. 2015;49:129–32. https://doi.org/10.1016/j.jbtep.2015.10.006.
12. Masten AS. Global perspectives on resilience in children and youth. Child Dev. 2014;85(1):6–20. https://doi.org/10.1111/cdev.12205.
13. Mataix-Cols D, do Rosario-Campos MC, Leckman JF. A multidimensional model of obsessive-compulsive disorder. Am J Psychiatry. 2005;162(2):228–38. https://doi.org/10.1176/appi.ajp.162.2.228.
14. Abed RT, de Pauw KW. An evolutionary hypothesis for obsessive compulsive disorder: a psychological immune system? Behav Neurol. 1999;11(4):245–50. https://doi.org/10.1155/1999/657382.
15. Maas CJM, Hox JJ. Robustness issues in multilevel regression analysis. Stat Neerl. 2004;58(2):127–37. https://doi.org/10.1046/j.0039-0402.2003.00252.x.

16. Maas CJM, Hox JJ. Sufficient sample sizes for multilevel modeling. Methodology. 2005;1(3):86–92. https://doi.org/10.1027/1614-2241.1.3.86.

17. Kanacri BPL, Pastorelli C, Eisenberg N, Zuffianò A, Castellani V, Caprara GV. Trajectories of prosocial behavior from adolescence to early adulthood: associations with personality change. J Adolesc. 2014;37(5):701–13. https://doi.org/10.1016/j.adolescence.2014.03.013.

18. Fontanelle LF, Hasler G. The analytical epidemiology of obsessive-compulsive disorder: risk factors and correlates. Prog Neuropsychopharmacol Biol Psychiatry. 2008;32(1):1–15. https://doi.org/10.1016/j.pnpbp.2007.06.024.

19. Hopkins JR. Adolescence: the transitional years. Cambridge: Academic Press; 2014.

20. Stavropoulos V, Gentile D, Motti-Stefanidi F. A multilevel longitudinal study of adolescent Internet addiction: the role of obsessive-compulsive symptoms and classroom openness to experience. Eur J Dev Psychol. 2016;13:99–114. https://doi.org/10.1080/17405629.2015.1066670.

21. Heyman I, Fombonne E, Simmons H, Ford T, Meltzer H, Goodman R. Prevalence of obsessive-compulsive disorder in the British nationwide survey of child mental health. Int Rev Psychiatry. 2003;15(1–2):178–84. https://doi.org/10.1192/bjp.179.4.324.

22. Fineberg NA, Baldwin DS, Menchon JM, Denys D, Grünblatt E, Pallanti S, Network RDR. Manifesto for a European research network into obsessive-compulsive and related disorders. Eur Neuropsychopharmacol. 2013;23(7):561–8. https://doi.org/10.1016/j.euroneuro.2012.06.00.

23. Cherian AV, Narayanaswamy JC, Viswanath B, Guru N, George CM, Math SB, Reddy YJ. Gender differences in obsessive-compulsive disorder: findings from a large Indian sample. Asian J Psychiatry. 2014;9:17–21. https://doi.org/10.1016/j.ajp.2013.12.012.

24. Mathis MAD, Alvarenga PD, Funaro G, Torresan RC, Moraes I, Torres AR, Hounie AG. Gender differences in obsessive-compulsive disorder: a literature review. Revista Brasileira de Psiquiatria. 2011;33(4):390–9. https://doi.org/10.1590/S1516-44462011000400014.

25. Valleni-Basile LA, Garrison CZ, Jackson KL, Waller JL, Mc Keown RE, Addy CL, Cuffe SP. Frequency of obsessive-compulsive disorder in a community sample of young adolescents. J Am Acad Child Adolesc Psychiatry. 1994;33(6):782–91. https://doi.org/10.1097/00004583-199407000-00002.

26. McLean CP, Anderson ER. Brave men and timid women? A review of the gender differences in fear and anxiety. Clin Psychol Rev. 2009;29(6):496–505. https://doi.org/10.1016/j.cpr.2009.05.003.

27. Zohar AH, Ratzoni G, Pauls DL, Apter A, Bleich A, Kron S, Cohen DJ. An epidemiological study of obsessive-compulsive disorder and related disorders in Israeli adolescents. J Am Acad Child Adolesc Psychiatry. 1992;31(6):1057–61. https://doi.org/10.1097/00004583-199211000-00010.

28. Moser JS, Moran TP, Kneip C, Schroder HS, Larson MJ. Sex moderates the association between symptoms of anxiety, but not obsessive compulsive disorder, and error-monitoring brain activity: a meta-analytic review. Psychophysiology. 2016;53(1):21–9. https://doi.org/10.1111/psyp.12509.

29. Hofmeijer-Sevink MK, van Oppen P, van Megen HJ, Batelaan NM, Cath DC, van der Wee NJ, van Balkom AJ. Clinical relevance of comorbidity in obsessive compulsive disorder: the Netherlands OCD Association study. J Affect Disord. 2013;150(3):847–54. https://doi.org/10.1016/j.jad.2013.03.014.

30. Snyder HR, Kaiser RH, Warren SL, Heller W. Obsessive-compulsive disorder is associated with broad impairments in executive function a meta-analysis. Clin Psychol Sci. 2014;. https://doi.org/10.1177/2167702614534210.

31. Doron G, Kyrios M. Obsessive–compulsive disorder: a review of possible specific internal representations within a broader cognitive theory. Clin Psychol Rev. 2005;25:415–32. https://doi.org/10.1016/j.cpr.2005.02.002.

32. Furnham A, Hughes DJ, Marshall E. Creativity, OCD, narcissism and the Big Five. Think Skills Creat. 2013;10:91–8. https://doi.org/10.1016/j.tsc.2013.05.003.

33. Hur YM. Genetic and environmental covariations among obsessive–compulsive symptoms, neuroticism, and extraversion in South Korean adolescent and young adult twins. Twin Res Human Genet. 2009;12(02):142–8. https://doi.org/10.1375/twin.12.2.142.

34. Rees CS, Roberts LD, van Oppen P, Eikelenboom M, Hendriks AAJ, van Balkom AJLM, van Megen H. Personality and symptom severity in obsessive-compulsive disorder: the mediating role of depression. Personal Individ Differ. 2014;2014(71):92–7. https://doi.org/10.1016/j.paid.2014.07.025.

35. Samuel DB, Widiger TA. Conscientiousness and obsessive-compulsive personality disorder. Person Disord Theory Res Treat. 2011;2(3):161. https://doi.org/10.1037/a0021216.

36. Tops M. Slow life history strategies and slow updating of internal models: the examples of conscientiousness and obsessive-compulsive disorder. Psychol Inq. 2014;25(3–4):376–84. https://doi.org/10.1080/1047840X.2014.916194.

37. Cheng H, Furnham A. The big-five personality traits, maternal smoking during pregnancy, and educational qualifications as predictors of tobacco use in a nationally representative sample. PLoS ONE. 2016;11(1):e0145552. https://doi.org/10.1371/journal.pone.0145552.

38. Hwang JY, Shin YC, Lim SW, Park HY, Shin NY, Jang JH, Kwon JS. Multidimensional comparison of personality characteristics of the Big Five model, impulsiveness, and affect in pathological gambling and obsessive-compulsive disorder. J Gambl Stud. 2012;28(3):351–62.

39. Rector NA, Hood K, Richter MA, Bagby RM. Obsessive-compulsive disorder and the five-factor model of personality: distinction and overlap with major depressive disorder. Behav Res Ther. 2002;40(10):1205–19. https://doi.org/10.1016/S0005-7967(02)00024-4.

40. Twenge JM. The age of anxiety? The birth cohort change in anxiety and neuroticism, 1952–1993. J Pers Soc Psychol. 2000;79(6):1007. https://doi.org/10.1037/0022-3514.79.6.1007.

41. Bergin J, Verhulst B, Aggen SH, Neale MC, Kendler KS, Bienvenu OJ, Hettema JM. Obsessive compulsive symptom dimensions and neuroticism: an examination of shared genetic and environmental risk. Am J Med Genet Part B Neuropsychiatr Genet. 2014;165(8):647–53. https://doi.org/10.1002/ajmg.b.32269.

42. Fullana MÀ, Mataix-Cols D, Trujillo JL, Caseras X, Serrano F, Alonso P, Torrubia R. Personality characteristics in obsessive-compulsive disorder and individuals with subclinical obsessive-compulsive problems. Br J Clin Psychol. 2004;43(4):387–98. https://doi.org/10.1348/0144665042388937.

43. Grisham JR, Fullana MA, Mataix-Cols D, Moffitt TE, Caspi A, Poulton R. Risk factors prospectively associated with adult obsessive–compulsive symptom dimensions and obsessive–compulsive disorder. Psychol Med. 2011;41(12):2495–506. https://doi.org/10.1017/S0033291711000894.

44. Paulus DJ, Vanwoerden S, Norton PJ, Sharp C. Emotion dysregulation, psychological inflexibility, and shame as explanatory factors between neuroticism and depression. J Affect Disord. 2016;190:376–85. https://doi.org/10.1016/j.jad.2015.10.014.

45. Costa PT, McCrae RR. Revised NEO Personality Inventory (NEO-PI-R) and NEO Five-Factor Inventory (NEO-FFI) professional manual. Odessa: Psychol Assess Resour; 1995.

46. Hendriks AAJ, Hofstee WKB, De Raad B. The five-factor personality inventory (FFPI). Person Individ Differ. 1999;27:307–25. https://doi.org/10.1016/S0191-8869(98)00245-1.

47. Eysenck HJ, Eysenck SBG. Manual of the Eysenck Personality Scales. London: Hodder & Stoughton; 1991.

48. Hodgen RJ, Rachman S. Obsessional-compulsive complaints. Behav Res Ther. 1977;15:389–95. https://doi.org/10.1016/0005-7967(77)90042-0.

49. Foa EB, Huppert JD, Leiberg S, Langner R, Kichic R, Hajcak G, et al. The Obsessive-Compulsive Inventory: development and validation of a short version. Psychol Assess. 2002;14:485–96. https://doi.org/10.1037/1040-3590.14.4.485.

50. Goodman WK, Price LH, Rasmussen SA, Mazure C, Delgado P, Heninger GR, et al. The Yale-Brown Obsessive Compulsive Scale 11. Validity. Arch General Psychiatry. 1989;46:1012–6. https://doi.org/10.1001/archpsyc.1989.01810110054008.

51. Bleidorn W, Klimstra TA, Denissen JJ, Rentfrow PJ, Potter J, Gosling SD. Personality maturation around the world a cross-cultural examination of social-investment theory. Psychol Sci. 2013;. https://doi.org/10.1177/0956797613498396.

52. Ikeda S, Mizuno-Matsumoto Y, Canuet L, Ishii R, Aoki Y, Hata M, Asakawa T. Emotion regulation of neuroticism: emotional information processing related to psychosomatic state evaluated by electroencephalography and exact low-resolution brain electromagnetic tomography. Neuropsychobiology. 2015;71(1):34–41. https://doi.org/10.1159/000368119.

53. Zimmermann P, Iwanski A. Emotion regulation from early adolescence to emerging adulthood and middle adulthood Age differences, gender differences, and emotion-specific developmental variations. Int J Behav Dev. 2014;38(2):182–94. https://doi.org/10.1177/0165025413515405.

54. Geller D, Biederman J, Jones J, Park K, Schwartz S, Shapiro S, Coffey B. Is juvenile obsessive-compulsive disorder a developmental subtype of the disorder? A review of the pediatric literature. J Am Acad Child Adolesc Psychiatry. 1998;1998(37):420–7. https://doi.org/10.1097/00004583-199804000-00020.

55. Roberts BW, Walton KE, Viechtbauer W. Patterns of mean-level change in personality traits across the life course: a meta-analysis of longitudinal studies. Psychol Bull. 2006;132(1):1. https://doi.org/10.1037/0033-2909.132.1.1.

56. Wood D, Denissen JJ. A functional perspective on personality trait development. In: Reynolds KL, Branscombe NR editors. Psychology of change. Life contexts, experiences, and identities. New York, US: Psychology Press; 2015. p. 97–115.

57. Del Giudice M, Ellis BJ, Shirtcliff EA. The adaptive calibration model of stress responsivity. Neurosci Biobehav Rev. 2011;35(7):1562–92. https://doi.org/10.1016/j.neubiorev.2010.11.007.

58. Derogatis LR, Savitz KL. The SCL-90-R, brief symptom inventory, and matching clinical rating scales. In: Maruish ME, editor. The use of psychological testing for treatment planning and outcomes assessment. Mahwah, NJ: Lawrence Erlbaum Associates; 1999. p. 679–724.

59. Donias S, Karastergiou A, Manos N. Standardization of the symptom checklist-90-R rating scale in a Greek population. Psychiatriki. 1991;2(1):42–8.

60. Floros G, Siomos K, Stogiannidou A, Giouzepas I, Garyfallos G. The relationship between personality, defense styles, internet addiction disorder, and psychopathology in college students. Cyberpsychol Behav Soc Netw. 2014;17(10):672–6. https://doi.org/10.1089/cyber.2014.0182.

61. Asendorpf JB, Van Aken MA. Validity of big five personality judgments in childhood: a 9 year longitudinal study. Eur J Pers. 2003;17(1):1–17. https://doi.org/10.1002/per.460.

62. Raudenbush SW, Bryk AS, Congdon RT. Hierarchical linear modeling. Thousands Oaks: Sage; 2002.

63. Newman DA. Longitudinal modeling with randomly and systematically missing data: a simulation of ad hoc, maximum likelihood, and multiple imputation techniques. Org Res Methods. 2003;6(3):328–62. https://doi.org/10.1177/1094428103254673

64. Motti-Stefanidi F, Asendorpf JB, Masten AS. The adaptation and well-being of adolescent immigrants in Greek schools: a multilevel, longitudinal study of risks and resources. Dev Psychopathol. 2012;24(02):451–73. https://doi.org/10.1017/S0954579412000090.

65. Mataix-Cols D, Rauch S, Baer L, et al. Symptom stability in adult obsessive-compulsive disorder: data from a naturalistic two-year follow-up study. Am J Psychiatry. 2002;159:263–8. https://doi.org/10.1176/appi.ajp.159.2.263.

66. Stewart S, Geller D, Jenike M, et al. Long-term outcome of pediatric obsessive-compulsive disorder: a meta-analysis and qualitative review of the literature. Acta Psychiatr Scand. 2004;110:4–13. https://doi.org/10.1111/j.1600-0447.2004.00302.x.

67. Gershon J, Gershon J. A meta-analytic review of gender differences in ADHD. J Atten Disord. 2002;5(3):143–54. https://doi.org/10.1177/108705470200500302.

68. Diamantopoulou S, Henricsson L, Rydell AM. ADHD symptoms and peer relations of children in a community sample: examining associated problems, self-perceptions, and gender differences. Int J Behav Dev. 2005;29(5):388–98. https://doi.org/10.1177/01650250500172756.

69. Simos G. Cognitive behaviour therapy: a guide for the practicing clinician, vol. 1. Hove: Psychology Press; 2002.

70. Siomos KE, Mouzas OD, Angelopoulos VN. Addiction to the use of internet and psychopathology in Greek adolescents: a preliminary study. Ann Gen Psychiatry. 2008;7(Suppl 1):S120.

71. Angst J, Gamma A, Endrass J, Goodwin R, Ajdacic V, Eich D, Rössler W. Obsessive-compulsive severity spectrum in the community: prevalence, comorbidity, and course. Eur Arch Psychiatry Clin Neurosci. 2004;254(3):156–64.

72. Baumgartner H, Homburg C. Applications of structural equation modeling in marketing and consumer research: a review. Int J Res Mark. 1996;13(2):139–61. https://doi.org/10.1016/0167-8116(95)00038-0.

73. Micceri T. The unicorn, the normal curve, and other improbable creatures. Psychol Bull. 1989;105(1):156–66. https://doi.org/10.1037/0033-2909.105.1.156.

10

Is low total cholesterol levels associated with suicide attempt in depressive patients?

A. Messaoud[1]* ⓘ, R. Mensi[1,2], A. Mrad[1], A. Mhalla[1], I. Azizi[1,2], B. Amemou[1], I. Trabelsi[3], M. H. Grissa[3], N. Haj Salem[4], A. Chadly[4], W. Douki[1,2], M. F. Najjar[2] and L. Gaha[1]

Abstract

Background: Patients with major depressive disorder (MDD) have a high risk of suicide. Many pathophysiological factors involved in MDD and suicide such us a low cholesterol levels have been associated with MDD and increased vulnerability to suicide. In this study, we investigate the relation between lipid parameters and suicide risk in patients with MDD.

Methods: Plasma levels of total cholesterol, triglycerides, and high-density lipoprotein cholesterol (HDL-c) and low-density lipoprotein cholesterol (LDL-c) were determined in 160 patients meeting the DSM-IV-TR criteria for MDD (110 patients without suicidal behavior and 52 suicidal attempters) and 151 healthy controls.

Results: A significant decrease in plasma cholesterol levels was observed in the group of suicidal depressive patients compared to those without suicidal behavior ($p < 0.001$). For the other lipid levels (triglycerides, HDL cholesterol, and LDL cholesterol), there were no significant differences between suicidal and non-suicidal patients.

Conclusions: Our study showed a significant decrease in plasma cholesterol levels in suicidal patients. This result support the hypothesis of the association of low plasma cholesterol level and suicidal behavior in patients with major depressive disorder.

Keywords: Depression, Suicide, Cholesterol, Biological marker

Background

Major depressive disorder is a common, recurrent, and chronic psychiatric illness. Several factors seem to be implicated in the pathophysiology of depression, and a contribution of genetic, environmental, and social factors is greatly discussed [1]. In a report on the Tunisian Health System [2], the Tunisian Ministry of the Public Health estimated that more than 8.2% of the population suffers from depression.

Severity of depression is accompanied by a high suicidal risk. Indeed, studies using the technique of psychological autopsy found that more than 90% of suicidal patients are affected by one or more psychiatric disorders, such as major depressive disorder (MDD), at the time of the suicidal act [3]. In this same context, Roy [4] found that 45–75% of suicide victims suffered from depression at the time of their death.

In Tunisia, especially after the revolution of January 14th, 2011, suicide rates continue to increase. In 2015, FTDES [5] recorded 549 cases of suicide and suicide attempts with an increase of 170.4% compared to 2014. This is an alarming and worrying phenomenon requiring an improvement in the strategies of prevention of this tragedy.

Many researchers have been interested in identifying biological markers that could be associated with depressive disorder and suicidal behavior, and could be used as an additional tool for prevention actions [6–8].

Several studies have suggested that an alteration in the lipid profile can occur to people with these kinds of disorders [9–13]. Some researches have concentrated on the relationship between plasma or serum cholesterol levels and suicide; however, conflicting results have been

*Correspondence: messaood.amel@yahoo.com
[1] Research Laboratory 'Vulnerability to psychotic disorders LR 05 ES 10', Department of Psychiatry, Monastir University Hospital, University of Monastir, Monastir, Tunisia
Full list of author information is available at the end of the article

reported [14–16]. Some of these studies have found an association between low cholesterol levels and increased risk of suicide [17–19], and others have reported negative association of cholesterol with suicidal ideation [20, 21], current parasuicide [15, 22], history of attempted suicide [23], and completed suicide [24].

Besides total cholesterol, other researches have investigated the link between triglycerides, HDL cholesterol, LDL cholesterol, depression, and suicidal behavior [25–27]. Some studies have documented that lower triglyceride levels were significantly associated with suicidal tendency in patients with depression [25, 26]. However, for HDL cholesterol or LDL cholesterol, Cantarelli et al. did not find any difference between depressed patients with or without suicidal behaviors [26].

In the present study, we examined the lipid and lipoprotein profiles in Tunisian adults with major depressive disorder and with or without suicide attempt. We aimed to verify whether an alteration in lipid profile increases the risk of suicide in patients with major depressive disorder or not.

Methods

Subjects

This study has included 162 patients with major depressive disorder according to DSM-IV and 151 controls.

Patients were classified into two groups: 110 patients with a major depressive episode (MDD) without suicidal behavior recruited during the consultations in the Department of Psychiatry of the University Hospital of Monastir; and 52 MDD suicide attempters recruited when admitted to the emergency department after a suicide attempt. Data were collected using a data sheet containing socio-demographic, clinical, and therapeutic information of the patient. Only patients between 20 and 60 years of age were involved in this study. We excluded from this study patients treated for dyslipidemia, hypertension, or diabetes. The majority of patients received antidepressant treatment according to their individual clinical needs.

The control group consisted of 151 volunteer subjects without psychiatric or endocrinological diagnoses matched for age, gender, BMI, tobacco, and alcohol addiction. Those with a history of suicidal act or major medical illness were excluded from this group. General characteristics of the subjects are shown in Table 1. Our study was approved by the Ethical Committee of the University Hospital of Monastir.

Psychiatric assessment

The diagnosis of the MDD was made using the Diagnostic and statistical manual of mental disorders (DSM-IV).

Table 1 General characteristics of the study population

Characteristics	Non-suicidal MDD patients($N = 110$)	MDD suicide attempters ($N = 52$)	Normal controls ($N = 151$)	p
Gender (men/women)	35/75	19/33	50/101	0.837
Age (years)	44.33 ± 10.50	29.84 ± 8.78	38.92 ± 13.28	0.000
BMI	26.24 ± 2.57	25.65 ± 3.61	25.58 ± 4.10	0.440
Addiction				
Cigarette smoking				
Smokers	20 (19.19%)	14 (38.9%)	24 (15.9%)	0.034
Non-smokers	90 (81.81%)	36 (61.1%)	127 (84.1%)	
Alcoholic beverages				
Consumers	12 (10.9%)	11 (21.6%)	16 (10.5%)	0.079
Non-consumers	98 (89.1%)	40 (78.4%)	135 (89.5%)	
Diagnosis (DSM-IV)				
Major depressive disorder, single episode	31(28.2%)	30 (57.7%)	–	–
Major depressive disorder, recurrent	97 (71.8%)	22 (42.3%)	–	–
Treatment				
ISRS	47 (42.7%)	18 (34.6%)	–	–
Tricyclics	42 (38.2%)	12 (23.1%)	–	
Mood stabilizers	31 (28.2%)	15 (28.9%)	–	
Antipsychotics	17 (15.5%)	5 (9.6%)	–	
Benzodiazepine	19 (17.3%)	8 (15.4%)		

Plasma levels of total cholesterol, triglycerides, HDL-c, and LDL-c are presented in Fig. 1

We have also used other scales such as Hamilton Depression Rating Scale (HDRS) and the Beck's Suicidal Ideation Scale (SSI) to rate the severity of depressive symptoms.

Biochemical measurements

Blood samples were drawn after overnight fasting. For suicidal patients, samples were collected within 24 h after the suicide attempt. Plasma levels of total cholesterol (TC), triglycerides (TG), and high-density lipoprotein cholesterol (HDL-c) were determined by enzymatic methods, and low-density lipoprotein cholesterol (LDL-c) was calculated by the Friedewald equation.

Statistical analysis

The statistical analyses were performed using SPSS 21.0 for Windows. All variables were presented as mean ± standard deviation (SD). Categorical variables were presented as the raw number and percentage (%). To compare total cholesterol, LDL-c, HDL-c. and triglycerides, we used the analysis of covariance (ANCOVA) and the student t test. ROC analysis for biological variables was used to find cutoff points, sensitivity, specificity, and positive and negative predictive values. Odds ratios were calculated. The Pearson's and Spearman's correlation coefficients were calculated to evaluate the correlations between biological and clinical (HDRS and SSI) variables. Differences were considered as significant if the p value was <0.05.

Results

Demographic characteristics of patients and controls groups are presented in Table 1. Suicidal patients with major depressive disorder were significantly younger than patients without suicidal behavior ($p < 0.001$). Most of the suicide attempters were women ($p \leq 0.05$). The majorities of our participants were not smokers and do not consume alcohol. There was no significant difference between patients regarding BMI (Table 1).

The mean plasma level of cholesterol was significantly lower among the suicide attempters than the depressive group (3.47 ± 0.95 vs 4.15 ± 0.75 mmol/L) and the control group (4.27 ± 1.01 mmol/L). The difference between the MDD suicidal patients group, non-suicidal patients, and control groups was significant ($p < 0.001$), but not between non-suicidal patients and control group ($p = 0.211$). The increase in the mean plasma values of triglycerides in all depressed patients, regardless to suicidal behaviors, compared to controls was statistically not significant ($p > 0.05$) (Fig. 1). However, the increase in the mean plasma concentration of LDL-c in depressive group, attempters and non-attempters, was statistically significant when compared with controls subjects ($p < 0.05$). For the HDL cholesterol level, we observed

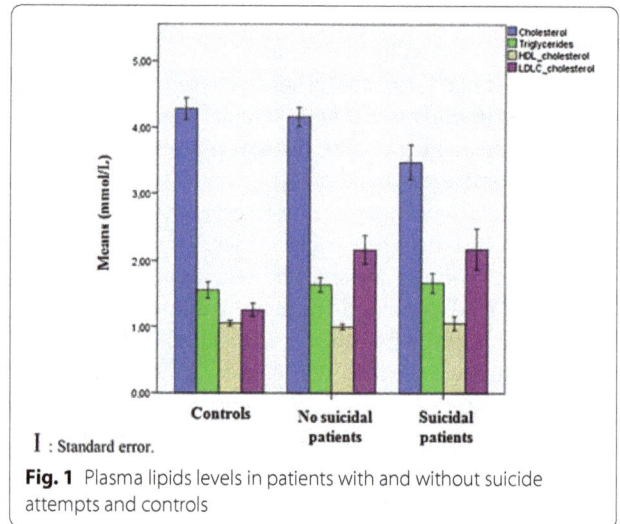

Fig. 1 Plasma lipids levels in patients with and without suicide attempts and controls

a slight decrease in all patients with major depressive disorder which is not significant when compared to the control group ($p < 0.05$). No significant difference, after adjusting for age and cigarette smoking, in all lipids parameters was noticed between the suicide attempts and completions groups.

The analysis of ROC curves of these four lipid parameters in the non-suicidal patients (a) showed that the cholesterol curve was near the diagonal with an area under the curve on the order of 0.511. The significant difference in LDL cholesterol level between depressive and control group did not appear in the ROC curve. However, in the suicidal patients (b), the curve of cholesterol was the most discriminant. The area under the curve of cholesterol was the highest compared with the other lipid parameters (Fig. 2).

For total cholesterol, a threshold value of 3.47 mmol/L was chosen for the subsequent analyses. The frequencies of distribution of lipid parameters showed that more than the half of MDD suicidal patients (55.7%) had a mean level of total cholesterol below 3.47 mmol/L. For these patients, the risk to commit a suicide attempt is increased five times with a plasma total cholesterol level less than 3.47 mmol/L. Similarly for HDL-c, patients with plasma level lower then 1.17 mmol/L have a suicidal risk multiplied by two than those with a level higher than this threshold value. Regarding triglycerides and LDL-c, no significant difference in the frequency of disturbance was observed between the patients with and without suicidal behaviors (Table 2).

When patients were classified according to gender, BMI, tobacco, smoking, and alcohol addiction, there were no statistically significant differences between the plasma triglycerides, HDL cholesterol, and LDL cholesterol in

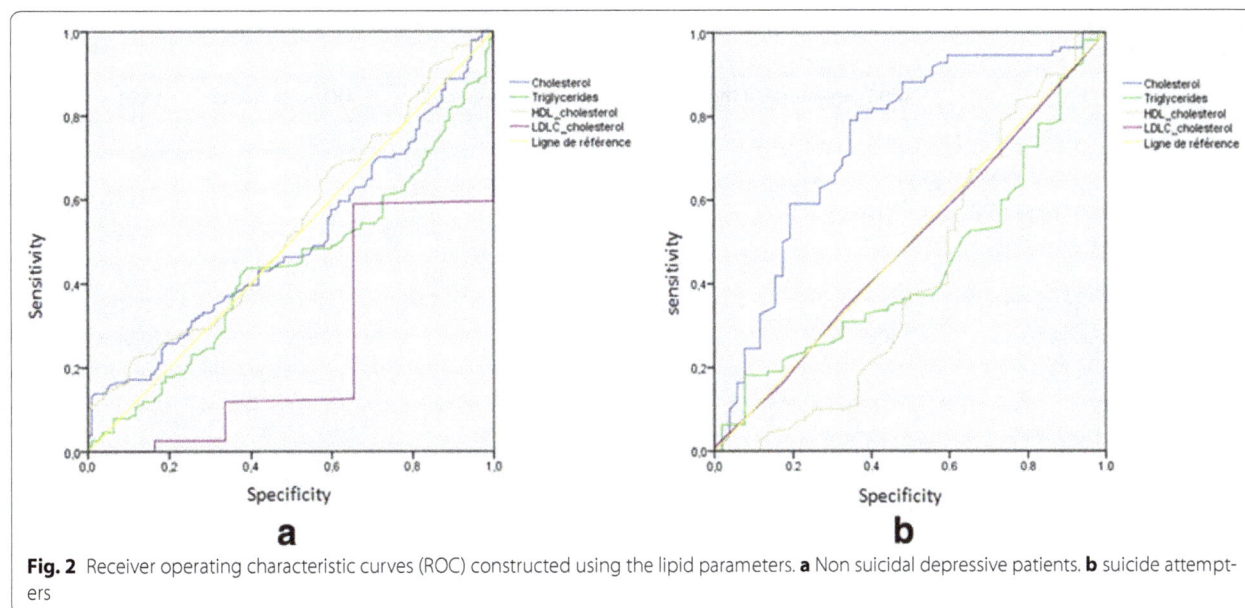

Fig. 2 Receiver operating characteristic curves (ROC) constructed using the lipid parameters. **a** Non suicidal depressive patients. **b** suicide attempters

Table 2 Association between disturbances in lipid parameters and the suicidal behavior in the study population

Parameters	Patients without suicide attempt		Patients with suicide attempt		p	Odds ratio	IC 95%
	N	%	N	%			
Total cholesterol (mmol/L)							
<3.47	19	17.3	29	55.7	0.000	5.039	2.889–12.620
≥3.47	91	82.7	23	54.3			
Triglycerides (mmol/L)							
<1.70	72	65.4	29	55.7	0.155	0.665	0.579–1.305
≥1.70	38	34.6	23	44.3			
HDL-c (mmol/L)							
<1.17	26	23.6	23	54.3	0.007	2.562	1.270–5.171
≥1.17	84	76.4	29	55.7			
LDL-c (mmol/L)							
<2.50	37	33.6	17	32.7	0.527	0.958	0.475–1.933
≥2.50	73	66.4	35	67.3			

suicidal and non-suicidal MDD patients. Yet, the mean plasma cholesterol concentration was significantly reduced in suicidal women when compared with corresponding value in MDD non-suicidal women (Table 3).

With regard to episodes of depression, the patients were classified into two categories: single and recurrent episode(s). We did not find significant differences in lipid concentrations among suicidal and non-suicidal MDD patients. As far as concerned about the severity of depression, there were no significant changes in the

plasma lipid levels between mild, moderate, and severe depression in all depressed patients. Also there were no significant differences of the plasma lipid levels in relation to the treatment (Table 3).

As shown in Table 4, plasma lipid and lipoprotein levels did not correlate with Hamilton Depression scores (HDRS) and the Beck's suicidal ideation scale (SSI) in non-suicidal patients. However, negative correlation between plasma levels of total cholesterol and the suicidal ideation (SSI) was found in suicidal patients.

Table 3 Plasma lipid levels according to demographic, clinical, and therapeutic data of MDD patients with or without suicide attempt

Parameters	Total cholesterol (mmol/L)	Triglycerides (mmol/L)	HDL-c (mmol/L)	LDL-c (mmol/L)
Gender				
Men				
Patients without suicide attempt	4.0 ± 0.79	1.67 ± 0.60	1.01 ± 0.23	2.17 ± 1.07
Patients with suicide attempt	3.59 ± 0.92	1.65 ± 0.41	1.10 ± 0.28	2.36 ± 1.01
Women				
Patients without suicide attempt	4.22 ± 0.73	1.62 ± 0.59	0.98 ± 0.21	2.16 ± 1.11
Patients with suicide attempt	3.40 ± 0.97*	1.67 ± 0.59	1.01 ± 0.41	2.06 ± 1.11
BMI (kg/m^2)				
<25				
Patients without suicide attempt	4.12 ± 0.65	1.63 ± 0.60	0.99 ± 0.20	2.00 ± 1.07
Patients with suicide attempt	3.51 ± 0.68	1.66 ± 0.56	1.09 ± 0.58	2.32 ± 1.10
[25–30]				
Patients without suicide attempt	4.13 ± 0.76	1.65 ± 0.60	0.99 ± 0.22	2.29 ± 1.09
Patients with suicide attempt	3.46 ± 1.10	1.68 ± 0.59	1.04 ± 0.42	2.17 ± 1.08
≥30				
Patients without suicide attempt	4.04 ± 1.24	1.59 ± 0.56	1.07 ± 0.162	1.71 ± 1.11
Patients with suicide attempt	3.80 ± 0.99	1.58 ± 0.24	0.93 ± 0.32	1.80 ± 1.09
Tabac				
Non-smokers				
Patients without suicide attempt	4.19 ± 0.76	1.62 ± 0.58	0.99 ± 0.20	2.12 ± 1.11
Patients with suicide attempt	3.48 ± 0.96*	1.69 ± 0.59	1.08 ± 0.38	2.02 ± 1.05
Smokers				
Patients without suicide attempt	4.10 ± 0.77	1.77 ± 0.65	0.98 ± 0.26	2.35 ± 1.08
Patients with suicide attempt	3.45 ± 0.91*	1.60 ± 0.36	0.97 ± 0.34	2.50 ± 1.16
Alcohol				
Non-consumers				
Patients without suicide attempt	4.19 ± 0.74	1.64 ± 0.60	0.99 ± 0.21	2.18 ± 1.13
Patients with suicide attempt	3.60 ± 0.89*	1.66 ± 0.58	1.04 ± 0.34	2.12 ± 1.09
Consumers				
Patients without suicide attempt	3.84 ± 0.80	1.60 ± 0.50	1.00 ± 0.24	2.00 ± 0.73
Patients with suicide attempt	3.03 ± 1.13*	1.67 ± 0.28	1.04 ± 0.48	2.36 ± 1.12
Clinical subtypes				
Patients without suicide attempt				
Single episode	4.02 ± 0.74	1.64 ± 0.76	0.99 ± 0.21	2.20 ± 1.04
Recurrent episode	4.20 ± 0.75	1.64 ± 0.61	0.99 ± 0.22	2.14 ± 1.11
Patients with suicide attempt				
Single episode	3.47 ± 0.98	1.62 ± 0.35	1.03 ± 0.41	2.06 ± 1.04
Recurrent episode	3.47 ± 0.94	1.75 ± 0.62	1.07 ± 0.32	2.31 ± 1.12
Severity of MDD				
Patients without suicide attempt				
Mild	4.10 ± 0.73	1.69 ± 0.69	1.00 ± 0.21	2.16 ± 1.08
Moderate	4.18 ± 0.76	1.59 ± 0.59	0.99 ± 0.22	2.20 ± 1.12
Severe	4.27 ± 0.90	1.83 ± 1.22	0.93 ± 0.26	1.50 ± 0.57
Patients with suicide attempt				
Mild	–	–	–	–
Moderate	3.51 ± 0.71	1.62 ± 0.86	0.98 ± 0.63	2.08 ± 0.98
Severe	3.45 ± 0.98	1.69 ± 0.94	1.11 ± 0.47	2.24 ± 1.10
Treatments				

Table 3 continued

Parameters	Total cholesterol (mmol/L)	Triglycerides (mmol/L)	HDL-c (mmol/L)	LDL-c (mmol/L)
Patients without suicide attempt				
ISRS	4.06 ± 0.84	1.58 ± 0.55	0.98 ± 0.19	2.21 ± 1.06
Tricyclics	4.28 ± 0.70	1.66 ± 0.68	0.99 ± 0.23	2.23 ± 1.20
Others	4.09 ± 0.46	2.17 ± 1.06	0.98 ± 0.22	2.00 ± 0.81
Patients with suicide attempt				
ISRS	3.49 ± 0.21	1.57 ± 0.62	1.05 ± 0.27	2.15 ± 1.13
Tricyclics	3.64 ± 0.75	1.94 ± 0.83	0.95 ± 0.64	2.52 ± 0.67
Others	3.25 ± 0.06	1.65 ± 0.33	1.29 ± 0.14	1.50 ± 0.70

$* p < 0.05$

Discussion

Table 4 Correlation between lipids levels and clinical scales scores (HDRS and SSI)

	CT	TG	HDL-c	LDL-c
MDD no suicidal patients				
HDRS				
−r	0.119	0.067	0.064	−0.045
−p	0.215	0.485	0.508	0.637
SSI				
−r	0.008	0.077	−0.023	−0.071
−p	0.936	0.423	0.808	0.462
MDD suicidal patients				
HDRS				
−r	0.101	−0.040	0.215	0.059
−p	0.563	0.817	0.215	0.737
SSI				
−r	−0.355*	−0.149	0.160	0.215
−p	0.037	0.394	0.359	0.215

r Spearmen coefficient correlation

$* p < 0.05$

According to our results, total plasma cholesterol levels among suicidal depressive patients were significantly lower than those among control depressive patients or control subjects. The low plasma total cholesterol level was significantly related to suicidal behavior. We did not find a difference in the level of plasma cholesterol between the suicide attempters and suicide death groups. This finding agrees with those of previous studies [28–30] but not with those of Baek et al. [31] and Bartoli et al. [32]. The mechanisms of action adduced by these studies show the direct relationship between low cholesterol levels and poor serotonin uptake and the decrease in brain-cell-membrane viscosity. So it seems possible that cholesterol can be used clinically to predict suicide risk in patients with MDD. We employed ROC analysis to test plasma total cholesterol as a discriminate parameter between suicidal and non-suicidal patients. Since the area under the curve is 0.742, cholesterol plasma level can discriminate between these two groups. According to the curve, the plasma total cholesterol level of 3.47 mmol/L is a good cutoff for possible risk of suicide for patients with MDD. So for patients with depression, a plasma cholesterol level less than 3.47 mmol/L indicates a possible risk of suicide and we must take preventive measures in order to anticipate the passage to the suicidal act.

Our data showed also that the significant difference in the level of cholesterol between suicidal and non-suicidal depressive patients existed with regard to the demographic characteristics, witch means that these characteristics did not interfere in this alteration of plasma cholesterol level in suicidal patients. Cantarelli et al. [26], for example, did not also find correlation between BMI and lipid parameters of mood disorder subjects with and without history of suicide. It has been reported also by some studies, related to the gender, that male gender is associated with lower cholesterol levels in various psychiatric disorders [33] and this can be explained by the fact that substance abuse, including alcoholism, may be associated with altered cholesterol serum levels [34]. We reported also that although smokers suffer from depression more than non-smokers and that smokers are twice more likely to commit suicide than non-smokers, we noticed the same difference in lipid profile between suicidal and non-suicidal patients regardless of their smoking addiction.

Our study noticed also that there was no significant changes in triglycerides and HDL-c levels between the depressed patients with and without suicide behavior and the control group. These data are in agreement with some other studies in the literature [35–37] but not with others who found a significant decrease in serum triglycerides in suicide attempters more than non-attempters [26]. In their study, Cantarelli et al. [26] found that serum triglycerides and leptin may act as a suicidal marker in patients with mood disorders. For HDL-c, a significant association between low HDL-c and increased prevalence of suicide attempts was observed in women [38].

The increase of LDL cholesterol level observed in all depressive patients, with or without suicide attempt, is in agreement with some studies [39]. However, Huang [40] did not find an association between plasma LDL-c and depression or suicidality. In our study, this increase in LDL-c plasma level was associated with depressive illness but not suicidal behavior. We noted that Fischer et al. [41] had found an association between higher LDL-c levels and the long allele coding for serotonin transporter gene in women.

With regard to demographic parameters taken into consideration in our study, the result showed that the risk of suicide attempt is higher in females. Our sample included more females than males with a history of attempted suicide. These data were confirmed by Onuegbu et al. [42]. It is important to mention that the total plasma cholesterol level measured in women after a suicide attempt is significantly lower than women who had not attempted suicide. This result was found also by Guillem et al. [22].

Regarding the way used to commit suicide, in our study, drug poisoning and/or raticide were the most common modes used by suicide attempters (83.3%). On the other hand, the majority of suicide deaths commit suicide by hanging (50%) or by immolation (30%). These results agree with those of Ghachem et al. [3] where suicide deaths use more decisive, fatal, and violent methods.

We did not find any difference in lipid concentrations depending on the kind of antidepressants used. Vuksan–Cusa et al. [25] have reported that medication is not the only contributor to changes in lipid profile.

No correlation was found in non-suicidal patients between lipid plasma levels and clinical assessments of depression and suicidal behavior. This result is in agreement with data of Onuegbu et al. [42]. In suicidal patients, we found a negative correlation between total cholesterol levels and SSI score, meaning that suicidal ideations are present more in patients with low total cholesterol levels.

Some methodological limitations should be considered in the interpretation of our results: the small sample size of the groups studied, especially the suicidal deaths, which lead to a limitation on the amount of independent variables we could use. Also the significant difference in age between suicidal and no suicidal patients can also confound the results.

Conclusion

In conclusion, our study's result adds to a majority of research showing the association between suicidal behavior and lower total plasma cholesterol levels. So we support the role of plasma cholesterol as a biological state

marker for the assessment of suicide risk in patients with a major depressive episode. We recommend to check if an increase of the cholesterol supplement in the diet can reduce the suicide risk in depressive patients.

Abbreviations
MDD: major depressive disorder; TC: total cholesterol; TG: triglycerides; HDL-c: high-density lipoprotein cholesterol; LDL-c: low-density lipoprotein cholesterol; BMI: body mass index; HDRS: Hamilton depression rating scale; SSI: scale of suicidal ideation.

Authors' contributions
The authors belonging to the psychiatric unit contributed by the interpretation of clinical parameters; those in the biochemistry department have facilitated us with bioassays, and other authors participated in the recruitment of patients in these services. All authors read and approved the final manuscript.

Author details
[1] Research Laboratory 'Vulnerability to psychotic disorders LR 05 ES 10', Department of Psychiatry, Monastir University Hospital, University of Monastir, Monastir, Tunisia. [2] Laboratory of Biochemistry-Toxicology, Monastir University Hospital, University of Monastir, Monastir, Tunisia. [3] Department of Emergency, Monastir University Hospital, University of Monastir, Monastir, Tunisia. [4] Department of Forensic Medicine, Monastir University Hospital, University of Monastir, Monastir, Tunisia.

Acknowledgements
Not applicable.

Competing interests
The authors declare that they have no competing interests.

Consent for publication and ethics approval
Our study was approved by the Ethical Committee of the University Hospital of Monastir. Patients have participated in this study freely.

Funding
This work is supported by the University of Monastir, Research Laboratory "Vulnerability to Psychotic disorders" and the Laboratory of Biochemistry and Toxicology, Monastir University Hospital, Tunisia.

References
1. Caspi A, Sugden K, Moffitt TE, Taylor A, Craig IW, Harrington H, McClay J, Mill J, Martin J, Braithwaite A, Poulton R. Influence of life stress on depression: moderation by a polymorphism in the 5-HTT gene. Sciences. 2003;301:386–9.
2. The Tunisian Health System (http://www.unfpa-tunisie.org/). Accessed Sept 2011.
3. Ghachem R, Boussetta A, Benasr A, Oumaya N. Suicide et pathologie mentale à Tunis: étude rétrospective sur 12 ans à l'hôpital Razi. L'Inf psychiatr. 2009;85:281–95.
4. Roy A. Suicide in recurrent affective disorder patients. Can J Psychiatry. 1984;29:319–22.
5. FTDES (http://ftdes.net/). Accessed Feb 2015.
6. Asellus P, Nordstrom P, Jokinen J. Cholesterol and CSF 5-HIAA in attempted suicide. J Affect Disord. 2010;125:388–92.
7. Lee BH, Kim YK. Potential peripheral biological predictors of suicidal behavior in major depressive disorder. Prog Neuropsychopharmacol Biol Psychiatry. 2011;35:842–7.
8. Pandey GN. Biological basis of suicide and suicidal behavior. Bipolar Disord. 2013;15:524–41.
9. Chang SS, Wen CP, Tsai MK, Lawlor DA, Yang YC, Gunnell D. Adiposity, its related biologic risk factors and suicide: a cohort study of 542,088 taiwanese adults. Am J Epidemiol. 2012;175:804–15.

10. Jee SH, Kivimaki M, Kang HC, Park IS, Samet JM, Batty GD. Cardiovascular disease risk factors in relation to suicide mortality in Asia: prospective cohort study of over one million Korean men and women. Eur Heart J. 2011;32:2773–80.

11. Jokinen J, Nordstrom AL, Nordstrom P. Cholesterol, CSF 5-HIAA, violence and intent in suicidal men. J Psychiatry Res. 2010;178:217–9.

12. Olie E, Picot MC, Guillaume S, Abbar M, Courtet P. Measurement of total serum cholesterol in the evaluation of suicidal risk. J Affect Disord. 2011;133:234–8.

13. Papadopoulou A, Markianos M, Christodoulou C, Lykouras L. Plasma total cholesterol in psychiatric patients after a suicide attempt and in follow-up. J Affect Disord. 2013;148:440–3.

14. Golomb BA, Stattin H, Mednick S. Low cholesterol and violent crime. J Psychiatry Res. 2000;34:301–9.

15. Kim YK, Lee HJ, Kim JY, Yoon DK, Choi SH, Lee MS. Low serum cholesterol is correlated to suicidality in a Korean sample. Acta Psychiatr Scand. 2002;105:141–8.

16. Takei N, Kunugi H, Nanko S, Aoki H, Iyo R, Kazamatsuri H. Low serum cholesterol and suicide attempts. Br J Psychiatry. 1994;164:702–3.

17. Lindberg G, Rastam L, Gullberg B, Eklund GA. Low serum cholesterol concentration and short term mortality from injuries in men and women. BMJ. 1992;305:277–9.

18. Muldoon MF, Manuck SB, Matthews KA. Lowering cholesterol concentrations and mortality: a quantitative review of primary prevention trials. BMJ. 1990;301:309–14.

19. Zureik M, Courbon D, Ducimetiere P. Serum cholesterol concentration and death from suicide in men: Paris prospective study I. BMJ. 1996;313:649–51.

20. Sullivan PF, Joyce PR, Bulik CM, Mulder RT, Oakley- Browne M. Total cholesterol and suicidality in depression. Biol Psychiatry. 1994;36:472–7.

21. Papassotiropoulos A, Hawellek B, Frahnert C, Rao GS, Rao ML. The risk of acute suicidality in psychiatric inpatients increases with low plasma cholesterol. Pharmacol psychiatry. 1999;32:1–4.

22. Guillem E, Pe´lissolo A, Notides C, Le´pine JP. Relationship between attempted suicide, serum cholesterol level and novelty seeking in psychiatric in-patients. Psychiatry Res. 2002;112:83–8.

23. Modai I, Valevski A, Dror S, Weizman A. Serum cholesterol levels and suicidal tendencies in psychiatric inpatients. J Clin Psychiatry. 1994;55:252–4.

24. Ellison LF, Morrison HI. Low serum cholesterol concentration and risk of suicide. Epidemiology. 2001;12:168–72.

25. Vuksan-Cusa B, Marcinko D, Nad S, Jakovljevic M. Differences in cholesterol and metabolic syndrome between bipolar disorder men with and without suicide attempts. Prog Neuropsychopharmacol Biol Psychiatry. 2009;33:109–12.

26. Cantarelli MG, Nardin P, Buffon A, Eidt MC, Godoy LA, Fernandes BS, Gonçalves CA. Serum triglycerides, but not cholesterol or leptin, are decreased in suicide attempters with mood disorders. J Affect Disord. 2015;172:403–9.

27. Eberhard A, Kramer-Reinstadler DK, Dietmar L, Georg K, Hartmann H, Wolfgang W, Fleischhacker G, Hickey D, Corvin A. No evidence for an association between serum cholesterol and the course of depression and suicidality. Psychiatry Res. 2004;121:253–61.

28. Golden J, Fitzpatrick P, Cunningham S, Walsh N. Total serum cholesterol in relation to psychological correlates in parasuicide. Br J Psychiatry. 2000;177:77–83.

29. Huang TL. Serum cholesterol levels in mood disorders associated with physical violence or suicide attempts in Taiwanese. Chang Gung Med J. 2001;24:563–8.

30. Terao T, Iwata N, Kanazawa K, Takano T, Takahashi N, Hayashi T, Sugawara Y. Low serum cholesterol levels and depressive state in human dock visitors. Acta Psychiatr Scand. 2000;101:231–4.

31. Baek JH, Kang ES, Fava M, Mischoulon D, Nierenberg AA, Yu BH, Lee D, Jeon HJ. Serum lipids, recent suicide attempt and recent suicide stat usin patients with major depressive disorder. Prog Neuropsychopharmacol Biol Psychiatry. 2014;51:113–8.

32. Bartoli F, Crocamo C, Dakanalis A, Riboldi I, Miotto A, Brosio E, Clerici M, Carrà G. Association between total serum cholesterol and suicide attempts in subjects with major depressive disorder: exploring the role of clinical and biochemical confounding factors. Clin Biochem. 2016;11.035.

33. Borgherini G, Dorz S, Conforti D, Scorse C, Magni G. Serum cholesterol and psychological distress in hospitalized depressed patients. Acta Psychiatr Scand. 2002;105:149–52.

34. Carmen DS, Enrique BG, Maria MPR, Eloy GR, Antonio C, Jeronimo SR, Maria AO, de Leon J. Low plasma cholesterol levels in suicidal males: a gender- and body mass. Prog Neuropsychopharmacol Biol Psychiatry. 2007;31:901–5.

35. Paplos K, Havaki-Kontaxaki B, Ferentinos P, Dasopoulou M, Kontaxakis V. Alexithymia, depression and serum lipids in suicide attempters. Psychiatr Psychiatriki. 2012;23:149–52.

36. Park S, Yi KK, Na R, Lim A, Hong JP. No association between serum cholesterol and death by suicide in patients with schizophrenia, bipolar affective disorder, or major depressive disorder. Behav Brain Funct. 2013;9:45.

37. Persons JE, Coryell WH, Fiedorowicz JG. Cholesterol fractions, symptom burden, and suicide attempts in mood disorders. Psychiatry Res. 2012;200:1088–9.

38. Jian Z, Robert EM, James RH, Shirley JT, John RW, Barbara EA. Low HDL cholesterol is associated with suicide attempt among young healthy women: the Third National Health and Nutrition Examination Survey. J Affect Disord. 2005;89:25–33.

39. Huang TL, Chen JF. Lipid and lipoprotein levels in depressive disorders with melancholic feature or atypical feature and dysthymia. Psychiatry Clin Neurosci. 2004;58:295–9.

40. Huang TL. Serum lipid profiles in major depression with clinical subtypes, suicide attempts and episodes. J Affect Disord. 2005;86:75–9.

41. Fischer P, Gruenblatt E, Pietschmann P, Tragl KH. Serotonin transporter polymorphism and LDL-cholesterol. Mol Psychiatry. 2006;11:707–9.

42. Onuegbu AJ, Agbedana EO, Baiyewu O, Olisekodiaka MJ, Ebesunun MO, Adebayo K, Ayelagbe OG, Adegoke OD. Evaluation of plasma lipids and lipoproteins in Nigerians suffering from depressive illness. Afr J Biomed Res. 2007;10:133–9.

11

Maternal bonding styles in smokers and non-smokers

Iren Csala[1,2], Monika Elemery[1], Fruzsina Martinovszky[2], Peter Dome[1,3], Balazs Dome[4,5,6,7], Gabor Faludi[1], Imola Sandor[2], Zsuzsa Gyorffy[2], Emma Birkas[2] and Judit Lazary[1*]

Abstract

Background: Parental bonding has been implicated in smoking behavior, and the quality of maternal bonding (MB) has been associated with poor mental health and substance use. However, little is known about the association of MB and the smoking of the offspring.

Methods: In our study, 129 smokers and 610 non-smoker medical students completed the parental bonding instrument, which measures MB along two dimensions: care and overprotection. Four categories can be created by high and low scores on care and overprotection: optimal parenting (OP; high care/low overprotection); affectionless control (ALC; low care/high overprotection); affectionate constraint (AC; high care/high overprotection), and neglectful parenting (NP; low care/low overprotection). Nicotine dependence was assessed by the Fagerstrom Nicotine Dependence Test, exhaled CO level, and daily cigarette consumption (CPD).

Results: Higher CPD was significantly associated with lower overprotection ($p = 0.016$) and higher care ($p = 0.023$) scores. The odds for being a smoker were significantly higher in the neglectful maternal bonding style compared to the other rearing styles ($p = 0.022$). Besides, smokers showed significantly higher care and lower overprotection scores with the Mann–Whitney U-test than non-smokers, although these associations did not remain significant in multiple regression models.

Conclusion: Our results indicate that focusing on early life relationship between patient and mother can be important in psychotherapeutic interventions for smoking.

Registration trials retrospectively registered

Keywords: Parental bonding style, Nicotine dependence, Smoking onset, Depression

Background

Smoking is the leading cause of premature death, preventable morbidity, and disability worldwide [1–3]. Despite the huge effort for decreasing the health consequences of smoking, it is still an unsolved problem. In order to reduce smoking initiation and to conduct an efficient and successful quitting therapy, it is important to know the psychosocial risk factors for smoking initiation, nicotine dependence, and failing to quit. Earlier studies have identified several of those factors such as low socioeconomic status, low educational level, peer smoking, and family influences [4–6].

The majority of studies on the effect of the smoker's parents on their tobacco use focused on the parents' smoking behavior, the parent's beneficial attitudes toward smoking, and parental practices against smoking. Those studies found that all these factors are related to the offspring's smoking outcomes [5–7]. Less is known about the effect of parental bonding and attachment, and even less about the effect of maternal parenting style.

Adult smoking often starts at the adolescent age, and almost all adult smokers have their first smoking experiment by the age of 16 [8, 9]. By the age of 18, they are regular smokers already [10]. Therefore, the experience of the first 16 years, including the parents' influence such

*Correspondence: lazaryjudit@gmail.com
[1] Department of Psychiatry and Psychotherapy, Semmelweis University, Budapest, Hungary
Full list of author information is available at the end of the article

as parental bonding as the parental bonding instrument measures it, is suggested to play an important role in the development of smoking behavior.

There is a large body of evidence suggesting that parental warmth, closeness, acceptance, emotional support, and emotional availability are associated with decreased chance of smoking or substance use [11–16]. However, the association between parental control and smoking behavior is inconsistent in the literature. Most studies reported that parental behavior control and parental monitoring relate inversely to smoking [12, 14, 17], but not all studies could confirm these findings [13, 15, 18]. Other studies even found a direct association between substance use and parental control [19, 20]. There are studies which distinguish strict control from psychological control and emphasize that the quality of control is determinant, i.e., while moderate and consistent strict control is beneficial, psychological control does not serve the offspring's healthy mental development [18, 21]. Another aspect of parenting was also investigated, namely encouraged autonomy by the parents which partially faces the psychological control, and it was also suggested to be beneficial against smoking initiation and related to better quitting outcomes [22].

The results described above propound that there might be an optimal combination of parenting techniques and there might be a worst case scenario for smoking development. The literature confirms this expectation: authoritative parenting style, which is labeled as high warmth and high control from the parents, has been documented consistently to show the best substance use and smoking outcomes [23–27]. On the other hand, parental neglect, the combination of low care and low control has been found to be the greatest risk of smoking among examined parenting styles [21, 23, 27].

As regards maternal bonding, there are only sporadic results. Most studies only investigated parental rearing style, and only a few of them examined the effect of maternal bonding separately. The results of these studies are inconsistent. Some studies reported an inverse relation between high maternal care and smoking or substance use [15, 27, 28], while other researchers have not found such a correspondence [13]. In addition, the degree of maternal control has been implicated in substance use including smoking, but the direction of the relationship is not clear [19, 27].

Thus, the main purpose of the current study was to reveal and compare the maternal bonding styles in samples of smokers and non-smokers.

Methods
Study subjects
A dataset of 831 subjects was examined in our study, including 221 treatment-seeker smokers (112 males and 108 females with mean age of 51.2 ± 12.4 years) from 5 Hungarian quitting centers and 610 non-smoker medical students (198 males and 610 females with mean age of 22.4 ± 2.1).

The control non-smoker volunteers were all medical student volunteers (198 males and 412 females) from the medical faculties of the four medical universities in Hungary: Semmelweis University (Budapest), and Universities of Pécs, Debrecen, and Szeged. The mean age of this group was 22.4 ± 2.1. In order to avoid bias resulting from the educational differences between the two subgroups, only those smoker individuals were selected for this analysis who had high school graduation or degree. This moderately or highly qualified smoker group consists of 129 individuals (61 males and 68 females), with a mean age of 52.4 ± 12.8.

The difference in the mean age of smokers and non-smoker controls in our study sample is notable. However, it has no effect on the individuals' perception of their mother's behavior as it is measured by the PBI, since it is proven to be stable in time [29]. Besides, according to the literature, the mean age of smoking initiation is below 18 years [10], which suggests that non-smokers of the medical students will not become a smoker later.

Smoker participants were adult tobacco users who were committed to quitting. This study presents the data of their pre-quitting, first examination. The control group consisted of 610 psychiatrically healthy non-smoker medical student volunteers. Smoking was confirmed or excluded based on the scores of the Fagerstrom Test for Nicotine Dependence and daily cigarette consumption.

Measures
Smoking variables
Nicotine dependence was assessed using the Fagerstrom Test for Nicotine Dependence (FTND), a widely used and validated 6-item measurement scoring from 0 to 10 [30]. Besides, the average daily number of cigarettes (cigarettes per day, CPD) and the exhaled carbon monoxide level (CO) were also obtained.

Treatment-seeking smoker participants were included in this study if all of the following criteria were fulfilled: above four points of FTND, above 10 ppm CO concentration in exhaled air, and at least 10 smoked cigarettes per day in the last month. The heavy smoker subgroup (HS) was defined as smokers with a daily consumption of over 20 cigarettes, and the light smoker subgroup (LS) was defined as those with a daily consumption of 20 or below, which is a common criteria of the intensity of smoking in the literature [31, 32].

Participants were selected into the control group only if they did not fit the described smoking criteria.

Parental bonding instrument (PBI)

The maternal version of the parental bonding instrument (PBI) [33, 34] was used to explore the individuals' perceived maternal bonding patterns. This 25-item self-report questionnaire examines retrospectively the maternal rearing style from the subject's view in their first 16 years on a 4-point Likert scale scoring from 0 to 3. In this study, we used only the maternal part of the instrument, where each item is a statement about the mother's attitude and behavior. The maternal PBI measures the maternal bonding style along two dimensions: care (13 items) and overprotection (12 items). Both dimensions have two poles: maternal care is defined by emotional warmth, affection, trust, empathy, and closeness (high scores) or emotional coldness, neglect, and rejection (low scores), while maternal overprotection is characterized by the discouragement of autonomy and independence, excessive control, and intrusion (high scores) or reassuring independence and autonomy (low scores). Values from these dimensions can be used separately and can be divided into high and low scores according to the defined cut-off points: 13.5 points for maternal overprotection (high overprotection: HOP; low overprotection: LOP) and 27.0 points for maternal care (high care: HC; low care: LC).

The subgroups of the care and the overprotection scales can be combined by creating four specific maternal rearing styles: optimal parenting (OP; high care and low overprotection), affectionless control (ALC; low care and high overprotection), neglectful parenting (NP; low care and low overprotection), and affectionate constraint (AC; high care and high overprotection).

Mood and age only have a slight effect on the perception of parenting assessed by the PBI, since it is stable across time [29, 35].

Statistical analysis

The Kolmogorov–Smirnov test was performed to analyze the distribution of our variables. The differences of the PBI variables in the smoker and non-smoker groups were compared with the Mann–Whitney U-test and binary logistic regression. Besides these methods, linear regression was also used for revealing the association between continuous smoking and PBI variables. All regression analyses were adjusted for age and gender, except for the gender analyses, which were only adjusted for age. Besides, the gender differences in the frequency of the four PBI categories were tested with Chi-square test. Data were analyzed using SPSS version 20.0 software (IBM corp.) and are presented as mean (M) ± standard deviation (SD). Significance level was set at $p < 0.05$.

Results

Characteristics of the studied population

A sample of 729 individuals participated in this study including 129 smokers (61 males and 68 females) and 610 non-smoker volunteers (412 females and 198 males), with a mean age of 52.4 ± 12.8 and of 22.4 ± 2.1, respectively.

Among smokers, the mean value of FTND was 6.4 ± 1.2, the average daily number of cigarettes smoked was 21.0 ± 7.1, and exhaled CO concentration was 18.6 ± 7.6 ppm. The ratio of heavy smokers was significantly higher among male smokers (66.7%) compared to that among female smokers (47.1%; $p = 0.020$). No other gender differences were found regarding the smoking features (Table 1).

The average care and overprotection scores were 29.7 ± 6.6 and 13.1 ± 7.8 in the total sample, respectively. The most frequent maternal bonding subtype in the total population was the optimal parenting subtype (50.1%) followed by the affectionate constraint (25.4%), the affectionless control (17.1%), and the neglectful parenting (7.4%) subtypes. Several gender differences were found in PBI variables. First, the care score was significantly higher among males than among females, but only in the smoker subgroup ($Care_{males} = 28.9 ± 6.2$, $Care_{females} = 25.3 ± 8.7, p = 0.011$).

The ratio of affectionate constraint was slightly higher among males in the total sample ($AC_{males} = 30.2\%$, $AC_{females} = 22.9\%$, $p = 0.019$) and also in the non-smoker cohort ($AC_{males} = 32.8\%$, $AC_{females} = 24.0\%$, $p = 0.025$). In the smoker group, optimal parenting and high care showed significantly higher proportion among males ($OP_{males} = 48.3\%$, $OP_{females} = 29.4\%$, $p = 0.022$; $HC_{males} = 70.0\%$, $HC_{females} = 45.6\%$, $p = 0.004$), while affectionless control and high overprotection were more frequent among females ($ALC_{males} = 15.0\%$, $ALC_{females} = 38.2\%$, $p = 0.003$; $HOP_{males} = 36.7\%$, $HOP_{females} = 54.4\%, p = 0.033$) (Table 2).

Table 1 Smoking characteristics of the study population

Smoking properties	Total	Males	Females
FTND	6.4 ± 1.2	6.4 ± 1.2	6.4 ± 1.1
CO level (ppm)	18.6 ± 7.6	18.9 ± 7.5	18.5 ± 7.8
CPD	21.0 ± 7.1	21.8 ± 7.1	20.3 ± 7.2
HS (≥20 CPD)	55.8%	66.7%	47.1%[a]

[a] Statistically significant difference between males and females, [a]<0.01

FTND Fagerstrom Nicotine Dependence Test; CPD cigarette per day; HS heavy smoker

Table 2 Demographic and maternal bonding characteristics of the study population

	Smokers			Non-smokers		
	Total	Males	Females	Total	Males	Females
N	129	61 (47.3%)	68 (52.7%)	610	198 (32.5%)	412 (67.5%)
Age (M ± SD)	52.4 ± 12.8	52.0 ± 14.2	52.8 ± 11.4	22.4 ± 2.1	22.5 ± 2.3	22.3 ± 2.1
MB						
Care (M ± SD)	27.0 ± 7.7	28.9 ± 6.2	25.3 ± 8.7[b]	30.3 ± 6.2	30.3 ± 5.4	30.2 ± 6.6
Protection (M ± SD)	14.6 ± 8.6	13.2 ± 8.1	15.8 ± 8.9	12.8 ± 7.6	13.4 ± 7.3	12.6 ± 7.7
AC	18.6%	21.7%	16.2%	26.9%	32.8%	24.0%[b]
OP	38.8%	48.3%	29.4%[b]	52.5%	50.0%	53.6%
ALC	27.1%	15.0%	38.2%[b]	14.9%	13.6%	15.5%
NP	15.5%	15.0%	16.2%	5.7%	3.5%	6.8%
HC/LC	57.4%/42.6%	70.0%/30.0%	45.6%/54.4%[a]	79.3%/20.7%	82.8%/17.2%	77.7%/22.3%
HOP/LOP	45.7%/54.3%	36.7%/63.3%	54.4%/45.6%[b]	41.8%/58.2%	46.5%/53.5%	39.6%/60.4%

[a,b] Statistically significant difference between males and females, [a]<0.01, [b]<0.05)

MB maternal bonding; *AC* affectionate constraint; *OP* optimal parenting; *ALC* affectionless control; *NP* neglectful parenting; *HC* high care; *LC* low care; *HOP* high overprotection; *LOP* low overprotection; *M* mean; *SD* standard deviation

The effect of maternal bonding on smoking variables

The 129 treatment-seeker smokers were included in an association analysis of maternal bonding and smoking behavior.

First, we analyzed the smoking variables in the four maternal bonding subtypes and obtained no significant differences between the maternal bonding subtypes regarding the FTND score and the CO level. Similarly, care and overprotection scores had no effect on any of the latter smoking variables, as categorical variables of care and overprotection scores (high care, low care, high overprotection, and low overprotection) were not associated with the FTND score and the CO level either. As regards the daily cigarette consumption, higher maternal Care was associated with reduced CPD ($p = 0.050$), and higher maternal overprotection was associated with increased CPD in total sample ($p = 0.016$). Besides, the average CPD was significantly higher in the low care subgroup than in the high-care subgroup, but only among females ($\text{CPD}_{\text{LC}} = 21.8$, $\text{CPD}_{\text{HC}} = 20.2$, $p = 0.014$). We also found that in the low care subgroup, the odds of being a heavy smoker were significantly higher compared to those in the high care subgroup in the total sample ($p = 0.050$, $\text{Exp(B)} = 2.2$) and a similar difference appeared within the female smoker cohort ($p = 0.021$, $\text{Exp(B)} = 3.4$).

Differences of maternal care and overprotection between smokers and non-smokers

We compared the maternal bonding scales and subscales of the PBI between treatment-seeker smokers and non-smokers. Basic data of the PBI variables for each separate group, including gender subgroups, are shown in Table 2.

First, comparison tests of continuous variables were performed with the Mann–Whitney U-test in the total sample and also in gender subgroups.

Care score was significantly higher among non-smokers in the total sample ($p < 0.001$) and among females ($p < 0.001$), while among males this association showed only marginal significance ($p = 0.066$). As regards maternal overprotection, smokers had significantly higher scores on this scale, but only among females ($p = 0.005$).

After running these statistical analyses, we also tested the differences of care and overprotection scores between smokers and non-smokers with binary logistic regression adjusted for age and gender. In this case, significant association was not obtained in the total sample, not even in gender subgroups.

Binomial variables of the care and overprotection scales did not significantly differ either between smoker and non-smoker individuals.

The four categories of the PBI in smokers and non-smokers

Exploring the association between smoking and maternal bonding, the distribution of the four maternal bonding subtypes were examined separately in smokers and in non-smokers with binary logistic regression adjusted for age and gender. Detailed data about the distribution of maternal bonding subtypes in each group are presented in Table 2.

Only one maternal bonding subtype showed significant association with smoking: the neglectful parenting style, which is defined as the combination of low care and low overprotection of the mother. The odds for being a smoker were significantly higher among individuals who perceived neglectful parenting from their mothers ($\text{Exp(B)} = 32.5$, $p = 0.020$).

Within the affectionate constraint, the optimal parenting and the affectionless control subgroups, no significant differences were detected between smokers and non-smokers.

Discussion

Our findings confirmed that neglectful maternal bonding style (low care and low overprotection) has an important effect on whether an individual becomes a smoker, but it has no effect on smoking quantity or the level of nicotine dependence.

In the literature, most of the studies on the relationship between parental bonding and smoking did not separate the behavior of the mother and the father. Foxcroft et al. investigated adolescents (between the ages of 12 and 16) in 'neglecting families' and found that the ratio of adolescent smokers was higher in these types of families [21]. Similar results were reported by Chassin et al. about adolescents from families with low control and acceptance, which is very similar to the definition of neglectful parenting, showing a higher rate of smoking initiation [25]. In line with these results, Adalbjarnardottir et al. found that adolescents' experimentation with smoking at age of 14 was more frequent among adolescents of neglectful parents [24].

A recent large-sample study among adolescents in China conducted by Wang et al. investigated the effect of maternal and paternal bonding, separately on smoking. They reported that maternal neglect was strongly related to higher odds for current smoking, while paternal neglect did not show association with current smoking [27].

These results suggest that maternal neglectful parenting might have an effect on experimentation and early stage of smoking initiation, and on the intensity of smoking. Besides, it might be more relevant in the development of smoking than paternal neglectful parenting.

The underlying biological mechanism of the connection between smoking and maternal neglect might be associated with the dopaminergic system [36]. There is some evidence that the quality of maternal attachment has an important effect on the development of the dopaminergic pathways, which plays a crucial role in nicotine dependence [37, 38] and in regulating maternal behavior as well [39]. An animal study by Meaney et al. examined rat pups after prolonged maternal separation and found that later, when these animals were already adult animals, these animals showed increased behavioral sensitivity to cocaine, which causes dopamine release in mesocorticolimbic dopaminergic neurons, suggesting that prolonged maternal separation is connected to higher susceptibility to addiction later in life through the altered development of the mesocorticolimbic dopaminergic system [40]. It confirms our assumption that maternal neglectful parenting has an important role in the development of smoking.

The perceived maternal bonding predicts the later maternal behavior of the female offspring [36, 41], which means that the maternal attachment style could transmit to the next generation causing a persistent cyclic problem in 'neglectful families.'

In our study, childhood experience of maternal care and overprotection was associated with daily cigarette consumption. No data in the literature were found about the relationship between maternal bonding and the intensity of smoking.

Our findings on the effect of maternal care and overprotection on smoking behavior were not convincing as it did not remain significant after adjusting the test for age and gender. However, based on the literature, maternal care and overprotection are related to smoking [15, 27]. Probably, the notable difference in age between smoker and non-smoker subgroups of our study accounted for the confounded results. Further investigations are required to clarify this discrepancy.

The early relation to the mother seems essential in later mental health. The lack of love, warmth, care, and affection and the complete absence of control and protection at the same time might be the most harmful maternal rearing style. However, it is a perceived maternal bonding, which not necessarily reflects the real behavior of the mother.

There are several limitations to our study. First, the non-smoker subgroup consists of only medical students, which causes notable differences in age and occupation from the smoker subgroup. Besides, the smoker subgroup has only individuals with high school graduation or degree. The low sample size of the smoker subgroup is also an important limitation to our study.

Conclusion

In conclusion, our data confirmed the importance of the maternal behavior in the development of smoking. Therefore, focusing on the early life relationship between the patient and his/her mother can be helpful in psychotherapy. As negative parenting behavior has a pathological effect during the early age on the onset of smoking in the adolescence, the education of parents about dysfunctional attitude can be an additional element of the preventive programs in the mental health systems.

Abbreviations

AC: affectionate constraint; ALC: affectionless control; CO: carbon monoxide; CPD: cigarettes per day; FTND: Fagerstrom Test for Nicotine Dependence; HC: high care; HOP: high overprotection; HS: heavy smoker; LC: low care; LOP: low overprotection; LS: light smoker; M: mean; MB: maternal bonding; NS: non-smoker; NP: neglectful parenting; OP: optimal parenting; PBI: parental bonding instrument; S: smoker; SD: standard deviation.

Authors' contributions

CSI contributed to the statistical analyses, data recording, and manuscript preparation. EM contributed to the sample collection and manuscript preparation. MF, SI, GZ, and BE contributed to the sample collection and data recording. DP, DB, and FG contributed to the study design. LJ contributed to the study design, statistical analyses, and interpretation of data and review of the manuscript. All authors read and approved the final manuscript.

Author details

[1] Department of Psychiatry and Psychotherapy, Semmelweis University, Budapest, Hungary. [2] Institute of Behavioral Sciences, Semmelweis University, Budapest, Hungary. [3] National Institute of Psychiatry and Addiction, Budapest, Hungary. [4] Department of Tumor Biology, National Koranyi Institute of Pulmonology, Budapest, Hungary. [5] Department of Thoracic Surgery, Medical University of Vienna, Vienna, Austria. [6] Department of Thoracic Surgery, National Institute of Oncology and Semmelweis University, Budapest, Hungary. [7] Division of Molecular and Gender Imaging, Department of Biomedical Imaging and Image-guided Therapy, Medical University of Vienna, Vienna, Austria.

Acknowledgements

The authors would like to thank J. Breuer for his supporting work.

Competing interests

The authors declare that they have no competing interests.

Consent for publication

A written consent form was obtained from all participants.

Funding

This study was funded by the Norwegian Financial Mechanism (HU0125). Zsuzsa Gyorffy and Peter Dome were supported by the Hungarian Academy of Sciences Janos Bolyai Research Grant.

References

1. Schmitz N, Kruse J, Kugler J. Disabilities, quality of life, and mental disorders associated with smoking and nicotine dependence. Am J Psychiatry. 2003;160(9):1670–6.
2. Lim SS, Vos T, Flaxman AD, Danaei G, Shibuya K, Adair-Rohani H, et al. A comparative risk assessment of burden of disease and injury attributable to 67 risk factors and risk factor clusters in 21 regions, 1990-2010: a systematic analysis for the Global Burden of Disease Study 2010. Lancet (London, England). 2012;380(9859):2224–60. doi:10.1016/s0140-6736(12)61766-8.
3. Bauer UE, Briss PA, Goodman RA, Bowman BA. Prevention of chronic disease in the 21st century: elimination of the leading preventable causes of premature death and disability in the USA. Lancet (London, England). 2014;384(9937):45–52. doi:10.1016/s0140-6736(14)60648-6.
4. Conrad KM, Flay BR, Hill D. Why children start smoking cigarettes: predictors of onset. Br J Addict. 1992;87(12):1711–24.
5. Mayhew KP, Flay BR, Mott JA. Stages in the development of adolescent smoking. Drug Alcohol Depend. 2000;59(Suppl 1):S61–81.
6. Leonardi-Bee J, Jere ML, Britton J. Exposure to parental and sibling smoking and the risk of smoking uptake in childhood and adolescence: a systematic review and meta-analysis. Thorax. 2011;66(10):847–55. doi:10.1136/thx.2010.153379.
7. Nolte AE, Smith BJ, O'Rourke T. The relative importance of parental attitudes and behavior upon youth smoking behavior. J Sch Health. 1983;53(4):264–71.
8. Nelson DE, Giovino GA, Shopland DR, Mowery PD, Mills SL, Eriksen MP. Trends in cigarette smoking among US adolescents, 1974 through 1991. Am J Public Health. 1995;85(1):34–40.
9. Pierce JP, Choi WS, Gilpin EA, Farkas AJ, Merritt RK. Validation of susceptibility as a predictor of which adolescents take up smoking in the United States. Health Psychol. 1996;15(5):355–61.
10. Filippidis FT, Agaku IT, Vardavas CI. The association between peer, parental influence and tobacco product features and earlier age of onset of regular smoking among adults in 27 European countries. Eur J Pub Health. 2015. doi:10.1093/eurpub/ckv068.
11. Fleming CB, Kim H, Harachi TW, Catalano RF. Family processes for children in early elementary school as predictors of smoking initiation. J Adolesc Health. 2002;30(3):184–9.
12. Picotte DM, Strong DR, Abrantes AM, Tarnoff G, Ramsey SE, Kazura AN, et al. Family and peer influences on tobacco use among adolescents with psychiatric disorders. J Nerv Ment Dis. 2006;194(7):518–23. doi:10.1097/01.nmd.0000224927.64723.f6.
13. Foster SE, Jones DJ, Olson AL, Forehand R, Gaffney CA, Zens MS, et al. Family socialization of adolescent's self-reported cigarette use: the role of parents' history of regular smoking and parenting style. J Pediatr Psychol. 2007;32(4):481–93. doi:10.1093/jpepsy/jsl030.
14. Choquet M, Hassler C, Morin D, Falissard B, Chau N. Perceived parenting styles and tobacco, alcohol and cannabis use among French adolescents: gender and family structure differentials. Alcohol Alcohol. 2008;43(1):73–80. doi:10.1093/alcalc/agm060.
15. Gau SSF, Lai MC, Chiu YN, Liu CT, Lee MB, Hwu HG. Individual and family correlates for cigarette smoking among Taiwanese college students. Compr Psychiatry. 2009;50(3):276–85.
16. Scherrer JF, Xian H, Pan H, Pergadia ML, Madden PA, Grant JD, et al. Parent, sibling and peer influences on smoking initiation, regular smoking and nicotine dependence. Results from a genetically informative design. Addict Behav. 2012;37(3):240–7. doi:10.1016/j.addbeh.2011.10.005.
17. Biglan A, Duncan TE, Ary DV, Smolkowski K. Peer and parental influences on adolescent tobacco use. J Behav Med. 1995;18(4):315–30.
18. Huver RM, Engels RC, Vermulst AA, de Vries H. Is parenting style a context for smoking-specific parenting practices? Drug Alcohol Depend. 2007;89(2–3):116–25. doi:10.1016/j.drugalcdep.2006.12.005.
19. Bernardi E, Jones M, Tennant C. Quality of parenting in alcoholics and narcotic addicts. Br J Psychiatry. 1989;154:677–82.
20. Raudino A, Fergusson DM, Horwood L. The quality of parent/child relationships in adolescence is associated with poor adult psychosocial adjustment. J Adolesc. 2013;36(2):331–40.
21. Foxcroft DR, Lowe G. Adolescent drinking, smoking and other substance use involvement: links with perceived family life. J Adolesc. 1995;18(2):159–77.
22. O'Byrne KK, Haddock CK, Poston WS. Parenting style and adolescent smoking. J Adolesc Health. 2002;30(6):418–25.
23. Radziszewska B, Richardson JL, Dent CW, Flay BR. Parenting style and adolescent depressive symptoms, smoking, and academic achievement: ethnic, gender, and SES differences. J Behav Med. 1996;19(3):289–305.
24. Adalbjarnardottir S, Hafsteinsson LG. Adolescents' perceived parenting styles and their substance use: concurrent and longitudinal analyses. J Res Adolesc. 2001;11(4):401–23.
25. Chassin L, Presson CC, Rose J, Sherman SJ, Davis MJ, Gonzalez JL. Parenting style and smoking-specific parenting practices as predictors of adolescent smoking onset. J Pediatr Psychol. 2005;30(4):333–44. doi:10.1093/jpepsy/jsi028.
26. Piko BF, Balazs MA. Authoritative parenting style and adolescent smoking and drinking. Addict Behav. 2012;37(3):353–6. doi:10.1016/j.addbeh.2011.11.022.
27. Wang Y, Ho SY, Wang MP, Lo WS, Lai HK, Lam TH. Hong Kong Chinese adolescents' self-reported smoking and perceptions of parenting styles. Int J Behav Med. 2015;22(2):268–75. doi:10.1007/s12529-014-9436-0.
28. Gerra G, Leonardi C, Cortese E, Zaimovic A, Dell'Agnello G, Manfredini M, et al. Childhood neglect and parental care perception in cocaine addicts: relation with psychiatric symptoms and biological correlates. Neurosci Biobehav Rev. 2009;33(4):601–10.
29. Murphy E, Wickramaratne P, Weissman M. The stability of parental bonding reports: a 20-year follow-up. J Affect Disord. 2010;125(1–3):307–15. doi:10.1016/j.jad.2010.01.003.
30. Heatherton TF, Kozlowski LT, Frecker RC, Fagerstrom KO. The Fagerstrom Test for Nicotine Dependence: a revision of the Fagerstrom Tolerance Questionnaire. Br J Addict. 1991;86(9):1119–27.
31. Mucha L, Stephenson J, Morandi N, Dirani R. Meta-analysis of disease risk associated with smoking, by gender and intensity of smoking. Gend Med. 2006;3(4):279–91.

32. Husten CG. How should we define light or intermittent smoking? Does it matter? Nicotine Tob Res. 2009;11(2):111–21. doi:10.1093/ntr/ntp010.

33. Parker G, Tupling H, Brown LB. A parental bonding instrument. Br J Med Psychol. 1979;52:1–10. doi:10.1111/j.2044-8341.1979.tb02487.x.

34. Tóth I, Gervai J. Perceived parental styles: the Hungarian version of the parental bonding instrument (PBI). Magy Pszichol Szle. 1999;54:551–66.

35. Wilhelm K, Niven H, Parker G, Hadzi-Pavlovic D. The stability of the parental bonding instrument over a 20-year period. Psychol Med. 2005;35(3):387–93.

36. Strathearn L. Maternal neglect: oxytocin, dopamine and the neurobiology of attachment. J Neuroendocrinol. 2011;23(11):1054–65. doi:10.1111/j.1365-2826.2011.02228.x.

37. Balfour DJ, Wright AE, Benwell ME, Birrell CE. The putative role of extra-synaptic mesolimbic dopamine in the neurobiology of nicotine dependence. Behav Brain Res. 2000;113(1–2):73–83.

38. Dani JA, Bertrand D. Nicotinic acetylcholine receptors and nicotinic cholinergic mechanisms of the central nervous system. Ann Rev Pharmacol Toxicol. 2007;47:699–729. doi:10.1146/annurev.pharmtox.47.120505.105214.

39. Mileva-Seitz VR, Bakermans-Kranenburg MJ, van Ijzendoorn MH. Genetic mechanisms of parenting. Horm Behav. 2016;77:211–23. doi:10.1016/j.yhbeh.2015.06.003.

40. Meaney MJ, Brake W, Gratton A. Environmental regulation of the development of mesolimbic dopamine systems: a neurobiological mechanism for vulnerability to drug abuse? Psychoneuroendocrinology. 2002;27(1–2):127–38.

41. Van Ijzendoorn MH. Intergenerational transmission of parenting: a review of studies in nonclinical populations. Dev Rev. 1992;12(1):76–99. doi:10.1016/0273-2297(92)90004-L.

12

An association study of *Taq1A ANKK1* and *C957T* and − *141C DRD2* polymorphisms in adults with internet gaming disorder

Soo-Hyun Paik, Mi Ran Choi, Su Min Kwak, Sol Hee Bang, Ji-Won Chun, Jin-Young Kim, Jihye Choi, Hyun Cho, Jo-Eun Jeong and Dai-Jin Kim*

Abstract

Background: Though Internet gaming disorder (IGD) is considered to share similar genetic vulnerability with substance addictions, little has been explored about the role of the genetic variants on IGD. This pilot study was designed to investigate the association of the *Taq1A* polymorphism of the ankyrin repeat and kinase domain containing 1 (*ANKK1*) gene and *C957T* and − *141C* of the dopamine D2 receptor (*DRD2*) with IGD and their role on the personality and temperament traits in IGD among adult population.

Methods: Sixty-three subjects with IGD and 87 control subjects who regularly played Internet games were recruited. Self-administered questionnaires on self-control, dysfunctional impulsivity, and temperament and character domains were done. The *Taq1A ANKK1* and the *C957T* and − *141C ins/del* from the *DRD2* genes were genotyped using the specific TaqMan PCR assay.

Results: The distributions of allele and genotype frequencies were not significantly different between the IGD and control groups in both genders. In male, excessive gaming and use of gaming to escape from a negative feeling were associated with the *del−* genotype of the − *141C*. Among IGD, the *del+* genotype was associated with higher novelty seeking. Logistic regression showed no predictive value of these polymorphisms for IGD when using age and gender as covariates.

Conclusions: Though no direct association of the *Taq1A ANKK1* and *C957T DRD2* variants with IGD were observed, the − *141C* polymorphism may play a role in IGD via mediating symptoms or temperament traits.

Keywords: Internet gaming disorder, Dopamine D2 receptor, ANKK1, TaqMan assay, Personality and temperament

Introduction

Internet gaming disorder (IGD) is conceptualized as a behavioral addiction that excessive preoccupation and loss of control over Internet gaming eventually leads to the functional impairment [1]. Growing evidence suggested that IGD resembles substance additions in phenomenology, genetic and environmental risk factors, and

*Correspondence: kdj922@catholic.ac.kr
Department of Psychiatry, Seoul St. Mary's Hospital, The Catholic University of Korea College of Medicine, Seoul, 222, Banpo-daero, Seocho-gu, Seoul 06591, South Korea

neurobiological mechanisms [2]. Individuals with IGD showed impulsivity and response disinhibition in Go/No-Go tasks [3], tendency to make risky decision in Cups tasks [4], and increased craving when gaming-related cues were presented [5]. Furthermore, dysregulation of the dopamine D2 receptors in the striatum was observed in Internet addiction [6]. On account of this, a previous study revealed the association of the *Taq1A* polymorphism of the ankyrin repeat and kinase domain containing 1 (*ANKK1*) gene, which was associated with altered availability of dopamine D2 receptor, with IGD in male adolescents [7]. Family and twin studies have shown that the genetic factors accounted for 41–66% of the variance of the Internet addiction [8–10], which was comparable to that of substance addictions [11]. Accordingly, the identification of genetic vulnerabilities is considered as providing better understanding of the neurobiology of IGD and improving intervention outcomes. However, little has been explored on the role of the genetic variants on IGD.

The genetic polymorphisms that potentially alter the availability and expression of the dopamine D2 receptor have been known to be associated with both substance and behavioral addictions [12, 13]. The *Taq1A* polymorphism (SNP ID: rs1800497), which is located in exon 8 of *ANKK1*, adjacent to the terminal codon of the *DRD2* (OMIM*126450; gene map locus 11q23.2), is known to alter binding specificity and reduce DRD2 expression in striatum and associated structures. A significant number of genetic studies have found the association of the *Taq1A* polymorphism with substance addiction and impulsivity and psychopathic traits in alcohol dependence [14–16]. The *C957T* polymorphism (SNP ID: rs1799732), which is located on exon 7 of the *DRD2* (gene map locus 11q23), is known to alter DRD2 availability and be associated with alcoholism with higher prevalence of the CC genotype [17, 18]. The − *141C Ins/Del* polymorphism (SNP ID: rs6277), which is located on promoter of the *DRD2* (gene map locus 11q23), alters striatal D2 receptor binding potentials, and is associated with alcoholism [16, 19, 20]. Given the gene performance and the association with substance addiction, the three polymorphisms may play a crucial role in IGD. To date, however, no study has investigated the association of these polymorphisms with IGD.

Personality and temperament traits such as high neuroticism, psychoticism, sensational seeking, and reward dependence and low self-directedness and cooperativeness were associated with IGD [21–24]. Personality traits are strongly influenced by genetics. Twin studies which reported individual differences in personality showed about 50% of heritability, which means that about half of the variation in personality traits is affected by genetics [25, 26]. Though this assumption is oversimplified and several studies performed in healthy volunteers have reported no association between the variants of *DRD2* gene and personality and temperament traits [27, 28], relations were found in substance and behavioral addiction. For example, the *Taq1A* A1 carriers of pathological gambling had higher harm avoidance and lower self-directedness than non-A1 carriers, and the *C957T* T carriers of alcohol dependence had higher psychopathic tendency [18, 29]. Given that genetics could influence addictive disorders either directly or mediated via personality traits [27], genetics may better account for the vulnerability for IGD when personality and

character traits are taken into account. At present, two studies have investigated the association of genetic variants with temperament traits in excessive Internet users: the *Taq1A* polymorphism with higher reward dependence and the short allelic variant of the serotonin transporter gene (SS-5HTTLPR) with higher harm avoidance [7, 30]. Despite, these studies only included male adolescents who normally manifested higher sensation seeking and risk taking behavior, used rather subjective definition of excessive Internet users, and represented only personality dimensions of interest. Accordingly, a need to investigate the genetics of IGD with consideration of the temperament and personality traits in adults, who have more stable personality structure than adolescents, is emerging.

The present pilot study was designed to investigate the association of the genetic polymorphisms of *DRD2* (− *141C* and *C957T*) and *ANKK1* (*Taq1A*) with IGD and its symptoms, and the role of these polymorphisms on IGD and various personality and temperament traits of IGD.

Materials and methods
Participants
We recruited volunteers who agreed with and were able to follow the study design from three online surveys conducted in 2015 and 2016 regarding the Internet gaming behaviors. All participants were assessed using the diagnostic criteria for IGD of the Diagnostic and Statistical Manual of Mental Disorder, 5th edition [31]. The IGD group was defined by endorsement of at least five or more of the nine criteria over a 12-month period. The control subjects were determined as individuals who played the Internet games regularly but were not considered as having IGD. All participants aged 19 or over and had at least 12 years of education.

We interviewed all subjects for the history of neurological or severe medical illness and assessed intellectual function using the Korean version of the Wechsler Adult Intelligence Scale version IV (K-WAIS-IV) to exclude intellectual disability. After excluding four subjects with intellectual disability and one with a history of neurological illness (brain tumor, postoperative status), 63 IGD and 87 control subjects were included in this study. The general characteristics were as follows: age range of 19–47 years old; mean age 30.09 years [standard deviation (SD): 6.343]; number of male participants 115 (76.7%); time spent gaming on weekdays 2.03 h (SD: 1.35); and time spent gaming on weekends 3.28 h (SD: 1.94).

The study protocol was approved by Institutional Review Boards of Seoul St. Mary's Hospital (IRB number: KC15EISI0103). This study met the ethical standards of the Declaration of Helsinki, including obtaining informed consent from all participants and adhering to the privacy rights of participants.

Measures
Participants were asked to fill out questionnaires regarding personality and temperament traits as follows: the brief self-control scale (BSCS), the Dickman dysfunctional impulsivity inventory (DII), and the temperament and character inventory-revised short (TCI-RS). Questions about time spent gaming on weekdays and weekends were asked separately.

The BSCS measures the ability to override or change one's inner response as well as to interrupt undesired behavioral tendencies and refrain from acting on them [32]. The BSCS is a 13-item questionnaire with a 5-point Likert scale, and higher scores indicate lower self-control.

The DII is composed of 12 out of 23 items of the Dickman functional and dysfunctional inventory [33]. In DII, dysfunctional impulsivity refers to the tendency to act with less forethought than most people of equal ability when this tendency is a source of difficulty. Items are rated true (1) or false (0) and higher scores indicate higher dysfunctional impulsivity.

The temperament and character inventory (TCI) has been widely used in the investigations of human psychobiological behaviors [34]. TCI measures four temperament dimensions: novelty seeking (NS), harm avoidance (HA), reward dependency (RD), and persistence (P), and three character dimensions: self-directedness (SD), cooperativeness (C), and self-transcendence (ST). We used a shortened TCI-R inventory (TCI-RS), which was consisted of 140 questions [35]. Items on the TCI-RS are rated on a 5-point Likert scale, and higher scores indicate higher prominence of the dimensions.

Genotyping: a specific TaqMan PCR assay
DNA was isolated from the whole blood using a Wizard Genomic DNA Purification Kit (Promega, Madison, WI, USA) according to the manufacturer's instructions. Genotypes for *Taq1A* (SNP ID: rs1800497), − *141C Ins/Del* (SNP ID: rs1799732), and *C957T* (SNP ID: rs6277) polymorphic loci were assessed using the TaqMan SNP genotyping assays (Thermo Fisher Scientific, Carlsbad, CA, USA) on a ViiA 7 Real-Time PCR System (Thermo Fisher Scientific, Foster City, CA, USA). All genotypes were reported using the allelic discrimination program in QuantStudioTM Real-Time PCR Software v1.1 (Thermo Fisher Scientific, Foster City, CA, USA). Only one − *141C* genotype of a male control subject was missing. After genotyping, the *Taq1A* was grouped as the A1+ (homozygous and heterozygous for the A1 allele) and the A1− genotypes (homozygous for the A2 allele), the *C957T* as the T+ (homozygous and heterozygous for the T allele) and the T− genotypes (homozygous for the C allele), and the − *141C Ins/Del* as the del+ (homozygous and heterozygous for the deletion allele) and *del* − genotypes (homozygous for the insertion allele).

Statistical analysis
χ^2 tests were done to investigate the association of polymorphisms with IGD and its symptoms. Independent *t* tests were carried out to compare the clinical and personality variables between the IGD and control groups except the TCI-RS. Analyses of covariance (ANCOVA) were performed using age as a covariate to explore the TCI-RS profiles between groups since TCI may vary with age [36]. When age had significant interactions with the TCI variables, the results of the independent *t* tests were present. Subgroup analyses in the IGD group were performed to investigate the associations of the polymorphisms with temperament and personality predispositions in IGD. Binary logistic regression analysis was conducted to calculate the predictive value of each genotype using age and gender as covariates and odds ratio (OR) and 95% confidential interval (CI) were present. χ^2 goodness-of-fit tests were performed in order to calculate the correspondence between the observed number of homozygous and heterozygous individuals and the numbers expected based on Hardy–Weinberg equilibrium. All statistical analyses were performed using SPSS 24.0 (SPSS Inc., Chicago, IL, USA).

Results
Clinical characteristics and personality traits
As shown in Table 1, participants with IGD were older (IGD: 32.03 ± 6.528, control: 28.68 ± 5.812, $t = − 3.398$, $p = .001$) and had higher prevalence of male (IGD: 87.4%, control: 61.9%, $\chi^2 = 13.232$, $p = .000$). IGD spent more time on gaming both weekdays and weekends and had higher scores on the BSCS and DII, indicating lower self-control ability and higher dysfunctional impulsivity, than the control subjects. As for the TCI-RS, the scores of NS, P, and ST were higher in IGD in independent *t* tests. However, since these three variables had significant interaction effect between group and age, ANCOVA was not performed for them (see Additional file 1 for the scatter plot of ANCOVA and regression slope of NS, P, and ST). Other TCI domains showed no significant differences between groups in ANCOVA. Additional subgroup analyses which divided the sample into two groups (age < 30 vs age ≥ 30) showed no significant differences in TCI-RS domains between groups (results not shown).

Table 1 Comparisons of clinical and personality variables

	Control ($n = 87$)	IGD ($n = 63$)	χ^2/t/F	P
Age (years old)	28.58 ± 5.812	32.03 ± 6.528	− 3.398	.001
Male proportion (%)	76 (87.4%)	39 (61.9%)	13.232	.000
Weekday gaming hours	1.66 ± 1.19	2.57 ± 1.40	− 2.805	.007
Weekend gaming hours	2.88 ± 1.88	3.86 ± 1.90	− 2.055	.044
BSCS	36.17 ± 6.547	41.44 ± 5.482	− 5.196	.000
DII	4.16 ± 3.429	6.57 ± 2.988	− 4.498	.000
Novelty seeking	31.59 ± 8.997	37.54 ± 8.561	− 2.689[a]	.009
Harm avoidance	33.104 ± 2.071	33.666 ± 1.642	.044	.834
Reward dependence	42.046 ± 1.355	44.967 ± 1.709	1.760	.189
Persistence	43.05 ± 10.538	49.46 ± 8.659	− 2.595[a]	.012
Self-directedness	49.368 ± 1.371	50.727 ± 1.730	.372	.544
Cooperativeness	52.759 ± 1.448	55.534 ± 1.827	1.391	.243
Self-transcendence	18.51 ± 8.775	24.92 ± 10.311	− 2.725[a]	.008

IGD Internet gaming disorder, *BSCS* brief self-control scale, *DII* Dickman dysfunctional impulsivity scale

* $p < .05$, ** $p < .005$

[a] Results of t tests

Association of polymorphisms with IGD and its symptoms

Genotype and allele distributions of three polymorphisms were not significantly different between the IGD and control groups (Table 2). The results were similar when analyzed male and female separately. The observed frequencies of homozygous, heterozygous, and non-carriers of the minor alleles were in Hardy–Weinberg equilibrium (Taq1A ANKK1 SNP: $\chi^2 = 0.44$, $p = .51$; C957T DRD2: $\chi^2 = 0.84$, $p = .36$, − *141C* DRD2: $\chi^2 = 0.74$, $p = .39$).

The association of each genotype with symptoms of IGD was not evident in whole sample (Additional file 2). Subgroup analyses performed in male showed that male with the *del−* genotype showed higher prevalence of the presence of G6 (Continued excessive use of Internet games despite knowledge of psychosocial problems) and G8 (Use of Internet games to escape or relieve a negative mood) than male with the *del+* (Table 3). No association of the genotypes with IGD symptoms was found in female.

Role of ANKK1/DRD2 polymorphisms on IGD and personality and temperament predispositions

In the IGD group, the *t* tests showed the association of the *del+* of the − 141C with higher NS (*del+*: 44.71 ± 9.050, *Del−*: 34.86 ± 6.863, $t = − 2.973$, $p = .007$) (Additional file 3). However, ANCOVA was inapplicable for the investigation of the association of the *del* genotype and NS due to the significant interaction effect (Additional

file 1). In subgroup analyses (age < 30 vs. age ≥ 30), no significant association between genotypes and TCI in the IGD group was found. The *Taq1A* and *C957T* polymorphisms were not significantly associated with personality and temperament predispositions in IGD.

Table 4 showed results of the binary logistic regression to predict the risk for IGD using age, gender, and each genotype as covariates. Overall classification accuracy was 72.3% and Nagelkerke R square was 23.0%. Being male (OR = 4.205, 95% CI 1.776–9.956, $p = .001$) and older age (OR = 1.098, 95% CI 1.034–1.166, $p = .002$) were considered as risk factors for IGD. However, any genotype had no predictive value for being IGD.

Discussion

The purpose of this preliminary study was to explore the role of the *Taq1A ANKK1 and − 141C Ins/Del* and *C957T DRD2* polymorphisms on IGD. Our results suggested that though these polymorphisms had no association with occurrence and the personality and temperament predispositions in adults with IGD, some symptoms of IGD were associated with the − *141C Ins/ Del* polymorphism in male population.

When compared between the IGD and control groups, IGD subjects had unique clinical and TCI characteristics. First, IGD subjects had higher mean age. The prevalence of IGD across different age groups in adult population has not been investigated before. Given that characteristics of gaming behavior were different across age groups in adults [37], adults with IGD may have unique psychological antecedents that are different from those of adolescents IGD. Second, IGD subjects showed high persistence and self-transcendence as well as low self-control and high impulsivity and novelty seeking as reported before [7, 38–40]. Given that high persistence was associated with perfectionism and obsessive–compulsive disorder [36, 41], this may support the compulsive nature of IGD [42]. High self-transcendence may pose the possibility of psychopathology in IGD [43, 44]. On account of the distribution of allele distribution, our sample was nearly absent in the T allele of *C957T* and the del of − *141C DRD2*. According to the refSNP database (https://www. ncbi.nlm.nih.gov/projects/SNP/snp_ref.cgi?rs=1799732 and https://www.ncbi.nlm.nih.gov/projects/SNP/snp_ref. cgi?rs=6277), the prevalence of the T and del allele was quite low in East Asia, ranging from 0.0487 to 0.0625 and 0.136, which were comparable to that of our sample, 0.0747 and 0.209, respectively.

We found that none of the polymorphisms were associated to the occurrence of IGD, which was inconsistent with a previous finding in male adolescents with IGD [7]. Given that adolescents are more eager to take risks and seek for novelties and thus have been considered to be

Table 2 Allele and genotype frequencies of ANKK1 and DRD2 polymorphisms

Genotype	ANKK1 Taq 1A			DRD2 C952T			DRD2 − 141C Ins/Del		
	A1A1	A1A2	A2A2	TT	TC	CC	Del/Del	Del/Ins	Ins/Ins
Whole									
Control (n = 87)	15 (17.2)	43 (48.3)	30 (34.5)	0 (0.0)	15 (17.2)	72 (82.8)	1 (1.2)	29 (33.7)	56 (65.1)
IGD (n = 63)	12 (19.0)	26 (41.3)	25 (39.7)	0 (0.0)	6 (9.5)	57 (90.5)	2 (3.2)	17 (27.0)	44 (69.8)
	$\chi^2 = .731, p = .694$			$\chi^2 = 1.808, p = .179$			$\chi^2 = 1.386, p = .500$		
Male									
Control (n = 76)	14 (18.4)	35 (46.1)	27 (35.5)	0 (0.0)	12 (15.8)	64 (84.2)	1 (1.3)	26 (34.7)	48 (64.0)
IGD (n = 39)	7 (17.9)	17 (43.6)	15 (38.5)	0 (0.0)	4 (10.3)	35 (89.7)	0 (0.0)	8 (20.5)	31 (79.52)
	$\chi^2 = .099, p = .952$			$\chi^2 = .659, p = .417$			$\chi^2 = 3.132, p = .209$		
Female									
Control (n = 11)	1 (9.1)	7 (63.6)	3 (27.3)	0 (0.0)	3 (27.3)	8 (72.7)	0 (0.0)	3 (27.3)	8 (72.7)
IGD (n = 24)	5 (20.8)	9 (37.5)	10 (41.7)	0 (0.0)	2 (8.3)	22 (91.7)	2 (8.3)	9 (37.5)	13 (54.2)
	$\chi^2 = 2.155, p = .341$			$\chi^2 = 2.210, p = .137$			$\chi^2 = 1.580, p = .454$		

	ANKK1 Taq 1A		DRD2 C952T		DRD2 − 141C Ins/Del	
Allele	A1+	A1−	T+	T−	Del+	Del−
Whole						
Control (n = 87)	57 (65.5)	30 (34.1)	15 (17.2)	72 (82.8)	30 (34.5)	57 (65.5)
IGD (n = 63)	38 (60.3)	25 (39.7)	6 (9.5)	57 (90.5)	19 (30.2)	44 (69.8)
	$\chi^2 = .425, p = 514$		$\chi^2 = 1.808, p = .179$		$\chi^2 = .368, p = .544$	
Male						
Control (n = 76)	49 (64.5)	27 (35.5)	10 (16.9)	49 (83.1)	27 (36.0)	48 (64.0)
IGD (n = 39)	24 (61.5)	15 (38.5)	2 (5.6)	34 (94.4)	8 (20.5)	31 (79.5)
	$\chi^2 = .096, p = .757$		$\chi^2 = .659, p = .417$		$\chi^2 = .2.893, p = .089$	
Female						
Control (n = 11)	15 (51.7)	14 (48.3)	3 (27.3)	8 (72.7)	3 (27.3)	8 (72.7)
IGD (n = 24)	15 (55.6)	12 (44.4)	2 (8.3)	22 (91.7)	11 (45.8)	13 (54.2)
	$\chi^2 = .669, p = .413$		$\chi2 = 2.210, p = .137$		$\chi^2 = 1.083, p = .298$	

IGD Internet gaming disorder

more susceptible to IGD [45, 46], adolescents with risky genetic factors may be more vulnerable to become IGD while adults may be more affected by the complex interaction of genetic and environmental factors. Meanwhile, males with the *del−* genotype more frequently used Internet games excessively despite knowledge of psychosocial problems and to escape or relieve a negative mood. The *del−* genotype was associated with alcoholism, especially in male population, and alcoholic patients with the *del−* continued to drink despite they had protective *ALDH2*2* and *ADH1B*2* alleles [20, 47]. Meanwhile, the role of the − *141C* polymorphism in vivo is controversial; one study showed healthy volunteers with the *del+* had higher striatal D2 receptor binding potential while the other showed no significant differences between the *del+* and *del−* [19, 48]. It can be inferred that the − *141C* DRD2 polymorphism may influence specific behaviors observed in addictive disorders, such as excessive use and compensation of negative mood. Interestingly, this

finding was observed only in male subjects. Previous behavioral genetic studies have consistently suggested that alcohol and drug use in males was more determined by genetic factors, while that in female was more by environmental factors [27, 49]. In addition, male had markedly greater dopamine release than female in the ventral striatum in healthy volunteers, which could account for increased vulnerability of addictive disorders in male [50]. Likewise, gaming behaviors may be more influenced by genetic factors in males than in females due to the neurobiological differences between genders. Further studies are needed to determine different pathways to IGD between male and female.

We found that none of the polymorphisms were related with personality and temperament predispositions in IGD, except the association between the *del+* genotype and high novelty seeking. Though age had significant interaction effect, this poses a possibility of the role of the − *141C* polymorphism on IGD. In vitro, the

Table 3 Association of genotypes with symptoms of IGD in male

	A1+ (n = 73)	A1− (n = 42)	T+ (n = 16)	T− (n = 99)	Del+ (n = 35)	Del− (n = 79)
G1	20 (27.4%)	12 (28.6%)	4 (25.0%)	28 (28.3%)	8 (22.9%)	24 (30.4%)
	$\chi^2 = .018, p = .892$		$\chi^2 = .074, p = .786$		$\chi^2 = .680, p = .410$	
G2	16 (21.9%)	12 (28.6%)	3 (18.8%)	25 (25.3%)	6 (21.4%)	22 (27.8%)
	$\chi^2 = .641, p = .423$		$\chi^2 = .316, p = .574$		$\chi^2 = 1.500, p = .221$	
G3	22 (30.1%)	14 (33.3%)	3 (18.8%)	33 (33.3%)	8 (22.9%)	28 (35.4%)
	$\chi^2 = .127, p = .722$		$\chi^2 = 1.362, p = .243$		$\chi^2 = 1.778, p = .182$	
G4	27 (37.0%)	18 (42.9%)	7 (43.8%)	38 (37.4%)	11 (31.4%)	34 (43.0%)
	$\chi^2 = .386, p = .535$		$\chi^2 = .167, p = .683$		$\chi^2 = 1.368, p = .242$	
G5	24 (32.9%)	19 (45.2%)	7 (43.8%)	36 (36.4%)	10 (28.6%)	33 (41.8%)
	$\chi^2 = 1.740, p = .187$		$\chi^2 = .321, p = .571$		$\chi^2 = 1.779, p = .180$	
G6	21 (28.8%)	13 (31.0%)	5 (31.3%)	29 (29.3%)	6 (17.1%)	28 (35.4%)
	$\chi^2 = .061, p = .805$		$\chi^2 = .025, p = .874$		$\chi^2 = 3.881, p = .049*$	
G7	27 (37.0%)	18 (42.9%)	5 (31.3%)	40 (40.4%)	11 (31.4%)	34 (43.0%)
	$\chi^2 = .386, p = .535$		$\chi^2 = .485, p = .486$		$\chi^2 = .368, p = .242$	
G8	20 (27.4%)	15 (35.7%)	5 (31.3%)	30 (30.3%)	6 (17.1%)	29 (36.7%)
	$\chi^2 = .871, p = .351$		$\chi^2 = .006, p = .939$		$\chi^2 = 4.364, p = .037*$	
G9	14 (19.2%)	10 (23.8%)	2 (12.5%)	22 (22.2%)	4 (11.4%)	20 (25.3%)
	$\chi^2 = .346, p = .556$		$\chi^2 = .788, p = .375$		$\chi^2 = 2.815, p = .093$	

G1–G9 represented DSM-5 IGD criteria (Additional file 2)

* $p < .05$

Table 4 Predictive values for Internet gaming disorder

Variables	B	S.E.	OR	95% CI	p
Male gender	1.436	.440	4.205	1.776–9.956	.001**
Age	.094	.031	1.098	1.034–1.166	.002**
A1+ of Taq1A ANKK1	− .534	.399	.586	.268–1.281	.180
T+ of C957T DRD2	− 1.161	.607	.559	.255–1.225	.146
Del+ of − 141C DRD2	− 2.797	.950	.313	.095–1.028	.056

CI confidential interval

** $p < .005$, * $p < .05$

del allele-containing construct showed marked reduction in promoter activity, manifesting only 21–43% of the reporter gene expression level attributed to the ins allele-containing construct [16]. In addition, the del+ genotype showed differential neural response when performing the Go/No-go task in alcohol-abusing adults [51], suggesting the role of − 141C polymorphism in important neurocognitive function. A recent study on the heritability of Internet addiction (IA) suggested that genetic factors accounted for 20–65% of a part of variance of specific IA factors such as personality factor self-directedness; they had negligible influence on generalized facets of IA [52]. Likewise, genetic factors may account for a certain part of the variance of temperament and personality traits observed in IGD. Though the del− genotype itself has been associated with alcohol dependence [20, 47, 53], the

− 141C polymorphism may have different roles in IGD possibly by mediating temperament traits.

Neither univariate and multivariate logistic regression analyses showed predictive value of polymorphisms of interest for the occurrence of IGD in adult population. Though we could not find the direct association of these polymorphisms with IGD, it is too hasty to draw final conclusion that these polymorphisms have no role in IGD. Given that genes interact with other genes as well as environmental factors and modify gene or protein expression levels even not altering DNA sequences, further researches using high-throughput technologies would give opportunities to explore these epistatic or epigenetic changes made in IGD.

This study had several limitations that should be noted. First, the sample size was relatively small given the possibility of false-positive findings in studies with small samples. However, this is a preliminary study to explore the role of the DRD2 and ANKK1 polymorphisms on IGD and would give an insight to the theme. Second, the IGD and control group had different mean age and gender distribution, which may confound the results. However, subgroup analyses in both genders and different age groups (age < 30 vs. age ≥ 30) showed comparable results with the original analyses. Third, psychiatric comorbidities such as depression or anxiety disorder and substance addictions were not screened. Nevertheless, since our sample was composed of non-clinical population and subjects with comparable intelligence levels, the proportion of psychiatric comorbidities is supposed to be small.

Despite the limitations, this study had some methodological strengths. First, our study focused on the adult population, which was a remarkable departure from previous studies that mainly focused on male adolescents. Since adolescents are susceptible to addictive disorder [46], the investigation of genetic predispositions in adult population would give more accurate perspectives by regressing out the contribution of characteristics of adolescents in the development of IGD. Second, we compared the IGD subjects with casual gamers. Considering that only a small portion of gamers become IGD out of casual gamers, this method had an advantage to investigate the neurobiological mechanisms that differentiate IGD from casual gamers. Third, the sample was homogeneous with respect to the ethnicity, education, and intellectual levels. By using interviews and objective measures, we excluded participants with neurological disorders and intellectual disabilities which may severely affect the personality and temperament traits.

Conclusions

Our findings suggest that the genetic variations of the − 141C DRD2 may play a role on IGD via mediating specific symptoms or temperament traits in adult population, especially in male gender, though no direct association was observed. The neurobiological mechanisms of IGD may be different between adults and adolescents and between male and female. Further researches are necessary to investigate the interaction between genes and environmental factors and the differences across genders and age groups in neurobiological and psychological antecedents of IGD.

Authors' contributions
All the authors contributed to the design of the study. S-HP, MRC, J-WC, HJ, J-EJ, and D-JK contributed to study planning and advised to the course of study. J-WC, J-YK, J-HC, HJ, and J-EJ conducted the data collection from participants. S-HP conducted the literature search and provided summaries of previous research studies. MRC, SMK, and SHB conducted the genotyping. S-HP and MRC conducted the statistical analysis and wrote the first draft of the manuscript. All authors contributed to the development of the manuscript and revised it critically. All authors read and approved the final manuscript.

Acknowledgements
Not applicable.

Competing interests
The authors declare that they have no competing interests. The authors alone are responsible for the content and writing of this paper.

Funding
This research was supported by a grant from the Brain Research Program through the National Research Foundation of Korea (NRF) funded by the Ministry of Science, ICT, & Future Planning (NRF-2014M3C7A1062893). The funding source had no role in the study design, collection, analysis or interpretation of data, writing of the manuscript, or the decision to submit the paper for publication.

References
1. American Psychiatry Association. Diagnostic and statistical manual of mental disorders. 5th ed. Arlington, VA: American Psychiatric Association; 2013.
2. Grant JE, Potenza MN, Weinstein A, Gorelick DA. Introduction to behavioral addictions. Am J Drug Alcohol Abuse. 2010;36(5):233–41.
3. Zhou Z, Yuan G, Yao J. Cognitive biases toward Internet game-related pictures and executive deficits in individuals with an Internet game addiction. PLoS ONE. 2012;7(11):e48961.
4. Yao Y-W, Chen P-R, Li S, Wang L-J, Zhang J-T, Yip SW, Chen G, Deng L-Y, Liu Q-X, Fang X-Y. Decision-making for risky gains and losses among college students with Internet gaming disorder. PLoS ONE. 2015;10(1):e0116471.
5. Yao Y-W, Wang L-J, Yip SW, Chen P-R, Li S, Xu J, Zhang J-T, Deng L-Y, Liu Q-X, Fang X-Y. Impaired decision-making under risk is associated with gaming-specific inhibition deficits among college students with Internet gaming disorder. Psychiatr Res. 2015;229(1):302–9.
6. Tian M, Chen Q, Zhang Y, Du F, Hou H, Chao F, Zhang H. PET imaging reveals brain functional changes in Internet gaming disorder. Eur J Nucl Med Mol Imaging. 2014;41(7):1388–97.
7. Han DH, Lee YS, Yang KC, Kim EY, Lyoo IK, Renshaw PF. Dopamine genes and reward dependence in adolescents with excessive Internet video game play. J Addict Med. 2007;1(3):133–8.
8. Li M, Chen J, Li N, Li X. A twin study of problematic Internet use: its heritability and genetic association with effortful control. Twin Res Hum Genet. 2014;17(4):279–87.
9. Long EC, Verhulst B, Neale MC, Lind PA, Hickie IB, Martin NG, Gillespie NA. The genetic and environmental contributions to Internet use and associations with psychopathology: a twin study. Twin Res Hum Genet. 2016;19(1):1–9.
10. Vink JM, Beijsterveldt TC, Huppertz C, Bartels M, Boomsma DI. Heritability of compulsive Internet use in adolescents. Addict Biol. 2016;21(2):460–8.
11. Kreek MJ, Nielsen DA, Butelman ER, LaForge KS. Genetic influences on impulsivity, risk taking, stress responsivity and vulnerability to drug abuse and addiction. Nat Neurosci. 2005;8(11):1450.
12. Comings DE, Blum K. Reward deficiency syndrome: genetic aspects of behavioral disorders. Prog Brain Res. 2000;126:325–41.
13. Noble EP. The DRD2 gene in psychiatric and neurological disorders and its phenotypes. Pharmacogenomics. 2000;1(3):309–33.
14. Doehring A, Kirchhof A, Lötsch J. Genetic diagnostics of functional variants of the human dopamine D2 receptor gene. Psychiatr Genet. 2009;19(5):259–68.
15. Neville MJ, Johnstone EC, Walton RT. Identification and characterization of ANKK1: a novel kinase gene closely linked to DRD2 on chromosome band 11q23. 1. Hum Mutat. 2004;23(6):540–5.
16. Arinami T, Gao M, Hamaguchi H, Toru M. A functional polymorphism in the promoter region of the dopamine D2 receptor gene is associated with schizophrenia. Hum Mol Genet. 1997;6(4):577–82.
17. Seeman P, Ohara K, Ulpian C, Seeman MV, Jellinger K, Van Tol HH, Niznik HB. Schizophrenia: normal sequence in the dopamine D2 receptor region that couples to G-proteins. DNA polymorphisms in D2. Neuropsychopharmacology. 1993;8(2):137–42.
18. Ponce G, Hoenicka J, Jimenez-Arriero M, Rodriguez-Jimenez R, Aragüés M, Martin-Sune N, Huertas E, Palomo T. DRD2 and ANKK1 genotype in alcohol-dependent patients with psychopathic traits: association and interaction study. Br J Psychiatr. 2008;193(2):121–5.
19. Jönsson E, Nöthen M, Grünhage F, Farde L, Nakashima Y, Propping P, Sedvall G. Polymorphisms in the dopamine D2 receptor gene and their relationships to striatal dopamine receptor density of healthy volunteers. Mol Psychiatry. 1999;4(3):290–6.
20. Konishi T, Luo HR, Calvillo M, Mayo MS, Lin KM, Wan YJY. ADH1B* 1, ADH1C* 2, DRD2 (-141C Ins), and 5-HTTLPR are associated with alcoholism in Mexican American men living in Los Angeles. Alcohol Clin Exp Res. 2004;28(8):1145–52.
21. Montag C, Flierl M, Markett S, Walter N, Jurkiewicz M, Reuter M. Internet addiction and personality in first-person-shooter video gamers. Media Psychol. 2011;23:163–73.

22. Montag C, Jurkiewicz M, Reuter M. Low self-directedness is a better predictor for problematic Internet use than high neuroticism. Comput Human Behav. 2010;26(6):1531–5.

23. Ha JH, Kim SY, Bae SC, Bae S, Kim H, Sim M, Lyoo IK, Cho SC. Depression and Internet addiction in adolescents. Psychopathology. 2007;40(6):424–30.

24. Cao F, Su L. Internet addiction among Chinese adolescents: prevalence and psychological features. Child Care Health Dev. 2007;33(3):275–81.

25. Jang KL, Livesley WJ, Vemon PA. Heritability of the big five personality dimensions and their facets: a twin study. J Pers. 1996;64(3):577–92.

26. Polderman TJ, Benyamin B, De Leeuw CA, Sullivan PF, Van Bochoven A, Visscher PM, Posthuma D. Meta-analysis of the heritability of human traits based on 50 years of twin studies. Nat Genet. 2015;47(7):702–9.

27. Munafo MR, Clark TG, Moore LR, Payne E, Walton R, Flint J. Genetic polymorphisms and personality in healthy adults: a systematic review and meta-analysis. Mol Psychiatry. 2003;8(5):471.

28. Gebhardt C, Leisch F, Schüssler P, Fuchs K, Stompe T, Sieghart W, Hornik K, Kasper S, Aschauer H. Non-association of dopamine D4 and D2 receptor genes with personality in healthy individuals. Psychiatr Genet. 2000;10(3):131–7.

29. Kwon YS, Lim S, Shin YC. An association study of the dopamine D2 receptor Taq1A polymorphism and temperament in Korean pathological gamblers. Korean J Biol Psychiatry. 2011;18(3):119–25.

30. Lee YS, Han DH, Yang KC, Daniels MA, Na C, Kee BS, Renshaw PF. Depression like characteristics of 5HTTLPR polymorphism and temperament in excessive Internet users. J Affect Disord. 2008;109(1):165–9.

31. Pontes HM, Kiraly O, Demetrovics Z, Griffiths MD. The conceptualisation and measurement of DSM-5 Internet gaming disorder: the development of the IGD-20 test. PLoS ONE. 2014;9(10):e110137.

32. Tangney JP, Baumeister RF, Boone AL. High self-control predicts good adjustment, less pathology, better grades, and interpersonal success. J Pers. 2004;72(2):271–324.

33. Dickman SJ. Functional and dysfunctional impulsivity: personality and cognitive correlates. J Pers Soc Psychol. 1990;58(1):95.

34. Cloninger CR, Svrakic DM, Przybeck TR. A psychobiological model of temperament and character. Arch Gen Psychiatry. 1993;50(12):975–90.

35. Farmer RF, Goldberg LR. A psychometric evaluation of the revised temperament and Character Inventory (TCI-R) and the TCI-140. Psychol Assess. 2008;20(3):281.

36. Josefsson K, Jokela M, Cloninger CR, Hintsanen M, Salo J, Hintsa T, Pulkki-Råback L, Keltikangas-Järvinen L. Maturity and change in personality: developmental trends of temperament and character in adulthood. Dev Psychopathol. 2013;25(3):713–27.

37. Korea Creative Content Agency (KCCA): a survey on game usage 2016. http://portal.kocca.kr/cop/bbs/view/B0000147/1831102.do?menuNo=200904. Accessed Feb 22, 2017.

38. Lin SS, Tsai C-C. Sensation seeking and Internet dependence of Taiwanese high school adolescents. Comput Hum Behav. 2002;18(4):411–26.

39. Dalbudak E, Evren C, Aldemir S, Coskun KS, Ugurlu H, Yildirim FG. Relationship of Internet addiction severity with depression, anxiety, and alexithymia, temperament and character in university students. Cyberpsychol Behav Soc Netw. 2013;16(4):272–8.

40. Kim EJ, Namkoong K, Ku T, Kim SJ. The relationship between online game addiction and aggression, self-control and narcissistic personality traits. Eur Psychiatry. 2008;23(3):212–8.

41. Mulder RT, Joyce PR. Temperament and the structure of personality disorder symptoms. Psychol Med. 1997;27(1):99–106.

42. Van Rooij AJ, Schoenmakers TM, Van de Eijnden RJ, Van de Mheen D. Compulsive Internet use: the role of online gaming and other Internet applications. J Adol Health. 2010;47(1):51–7.

43. Cloninger CR, Zohar AH. Personality and the perception of health and happiness. J Affect Disord. 2011;128(1):24–32.

44. Cloninger CR, Zohar AH, Cloninger KM. Promotion of well-being in person-centered mental health care. Focus. 2010;8(2):165–79.

45. Griffiths M, Wood RT. Risk factors in adolescence: the case of gambling, videogame playing, and the Internet. J Gambl Stud. 2000;16(2):199–225.

46. Crews F, He J, Hodge C. Adolescent cortical development: a critical period of vulnerability for addiction. Pharmacol Biochem Behav. 2007;86(2):189–99.

47. Ishiguro H, Arinami T, Saito T, Akazawa S, Enomoto M, Mitushio H, Fujishiro H, Tada K, Akimoto Y, Mifune H. Association study between the 441c ins/del and taqi a polymorphisms of the dopamine d2 receptor gene and alcoholism. Alcohol Clin Exp Res. 1998;22(4):845–8.

48. Pohjalainen T, Någren K, Syvälahti E, Hietala J. The dopamine D2 receptor 5′-flanking variant, -141C Ins/Del, is not associated with reduced dopamine D2 receptor density in vivo. Pharmacogenet Genom. 1999;9(4):505–9.

49. Jang KL, Livesley W, Vernon PA. Gender-specific etiological differences in alcohol and drug problems: a behavioural genetic analysis. Addiction. 1997;92(10):1265–76.

50. Munro CA, McCaul ME, Wong DF, Oswald LM, Zhou Y, Brasic J, Kuwabara H, Kumar A, Alexander M, Ye W. Sex differences in striatal dopamine release in healthy adults. Biol Psychiatry. 2006;59(10):966–74.

51. Filbey FM, Claus ED, Morgan M, Forester GR, Hutchison K. Dopaminergic genes modulate response inhibition in alcohol abusing adults. Addict Biol. 2012;17(6):1046–56.

52. Hahn E, Reuter M, Spinath FM, Montag C. Internet addiction and its facets: the role of genetics and the relation to self-directedness. Addict Behav. 2017;65:137–46.

53. Prasad P, Ambekar A, Vaswani M. Dopamine D2 receptor polymorphisms and susceptibility to alcohol dependence in Indian males: a preliminary study. BMC Med Genet. 2010;11(1):24.

13

Lower suicide intention in patients with personality disorders admitted for deliberate self-poisoning than in patients with other diagnoses

T. K. Grimholt[1*], D. Jacobsen[1], O. R. Haavet[2] and Ø. Ekeberg[3,4]

Abstract

Background: People with deliberate self-poisoning and personality disorders are in increased risk for suicide. Intention and psychiatric features are important factors in a psychiatric evaluation and for planning aftercare.

Methods: Patients admitted to medical departments after deliberate self-poisoning were studied ($n = 117$). Patients with personality disorder according to (ICD-10, F.60-69) were compared to patients with affective disorders, substance use disorders, and unknown psychiatric diagnosis on Beck Suicide Intention Scale (SIS), Beck Suicide Ideation Scale (BSI), Beck Hopelessness Scale (BHS), and Beck Depression Inventory (BDI).

Results: The mean suicide intention score (SIS) was significantly lower among patients with personality disorders compared with patients with other psychiatric diagnoses 10.2 (95% CI 8.1–12.4) vs. 14.6 (95% CI 12.7–16.4) ($p = 0.040$). The hopelessness scores (BHS) were significantly higher among patients with personality disorders 13.0 (95% CI 10.9–15.2) compared with patients with affective disorders 8.2 (95% CI 6.1–10.3) and substance use disorders 9.9 (95% CI 5.2–14.6) ($p = 0.0014$) and unknown psychiatric diagnoses 10.6 (95% CI 9.1–12.2). There were no significant differences between the groups on suicide ideation (BSI) and depression (BDI).

Conclusions: Although patients with personality disorders had lower suicide intention compared to patients with other psychiatric diagnoses, they reported significantly more hopelessness. This distinction is an important implication in the clinical assessment and planning of further treatment of DSP patients.

Keywords: Deliberate self-poisoning, Depression, Hopelessness, Intention

Background

Deliberate self-poisoning (DSP) is associated with a high risk of further suicidal behaviour [24] and increased risk of premature death [7]. Patients with personality disorders are at greater risk of repeated suicide attempts [17]. The intention among patients admitted to acute medical wards after an episode of deliberate self-poisoning varies from a "cry for help" up to a serious wish to die [8]. The degree of a wish to die at the time an episode

of self-poisoning is associated with higher risk of subsequent suicide [15]. Since higher suicide risk among patients with personality disorders has been demonstrated with an OR of 2.0 (1 95% CI 1.38–2.95) [2], the assessment in the hospital plays a crucial role after an episode of deliberate self-poisoning. Most studies have not measured intention [16]. It is important to provide thorough assessment and a plan for appropriate care before discharge from general hospital. Especially, one of the recognized risk factor for suicide in patients with personality disorders is the less likelihood to ask for, or receive help [19].

The aim was to study suicide intention and psychiatric symptoms, such as hopelessness, suicidal ideation,

*Correspondence: tinegrim@yahoo.no
[1] Department of Acute Medicine, Oslo University Hospital, Nydalen, Pb 4950, Oslo, Norway
Full list of author information is available at the end of the article

and depression in patients with personality disorders compared with patients with other psychiatric diagnoses admitted to hospital after an episode of deliberate self-poisoning. We also compared subgroups of patients with affective disorders, substance use disorders, and unknown psychiatric diagnoses.

Methods

We included patients admitted to acute medical wards in Oslo and Akershus hospital in the period between 2009 and 2014 in accordance with the definition of deliberate self-poisoning [26]. In total, 117 patients were included as a part of baseline data from a multicenter, randomized trial conducted at five hospitals and General Practitioners (GP) in Oslo and Akershus County [13, 14].

A total of 636 patients were assessed for eligibility at the two hospitals Oslo University Hospital and Diakonhjemmet Hospital, whereas 124 were included. The process of inclusion is thoroughly described in the original papers. The patients and the assigning staff were blinded to the treatment category at the time of inclusion to prevent selection bias and baseline data are not biased, because the intervention was carried out after discharge from the hospital.

The inclusion criteria were: adults aged 18–75 years, hospitalized in acute medical wards. Patients with present psychosis, admitted to further psychiatric inpatient treatment, not registered with a GP, with mental retardation or organic cognitive impairment were excluded. Patients that were not able to participate in a clinical interview or fill out a self-report questionnaire because of foreign language were also excluded. Demographic and clinical variables were registered in a form by a study coordinator in each hospital. Patients with personality disorder in accordance with the ICD-10 diagnoses F60-69 were registered. The diagnoses were based on psychiatric assessment and on information from the patients during the assessment plus a review of the medical chart. The groups were analysed based on a classification depending on whether one of the diagnoses was registered in the following order: (1) F60-69 personality; (2) F30-39 affective disorders; (3) F10-19 substance use disorders; and (4) unknown psychiatric diagnosis (in cases of comorbidity where a patient had more than one of the diagnoses, the first in this order was chosen). For the other patients, the diagnoses were less reliable, but most often in the F-40-49 group *adjustment disorder* or *anxiety disorder*. We decided to classify this group as *unknown diagnosis* as we would need a more extensive diagnostic interview to conclude whether a patient had an F 43 diagnosis: reaction to severe stress and adjustment disorders as a reaction to stressful life events or dissociative or somatoform disorders.

We registered gender, age, educational level, and living status. Clinical variables were previous deliberate self-harm, self-poisoning, self-cutting, hospital treatment and received health care before the current episode that leads to hospitalization. In addition, Beck's scales for intention, suicide ideation, depression, and hopelessness were assessed.

Beck Suicide Intention Scale (SIS) is based on a clinical interview of an instrument with 15 items referring to the patient's precautions and beliefs of the act. Each item is scored on a scale from 0 to 2, with a possible total score of 30 indicating the highest intention of suicide and a wish to die. The questionnaire covers precautions, planning, communication, and expectations regarding the medication load, the degree of planning, and wish to die or live. It is divided into two sections: the first eight items constitute the 'circumstances' section (part 1) and are concerned with the objective circumstances of the act of self-harm; the remaining seven items, the 'self-report' section (part 2), are based on the patients' own reconstruction of their feelings and thoughts at the time of the act [6].

Beck Suicide Ideation Scale (BSI) is a 19-item instrument that measures the intensity, duration, and specificity of a patient's thoughts about committing suicide. The scores range from 0 to 38. If the patient scores 0 on both items four and five, which indicates active suicidal desire, the instruction is to skip the next 14 items which address specific suicide plans and attitudes [4].

Beck Hopelessness Scale (BHS) is a 20-item scale with true/false statements for measuring positive and negative expectations about the future. The total BHS score ranges from 0 (no hopelessness) to 20 (maximum hopelessness). The classification of scores is: 0–3, minimal; 4–8, mild; 9–14, moderate; and 15–20, severe hopelessness [5].

Beck Depression Inventory (BDI) measures the severity of depression during the previous week. It is composed of 21 items related to depressive symptoms. Each item has a set of at least four possible answers, varying in intensity. The standard cut-offs are: scores of 0–9 indicate that a person is not depressed, 10–18 indicates mild-to-moderate depression, 19–29 indicates moderate-to-severe depression, and 30–63 indicates severe depression [3].

Statistical analyses

Means and frequencies describe demographical and clinical data for the group personality disorders compared with all the other groups combined in Table 1. Chi-square test was used to compare categorical data. Independent sample *t* test and ANOVA were used for normally distributed continuous data to compare groups. To compare all the diagnostic groups on the SIS, BSI, BHS, and BDI, ANOVA was used. To compare the group personality disorders with

Table 1 Demographic and clinical variables

(N = 117)	F60-69 personality disorder (n = 25)	Other diagnoses (F30-39 affective disorders, F10-19 substance use disorders, F40-49 anxiety disorders and unknown psychiatric diagnoses combined)	p value
Male	16%	34%	
Female	84%	66%	0.087
Mean age, years (SD)	34.6 (11.6)	40.2 (15.4)	0.099[a]
Living alone	30%	70%	0.111
Educational level			
Elementary school	40%	44%	0.772
College	36%	29%	
Higher education/University	24%	28%	
Previously hospitalized with DSP	29%	71%	0.047*
Contact with health care services because of any DSH *last week* before current episode[b]	65%	36%	0.015*
Previous self-poisoning			
No	12%	37%	0.71
Once	20%	22%	
2–3 times	40%	27%	
4 times or more	28%	14%	
Previous cutting			
No	37%	59%	0.023*
Once	16%	12%	
2–3 times	–	11%	
4 times or more	47%	18%	

The numbers in the table vary from 113 to 117 due to missing responses on single questions

* Significant p-value

[a] Independent samples *t* test, the other *p* values are calculated from a Chi-square test

[b] Not all the columns in the Chi-square test are displayed here, only less than 1 week category

the other groups combined on the 15 items in the Beck Suicide Intention Questionnaire, the Chi-square test was used. Significance level was set at *p* values <0.05. SPSS vs. 21.0 Chic Il. was used to analyse the data.

Ethics

The participants were informed at the hospital, received written information, and written consent was obtained in line with the Personal Protection Agency at Oslo University Hospital manual and the Norwegian ethic's committee that approved the project (ID: S-08708b).

Results

In total, it was possible to if verify one or more diagnoses in 117 of the 173 included patients; F60-69 personality disorder was registered in 25. The comparison group with other diagnoses consisted of; F30-39 affective disorders (*n* = 35), F10-19 substance use disorders (*n* = 12) and with unknown psychiatric diagnoses (*n* = 45). Demographical and clinical data in the sample are shown in Table 1. There were no significant differences between the patients with personality disorders compared with the group with all the other diagnostic categories combined on the demographic variables. The patients with other or no diagnoses had significantly more often been hospitalized with of deliberate self-poisoning. However, the personality disorder group had been significantly more frequently treated in emergency medical outpatient clinic or with their general practitioner because of deliberate self-harm during the last week before the current episode. There were no significant differences in reported previous episodes of deliberate self-poisoning, but the patients with personality disorders had significantly more often been engaged in self-cutting.

Table 2 shows that the mean score on the Beck Suicide Intention Scale (SIS) was significantly lower in the personality disorder group 10.2 (95% CI 8.1–12.4) compared with the other groups, and highest in the group with unknown psychiatric diagnoses 14.6 (95% CI 12.7–16.4) (*p* = 0.040).

There were no significant differences between the groups on suicide ideation and depression; however, the

Table 2 Suicide intention, suicide ideation, hopelessness, and depression according to diagnostic groups

	F60-69 personality disorders ($n = 25$) Mean (95% CI)	Unknown psychiatric diagnoses ($n = 45$) Mean (95% CI)	F30-39 affective disorders ($n = 35$) Mean (95% CI)	F10-19 substance use disorders ($n = 12$) Mean (95% CI)	p value
Beck Suicide Intention Scale[a]	10.2 (8.1–12.4)	14.6 (12.7–16.4)	12.5 (10.1–14.9)	11.3 (6.5–16.1)	0.040*
Beck Suicide Ideation Scale	19.0 (14.6–23.4)	16.1 (12.7–19.5)	16.5 (12.6–20.3)	16.3 (4.0–29.0)	0.680
Beck Hopelessness Scale	13.0 (10.9–15.2)	10.6 (9.1–12.2)	8.2 (6.1–10.3)	9.9 (5.2–14.6)	0.014*
Beck Depression Inventory	27.8 (22.6–33.0)	26.1 (22.4–29.8)	23.0 (20.1–29.0)	21.9 (12.6–31.2)	0.532

ANOVA used to compare all the four diagnoses groups. In this table, the total group used for comparison is split into three subgroups: unknown psychiatric diagnoses, affective disorders, and substance use disorders

* Significant p-value

[a] Score ranges from 0 = lowest intention up to 30 = highest intention

levels were all severe. The hopelessness scores (BHS) were significantly higher among patients with personality disorders 13.0 (95% CI 10.9–15.2) compared with patients with unknown psychiatric diagnoses 10.6 (95% CI 9.1–12.2), affective disorders 8.2 (95% CI 6.1–10.3), and substance use disorders 9.9 (95% CI 5.2–14.6) ($p = 0.0014$) (Table 2).

In the first section of the Beck Suicide Intention Scale related to the circumstances, there was no significant difference [mean score 5.7 (personality disorder) vs. 5.5 (all other psychiatric diagnoses combined), $p = 0.806$]. In the last section related to intentions and expectations about the outcome of the overdose, there was a significant difference [mean score 5.0 (personality disorder) vs. 7.9 (all other psychiatric diagnoses combined), $p = 0.003$].

In Table 3, the comparison on each of the 15 items showed that the personality disorder patients had communicated the impending action more clearly the last year. Their intention was more often a wish to influence others and to a lower degree wanted to die by the poisoning. Furthermore, they did not to the same degree perceive death as a probable outcome of the act or that the ingested substances were lethal.

Discussion

The main finding was a significantly lower degree of suicide intention in patients with personality disorders compared to all the other diagnoses groups combined and this was especially related to the intention to influence significant others and less expected lethality of the act.

In line with previous research, the patients with personality disorders also reported a significantly more hopeless view of the future [22]. Taken together, these findings are interesting for clinical practice, as both higher intention [15], and level of hopelessness has been demonstrated as predictors for further suicide attempts and subsequent suicide [18, 30].

Furthermore, this distinction is important, because when the clinician assess intention (as is a recommended part of a psychiatric interview in the hospital) and find low intention, this could mask the total picture of the patients state, as the level of hopelessness, and thus, further suicide risk might be underestimated. Hopelessness was predictive of all types of suicidal behaviors in a 13-year follow-up study, where those who expressed hopelessness were 11.2 times as likely to have completed suicide [18].

As demonstrated in previous research, patients with lower levels of suicidal intention received less planned follow-up at the time of discharge from general hospital after self-poisoning [8]. However, the fact that the personality disorder group also had been significantly more frequently in contact with health care services the last week before they were hospitalized is interesting. This may indicate that they presented with suicidal ideation that was not addressed during the recent consultation.

For clinicians, especially in primary care, it is important to be aware if a crisis is emerging and the patient express suicidal ideation that, although the patient did not intend to die, the self-poisoning might under certain circumstances have a fatal outcome. It is, therefore, important to recognize altered illness behaviour in patients with personality disorders and give advice about, e.g., to avoid use of alcohol or substances of abuse that lower threshold to engage in suicidal behaviour and self-harm. Sher and colleagues found that about 50% of patients with borderline personality disorder had a history of comorbid substance use disorder and thus underpins the importance of being cautious [27]. Soloff et al. found no significant differences in the characteristics of suicide attempts between psychiatric inpatients with borderline personality disorder and those with major depressive episode. However, patients with both disorders had the greatest number of suicide attempts and the highest level of objective planning [28].

Table 3 Item scores on Beck Suicide Intention Scale according to diagnostic group

	F60-69 personality disorders (*n* = 25)%	Other diagnoses (F30-39 affective disorders, F10-19 substance use disorders, F40-49 anxiety disorders and unknown psychiatric diagnoses combined) (*n* = 86)%	*p* value
Part 1			
Circumstances section			
Isolation			
Someone present	12	22	
Someone nearby	8	29	
Alone	80	49	0.19
Arranged to avoid interference			
Probable	40	42	
Improbable	28	35	
Highly improbable	32	23	0.644
Precautions against being discovered			
None	68	57	
Passive	28	27	
Active (e.g. locked door)	4	16	0.277
Contacted someone to tell			
Contacted someone	71	45	
Contacted but did not tell	13	16	
Did not contact anyone	17	38	0.74
Pre-arrangements for death			
None	72	81	
Thought about it	16	14	
Performed pre-arrangements (will, gave away jewellery etc.)	12	5	0.381
Degree of planning			
None	68	66	
Minimal to moderate	32	29	
Detailed	0	5	0.541
Suicide note			
Did not write	64	63	
Thought about it	8	8	
Wrote note or letter	28	29	0.994
Communicated intention with the act			
None	48	61	
Unclear/indirectly	12	24	
Clearly	40	16	0.026*
Part 2			
Patients' own reconstruction of their feelings and thoughts			
Intention with the act			
Influence others	24	10.5	
Temporary rest/relief	52	37	
To die	24	52	0.029*
Expected consequences			
Death not probable or did not think about it	44	22	
Death possible	44	40	
Death probable	13	38	0.035*
Perceptions of lethality			
Less than lethal	54	33	

Table 3 continued

	F60-69 personality disorders (n = 25)%	Other diagnoses (F30-39 affective disorders, F10-19 substance use disorders, F40-49 anxiety disorders and unknown psychiatric diagnoses combined) (n = 86)%	p value
Uncertain	33	32	
Lethal	13	35	0.055
Seriousness of the attempt			
Not serious	30	21	
Uncertain	52	28	
Serious	17	51	0.013*
Ambivalence of living/dying			
Wanted to live	29	20	
Did not care	50	37	
Wanted to die	21	43	0.139
Perceptions of reversibility			
Death improbable if received help	54	33	
Uncertain	13	17	
Certain of dying or did not think about it	33	51	0.164
Degree of intention			
None, impulsive	67	60	
Planned less than 3 h before intake	17	19	
Planned more than 3 h before intake	17	21	0.831

The beck suicide intention interview was not performed for all the patients, and therefore, the numbers are lower in the comparison group

* Significant p-value

Additional psychopathology in the personality disorder group, such as depressive disorders or substance use disorders, could have affected the results in our study. However, due to the current design and the low numbers of patients included in this study, it was not possible to pursue any further analyses.

The findings in the current study show that the intention with the self-poisoning among patients with personality disorders was significantly different, as this group to a higher extent wanted to influence other persons. This supports previous research of this population, where interpersonal problems have been linked to suicidal behaviour [31].

Patients with borderline personality disorders and a history of suicide attempt have been described as more aggressive and affectively dysregulated compared with non-attempters [27].

According to the DSM-IV criteria [1], some of the essential features in borderline personality disorders are the impairments in personality functioning and presence of maladaptive personality traits such as neuroticism and easily prone to impulsivity, depression, and anxiety. Frequent feelings of hopelessness and a pessimistic view of the future together with suicide ideation and behaviour is common. In the current study, the levels of hopelessness

were significantly higher, while suicide ideation and depression were not significantly different but higher. However, although there are differences in phenomenology, longitudinal course among, e.g., bipolar disorders and borderline personality disorders, and the findings of comorbidity studies are equivocal [25], there is a need for further research into this in the current population.

Furthermore, because patients with personality disorders can exhibit a pattern of more rapid shifts in affect related to environmental events, in contrast to depressive disorders, it would have been interesting to further investigate whether there are differences in eventual changes of psychiatric symptoms across the diagnostic groups over time after discharge from the hospital.

As demonstrated by Lawn, patients with personality disorders found it challenging to seek help from hospital emergency departments during crises [19]. In the current study, there were significantly fewer patients with personality disorders that had been previously hospitalized with self-poisoning (29 vs. 71%), although the numbers of self-reported non hospitalized self-poisoning were higher. These results underpin Lawns findings and need to be further investigated. However, it could also indicate that although the reported frequency of previous self-harm was higher, the seriousness and lethality were lower and, therefore, could be treated at a lower level of health care, possibly without impairing treatment quality, in line with the policy in the Norwegian health care system [21].

Nevertheless, it is important to use the opportunity to provide sufficient follow-up at the time of discharge from hospital. Although evidence of effective treatment after deliberate self-harm from clinical trials is sparse in general, findings in a recent Cochrane review support a substantial role for psychotherapy in the treatment of people with borderline personality disorder [29].

In two studies of patients admitted to emergency departments after a suicide attempt, the mean Beck hopelessness score was 9.6 and 10.2, respectively [9, 11]. In a similar Swedish study, the mean scores of the Beck Hopelessness Scale for the total group were 10.4. For the diagnostic groups, the scores were 9.3 for patients with substance use disorders, 9.0 for depressive disorders, and lowest for the adjustment disorders 7.5 [23]. Lester, Beck, and Steer studied patients admitted to hospital for suicide attempts and found no differences on the depression inventory scores when they compared the depressive attempters with patients that described illicit activities or diagnosed with anti-social, drug, or alcohol personality disorders [20]. In concordance with our findings, the latter group also reported lower suicide intent than those diagnosed with depression, although there were no significant differences between the diagnostic groups on the depression inventory in our study.

Strengths and limitations

There are some limitations in this paper. The reliability of the personality disorder diagnoses would probably have been improved, and particularly if a structured interview had been used. All patients had a psychiatric assessment, and for most of them, there were access to records from previous hospitalizations. In addition, only major diagnostic groups were classified, which strengthens the validity. In addition, the diagnoses were like in similar studies [10, 12] registered from the patient's chart. Furthermore, it is more likely that the number of patients with personality disorder in the current sample is underreported rather than the other way, as the diagnosis was based on records from previous psychiatric and medical treatment. The frequency of personality disorders among deliberate self-poisoning was also similar to a comparable study, where clinicians found that 22.6% had a borderline personality disorder [10]. In a clinical setting, the assessing personnel will mainly have information available from the patients themselves and the medical records, and thus, our finding resembles the clinical

practice. Second, this method did not enable us to analyse any distinction between patients with borderline personality disorders and the other forms of personality disorder, as the first group in particular is known to have increased suicidal risk [16]. Third, our findings must be interpreted in the context of a somatic hospital setting and the severity of psychiatric symptoms found in other studies and the lethality of the overdose may differ from patients seen in, e.g., primary care out patient settings not requiring medical treatment and or patients treated in psychiatric inpatient care. It should also be noted that we due to the study design excluded the patients admitted to further psychiatric inpatient treatment.

Finally, people with or without personality disorder, which attempt suicide solely treated in primary care, is a possible confounding factor.

The strengths of this paper are that these findings to our knowledge have not previously been addressed, and are relevant for clinicians that treat a high number of deliberate self-poisoning patients in the hospitals. Furthermore, the high numbers included in each group make the comparisons in the statistical analysis more robust and thus the external validity and generalizability of the results in spite of the combination of the other or no diagnoses into one group. Finally, the use of validated scales strengthens the reliability of the results.

Conclusion

Patients with personality disorders reported significantly lower suicide intention compared to patients with affective, substance use disorders, unknown psychiatric diagnoses. This was mainly due to the expected outcome from the poisoning, as the personality disorder patients more often indented to influence others, and did not expect that the overdose was lethal. The patients with personality disorders also reported significantly more hopelessness, but not significant different levels of depression and suicide ideation. Taken together, this underlines the importance of carrying out a thorough assessment in the hospital and not only emphasizes suicidal intention when planning for aftercare.

Authors' contributions
TKG designed the study, analysed data, and wrote the manuscript. OE designed the study and wrote the manuscript. ORH and DJ contributed intellectually and critically to the manuscript. All authors read and approved the final manuscript.

Author details
[1] Department of Acute Medicine, Oslo University Hospital, Nydalen, Pb 4950, Oslo, Norway. [2] Department of General Practice, Institute of Health and Society, University of Oslo, Oslo, Norway. [3] Division of Mental Health and Addiction, Oslo University Hospital, Oslo, Norway. [4] Department of Behavioural Sciences in Medicine, Institute of Basic Medical Sciences, Faculty of Medicine, University of Oslo, Oslo, Norway.

Acknowledgements
The authors want to thank all the personnel that contributed to assign patients into this study.

Competing interests
All the authors declare that they have no competing interests.

Funding
This study was funded by the South-Eastern Norway Regional Health Authority, The Norwegian Extra Foundation for Health and Rehabilitation and the Norwegian Council for Mental Health.

References

1. APA, APA. DSM-IV-TR: diagnostic and statistical manual of mental disorders (4th edn, text tevision). Washington: American Psychiatric Association; 2000.
2. Arsenault-Lapierre G, Kim C, Turecki G. Psychiatric diagnoses in 3275 suicides: a meta-analysis. BMC Psychiatry. 2004;4:37. doi:10.1186/1471-244X-4-37.
3. Beck AT, Steer RA, Beck JS, Newman CF. Hopelessness, depression, suicidal ideation, and clinical diagnosis of depression. Suicide Life Threat Behav. 1993;23(2):139–45.
4. Beck AT, Steer RA, Ranieri WF. Scale for suicide ideation: psychometric properties of a self-report version. J Clin Psychol. 1988;44(4):499–505.
5. Beck AT, Weissman A, Lester D, Trexler L. The measurement of pessimism: the hopelessness scale. J Consult Clin Psychol. 1974;42(6):861–5.
6. Beck RW, Morris JB, Beck AT. Cross-validation of the suicidal intent scale. Psychol Rep. 1974;34(2):445–6. doi:10.2466/pr0.1974.34.2.445.
7. Bergen H, Hawton K, Waters K, Ness J, Cooper J, Steeg S, Kapur N. Premature death after self-harm: a multicentre cohort study. Lancet. 2012;380(9853):1568–74. doi:10.1016/S0140-6736(12)61141-6.
8. Bjornaas MA, Hovda KE, Heyerdahl F, Skog K, Drottning P, Opdahl A, Ekeberg O. Suicidal intention, psychosocial factors and referral to further treatment: a one-year cross-sectional study of self-poisoning. BMC Psychiatry. 2010;10:58. doi:10.1186/1471-244X-10-58.
9. Brown GK, Ten Have T, Henriques GR, Xie SX, Hollander JE, Beck AT. Cognitive therapy for the prevention of suicide attempts: a randomized controlled trial. JAMA. 2005;294(5):563–70. doi:10.1001/jama.294.5.563.
10. Cailhol L, Damsa C, Bui E, Klein R, Adam E, Schmitt L, Andreoli A. Is assessing for borderline personality disorder useful in the referral after a suicide attempt? Encephale. 2008;34(1):23–30. doi:10.1016/j.encep.2007.04.004.
11. Dieserud G, Roysamb E, Ekeberg O, Kraft P. Toward an integrative model of suicide attempt: a cognitive psychological approach. Suicide Life Threat Behav. 2001;31(2):153–68.
12. Ferreira AD, Sponholz A Jr, Mantovani C, Pazin-Filho A, Passos AD, Botega NJ, Del-Ben CM. Clinical features, psychiatric assessment, and longitudinal outcome of suicide attempters admitted to a tertiary emergency hospital. Arch Suicide Res. 2016;20(2):191–204. doi:10.1080/13811118.2015.1004491.
13. Grimholt TK, Jacobsen D, Haavet OR, Sandvik L, Jorgensen T, Norheim AB, Ekeberg O. Effect of systematic follow-up by general practitioners after deliberate self-poisoning: a randomised controlled trial. PLoS ONE. 2015;10(12):e0143934. doi:10.1371/journal.pone.0143934.
14. Grimholt TK, Jacobsen D, Haavet OR, Sandvik L, Jorgensen T, Norheim AB, Ekeberg O. Structured follow-up by general practitioners after deliberate self-poisoning: a randomised controlled trial. BMC Psychiatry. 2015;15(1):245. doi:10.1186/s12888-015-0635-2.
15. Harriss L, Hawton K, Zahl D. Value of measuring suicidal intent in the assessment of people attending hospital following self-poisoning or self-injury. Br J Psychiatry. 2005;186:60–6. doi:10.1192/bjp.186.1.60.
16. Hawton K, Heeringen KV. The international handbook of suicide and attempted suicide. Chichester: Wiley; 2000.
17. Johnsson Fridell E, Ojehagen A, Traskman-Bendz L. A 5-year follow-up study of suicide attempts. Acta Psychiatr Scand. 1996;93(3):151–7.
18. Kuo WH, Gallo JJ, Eaton WW. Hopelessness, depression, substance disorder, and suicidality—a 13-year community-based study. Soc Psychiatry Psychiatr Epidemiol. 2004;39(6):497–501. doi:10.1007/s00127-004-0775-z.
19. Lawn S, McMahon J. Experiences of care by Australians with a diagnosis of borderline personality disorder. J Psychiatr Ment Health Nurs. 2015;22(7):510–21. doi:10.1111/jpm.12226.
20. Lester D, Beck AT, Steer RA. Attempted suicide in those with personality disorders. A comparison of depressed and unsocialized suicide attempters. Eur Arch Psychiatry Neurol Sci. 1989;239(2):109–12.
21. Lund C, Bjornaas MA, Sandvik L, Ekeberg O, Jacobsen D, Hovda KE. Five-year mortality after acute poisoning treated in ambulances, an emergency outpatient clinic and hospitals in Oslo. Scand J Trauma Resusc Emerg Med. 2013;21:65. doi:10.1186/1757-7241-21-65.
22. MacLeod AK, Tata P, Tyrer P, Schmidt U, Davidson K, Thompson S, POP-MACT Group. Personality disorder and future-directed thinking in parasuicide. J Pers Disord. 2004;18(5):459–66. doi:10.1521/pedi.18.5.459.51329.
23. Nimeus A, Traskman-Bendz L, Alsen M. Hopelessness and suicidal behavior. J Affect Disord. 1997;42(2–3):137–44.
24. Owens D, Horrocks J, House A. Fatal and non-fatal repetition of self-harm. Systematic review. Br J Psychiatry. 2002;181:193–9.
25. Paris J. Borderline or bipolar? Distinguishing borderline personality disorder from bipolar spectrum disorders. Harv Rev Psychiatry. 2004;12(3):140–5. doi:10.1080/10673220490472373.
26. Platt S, Bille-Brahe U, Kerkhof A, Schmidtke A, Bjerke T, Crepet P, et al. Parasuicide in Europe: the WHO/EURO multicentre study on parasuicide. I. Introduction and preliminary analysis for 1989. Acta Psychiatr Scand. 1992;85(2):97–104.
27. Sher L, Fisher AM, Kelliher CH, Penner JD, Goodman M, Koenigsberg HW, Hazlett EA. Clinical features and psychiatric comorbidities of borderline personality disorder patients with versus without a history of suicide attempt. Psychiatry Res. 2016;246:261–6. doi:10.1016/j.psychres.2016.10.003.
28. Soloff PH, Lynch KG, Kelly TM, Malone KM, Mann JJ. Characteristics of suicide attempts of patients with major depressive episode and borderline personality disorder: a comparative study. Am J Psychiatry. 2000;157(4):601–8. doi:10.1176/appi.ajp.157.4.601.
29. Stoffers JM, Vollm BA, Rucker G, Timmer A, Huband N, Lieb K. Psychological therapies for people with borderline personality disorder. Cochrane Database Syst Rev. 2012;8:CD005652. doi:10.1002/14651858.CD005652.pub2.
30. Suominen K, Isometsa E, Ostamo A, Lonnqvist J. Level of suicidal intent predicts overall mortality and suicide after attempted suicide: a 12-year follow-up study. BMC Psychiatry. 2004;4:11. doi:10.1186/1471-244X-4-11.
31. Welch SS, Linehan MM. High-risk situations associated with parasuicide and drug use in borderline personality disorder. J Pers Disord. 2002;16(6):561–9.

14

The association between altered lipid profile and suicide attempt among Tunisian patients with schizophrenia

Rym Mensi[1,3]* , Amal Messaoud[1,3], Ahmed Mhallah[1,2], Islem Azizi[1,3], Walid Haj Salah[1,2], Wahiba Douki[1,3], Mohamed Fadhel Najjar[3] and Lotfi Gaha[1,2]

Abstract

Background: There have been many studies on psychiatric disorders, but very little is known about the biology of suicide with schizophrenia. In the present study, we are looking for a possible connection between altered lipid profile and suicidal behavior in schizophrenic Tunisian patients.

Methods: Assay of total cholesterol (TC), high-density lipoprotein cholesterol (HDL-c), low-density lipoprotein cholesterol (LDL-c), and triglycerides (TG) has been done for 126 schizophrenic patients with and without suicide attempts and 131 healthy controls recruited in the University Hospital of Monastir.

Results: TC and LDL-c levels were significantly higher in schizophrenic patients compared to controls. TC was significantly lower in schizophrenic patients with suicide attempt compared to those without suicide attempt. Depending to the sonority of suicide attempt, TC was significantly lower in patients with recent suicide attempt compared to those with lifetime suicide attempt and without suicide attempt ($p < 0.001$), and no significant differences between TG, LDL-c, and HDL-c were noted.

Conclusions: Results of this study showed that TC levels in schizophrenic patients after a recent suicide attempt are significantly lower than in patients without suicide attempt and with lifetime suicide attempts. TC can be one of biological markers defined suicidal risk for schizophrenic patients.

Keywords: Lipids, Cholesterol, Schizophrenia, Suicide

Background

Suicide, a public health problem of high complexity with different etiological factors, is causing annually a premature loss of approximately one million lives worldwide [4] Suicide is the third most common cause of death in various countries in the 15–44 years age group, and the second most common cause of death in the 10–24 years age group (OMS [28]), and is still poorly understood. New approaches are therefore needed to complement the fundamental of social influences, cultural and individual propensity to suicide. Suicide is the chief cause of premature

death among patients with schizophrenia [5]. The rate of suicide in schizophrenic patients is several times higher than in the general population. Identification of those at highest risk remains a problem for the clinician. Patients who have previously attempted suicide form a well-defined, high-risk group for suicide. It has been shown in other studies [16, 17, 39] that the prevalence of lifetime suicide attempts in females is almost twice than of males (7 vs. 4%, respectively), although the difference did not reach significant level.

In particular, improved prevention strategies are required in addition to extensive scientific study. Many researchers have focused on the search of biological markers that may be linked to suicidal behavior and can be used as an additional instrument for prevention and therapeutic action. It has been found that metabolic

*Correspondence: rim.mensi@gmail.com
[1] Research Laboratory "Vulnerability to Psychotic Disorders LR05ES10",
Faculty of Medicine, University of Monastir, 5012 Monastir, Tunisia
Full list of author information is available at the end of the article

deregulation, especially altered lipid profile including low total cholesterol (TC) and low-density lipoproteins-cholesterol (LDL-c) levels, may underlie higher suicide risk in patients with schizophrenia [1, 3]. A number of studies have investigated a possible link between low serum cholesterol and psychiatric symptoms, especially suicidal behavior [36]. These findings might be explained by the hypothesis that reduced cholesterol level contributes to decreased serotonergic transmission due to altered affinity and function of serotonin receptors and transporters [8]. It has been further hypothesized that low peripheral and central cholesterol levels may reduce lipid viscosity of neuronal cell membranes lowering the availability of pre-synaptic serotonin transporters and post-synaptic serotonin receptors [21, 38]. However, it should also be noted that some studies have failed to prove an association between lipid profile and suicide in patients with schizophrenia [20, 22, 29, 34]. In sum, cholesterol has received attention as a potentially meaningful biomarker for suicide.

Most previous studies with clinical population had small samples, and focused on total cholesterol as the measure of interest. Given that each lipoprotein subfraction has a different role in the human body, total cholesterol might not be sufficient to determine the relationship between lipids and suicidality. Additionally, it is not clear whether a lower lipid profile is either a state or trait marker for suicide. Other blood markers should be compared in the same population to investigate potential biomarkers equally and to evaluate group differences between suicide attempters and non-attempters.

Therefore, in the present study, we investigated the possible connection between serum cholesterol, triglycerides, HDL-c and LDL-c levels, and suicide for schizophrenic patients with and without suicide attempts and healthy controls.

Methods

Patients

The protocol of this study was approved by the ethical committees of the University Hospital in Monastir. After providing consent, 126 subjects (91 men and 35 women) with the age range of 20–65 years were recruited during 11 months (April 2013–March 2014) at the Department of psychiatry, in the University Hospital of Monastir, which is located in the Mid-eastern part of Tunisia. We recruited patients randomly but only those that met the inclusion criteria for our study. Socio-demographic and clinical data were collected by an information sheet and from the medical record of the patient. We excluded all patients with metabolic disorders. The blood sample of the control group was taken from the blood bank of University Hospital in Monastir Tunisia; 131 Healthy

controls (94 men and 37 women) did not have any mental or metabolic illness and they are in the same age range of patients (20–65 years). The suicide attempts were divided into two groups: lifetime suicide group (who had attempted suicide for more than 2 months) and recent suicide group (who had attempted suicide for less than 2 months). BMI was calculated as the weight (kilograms) divided by the square of the height (square meters).

Assessment

Venipuncture was performed for all subjects between 8 and 9 a.m. after a 12 h overnight fast. Approximately 5 ml of blood was collected. Immediately after collecting blood samples, serum concentration of total cholesterol (TC), high-density lipoprotein cholesterol (HDL-c), and triglycerides (TG) were determined using enzyme methods on COBAS 6000™ automates analyzer, and low-density lipoprotein cholesterol (LDL-c) was calculated with the *Friedewald* equation. Reference intervals for the measured parameters were as follows: TC <5.0 mmol/L, LDL <3.0 mmol/L, HDL >1.0 mmol/L, and TG <1.7 mmol/L.

Measurements

Table 1 shows comparison of socio-demographic details (age, gender, BMI, smoking status, and alcoholic status) between patients and controls.

The structured clinical interview for diagnostic and statistical manual of mental disorder-IV (DSM-IV) for schizophrenia was applied to assess the psychiatric status of individuals.

In the current study, we have two groups: schizophrenic patients and healthy controls. Schizophrenic patients are divided into schizophrenic patients without suicide attempts, schizophrenic patients with lifetime suicide attempts, and schizophrenic patients with recent suicide attempts.

Psychometric scales

For all patients, we conducted a psychometric assessment through psychometric scales: PANSS (*Positive and Negative Syndrome Scale*) which enables the assessment of positive symptoms, negative, and general psychopathology, CGI (*Clinical Global Impression*) which allows assessment of the severity, the therapeutic index, and improvise patients under treatment, EGF (*Global Assessment of Function*), BPRS (*Brief Psychiatric Rating Scale*), and CALGAGY (*Depression Scale For Schizophrenia*).

Data analysis methods

Data collected from medical, laboratory, and treatment records were noted and entered into a database: SPSS for the Windows 20.0 package program was used for analyses

Table 1 Demographic characteristics of different groups of study population

Demographic characteristics	±SD/freq. (%)		p
	Schizophrenia group (n = 126)	Controls group (n = 131)	
Gender			
Male	91 (72.2%)	94 (71.8%)	0.934
Female	35 (27.8%)	37 (28.2%)	
Sex ratio	2.6	2.54	
Age (year)	43.44 ± 10.60	40.81 ± 14.60	0.101
BMI (kg/m²)	26.25 ± 5.86	24.86 ± 3.82	*0.026*
Smoking status			
Smoking	73 (57.9%)	54 (41.2%)	0.713
No-smoking	51 (40.5%)	77 (58.8%)	
Weaned	2 (1.6%)	0 (0%)	
Alcoholic status			
Consumer	24 (19%)	14 (10.7%)	0.056
No-consumer	102 (81%)	117 (89.3%)	

to compare the clinical and demographic characteristics variables between patients and healthy subjects.

All data are presented as the mean ± standard deviation (SD) or as n (%). Analysis of various, Chi square test, independent simple *t* test, was used for the comparisons whenever appropriate. A result of $p < 0.05$ was accepted as significant.

Results and discussion

A total of 126 subjects with schizophrenic disorders were included in this study; 55 subjects had presented an episode of suicide attempt (15 had a recent suicide attempters and 40 had a lifetime suicide attempters) and 71 patients without any suicidal behavior. In this study, we have more males than females (Table 1).

BMI was significantly higher in schizophrenic patients compared to controls. The majorities of our patients smoke and do not consume alcohol.

Suicidal thoughts were reported by 37.4% of men and 60% of women with schizophrenia. The predominant type of schizophrenia was undifferentiated for patients without suicide attempt (47.88%) and paranoid for patients with suicide attempt (45.44%).The majority of the prescribed Antipsychotic Drugs are typical (83.1%). In this study, we found that differences in psychometric scores between patients with and without suicide attempt are significantly higher in schizophrenic patients with suicide attempts for PANSS (general, positive, and negative), CGI Severity and BPRS are significantly higher in schizophrenic patients with suicide attempts (Table 2).

Concentrations of total cholesterol and LDL-c were significantly higher in schizophrenic patients compared with controls. No relationship with HDL-c and triglycerides was found (Fig. 1).

Each lipid measure of the schizophrenic patients with recent suicide attempt, with lifetime suicide attempts, and without suicide attempt is shown in Table 3. The level of TC in the schizophrenic group with recent suicide attempts was significantly lower than schizophrenic groups with lifetime suicide attempts and without suicide attempts. There were no statistically significant differences in the LDL-c, HDL-c, and TG levels between these groups.

The comparison reveals no differences in concentrations of TC, TG, HDL-c, and LDL-c between patients treated with typical, atypical, and association between these two classes of Neuroleptics drug (Table 4).

Significant correlations between TC levels and EGF score as well as between the differences in TC levels and CALGARY score were found only for the subgroup of recent suicide attempters, indicating that TC levels may serve as a predictive factor for suicide attempts in patients with schizophrenia. There were also no associations between TC levels and score in PANSS (general, positive, and negative), CGI (severity, over all improvement, and therapeutic index), and BPRS (Table 5).

According to the threshold values represented by the Roc curve (Figs. 2 and 3), we divided our study of population to compare the effective of each interval. The results are summarized in Table 6.

In suicidal risk for patients with schizophrenia, the cutoff value of 3.76 mmol/L of TC was optimum, and at that point, sensitivity was 69% and specificity 31%. The area

Table 2 Clinical characteristics of schizophrenic patients with and without suicide attempts

	Patients without SA (n = 71)	Patients with SA (n = 55)	p
Psychometric evaluation			
PANSS general	35.25 ± 14.97	41.71 ± 15.86	0.021
PANSS positive	14.70 ± 6.83	19.80 ± 8.88	<0.001
PANSS negative	17.52 ± 8.93	20.76 ± 9.02	0.046
CGI severity	3.01 ± 1.61	3.31 ± 1.46	<0.001
CGI overall improvement	2.32 ± 1.20	2.22 ± 0.91	0.292
CGI therapeutic index	4.94 ± 3.49	5.20 ± 3.34	0.590
EGF	61.42 ± 18.21	53.27 ± 17.44	0.678
BPRS	53.49 ± 23.53	69.24 ± 25.24	0.012
Calgary	6.56 ± 10.11	8.31 ± 6.21	0.262
Type of schizophrenia			
Undifferentiated	35 (47.88%)	17 (30.90%)	0.113
Paranoid	23 (32.39%)	25 (45.44%)	
Disorganized	13 (18.30%)	13 (23.64%)	
Neuroleptics			
Typical	59 (83.1%)	47 (85.5%)	0.952
Typical and atypical	12 (16.9%)	8 (13.5%)	
Doses of chlorpromazine	990.07 ± 617.703	963.18 ± 652.663	0.814
Age at onset (year)	25.99 ± 8.39	25.26 ± 8.98	0.643

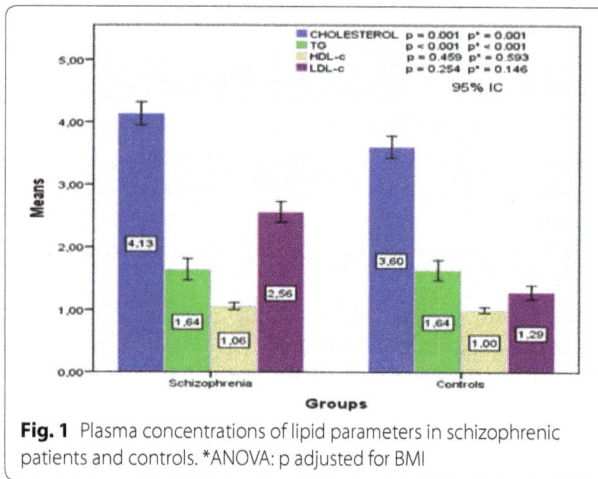

Fig. 1 Plasma concentrations of lipid parameters in schizophrenic patients and controls. *ANOVA: p adjusted for BMI

Schizophrenia is a serious mental disorder, and previous literature has reported that suicide was one of the main causes of premature death for sufferers from schizophrenia which was the major risk factor for complete suicide [32]. Cholesterol is a core component of the central nervous system (CNS), essential for the cell membrane stability, and the correct functioning of neurotransmission [33]. In our study, we found that TC was significantly higher among patients with schizophrenia compared to controls. Other studies have also shown that TC is higher among patients with schizophrenia compared to controls [25].

Considering the type of schizophrenia and according to our results and considering the type of schizophrenia, the majority of our patients with a suicide attempts are paranoid-type (41.81%), while the majority of patients without a suicide attempts are undifferentiated (46,47%), but the difference between the two types was not significant. The same results were found by Huang et al. [22].

under the curve was statistically significantly lower in patients with a recent suicide attempt than for patients without suicide attempt (p < 0.001).

Table 3 Comparison of lipid profile in schizophrenic patients depending on the seniority of suicide attempt

Blood levels	Recent suicide attempters Group 1 (n = 15)	Lifetime suicide attempters Group 2 (n = 40)	Never-suicide attempters Group 3 (n = 71)	p	[1] vs. [3] p	[1] vs. [4] p	[3] vs. [4] p
TC (mmol/L)	3.19 ± 1.00	4.02 ± 0.96	4.39 ± 0.98	0.000	0.007	0.000	0.063
HDL-C (mmol/L)	1.66 ± 0.94	1.64 ± 1.04	1.64 ± 0.93	0.995	0.935	0.920	0.994
LDL-C (mmol/L)	1.04 ± 0.36	1.04 ± 0.27	1.04 ± 0.27	0.921	0.947	0.848	0.691
TG (mmol/L)	2.60 ± 0.50	2.62 ± 1.11	2.62 ± 1.12	0.847	0.934	0.746	0.597

Table 4 Variations of lipid profile in schizophrenic patients according to the treatment

	Neuroleptics			p
	Typical [1]	Atypical [3]	Typical and atypical [4]	
TC (mmol/L)	4.16 ± 1.07	4.05 ± 0.25	4.05 ± 1.01	0.933
TG (mmol/L)	1.70 ± 1.41	1.41 ± 0.87	1.26 ± 0.64	0.210
HDL-C (mmol/L)	1.03 ± 0.28	1.21 ± 0.36	1.17 ± 0.48	0.145
LDL-C (mmol/L)	2.57 ± 0.98	2.25 ± 0.50	2.56 ± 0.72	0.797

Table 5 Correlation of lipid profile in schizophrenic patients according to the psychometric evaluation for patients with recent suicide attempt

	TC (mmol/L)	TG (mmol/L)	HDL-c (mmol/L)	LDL-c (mmol/L)
PANSS general				
r	−0.050	−0.19	−1.17	0.04
p	0.575	0.830	0.191	0.967
PANSS +				
r	−0.11	−0.014	−0.093	0.076
p	0.901	0.875	0.301	0.398
PANSS −				
r	0.073	0.018	−0.020	−0.006
p	0.418	0.844	0.824	0.946
CGI severity				
r	−0.036	0.029	−0.142	0.039
p	0.689	0.749	0.114	0.664
CGI improving patients under treatment				
r	−1.06	0.051	−0.075	−0.006
p	0.237	0.569	0.404	0.945
CGI therapeutic index				
r	−0.057	−0.075	−0.090	−0.06
p	0.523	0.406	0.315	0.502
EGF				
r	−0.186	−0.058	−0.0514	−0.119
p	0.037	0.515	0.550	0.184
Calgary				
r	0.222	−0.046	0.132	0.150
p	0.012	0.609	0.139	0.093

The gender difference regarding risk of suicide attempt is well known. The well-known risk of attempted suicide is higher in females [31]. Accordingly, our study included more males than females with a suicide attempt. Higher frequency of alcohol consumption is found for patients (19%) compared to healthy controls (10.7%). In this study, alcohol consumption is less frequent compared to the results of North America or European studies which found high rates of use alcohol (rang 21–51%) [12]. These differences may be linked to availability of alcohol or cultural factors, in particular to the social pressure for alcohol abstinence in Tunisia as in other Islamic countries (Table 7).

Therefore, the results obtained here corroborate most studies in which a relationship between suicidal behavior and low TC in schizophrenia patients was observed [26, 27]. Other studies did not find associations between serum cholesterol and death by suicide in patients with schizophrenia [35]. Some studies about attempted suicide mainly focused on patients suffering from major depression. Almeida-Montes et al. [2] found no significant difference in lipid profiles between patients who had attempted suicide and those who had not among patients with a diagnosis of a major depressive episode. No association between TC levels and suicidal act was shown in bipolar patients and those with major depressive disorder [8]. The same study showed that TG is significantly lower in those patients. The question has thus arisen as to why cholesterol levels have been found to be correlated with suicide attempts in some studies and not in others. Race differences in serum lipid profiles and lipoprotein lipase activity may be a culprit [15]; nutritional habits, life style, traditions, as well as seasons and climate may play a role in explaining these differences [10, 18, 19].

On the other hand, no association with Triglycerides, LDL cholesterol, and HDL cholesterol was observed in these patients for any lipidic parameter, which was also the case in the present study. However, Janusz et al. [23] have reported that total cholesterol, LDL cholesterol, total lipids, and triglycerides are significantly lower in patients with schizophrenia who had a suicidal attempt. In terms of gender differences, we must emphasize that females may be especially sensitive to dieting-induced changes in the central serotonin function [39].

Lower lipid levels in people with schizophrenia may also relate to the occurrence of metabolic syndrome. In relation to this, Vuksan-Cusa et al. [37] observed that the prevalence of metabolic syndrome in people with schizophrenia was lower in suicide attempters than in non-attempters. A post-mortem study reported down regulation of lipid metabolism mortem genes in the frontal cortex of suicide completers [24].

The aims of our study was to calculate the new cutoff value of total cholesterol according to the location of suicide in schizophrenic patients using Roc curve which was described by plotting the sensitivity on the y-axis against 1-specificity on the x-axis for each of several cutoffs. The results are interesting for total cholesterol in which 80% of patients with recent suicide attempt have a rate of TC ≤3.76 against 36.6% for patients without suicide attempt. Among patients who have not attempted suicide, 36.6% had rate of total cholesterol ≤3.76. Lipid profile of these patients should be controlled regularly to prevent suicide risk among them.

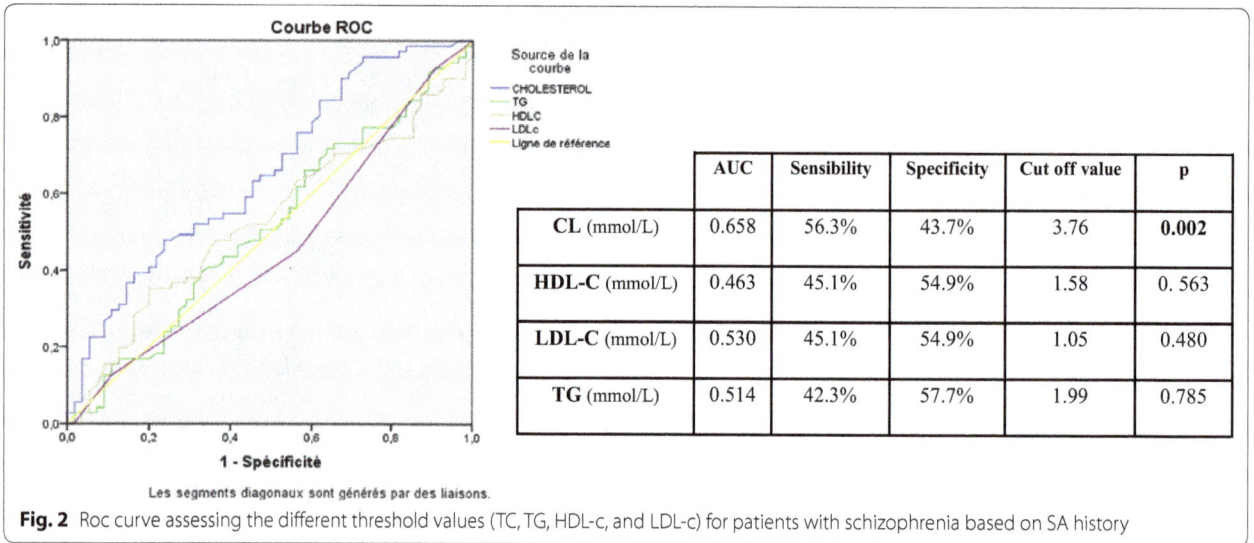

Fig. 2 Roc curve assessing the different threshold values (TC, TG, HDL-c, and LDL-c) for patients with schizophrenia based on SA history

	AUC	Sensibility	Specificity	Cut off value	p
CL (mmol/L)	0.658	56.3%	43.7%	3.76	**0.002**
HDL-C (mmol/L)	0.463	45.1%	54.9%	1.58	0. 563
LDL-C (mmol/L)	0.530	45.1%	54.9%	1.05	0.480
TG (mmol/L)	0.514	42.3%	57.7%	1.99	0.785

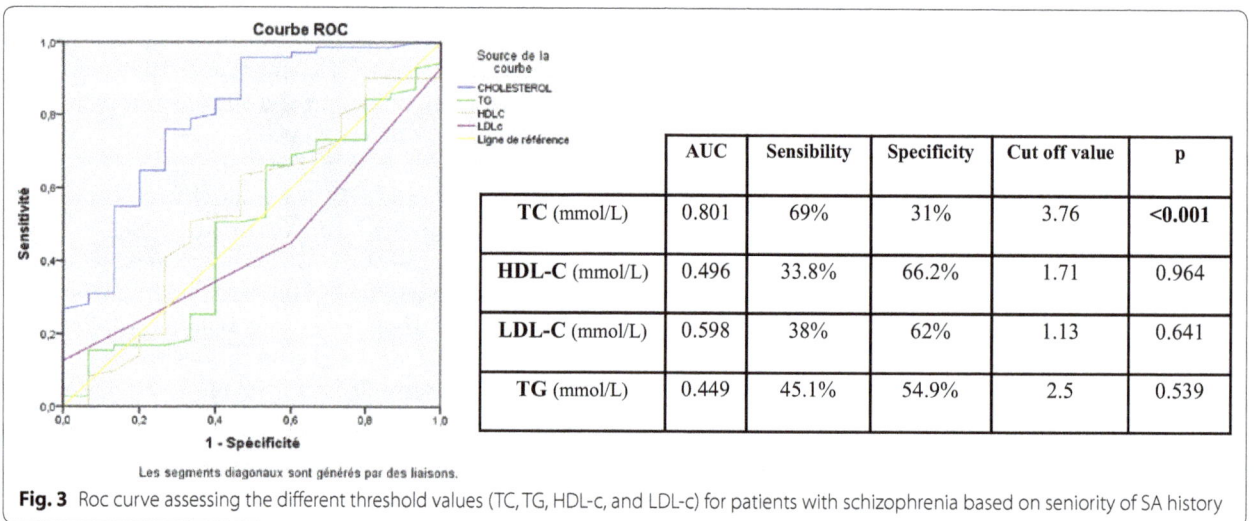

Fig. 3 Roc curve assessing the different threshold values (TC, TG, HDL-c, and LDL-c) for patients with schizophrenia based on seniority of SA history

	AUC	Sensibility	Specificity	Cut off value	p
TC (mmol/L)	0.801	69%	31%	3.76	**<0.001**
HDL-C (mmol/L)	0.496	33.8%	66.2%	1.71	0.964
LDL-C (mmol/L)	0.598	38%	62%	1.13	0.641
TG (mmol/L)	0.449	45.1%	54.9%	2.5	0.539

Table 6 Total cholesterol, triglycerides, HDL-c, and LDL-c levels in schizophrenic patients with and without suicide attempters

	Schizophrenia		OR	Confidence interval 95%	p
	Without SA N = 71	With SA N = 55			
TC (mmol/L)					
≤3.51	12 (16.9%)	21 (38.2%)	*3.037*	1.330–6.932	*0.002*
>3.51	59 (83.1%)	34 (61.8%)			
TG (mmol/L)					
≤1.61	41 (57.7%)	34 (61.8%)	0.844	0.411–1.733	0.785
>1.61	30 (42.3%)	21 (38.2%)			
HDL-C (mmol/L)					
≤1.10	39 (54.9%)	36 (65.5%)	0.643	0.311–1.330	0. 563
>1.10	32 (45.1%)	19 (34.5%)			
LDL-C (mmol/L)					
≤2.5	39 (54.9%)	24 (43.6%)	1.574	0.775–3.198	0.480
>2.5	32 (45.1%)	31 (56.4%)			

Table 7 Total cholesterol, triglycerides, HDL-c, and LDL-c levels in schizophrenic patients with schizophrenia based on seniority of SA

	Schizophrenia		OR	Confidence interval 95%	p
	Lifetime SA	Recent SA			
TC (mmol/L)					
≤3.76	26 (36.6%)	12 (80%)	6.923	1.787–26.816	<0.001
>3.76	45 (63.4%)	3 (20%)			
TG (mmol/L)					
≤1.71	46 (64.8%)	9 (60%)	1.227	0.392–3.843	0.964
>1.71	25 (35.2%)	6 (40%)			
HDL-c (mmol/L)					
≤1.13	44 (62%)	11 (73.3%)	0.593	0.171–2.049	0.641
>1.13	27 (38%)	4 (26.7%)			
LDL-c (mmol/L)					
≤2.50	39 (54.9%)	6 (40%)	1.828	0.588–5.681	0.539
>2.50	32 (45.1%)	9 (60%)			

However, a unique measure of TC level may not reflect patient's basic state. We cannot conclude if lower cholesterol is a state or a trait factor in suicide attempters. It is important to define an a priori biological threshold to distinguish subjects with low and high cholesterol. Additionally, since the study was conducted in a single university hospital, the finding may not be representative of all Tunisian patients with schizophrenia.

The absence of difference for triglyceride levels suggests that the association between cholesterol and suicidal risk is not influenced by nutritional status.

The effect of medication on cholesterol level is a potential confounder not taken into account in this study. Moreover, psychotropic drugs are usually associated with high cholesterol levels.

The relationship between low serum cholesterol levels and suicidal behavior is far from clear. There have been numerous hypotheses that have attempted to explain the mechanisms by which cholesterol levels may influence the risk of attempting suicide. The most widely held view is that there may be a link between serum cholesterol levels and the central nervous serotonergic system [7] via the reduction of brain serotonin activity [11]. Another hypothesis is that the phospholipids metabolism is disrupted, combining a deficit of incorporation of polyunsaturated fatty acids in the membrane with an increase their destruction [8]. Others have suggested that cholesterol may affect disease state and behaviors, as it plays a role in the production of the myelin sheath, in transmembrane exchange, enzyme function, in the synthesis of steroid hormones, and neurotransmitter receptor expression [14].

However, it should be stressed that an association between low cholesterol and suicidal behavior in schizophrenia was not confirmed in a number of studies [22, 30]. Recently, Freemantle et al. [13] analyzed brain *oxysterol* levels, which are enzymatic oxidation products of cholesterol, in the prefrontal cortex of suicide victims. Their results show a significant increase in 24-hydroxysterol, reflecting a higher turnover of cholesterol. They suggest that this metabolic process may be responsible for a reduction in central and peripheral cholesterol in these subjects. These authors also found altered phospholipids levels connected with increased activity of *cholesteryl ester hydrolase*, which may impair inhibitory neurotransmission in the prefrontal cortex of subjects with violent suicides [13].

In subsequent studies, we will aim for the study of genes implicated in the transition to the suicidal act in patients with schizophrenia. We hypothesize that an array of alteration in genes responsible for lipid regulation is incremented in the suicide for schizophrenic patients.

As most of the studies yielding negative results in this respect were performed in Asian populations, it can be speculated that ethnic differences may play a role.

Conclusion

The results show that total Cholesterol levels are low in suicide attempters after a recent suicide attempt, and remain lower than normal in a later time after the event.

Suicide prevention in patients with schizophrenia remains fundamental in the same way as the reduction of positive and negative symptoms, or improving the quality of life and reducing disability caused by the disease. We should automatically track a patient with schizophrenia suicidal risk factors or situations that promote their development.

One of the most important areas of research in suicide of schizophrenic patients should be based on the identification of biomarkers that may identify those patients prone to this risk of suicidal acts which is seemed important to focus on the specific involvement of fluidity membrane, and it is desirable to complete the analysis of lipid metabolism by assaying the various fractions of blood cholesterol to determine those included in this relationship.

Limitations

The limitations of our study are the following: First, the sample size in the recent suicide attempt subgroup was small. It would be interesting to increase the sample size for this subgroup. The data for the current study were obtained from the region of Monastir. Future studies on this research topic may be conducted in larger and more diverse samples. Some variables, such as lipid total, were not measured in the present study, and this issue would be considered in the future investigation.

Abbreviations
HDL-c: high-density lipoprotein cholesterol; LDL-c: low-density lipoprotein cholesterol; TC: total cholesterol; TG: triglycerides; SA: suicide attempt.

Authors' contributions
RM has made patient enrollment and dosage of biochemical parameters, and data analysis by SPSS. AM helped with the analyses using SPSS. AM conducted psychometric scales. IA helped with the dosage of biochemical parameters. WHS conducted interviews with patients. WD participated in the design of the study and performed the statistical analysis. MFN oversaw the dosage of lipidic profile. LG participated in the design of the study and its coordination, and helped to draft the manuscript. All authors read and approved the final manuscript.

Author details
[1] Research Laboratory "Vulnerability to Psychotic Disorders LR05ES10", Faculty of Medicine, University of Monastir, 5012 Monastir, Tunisia. [2] Department of Psychiatry, University Hospital in Monastir, Monastir, Tunisia. [3] Clinical Biochemistry and Toxicology Laboratory, University Hospital in Monastir, Monastir, Tunisia.

Acknowledgements
Not applicable.

Competing interests
The authors declare that they have no competing interests.

Funding
This work was supported by the Research Laboratory "Vulnerability to Psychotic disorders" University of Monastir, Tunisian Republic and by Clinical Biochemistry and Toxicology Laboratory, University Hospital in Monastir, Tunisian Republic.

References
1. Ainiyet B, Rybakowski JK. Suicidal behavior in schizophrenia may be related to low lipid levels. Med Sci Monit. 2014;20:1486–90.
2. Almeida-Montes LG, Valles-Sanchz V, Monero-Aguilar J, et al. Relation of serum cholesterol, lipid, serotonin and tryptophan levels to severity of depression and to suicide attempts. J Psychiatry Neurosci. 2000;25:371–7.
3. Atmaca M, Kuloglu M, Tezcan E, Ustundag B. Serum leptin and cholesterol levels in schizophrenic patients with and without suicide attempts. Acta Psychiatr Scand. 2003;108:208–14.
4. Bertolote JM, Fleischmann A. A global perspective in the epidemiology of suicide. Suicidology. 2002;7:6–8.
5. Caldwell CB, Gottesman II. Schizophreniaa high-risk factor for suicide: clues to risk reduction. Suicide Life Threat Behav. 1992;22:479–93.
6. Caldwell CB, Gotterman II. Schizophrenics kill themselves too: a review of risk factors for suicide. Schizophr Bull. 1990;16(4):571–89.
7. Diaz-Sastre Carmen, Baca-Garcia Enrique, Perez-Rodriguez Maria M, Garcia-Resa Eloy, Ceverino Antonio, Maria Jeronimo Saiz-Ruiz, Oquendo A, de Leon Jose. Low plasma cholesterol levels in suicidal males: a gender- and body mass index-matched case-control study of suicide attempters and non attempters. Prog Neuropsychopharmacol Biol Psychiatry. 2007;31:901–5.
8. De Graca Cantarelli M, Tramontina AC, Leite MC, Goncalves CA. Potential neuro-chemical links between cholesterol and suicidal behavior. Psychiatry Res. 2014;220:745–51.
9. De Leon J, Diaz FJ. A meta-analysis of worldwide studiesdemonstrates an association between schizophrenia and tobacco smoking behaviors. Schizophr Res. 2005;76:135–57.
10. De Leon J, Mallory P, Maw L, Susce MT, Perez-Rodriguez MM, Baca-Garcia E. Lack of replication of the association of low serum cholesterol and attempted suicide in another country raises more questions. Ann Clin Psychiatry. 2011;23:163–70.
11. De Leon J, Mallory P, Maw L, Susce MT, Perez-Rodriguez MM, Baca-Garcia E. Lack of replication of the association of low serum cholesterol and attempted suicide in another country raises more questions. Ann Clin Psychiatry. 2011;23:163–70.
12. Dervaux A, Baylé FJ, Laqueille X, Bourdel MC, Le Borgne MH, Olié JP, Krebs MO. Validity of the CAGE questionnaire in schizophrenic patientswith alcohol abuse and dependence. Schizophr Res. 2006;81:151–5.
13. Freemantle E, Chen GG, Cruceanu C, et al. Analysis of oxysterols and choles-terol in prefrontal cortex of suicides. Int J Neuropsychopharmacol. 2013;16:1241–9.
14. Golomb BA, Criqui MH, White HL, Dimsdale JE. The UCSD Statin Study: a randomized controlled trial assessing the impact of statins on selected noncardiac outcomes. Control Clin Trials. 2004;25:178–202.
15. Lee HJ, Kim YK. Serum lipid levels and suicide attempts. Acta Psychiatr Scand. 2003;108:215–21.
16. Jeon HJ, Lee JY, Lee YM, Hong JP, Won SH, Cho SJ, Kim JY, Chang SM, Lee D, Lee HW, Cho MJ. Lifetime prevalence and correlates of suicidal ideation, plan, and single and multiple attempts in a Korean nationwide study. J Nerv Ment Dis. 2010;198:643–6.
17. Jeon HJ, Lee JY, Lee YM, Hong JP, Won SH, Cho SJ, Kim JY, Chang SM, Lee HW, Cho MJ. Unplanned versus planned suicide attempters, precipitants, methods, and an association with mental disorders in a Korea based community sample. J Affect Disord. 2010;127:274–80.
18. Joffe YT, Collins M, Goedecke JH. The relationship between dietary fatty acids and inflammatory genes on the obese phenotype and serum lipids. Nutrients. 2013;5:1672–705.
19. Kamezaki F, Sonoda S, Tomotsune Y, Yunaka H, Otsuji Y. Seasonal variation in serum lipid levels in Japanese workers. J Atheroscler Thromb. 2010;17:638–43.
20. Kuo CJ, Tsai SY, Lo CH, Wang YP, Chen CC. Risk factors for completed suicide in schizophrenia. J Clin Psychiatry. 2005;66:579–85.
21. Lee BH, Kim YK. Potential peripheral biological predictors of suicidal behavior in major depressive disorder. Prog Neuropsychopharmacol Biol Psychiatry. 2011;35:842–7.
22. Huang T, Wu S. Serum cholesterol levels in paranoid and non-paranoid schizophrenia associated with physical violence or suicide attempts in Taiwanese. Psychiatry Res. 2000;96:175–8.
23. Ainiyet B, Rybakowski JK. Suicidal Behavior in schizophrenia may be related to low lipid levels. Med Sci Monit. 2014;20:1486–90.
24. Lalovic A, Klempan T, Sequeira A, Luheshi G, Turecki G. Altered expression of lipid metabolism and immune response genes in the frontal cortex of suicide completers. J Affect Disord. 2010;120:24–31.
25. Mechria Mabrouk HH, Hellara I, Ben Omrane C, Neffati F, Mechri A, Douki W, Gaha L, Najjar MF. Lipid profile and cardiovascular risk in 121 schizophrenic patients. Immuno Anal Biol Spéc. 2012;27(4):159–67.
26. Marcinko D, Popović-Knapić V, Franić T, et al. Association of cholesterol and socio-demographic parameters with suicidality in the male patients with schizophrenia. Psychiatr Danub. 2008;20:390–5.
27. Modai I, Valevski A, Dror S, Weizman A. Serum cholesterol levels and suicidal tendencies in psychiatric inpatients. J Clin Psychiatry. 1994;55:252–4.
28. OMS (2014) http://www.who.int/mediacentre/news/releases/2014/suicide-prevention-report/en/. Accessed 30 July 2016

29. Park S, Yi KK, Lim A, Hong JP. No association between serum cholesterol and death by suicide in patients with schizophrenia, bipolar affective disorder, or major depressive disorder. Behav Brain Funct. 2013;9:45.
30. Park S, Yi KK, Na R, Lim A, Hong JP. No association between serum cholesterol and death by suicide in patients with schizophrenia, bipolar affective disorder, or major depressive disorder. Behav Brain Funct. 2013;9:45.
31. Rihmer Z, Gonda X, Torzsa P, Kalabay L, Akiskal HS, Eory A. Affective temperament history of suicide attempt and family history of suicide in general practice patients. J Affect Disord. 2013;149:350–4.
32. Saha S, Chant D, McGrath J. A systematic review of mortality in schizophrenia: is the differential mortality gap worsening over time. Arch Gen Psychiatry. 2007;64:1123–31.
33. Ghaemi SN, Shields GS, Hegarty JD, Goodwin FK. Cholesterol levels in mood disorders: high or low. Bipolar Disord. 2000;2:60–4.
34. Steinert T, Woelfle M, Gebhardt RP. No correlation of serum cholesterol levels with measures of violence in patients with schizophrenia and non-psychotic disorders. Eur Psychiatry. 1999;14:346–8.

35. Park S, Yi KK, Na R, Lim A, Hong JP. No association between serum cholesterol and death by suicide in patients with schizophrenia, bipolar affective disorder, or major depressive disorder. Behav Brain Funct. 2013;9:45.
36. Troisi A. Cholesterol in coronary heart disease and psychiatric disorders: same or opposite effects on morbidity risk. Neurosci Biobehav Rev. 2009;33:125–32.
37. Vuksan-Cusa B, Marcinko D, Nad S, Jakovljevic M. Differences in cholesterol and metabolic syndrome between bipolar disorder men with and without suicide attempts. Prog Neuropsychopharmacol Biol Psychiatry. 2009;33:109–12.
38. Wallner B, Machatschke IH. The evolution of violence in men: the function of central cholesterol and serotonin. Prog Neuropsychopharmacol Biol Psychiatry. 2009;33:391–7.
39. Zhang J, McKeown RE, Hussey JR, Thompson SJ, Woods JR, Ainsworth BE. Low HDL cholesterol is associated with suicide attempt among young healthy women: the Third National Health and Nutrition Examination Survey. J Affect Disord. 2005;89(1–3):25–33.

15

Hospital nurses' attitudes, negative perceptions, and negative acts regarding workplace bullying

Shu-Ching Ma[1,2,5], Hsiu-Hung Wang[1] and Tsair-Wei Chien[3,4*] (iD)

Abstract

Background: Workplace bullying is a prevalent problem in today's work places that has adverse effects on both bullying victims and organizations. To investigate the predictors of workplace bullying is an important task to prevent bullying victims of nurses in hospitals.

Objective: This study aims to explore the relationships among nurses' attitudes, negative perceptions, and negative acts regarding workplace bullying under the framework of the theory of planned behavior (TPB).

Methods: A total of 811 nurses from three hospitals in Taiwan were surveyed. Nurses' responses to the 201 items of 10 scales were calibrated using Rasch analysis and then subjected to path analysis with partial least-squares structural equation modeling (PLS-SEM).

Results: The instrumental attitude was significant predictors of nurses' negative perceptions to be bullied in the workplace. Instead, the other TPB components of subjective norm and perceived behavioral control were not effective predictors of nurses' negative acts regarding workplace bullying.

Conclusions: The findings provided hospital nurse management with important implications for prevention of bullying, particularly to them who are tasked with providing safer and more productive workplaces to hospital nurses. Awareness of workplace bullying was recommended to other kinds of workplaces for further studies in future.

Keywords: Workplace bullying, Theory of planned behavior, Rasch measurement, Path analysis, Partial least squares structural equation modeling

Introduction

Workplace bullying occurs when an employee experiences a persistent pattern of mistreatment from others in the workplace that causes harm [1]. Likely, workplace bullying is persistent exposure to interpersonal aggression and mistreatment from colleagues, superiors, or subordinates [2, 3]. The form of bullying can include such expressions as verbal, nonverbal, psychological, physical abuse, humiliation and cyber [4]. Unlike the forms of school bullying in the workplace bullying, workplace bullying is in the majority of cases reported as having been

perpetrated by someone in authority over the target, sometimes from peers, and occasionally from subordinates [5].

Bullying can be covert or overt. It is frequently missed by superiors and well known by many employees throughout the organization. Researchers have done impressive studies investigating this problem by determining its frequency, identifying groups at risk in different occupational groups and sectors [6], addressing prevalence of bullying in different countries and among different occupational groups [7], reporting the impact on bullying in a workplace and the group-level processes that impact on the incidence and maintenance of bullying behavior [8], detecting the appropriateness of level of the bully scaling [9], testing a multidimensional model of

*Correspondence: smile@mail.chimei.org.tw
[3] Research Department, Chi-Mei Medical Center, 901 Chung Hwa Road, Yung Kung Dist., Tainan 710, Taiwan
Full list of author information is available at the end of the article

bullying in the nursing workplace [10], and even exploring a computer adaptive testing (CAT) tactic to examine hospital nurses' perception of workplace bullying [11]. However, they all have focused on only one aspect of assessment regarding bully attitudes or negative acts, or merely on a single correlation between attitudes and negative acts but failed to investigate the correlation between these variables under a sound theoretical framework, for instance, using theory of planned behavior (TPB) [12] to examine the relations of those variable domains.

PLS-SEM used for exploring the relationships between these variables

The counterproductively negative effects like bully are not limited to the targeted individuals but led to a decline in employee morale and a change in an organizational culture. None to date was to fill this gap through a comprehensively overall viewpoint by exploring the relationships among nurses' attitudes, negative perceptions, and negative acts regarding workplace bullying under the framework of the TPB, particularly, using the method of partial least squares structural equation modeling (PLS-SEM). The PLS-SEM is evolving as a statistical modeling technique and its use has increased exponentially in recent years within a variety of disciplines, due to the recognition that PLS-SEM's distinctive methodological features make it a viable alternative to the more popular covariance-based SEM approach [13] in social sciences.

Theory of planned behavior applied to this study

The TPB proposed by Ajzen [12, 14] is a rigorous theoretical framework to provide prediction and explanation of examinees' intentions to behavior. TPB has been successfully applied to provide a better interpretation of diverse behaviors in western settings [15]. According to TPB theory, three determinants—including attitude (i.e., whether I want to or not to support something), subjective norms (i.e., whether others encourage or limit me to support or not to support something), and perceived behavioral control (i.e., whether I have opportunities and resources to do or not to do something)—exert their effects on behavior through intentions [12] presented in Fig. 1.

In the current study, we applied the counterproductive TPB (CP-TPB for short in this study) concept to the bully negative acts through its underlying negative perceptions predicted by the other three determinants (i.e., attitude, subjective norms, and perceived behavioral control).

Attitude is denoted as the personal orientation with a positive or negative thinking. The orientation often contains two components: (1) affective and (2) instrumental attitude [12, 16]. The affective attitude is related to feelings or emotions positively or negatively toward a target; while instrumental attitude carries an appraisal

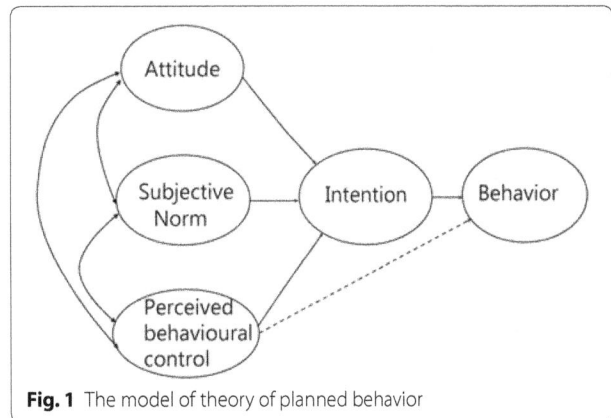

Fig. 1 The model of theory of planned behavior

of the consequences of the target. As such, a paper [17] reported that the negative Automatic Thoughts Questionnaires (ATQ) score [18] was positively correlated with the Liebowitz Social Anxiety Scale (LSAS) scores and the positive ATQ score was negatively correlated with the LSAS scores [17].

Subjective norm refers to perceived social pressure from others to perform (or not perform) the behavior. Perceived behavioral control refers to one's perception of the ability and control over the target. Self-efficacy is a perceived ability or a controllability, which refers to people's beliefs that they have the ability to resist any negative acts such as the bully behavior.

Negative acts might be perceived by a series of negative feelings such as poor mental health, burnout, and intention to resign. That is, one holding a negative attitude is possible to yield negative perceptions that might lead to a feeling of all negative acts around him or her. For more information about the definition of each study scale, we provide a couple of practical examples (e.g., original questions) on their specific meaning and implication in Additional file 1.

Generally, those with a favorable attitude, positive subjective norms, and a high level of perceived behavioral control (i.e., self-efficacy) will more likely earn a low probability of negative perceptions and negative acts. Similarly, a low degree of organizational subject norm and personal perceived behavioral control possibly links to negative acts through the negative perceptions. It is required to replace the TPB from need-to-do-it with the CP-TPB avoidance-to-do-it for interpreting the relationship of components with a study model.

Aims of the study

This study aims at examining the extent to which CP-TPB can predict and explain nurses' negative perceptions and negative acts of a bullied victim in a hospital. The following two specific hypotheses are tested in Fig. 1:

(1) Nurses' negative perceptions to negative acts can be predicted by attitude, subjective norm, and perceived behavioral control regarding workplace bullying; and (2) nurses' negative acts can be predicted by negative perceptions and perceived behavioral control regarding workplace bullying.

Methods
Study participants
The study sample was randomly selected and recruited using the last 3 digits of the identification card number from nurses of a group of hospitals with 2133 beds in southern Taiwan in the summer of 2012. As an incentive for participation, a gift consumer card for US$6.40 good for purchases at 7–11 convenience stores was offered to participants. A total of 811 nurses completed 201 items for 10 scales (e.g., each one illustrated by several items, see Additional file 1). This study was approved and monitored by the Research Ethics Review Board of the Chi-Mei Medical Center. Demographic data collected included gender, work tenure in hospitals of all types, age, marital status, and education level.

Instruments
A Nurse's Conceptions Regarding Workplace Bullying Questionnaire containing 201 item of 10 scales was developed to assess the five components in the TPB framework in Fig. 1. The scales included two parts: (A) negatively inversed scores (the higher scores, the more negative perceptions or acts): workplace bullying, intent to resign, nurse burnout, and personal mental disorder, (B) positively increased monotonically scores (the higher scores, the more positive effects on persons or organizations): job satisfactory, service spirit, authority distance, leadership of nurse superiors, organization culture, and personality. Participants were asked to rate each item on a 5-point scale with response options ranging from strongly disagree (1) to strongly agree (5). A higher score represents a higher level of the respective latent trait of the aforementioned two kinds of negative and positive scales under investigation.

The scale development procedure was guided by DeVellis' instruction [19] and item crafting was guided by Ajzen's principles [16] for TPB scale construction. The questions were constructed based on previous literature on workplace bullying [9–11], and consultative discussions with relevant experts (in the field of health care assessment) as well as frontline nurses who have had first-hand experiences in nursing care. The scales were then subjected to a pilot test on a small sample of nurses ($n = 32$) for the purpose of helping refine those questions by identifying ambiguities and anomalies in items of wording, as well as possible bias.

The scores on negatively worded items just in Authority distance scale were reversed before the data analysis so as to maintain the consistency of interpretation. The other three scales of mental disorder, burnout, and intent to resign with negatively worded items are kept with original codes for data analysis.

Data analysis
Two analytical methods, i.e., Rasch analysis [20] and path analysis, were used in the present study. Rasch rating scale analysis using Winsteps 3.7 [21] was used for examining the psychometric properties of the ten scales and for calibrating nurse' (person) measures on each of the ten latent traits. The Rasch estimated person measures were subsequently analyzed by path analysis using PLS-SEM [13] to investigate the relationships among components under CP-TPB model. This approach to data analysis differs from the conventional SEM method containing all indicators to fulfill the function of measurement model. In contrast, we applied Rasch analysis to PLS-SEM for measuring the latent (unobserved) traits using those ten underlying measures.

An inherent weakness associated with conventional analytical techniques based on classic test theory (CTT), such as factor analysis, is that they require linear, interval scale data input [22]. Raw data collected through Likert-type scales are always ordinal since their categories indicate its ordering without any proportional levels of meaning [23, 24]. Therefore, it is highly possible misleading conclusions if applying CTT to raw scores which are ordinal data (i.e., response from 1 to 5 ordered category) in nature.

The Rasch model overcomes this problem by converting ordinal data into interval measures which have a constant interval meaning and provide objective measurement from ordered category responses [24]. Once the interval metric is established, person measures and item difficulties are to be calibrated onto a single unidimensional latent trait continuum which facilitates direct comparisons between person measures and item difficulties. Empirically, Rasch analysis has been successfully applied in education and social sciences in addressing assessment issues [23, 25, 26].

Multiple criteria including Rasch person/item reliability, item fit statistics, the amount of variance explained by each of the scale measures, and step thresholds are used to examine the psychometric properties of those scales. Rasch person/item reliability estimates the replicability of person/item ordering along the latent trait metric [23]. Item fit statistics estimate the extent to which the data matches the measurement specifications of the Rasch model. Outfit and infit mean squares (MNSQ) are widely used indices of item fit statistics. The values of Outfit and Infit MNSQ (range from 0 to positive infinity) with 1.0 indicating the (unattainable) perfect fit to the Rasch model. Researchers [27] suggested that MNSQs falling in the range of 0.6 and 1.4 indicated a productive measurement for survey data with rating scales. This criterion (i.e., MNSQ in a range of 0.6 and 1.4) was used as the cut-off value of MNSQ fit statistics in this study. Variance explained by Rasch measures refers to the proportion of variance in the observed data which can be explained by the Rasch measures [25]. A higher proportion of variance indicates that the Rasch model better predicts both items and persons. Step threshold difficulties are examined to ensure the appropriate category functioning of the rating scales by Linacre suggested guidelines [28].

In path analysis, the PLS-SEM method [13, 29] was applied to investigate the correlation between components under the theoretical framework of CP-TPB model. The path coefficients between any two components under the CP-TPB using PLS-SEM were examined by the criterion of type I error at 0.05 level.

Results
Psychometric properties of the scales
The psychometric properties of the ten scales were investigated from a Rasch measurement perspective. Any item mis-fitting to the Rasch model (both infit and outfit MNSQ being higher than 1.4) was removed from the responding scale with an approach of one at a time (i.e., each run just for one deleted item) according to the misfit order [30], and re-applied Rasch analysis until all remaining items showed sufficient fit to the Rasch model. Table 1 presents the summary of psychometric properties of all scales.

It is shown in Table 1 that the Rasch person/item reliabilities for all scales are higher than 0.80 except the

person reliability for the intent to resign and authority distance scales due to a short length of items. Rasch measures explained over 40% of the variables observed in the data for all scales. The results indicated that all the ten scales had quite good psychometric properties at an acceptable scaling quality. Table 1 presents the summary of psychometric properties of all scales. The final sample items of the scales are illustrated in Additional file 1.

The category functioning of the rating scales were examined to determine whether respondents used all response opportunities appropriately. It can be seen that the step thresholds (the intersection point between consecutive categories) advanced monotonically with the category, indicating that the 5-point rating scale functioned rather well, and meaning higher performance categories corresponded to higher measures of the latent trait. In summary, the results showed that the scales were psychometrically robust enough for use with the sample in the current study.

Descriptive statistics
Descriptive statistics were undertaken to provide an overall viewpoint of the interval Rasch-calibrated measures of nurses on the ten constructs. Table 2 presents means (in a log odds unit) and standard deviations (SD) of nurses' measures on the scales as well as Pearson correlations among the constructs of interest. In Rasch analysis, the mean of item difficulties is arbitrarily set to zero and the interpretation of item difficulties and person measures are based on pair-wise comparisons between items and persons. Therefore, person measures higher than zero indicate a positive response, while person measures lower than zero that indicate a negative response (e.g., the first four scales with negatively inversed scores present not serious because scores are less than zero).

Table 1 Psychometric properties of measurement scales

Scale	No. of items	Rasch person/item reliability	Variance explained by measures (%)	Step threshold			
				Step 1	Step 2	Step 3	Step 4
A. The higher scores, the more negative perceptions or acts							
Bullying acts	22	0.90/0.98	41.90	−2.30	−0.13	0.44	1.99
Intent to resign	6	0.76/1.00	51.80	−1.36	−0.57	0.20	1.65
Burnout	11	0.90/1.00	61.40	−3.89	−1.00	1.76	3.13
Mental disorder	6	0.83/1.00	67.20	−4.19	−0.69	1.81	3.07
B. The higher scores, the more positive effects on persons or organizations							
Job satisfaction	20	0.92/0.99	51.30	−3.77	−2.52	0.89	5.39
Service spirit	17	0.92/1.00	56.90	−4.73	−2.63	1.49	5.78
Authority distance	6	0.75/0.99	43.90	−2.96	−0.53	0.95	2.54
Leadership	50	0.83/1.00	42.50	−2.30	−0.48	0.50	2.29
Organization culture	20	0.84/0.97	41.00	−2.32	−1.00	0.42	2.00
Personality	43	0.91/1.00	44.50	−2.97	−1.39	0.56	3.81

Table 2 Means, standard deviations, and correlations of the study components

	Component	Mean	SD	(1)	(2)	(3)	(4)	(5)	(6)	(7)	(8)	(9)
(1)	Bullying acts	−4.76	1.84	–								
(2)	Intent to resign	−0.76	0.89	0.23**	–							
(3)	Burnout	−1.64	2.08	0.26**	0.23**	–						
(4)	Mental disorder	−3.54	2.64	0.34**	0.14**	0.47**	–					
(5)	Job satisfaction	1.36	1.88	−0.32**	−0.29**	−0.39**	−0.3**	–				
(6)	Service spirit	3.13	2.20	−0.18**	−0.19**	−0.25**	−0.12**	0.61**	–			
(7)	Authority distance	1.31	1.26	0.02	0.01	0.03	0.00	−0.06	−0.06	–		
(8)	Leadership	1.55	0.49	−0.02	−0.02	0.00	0.04	−0.04	0.00	0.22**	–	
(9)	Organization culture	0.70	1.19	−0.02	−0.01	0.01	0.03	0.02	0.00	−0.07*	0.22**	–
(10)	Personality	2.76	0.92	−0.04	−0.04	−0.01	0.01	0.02	0.02	−0.02	0.10	0.33**

*$p < 0.05$; **$p < 0.01$

It is shown in Table 2 that, in general, nurses held a substantially low level of negative perceptions [i.e., scales (2)–(4)] to potentially be bullied victims [i.e., the scale (1)] with means less than zero. Attitude, both job satisfaction (mean = 1.36) and service spirit (=3.13), and subject norm with means of 1.31 and 1.55 regarding authority distance and leadership were quite positive, while perceived behavioral controls, i.e., organization culture (mean = 0.70) and personality (mean = 2.76), were positive.

It is worth noting that all of those respective latent traits were significantly related within the component (i.e., with a good convergent validity) and unrelated between components (i.e., with a good discriminant validity). Nurses had a slightly negative mean measure on bully acts (mean = −4.76). This indicates that, according to the direct effect from the nearby nurses' negative perceptions and the indirect effect from the three far-left components, a rather good hospital climate was evident and led to a lower negative perceptions and a very low negative acts of workplace bullying.

Results of path analysis

Nurses Rasch-calibrated measures on the CP-TPB components are subsequently subjected to path analysis, aiming at addressing the main research questions: to explore whether nurses' negative perceptions to negative acts can be predicted by attitude, subjective norm, and perceived behavioral control regarding workplace bullying. The results of path analysis showed that the standardized regression weight of the path (−0.40) from attitude to negative perceptions was significant ($p < 0.01$). The paths from subjective norm (=−0.006) and perceived behavioral control (=0.004) to negative perceptions were not significant. The correlations between the three far-left components were virtually zero. The standardized regression weight of the path from negative perceptions to negative acts (=0.38) was significant ($p < 0.01$), while the paths from perceived behavioral control component (=−0.03) were not significant.

The proposed model accounts for 16.4% of the variances in nurses' negative perceptions with a statistical power of 0.99 (calculated by 3 predictors, 813 sample size, probability level at 0.05, and observed $R^2 = 0.164$) and accounts for 14.9% of the variances with a statistical power of 0.99 (computed by 2 predictors, 813 sample size, probability level at 0.05, and observed $R^2 = 0.149$) in nurses' negative acts. The relationships among the latent traits in the CP-TPB are presented in Fig. 2.

The direct and indirect effect coefficients of predictors on workplace bullying are presented in Table 3. In the proposed model, negative perceptions (via direct effect) had a substantial positive effect (=0.38) on negative acts; attitude predictor (via indirect effect) had a moderate negative effect (=−0.16) on negative acts, while the other predictors had a far less than substantial effect on negative acts.

Discussion

This study used CP-TPB as a theoretical framework to verify that (1) nurses' negative perceptions to negative acts can be predicted by personal attitude; and (2) nurses'

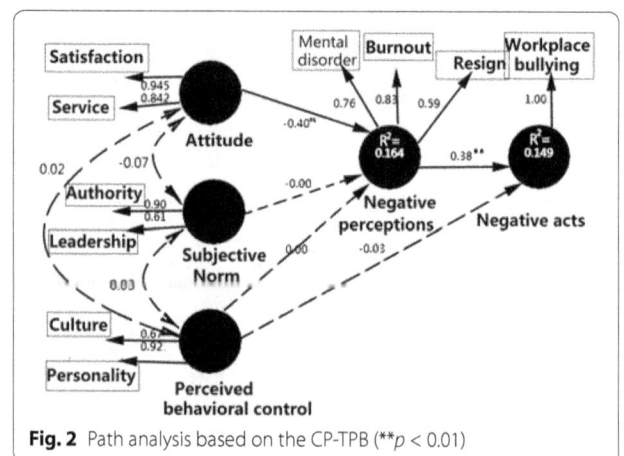

Fig. 2 Path analysis based on the CP-TPB (**$p < 0.01$)

Table 3 Effects of each latent variable on the bully behavior

Predictor components	Direct effect	Indirect effect	Total effect
Negative perceptions	0.38	–	0.38
Attitude	–	−0.16	−0.16
Subjective norm	–	−0.01	−0.01
Perceived behavioral control	−0.04	–	−0.04

negative acts regarding workplace bullying can be predicted by negative perceptions.

What this adds to what was known

Many previous pieces of research [5–11] have investigated the impact on bullying in a workplace and the group-level processes that impact on the incidence and maintenance of bullying behavior, but few attempts have been made to build a structural understanding of workplace bullying or of the relationships among variables which have influences on nurses' negative perceptions and negative acts of bullies.

The approach adopted for the analysis was a two-step process with Rasch analysis followed by path analysis. Rasch model can convert ordinal data into interval measures [24] and deal with missing data [31, 32] which are problematic in CTT approaches [33–35]. The Rasch person reliabilities for the intent to resign and authority distance scales are less than 0.80 in Table 1. It is because a shorter length of six items.

In path analysis, the PLS-SEM method has recently gained increasing attention, especially for the management information systems [36], as well as in marketing [37] and strategic management [38] disciplines, but also in accounting [39], family business research [40], operations management [41], and in organizational research [42]. The method is currently regarded as suitable and, to some extent, a favorable alternative to the more restrictive traditionally used covariance-based SEM (CB-SEM) method [43].

Among nurses, the prevalence of bullying was reported to be widespread [44, 45], with estimates suggesting 80% of nurses experience bullying at some point in their working lives [46]. The consequences of bullying include the following: severe psychological trauma [47]; lowered self-esteem [48]; depression and anxiety [49]; post-traumatic stress disorder [50]; physical illness [51]; financial loss; and the eventual inability to work [52]. The ripple effect of bullying also extends to family members who are liable to experience considerable stress from living with a family member who has been bullied [53]. The findings of this study can provide hospital nurse management with important implications for prevention of bullying,

particularly to them who are tasked with providing safer and more productive workplaces to hospital nurses.

What it implies and what should be changed?

The explanatory model of bullying resulting from this study in Fig. 2 identifies three components (low attitude → negative perceptions → negative acts) relations that contribute to bullying features, the relationship between bullying acts and the antecedent predictors. The model provides an insight into developing additional strategies to manage workplace bullying. In particular, the model may assist nurse managers to understand features of the work climate that perpetuate the bully behavior. Importantly, the model draws attention to personal attitude (i.e., satisfying nurse job and enjoying healthcare service) that contribute to reduce personal negative perceptions and negative acts regarding workplace bullying.

Strengths of this study

We applied Rasch model to detect data unidimensional, to establish interval metric for SEM modeling, and to interpret the relationship between components of latent traits. Empirically, Rasch analysis has been successfully applied in education and social sciences in addressing assessment issues [23, 25, 26] and worth applying to this study.

The Rasch estimated person measures were subsequently analyzed by path analysis using PLS-SEM [13] to investigate the relationships among components under CP-TPB model. The approach differs from the conventional SEM method containing all indicators to fulfill the function of the measurement model. We, on the other hands, applied Rasch analysis to PLS-SEM for measuring the latent (unobserved) traits using those ten underlying measures.

Structural equation modeling (SEM) has become the methodology of choice for many social science researchers investigating complex relationships between latent constructs, such as those ten components in this study. Compared with another commonly used approach of CB-SEM subjected to data normal distribution assumptions and to have a not-too-small sample size, there are many advantages in applying PLS-SEM [43].

Definitions of being bullied and engaging in bullying

This study sample was drawn from those frontline nurses who have had first-hand experiences in nursing care. All questions of the 22-item Negative Acts Questionnaire-Revised (NAQ-R) questionnaire [54] are pertaining to frequency of being bullied. We adopted the definition of bullying [55]: *when a person is teased repeatedly in a way he or she does not like... But it is not bullying when two students of about the same strength or power argue or fight. It is also not bullying when a student is teased in a friendly and playful way.*

Olweus [56] identified three prominent characteristics of bullying behavior: negative actions, repetition, and power imbalance. The negative perceptions were thus rated by victims of bullying instead of those nurses who engage in bullying behavior. Otherwise, those scale quality indices shown in Table 1 and Fig. 2 will be explicitly distorted and invalidated if nurses were confused in rating questions based on a distinct perspective of being bullied or engaging in bullying.

Limitations and future study

The interpretation and generalization of the conclusions of this study should be carried out with caution. First, the data of this study were collected in the context of a single hospital group in Taiwan. It is worth noting that any attempt to generalize the findings of this study, especially in the prediction of workplace bullying, should be made in healthcare systems with similar social and cultural contexts.

Second, although the participants were randomly and carefully selected in a unique hospital group to represent as much different as characteristics of samples, the generalization is not as strong as that sampling from a variety of hospital groups.

Third, nurses' perceptions were investigated by self-report data with response to such more 201 items at one moment. We cannot guarantee that all of them endorsed questionnaire with carefulness and without any cheating or guessing response.

Fourth, the 201 items of the study ten components were not included in the paper due to the space limitation. Interested readers are welcome to request the questionnaire if necessary.

The bully issue is a global problem in service-originated societies, especially among nurses in the healthcare setting [57, 58]. Our findings that nurses' negative perceptions can be predicted by attitude as an indirect effect to negative acts are required to further prove and to induce other researches in future. For instance, in a therapeutic or care process, patients with schizophrenia, caregivers practice body restraint for protecting the individual or the community, and to facilitate transportation to health facilities might be bullying behaviors if no compassion and love exist in healthcare.

Reviewing Olweus [54] identification of bullying behaviors with three prominent characteristics: negative actions, repetition, and power imbalance. It is interesting to hypothesize that when patients with schizophrenia were treated with body restraint (negative actions) frequently (repetition) by nurse authority to patients (power imbalance), giving patient family members hold negative attitudes (or thoughts) toward nurse treatments.

Comorbid mental disorders and negative perceptions will be caused, such as depression and substance drug abuse. Patient restraint will be considered as a kind of bullying behavior (i.e. negative acts).

Conclusions

This study contributes to the academic literature by applying both Rasch analysis and PLS-SEM to explore the relationships among nurses' attitudes, negative perceptions, and negative acts regarding workplace bullying under the framework of the TPB, which provides hospital nurse management with important implications for prevention of bullying, particularly to them who are tasked with providing safer and more productive workplaces to hospital nurses. Awareness of workplace bullying was recommended to other kinds of workplaces for further studies in future. Researchers and nurse superintendents should develop prevention and intervention programs directed at workplace bullying based on the perceived severity rather than only on the prevalence and frequency of bullying behaviors.

Abbreviations
ATQ: Automatic Thoughts Questionnaires; CP-TPB: counterproductively negative effects on theory of planned behavior; CTT: classic test theory; LSAS: Liebowitz Social Anxiety Scale; SAD: social anxiety disorder; SD: standard deviations; TPB: theory of planned behavior.

Authors' contributions
SCM developed the study concept and design. TWC and SCM analyzed and interpreted the data. HHW monitored the process of this study and help responded to the reviewers' advises and comments. TWC drafted the manuscript, and all authors provided critical revisions for important intellectual content. The study was supervised by TWC. All authors read and approved the final manuscript.

Author details
[1] College of Nursing, Kaohsiung Medical University, Kaohsiung, Taiwan. [2] Nursing Department, Chi-Mei Medical Center, Tainan, Taiwan. [3] Research Department, Chi-Mei Medical Center, 901 Chung Hwa Road, Yung Kung Dist., Tainan 710, Taiwan. [4] Department of Hospital and Health Care Administration, Chia-Nan University of Pharmacy and Science, Tainan, Taiwan. [5] Bachelor Program of Senior Services, Southern Taiwan University of Science and Technology, Tainan, Taiwan.

Competing interests
The authors declare that they have no competing interests.

Consent for publication
Not applicable.

Funding
There are no sources of funding to be declared.

References

1. Rayner C, Keashley L. Bullying at work: a perspective from Britain and North America. In: Fox S, Spector PE, editors. Counterproductive work behavior: investigations of actors and targets. Washington, DC: American Psychological Association; 2005. p. 271–96.

2. Einarsen S, Hoel H, Notelaers G. Measuring exposure to bullying and harassment at work: validity, factor structure and psychometric properties of the negative acts questionnaire-revised. Work Stress. 2009;23(1):24–44.

3. Leymann H. The content and development of mobbing at work. Eur J Work Organ Psychol. 1996;5(2):165–84.

4. Chen LM, Liu KS, Cheng YY. Validation of the perceived school bullying severity scale. Educ Psychol. 2012;32(2):169–82.

5. Rayner C, Cooper CL. Workplace bullying. In: Kelloway E, Barling J, Hurrell Jr J, editors. Handbook of workplace violence. Thousand Oaks: Sage; 2006. p. 47–90.

6. Zapf D, Einarsen S, Hoel H, Vartia M. Empirical findings on bullying in the workplace. In: Einarsen S, Hoel H, Zapf D, Cooper CL, editors. Bullying and emotional abuse in the workplace: international perspectives in research and practice. New York: Taylor & Francis; 2003.

7. Mikkelsen EG, Einarsen S. Bullying in Danish work-life: prevalence and health correlates. Eur J Work Organ Psychol. 2001;10(4):393–413.

8. Ramsay S, Troth A, Branch S. Work-place bullying: a group processes framework. J Occup Organ Psychol. 2010;84(4):799–816.

9. Tsuno K, Kawakami N, Inoue A, Abe K. Measuring workplace bullying: reliability and validity of the Japanese version of the negative acts questionnaire. J Occup Health. 2010;52(4):216–26.

10. Hutchinson M, Wilkes L, Jackson D, Vickers MH. Integrating individual, work group and organizational factors: testing a multidimensional model of bullying in the nursing workplace. J Nurs Manag. 2010;18(2):173–81.

11. Ma SC, Chien TW, Wang HH, Li YC, Yui MS. Applying computerized adaptive testing (CAT) to the negative acts questionnaire-revised (NAQ-R)—the Rasch analysis. J Med Internet Res. 2013;16(2):e50.

12. Ajzen I. The theory of planned behavior. Organ Behav Hum Decis Process. 1991;50(2):179–211.

13. Hair JF, Hult GTM, Ringle CM, Sarstedt M. A primer on partial least squares structural equation modeling (PLS-SEM). Thousand Oaks: Sage; 2014.

14. Ajzen I. From intentions to actions: a theory of planned behavior. In: Kuhl J, Beckmann J, editors. Action control: from cognition to behavior. Berlin: Springer; 1985. p. 11–39.

15. Yan Z, Cheng ECK. Primary teachers' attitudes, intentions and practices regarding formative assessment. Teach Teach Educ. 2015;45:128–36.

16. Ajzen I. Constructing a TpB questionnaire: conceptual and methodological considerations. http://www.unibielefeld.de/ikg/zick/ajzen%20construction%20a%20tpb%20questionnaire.pdf. Accessed 14 Mar 2015.

17. Hollon SD, Kendall PC. Cognitive self-statements in depression: development of an automatic thoughts questionnaire. Cogn Ther Res. 1980;4(4):383–95.

18. Iancu I, Bodner E, Joubran S, Lupinsky Y, Barenboim D. Negative and positive automatic thoughts in social anxiety disorder. Isr J Psychiatry Relat Sci. 2015;52(2):129–35.

19. DeVellis RF. Scale development: theory and applications. 3rd ed. Thousand Oaks: Sage Publications; 2012.

20. Rasch G. Probabilistic models for some intelligence and achievement test. Copenhagan: Danish Institute for Educational Research; Expanded ed. (1980). Chicago: The University of Chicago Press; 1960.

21. Linacre JM. Winsteps (Version 4.0.1) [Computer Software]. Beaverton, Oregon: Winsteps.com; 2011/9/3. Retrieved at http://www.winsteps.com/.

22. Wright BD. A history of social science measurement. Educ Meas Issues Pract. 1997;16(4):33–45.

23. Bond TG, Fox CM. Applying the Rasch model: fundamental measurement in the human sciences. 2nd ed. Mahwah: Lawrence Erlbaum; 2007.

24. Linacre JM. A user's guide to WINSTEPS/MINISTEP: Rasch-model computer programs. Chicago: Winsteps; 2015.

25. Panayides P, Robinson C, Tymms P. The assessment revolution that has passed England by: Rasch measurement. Br Educ Res J. 2010;36(4):611–26.

26. Tormakangas K. Advantages of the Rasch measurement model in analyzing educational tests: an applicator's reflection. Educ Res Eval Int J Theory Pract. 2011;17(5):307–20.

27. Wright BD, Linacre JM. Reasonable mean-square fit values. Rasch Meas Trans. 1994;8:370.

28. Linacre JM. Optimizing rating scale category effectiveness. J Appl Meas. 2002;3(1):85–106.

29. Haenlein M, Kaplan AM. A beginner's guide to partial least squares analysis. Underst Stat. 2004;3:283–97.

30. Hart DL, Wright BD. Development of an index of physical functional health status in rehabilitation. Arch Phys Med Rehabil. 2002;83(5):655–65.

31. Fisher WP Jr. Fuzzy truth and the Rasch model. Rasch Meas Trans. 1995;9(3):442.

32. Ludlow LH, O'Leary M. Scoring omitted and not-reached items: practical data analysis implications. Educ Psychol Meas. 1999;59(4):603–15.

33. Montiel-Overall P. Implications of missing data in survey research. Can J Inf Libr Sci. 2006;30(3):241–70.

34. Moulton M. One ruler, many tests: a primeron test equating. EDS Publications. http://www.eddata.com/resources/publications/EDS_APEC_Equating_Moulton.pdf. Accesssed 15 Mar 2015.

35. Peugh JL, Enders CK. Missing datain educational research: a review of reporting practices and suggestions for improvement. Rev Educ Res. 2004;74(4):525–56.

36. Ringle CM, Sarstedt M, Straub DW. A critical look at the use of PLS-SEM in MIS quarterly. MIS Q. 2012;36:iii–xiv.

37. Hair JF, Sarstedt M, Ringle CM, Mena JA. An assessment of the use of partial least squares structural equation modeling in marketing research. J Acad Mark Sci. 2012;40:414–33.

38. Hair JF, Sarstedt M, Pieper TM, Ringle CM. The use of partial least squares structural equation modeling in strategic management research: a review of past practices and recommendations for future applications. Long Range Plan. 2012;45:320–40.

39. Lee L, Petter S, Fayard D, Robinson S. On the use of partial least squares path modeling in accounting research. Int J Account Inf Syst. 2011;12:305–28.

40. Sarstedt M, Ringle CM, Smith D, Reams R, Hair JF. Partial least squares structural equation modeling (PLS-SEM): a useful tool for family business researchers. J Fam Bus Strategy. 2014;5:105–15.

41. Peng DX, Lai F. Using partial least squares in operations management research: a practical guideline and summary of past research. J Oper Manag. 2012;30:467–80.

42. Sosik JJ, Kahai SS, Piovoso MJ. Silver bullet or voodoo statistics? A primer for using the partial least squares data analytic technique in group and organization research. Group Organ Manag. 2009;34:5–36.

43. Astrachana CB, Patelb VK, Wanzenriedc G. A comparative study of CB-SEM and PLS-SEM for theory development in family firm research. J Fam Bus Strategy. 2014;5(1):116–28.

44. Farrell GA, Bobrowski C, Bobrowski P. Scoping workplace aggression in nursing: findings from an Australian study. J Adv Nurs. 2006;55(6):778–87.

45. Hutchinson M, Vickers M, Jackson D, Wilkes L. They stand you in a corner; you are not to speak': nurses tell of abusive indoctrination in work teams dominated by bullies. Contemp Nurse. 2006;21(2):228–38.

46. Lewis M. Nurse bullying: organizational considerations in the maintenance and perpetration of health care bullying cultures. J Nurs Manag. 2006;14(1):52–8.

47. Hallberg L, Strandmark M. Health consequences of workplace bullying: experiences from the perspective of employees in the public service sector. Int J Qual Stud Health Wellbeing. 2006;1(2):109–19.

48. Randle J. Bullying in the nursing profession. J Adv Nurs. 2003;43(4):395–401.

49. Quine L. Workplace bullying in nurses. J Health Psychol. 2001;6(1):73–84.

50. Mikkelsen EG, Einarsen S. Relationships between exposure to bullying at work and psychological and psychosomatic health complaints: the role of state negative affectivity and generalized self-efficacy. Scand J Psychol. 2002;43(5):397–405.

51. Kivimakia M, Virtanen M. Workplace bullying and the risk of cardiovascular disease and depression. Occup Environ Med. 2003;60:779–83.

52. Einarsen SE, Mikkelsen EG. Individual effects of exposure to bullying at work. In: Einarsen SE, Hoel H, Zapf D, Cooper CL, editors. Bullying and emotional abuse in the workplace. International perspectives in research and practice. London: Taylor & Francis; 2003. p. 127–44.

53. Kivimakia M, Elovainiob M, Vahterac J. Workplace bullying and sickness absence in hospital staff. Occup Environ Med. 2000;57:656–60.

54. Nielsen MB, Skogstad A, Matthiesen SB, Glasø L, Aasland MS, Notelaers G, et al. Prevalence of workplace bullying in Norway: comparisons across time and estimation methods. Eur J Work Organ Psychol. 2009;18(1):81–101.

55. Craig W, Harel-Fisch Y, Fogel-Grinvald H, Dostaler S, Hetland J, Simons-Morton B, Molcho M, de Mato MG, Overpeck M, Due P, Pickett W, HBSC Violence & Injuries Prevention Focus Group, HBSC Bullying Writing Group. A cross-national profile of bullying and victimization among adolescents in 40 countries. Int J Public Health. 2009;54(Suppl 2):216–24.

56. Olweus D. Bullying at school: what we know and what we can do. Oxford: Blackwell; 1993.

57. Karatza C, Zyga S, Tziaferi S, Prezerakos P. Workplace bullying and general health status among the nursing staff of Greek public hospitals. Ann Gen Psychiatry. 2016;15:7.

58. Ma SC, Wang HH, Chien TW. A new technique to measure online bullying: online computerized adaptive testing. Ann Gen Psychiatry. 2017;16:26.

16

Lifestyle factors and the metabolic syndrome in Schizophrenia

Adrian Heald[1,2], John Pendlebury[3], Simon Anderson[4], Vinesh Narayan[3], Mark Guy[5], Martin Gibson[2], Peter Haddad[3] and Mark Livingston[6*]

Abstract

Background: Cardiometabolic disease is more common in patients with schizophrenia than the general population.

Aim: The purpose of the study was to assess lifestyle factors, including diet and exercise, in patients with schizophrenia and estimate the prevalence of metabolic syndrome.

Methods: This is a cross-sectional study of a representative group of outpatients with schizophrenia in Salford, UK. An interview supplemented by questionnaires was used to assess diet, physical activity, and cigarette and alcohol use. Likert scales assessed subjects' views of diet and activity. A physical examination and relevant blood tests were conducted.

Results: Thirty-seven people were included in the study. 92% of men had central adiposity, as did 91.7% of women (International Diabetes Federation Definition). The mean age was 46.2 years and mean illness duration was 11.6 years. 67.6% fulfilled criteria for the metabolic syndrome. The mean number of fruit and vegetable portions per day was 2.8 ± 1.8. Over a third did not eat any fruit in a typical week. 42% reported doing no vigorous activity in a typical week. 64.9% smoked and in many cigarette use was heavy. The Likert scale showed that a high proportion of patients had insight into their unhealthy lifestyles.

Conclusions: Within this sample, there was a high prevalence of poor diet, smoking and inadequate exercise. Many did not follow national recommendations for dietary intake of fruit and vegetables and daily exercise. These factors probably contribute to the high prevalence of metabolic syndrome. Many had insight into their unhealthy lifestyles. Thus, there is potential for interventions to improve lifestyle factors and reduce the risk of cardiometabolic disease.

Keywords: Diet, Lifestyle, Schizophrenia, Metabolic syndrome

Background

People with schizophrenia suffer from increased morbidity and mortality compared with the general population, having a life expectancy that is approximately 20% shorter [1]. The excess mortality is largely due to cardiovascular disease (CVD). Furthermore, people with schizophrenia and other severe and enduring mental illnesses (SMI) are twice as likely to die from CVD compared with those in the general population [2–4], and the excess mortality is higher in younger individuals. Known risk factors for CVD include smoking, being overweight, inadequate exercise and a low intake of fruit and vegetables [5]. These lifestyle risk factors are more common in people with schizophrenia than in the general population [6–9].

In a North-American review, 42% of individuals with schizophrenia were reported to be obese [body mass index (BMI) ≥ 27 kg/m^2] compared with 27% of the general population [6]. McCreadie and colleagues [7, 8] showed that the diets of people with schizophrenia in Scotland were less healthy than those of the general

*Correspondence: mark.livingston@nhs.net
[6] Department of Blood Sciences, Walsall Manor Hospital, Walsall WS2 9PS, UK
Full list of author information is available at the end of the article

population on a range of parameters. Short-term efforts to improve diet in individuals with schizophrenia have been shown to be of only limited benefit [10] with the implication that any intervention must be long-term to be effective. Studies have repeatedly reported high rates of smoking in those with schizophrenia [8]. Information about exercise levels in schizophrenia is scanty, but clinical experience suggests it is often poor.

The high prevalence of poor diet, inadequate exercise and obesity in schizophrenia may partly reflect the associated socio-economic disadvantages of the illness, and many sufferers are unable to gain paid employment. In addition, core psychiatric symptoms including avolition and tiredness may contribute. Antipsychotic medication can cause metabolic derangements, including hyperglycemia and hyperlipidaemia [11, 12] as well as weight gain [12, 13] which if sustained can contribute to CVD. Other psychiatric medications, including mood stabilisers and some antidepressants, can also cause weight gain [2]. In summary, the excess of CVD in schizophrenia appears multifactorial.

Given the evidence of suboptimal lifestyle choices in people with SMI, the aims of this study were to determine the pattern of dietary intake and exercise in a representative group of individuals with schizophrenia in a UK inner city area and to determine whether age predicted the presence of metabolic syndrome in this group.

Methods

The study was carried out at two Community Mental Health Centres in Salford, an inner city area in North West England, UK. The study was approved by the local Salford Ethics Committee and the Trust Research and Development Department. All outpatients aged between 16 and 65 years of age who were prescribed a neuroleptic drug and had a diagnosis of schizophrenia or schizoaffective disorder were eligible to enter the study. A series of consecutive outpatients were asked to consider entering the study. The majority of participants (23 out of 37) were living alone.

With regard to the characteristics of responders vs non-responders, in relation to clinical variables, for those non-responders for whom data are available (21 service users), there was no significant difference in age, BMI, blood glucose, and cholesterol level between the groups.

Patients who consented attended for a single assessment in a fasted state (i.e. not having had anything to eat since 22.00 h the night before). They completed a short interview to assess diet and activity in the previous week (Additional file 1). Assessment of diet and exercise was based on validated assessment tools [14]. Activity was rated as vigorous or moderate using the definitions given in Additional file 1. Subjects also completed Likert scales

(rated 1–10) that assessed their views of diet, activity and medication compliance.

Each participant underwent basic anthropometric measurements, namely height, weight, and waist: hip ratio. Pulse and blood pressure were checked using a validated semi-automatic Omron HEM-705CP monitor (Omron Healthcare, Kyoto, Japan). The interviews and anthropometric measurements were undertaken by one of two trained research nurses. Socio-demographic details, details of psychiatric and medical history, and current prescribed medication were taken from the medical notes.

A fasting blood sample was taken for a variety of biochemical tests including serum glucose, lipids and prolactin. Apart from prolactin measurement, all assays were performed on the Roche Modular System (Burgess Hill, West Sussex, UK). Prolactin was assayed on the Siemens Immulite 2000 automated analyser (Siemens Healthcare Diagnostics, Frimley, Camberley, Surrey, UK).

Metabolic syndrome definition

According to the 2005 IDF definition [15], for a person to be defined as having the metabolic syndrome they must have the following:

Central obesity (defined as waist circumference ≥ 94 cm for European men and ≥ 80 cm for European women, with ethnicity specific values for other groups, specifically 90 cm for South Asian and Oriental origin men) plus any two of the following four factors (all but two of the participants in this study were of European origin):

- raised TG level: ≥ 150 mg/dL (1.7 mmol/L), or specific treatment for this lipid abnormality
- reduced HDL cholesterol: <40 mg/dL (1.03 mmol/L) in males and <50 mg/dL (1.29 mmol/L) in females, or specific treatment for this lipid abnormality
- raised blood pressure: systolic BP $\geq$ 130 or diastolic BP $\geq$ 85 mmHg, or treatment of previously diagnosed hypertension
- raised fasting plasma glucose (FPG) ≥ 100 mg/dL (5.6 mmol/L), or previously diagnosed type 2 diabetes if >5.6 mmol/L or 100 mg/dL.

Results
Sample characteristics

The response rate among those eligible to enter the study was 41%. Twenty-five men and twelve women participated in the study. All had schizophrenia or schizoaffective disorder.

The mean duration of illness was 11.6 years (95% confidence interval: 7.3–18.2). The mean age was 46.2 years (46.2–49.2). Of the group, 30 (81%) were unemployed, four were in paid employment, one was in voluntary employment, one was retired, and one was off work due to sickness at the time of interview. The majority of participants (35 out of 37) were of White European origin, with one of South Asian ethnicity, and one of Chinese ethnicity. In keeping with the protocol, all patients were taking neuroleptic medication. The key results are summarised in Table 1.

Of the participants, 20 out of 37 were taking oral atypical agents (eight were taking Clozapine) with 13 on depot neuroleptics (of which two were receiving depot Risperidone) and four on mood stabilisers as the primary psychotropic agent.

Smoking and alcohol use

Twenty-four out of 37 subjects (64.9%) were current smokers, six (16.2%) were ex-smokers with seven (18.9%) never having smoked. Of the current smokers, four smoked between 1 and 10 cigarettes per day, nine between 11 and 20 cigarettes per day, and eleven between 21 and 60 cigarettes per day. 15% of male subjects consumed above the recommended safe levels of alcohol in a week (21 units per week). No women consumed above the recommended safe levels of alcohol in a week (14 units per week). Of the total sample of 37 patients, 14 took no alcohol in a week.

Weight and related measurements

Within the group, BMI ranged from 18.4 to 52.4 kg/m^2 (normal range: 18.5–25.0 kg/m^2; World Health Organisation [16]). Mean (95% CI) BMI for men was 31.2 (28.2–34.3) kg/m^2, and for women was 31.8 (26.3–37.3) kg/m^2. 47.2% of the group had a BMI in the obese range ($\geq$30.0 kg/m^2). Thirty-two (86.5%) reported that they did not find it difficult to put on weight.

For men (all of White European origin), mean (95% CI) waist circumference was 106.9 (100.8–112.9) cm (Fig. 1). For Caucasian men, central adiposity is defined as waist $\geq$94 cm [15]. For men (one was South Asian), waist circumference was 96.5 (86.7–106.3) cm (Fig. 1). For women of European and South Asian ethnicity, central adiposity is defined as waist $\geq$80 cm [16]. 92.0% of men had central adiposity as defined, as did 91.7% of women.

Pulse and blood pressure

Mean ($\pm$SD) systolic blood pressure was 126 $\pm$ 19 mmHg and mean diastolic blood pressure was 80 $\pm$ 13 mmHg. 21.6% had a systolic blood pressure >140 mmHg and 45.9% a diastolic blood pressure >80 mmHg.

Laboratory results

Four out of 37 patients were known to have diabetes, and three of the 37 patients (8.1%) had a fasting glucose between 6.1 and 6.9 mmol/L [17]. Fasting total cholesterol was >5 mmol/L in 48% of individuals with fasting LDL-cholesterol >3 mmol/L in 43.3% of patients. 16.7% of the patients had a serum prolactin >1000 µL, the threshold agreed by local endocrine services as meriting further investigation.

Metabolic syndrome

Twenty-five patients (67.6%) would be categorised as having the metabolic syndrome using the International Diabetes Federation (IDF) Criteria [15]. This was more likely if the individual was older (odds ratio 1.4 (95% CI 1.32–1.48).

Diet

Thirty-two participants completed the dietary questionnaire. A total of 13.5% of participants ate $\geq$5 portions of fruit and vegetables per day. Mean ($\pm$SD) portions of fruit per day were 1.1 $\pm$ 1.0 and of vegetables were 1.7 $\pm$ 1.2. Total fruit and vegetable portions were 2.8 $\pm$ 1.8. For the group, oily fish was eaten on average on 0.5 $\pm$ 0.6 days of each week.

Fruit was only eaten on $\geq$3 days each week by 34.4% of the group, with 37.5% reporting not eating fruit on

Table 1 Details of sample and key results

Socio-demographic factors	Number and % of patients (unless otherwise specified)
Mean age (95% CI), yrs	46.2 (43.2–49.2)
Male (%)	25 (67.6)
Mean duration of illness (95% CI), yrs	11.6 (7.3–18.2)
Caucasian (%)	35 (94.6)
Lifestyle parameters	
5 portions or more of fruit and vegetables per day (%)	13.5
Fresh fruit at least once a week (%)	62.5
Vigorous exercise taken once a week for $\geq$10 min (%)	29
BMI $\geq$30 (%)	47.2
Current smoker (%)	64.9
Weekly alcohol > safe limits (%)	15
Blood parameters	
Fasting glucose elevated >6.0 mmol/L (%)	21.2
Cholesterol >5 mmol/L (%)	48
Prolactin elevated >1000 mu/L (%)	16.7
Miscellaneous	
Blood pressure >140/90 mmHg (%)	32.4
Metabolic syndrome (%)	67.6
Regard diet as unhealthy (%)	54.1
Regard themselves as physically inactive (%)	51.4

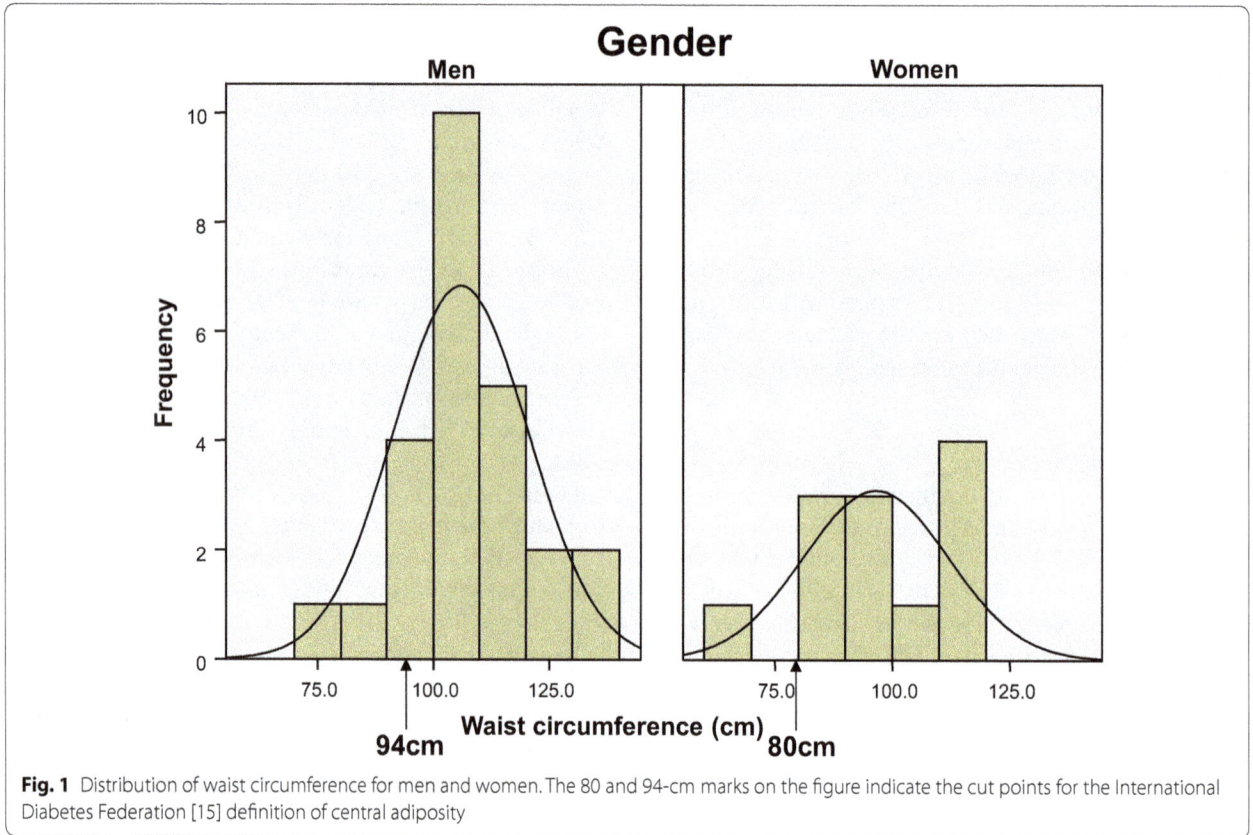

Fig. 1 Distribution of waist circumference for men and women. The 80 and 94-cm marks on the figure indicate the cut points for the International Diabetes Federation [15] definition of central adiposity

any day of the week (Table 2). Vegetables were eaten on ≥3 days of each week by 59.4% of individuals.

With regard to takeaway foods, twelve (37.5%) did not have any in the previous week, 18 (56.3%) had 1–2 takeaways and two (6.3%) had >2 takeaways. For ready meals, the breakdown was similar with 50% (16 out of 32) having none, 34.4% (11/32) having 1–2 ready meals, 9.4% (3 out of 32) having 3–4 ready meals but 6.3% (2 out of 32) having ≥7.

For crisps, 18 out of 32 (56.3%) had no crisps in the last week and for bread 56.3% (18 out of 32) had white bread, 13 wholemeal/granary bread/brown bread, and one had no bread.

Table 2 Breakdown of fruit and vegetable intake in a week for the whole group

Number of days eating vegetables	% of group	Number of days eating fruit	% of group
0	12.5	0	37.5
1–2	28.1	1–2	28.1
3–5	34.4	3–5	18.8
>5	25.0	>5	15.6

Activity

41.9% of participants reported doing no vigorous activity in the last week (see Additional file 1 for definition). 35.5% did <1 h of vigorous activity per week. Only 29% did ≥10 min of vigorous activity per week. 29% described doing no moderate activity in any week and 39% of patients did so for <1 h per week (Fig. 2). Of 31 responders, 21 walked for <1 h each day, 14 said that they walked for ≥10 min each day with five walking once or not at all in any week, and the remaining twelve walking 2–6 times each week for >10 min.

Likert scale ratings

The people studied displayed an understanding that their lifestyle was less healthy than might be achieved, in terms of both diet and exercise.

Diet

Patient ratings on a visual scale of 1–10 for the question 'Would you describe your diet as healthy (average over the last 3 months)?' gave a mean ± SD of 5.7 ± 2.2. The anchor points were 0 = very unhealthy, 10 = very healthy.

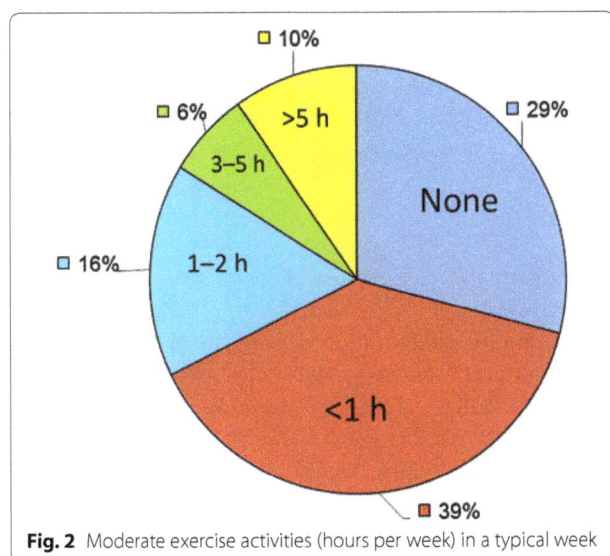

Fig. 2 Moderate exercise activities (hours per week) in a typical week

Activity

Patient ratings on a visual scale of 1–10 for the question 'Would you consider yourself fairly physically active (average over the last 3 months)?' gave a mean ± SD of 5.0 ± 2.9. The anchor points were 0 = very physically inactive, 10 = very physically active.

Medication compliance

Patient ratings on a visual scale of 1–10 for the question 'Are you compliant with medication prescribed for you to take (over the last 3 months)?' gave a mean ± SD of 9.8 ± 0.8. The anchor points were 0 = not compliant, 10 = very compliant.

If a score of <5.0 on the Likert scales is used to indicate that a patient does not think they have a healthy diet, and a score <5.0 as a patient regarding themselves as not physically active, then the percentage of patients who accepted that they had a problem in these two areas was 54.1 and 51.4%, respectively.

Discussion

We report three important findings from this study: (i) a high prevalence of metabolic syndrome; (ii) a high prevalence of poor diet, smoking and inadequate exercise; and (iii) that a high proportion of patients have insight into their unhealthy lifestyles. In relation to the third finding, we believe that an insight into lifestyle has not previously been reported. The fact that our subjects showed some degree of insight into their lifestyle problems indicates that there is potential for working with this group to improve the quality of diet and to increase the amount of exercise taken each day [10, 18].

In terms of methodology, the study sample was small but it is representative of patients with schizophrenia and schizoaffective disorder. In the current study, we approached a consecutive series of outpatients and just over 40% took part in the study. This is comparable with contemporary analysis of rates of screening in UK Primary Care [19].

If there is a sampling bias, it is likely that more motivated patients with healthier lifestyles took part. Patients were asked to attend in a fasted state and this was checked with them on the day that they attended. All anthropometric measurements were taken by one of two trained research nurses ensuring accuracy and consistency. The cut-offs that were used to define insight into lifestyle on the Likert scales have not been formally assessed; however, assessment of diet and exercise was based on validated assessment tools [14].

The prevalence of metabolic syndrome in our group was 67.6%. This is a major concern because metabolic syndrome is a strong predictor of CVD [15, 19, 20] and of cardiovascular death [21]. The rates of metabolic syndrome are similar to other studies. In terms of components of the metabolic syndrome, most patients had a BMI and waist circumference above normal thresholds, with 92% of both men and women having central adiposity. Perhaps surprisingly, only a fifth of patients had an elevated systolic blood pressure.

Many individuals did not follow the recommendations for dietary intake of fruit and vegetables [22]. A significant proportion did not exercise as much as is recommended [17]. Levels of smoking were high. These results mirrored the seminal work done on lifestyle in schizophrenia conducted by McCreadie et al. [7] in the 1990s and subsequently [8, 9]. It is of concern that there has been no improvement in the intervening period. In particular, the last decade has seen investment in strategies to reduce smoking in the general population which have been successful. In contrast, smoking levels remain high in those with SMI. Our data show that the problems noted by McCreadie [8] in a Scottish sample, namely high levels of smoking, poor diet and low levels of exercise are also seen in England, increasing the likelihood that these findings represent the national picture.

Regular health screening, including measurement of fasting lipids and glucose, is recommended for those with SMI and those treated with antipsychotics in many treatment guidelines [23]. In addition, it is generally agreed that lifestyle interventions are necessary to improve physical health of SMI patients [24, 25]. In non-psychiatric patients at high risk of developing diabetes, simple lifestyle adjustments have been shown to reduce diabetes risk. These interventions include decreasing calorific and fat content of food and increase fibre intake, increasing intake of fruit and vegetables, eating complex rather than simple carbohydrates (e.g. whole-wheat bread rather than refined white bread) and avoiding sugary drinks, as well as carrying out exercise for at least 10–15 min per day. Advice to the general population to improve fruit and vegetable intake has been shown to be successful, at least in the short term [26].

In an intervention study [9], the diet of people with schizophrenia improved when they were given free fruit and vegetables; however, this was not sustained after withdrawal of the intervention, although there was a trend for the return to pre-intervention consumption to be more gradual when the free food intervention was combined with dietary advice.

A significant proportion of patients in our study had hyperprolactinaemia. This is a recognised adverse effect of many antipsychotics [27, 28]. The propensity to cause hyperprolactinaemia varies significantly between different atypical antipsychotics. Raised prolactin can be asymptomatic, leading to various acute adverse effects, and can also result in long-term medical problems, including osteoporosis.

We do not have a direct comparison group from the general population. However, a detailed survey of the Salford UK population in terms of lifestyle is underway (www.citizenscientist.org.uk). The majority of the participants were living alone, so collection from someone cohabiting with them was not possible.

It could be argued that the quality of diet found in our study group is not significantly different from that of people in a similar socio-demographic situation [29]. However, the high rates of diabetes and cardiovascular events [2–4] in SMI define them as a high-risk group for cardiometabolic disease and, as such, there is the potential for targeted intervention to produce benefit.

We recommend the following principles of management to reduce cardiometabolic risk:

- Potential pre-diabetes states should be investigated and managed as per agreed guidelines for the general population but with annual screening for this recommended for those with psychosis receiving antipsychotic medications. The prescription of metformin for those not responding to or not adherent to intensive lifestyle interventions needs to be considered in the context of the individual service user.
- Diabetes should be managed by the family practitioner or a specialist physician where necessary.
- Dyslipidemia, especially in the context of a patient with diabetes, should be actively managed according to existing guidelines for the general population. There is no contra-indication to the prescription of a statin.

- Hypertension should be managed according to national guidelines. There is no contra-indication to prescription of antihypertensive medications.
- Smoking is an important additive risk factor for diabetes and cardiovascular disease and service users who smoke should be referred to smoking cessation services.

Our data show that there is scope to achieve a more healthy lifestyle in individuals with SMI. Such improvements require collaboration between local Mental Health providers and General practitioners plus specialist services, particularly dietetics, community health trainers and occupational therapy. It is likely that in many areas of the UK, and elsewhere, significant healthcare system redesign will be necessary to achieve this goal [30].

One of the founding principles of the NHS in 1948 was that it should strive to improve the health of the individual and the population and prevent disease. The needs of the service users lie at the heart of this fundamental mission and of other healthcare providers across the world responsible for the welfare of patients with schizophrenia and other forms of severe enduring illness.

Conclusions

Within this sample, there was a high prevalence of poor diet, smoking and inadequate exercise. Many did not follow national recommendations for dietary intake of fruit and vegetables and daily exercise. These factors probably contribute to the high prevalence of metabolic syndrome. Many had insight into their unhealthy lifestyles. Thus, there is potential for interventions to improve lifestyle factors and reduce the risk of cardiometabolic disease.

Abbreviations

BMI: body mass index; CVD: cardiovascular disease; FBG: fasting blood glucose; IDF: International Diabetes Federation; SMI: severe and enduring mental illnesses.

Authors' contributions

AHH and PH conceived the project. AHH, PH and ML were principal contributors to writing the manuscript. JP and VN recruited patients and assisted in the composition of the manuscript. MG performed the laboratory analyses. SGA carried out the statistical analysis. All authors read and approved the final manuscript.

Author details

[1] Department of Medicine, Leighton Hospital, Crewe CW1 4QJ, Cheshire, UK. [2] The School of Medicine and Manchester Academic Health Sciences Centre, University of Manchester, Manchester M13 9PT, UK. [3] Greater Manchester West Mental Health NHS Foundation Trust, Greater Manchester, UK. [4] Institute

of Cardiovascular Sciences, University of Manchester, Manchester, UK.
[5] Department of Clinical Biochemistry, Salford Royal Hospital, Salford M6 8HD, UK. [6] Department of Blood Sciences, Walsall Manor Hospital, Walsall WS2 9PS, UK.

Acknowledgements
None.

Competing interests
The authors declare that they have no competing interests.

Ethical approval
Full Ethics approval for the Study was given by the Salford Ethics Committee. All participants had given informed consent to be included in the study. All authors of the paper consent to publication of this paper. The data and other materials will be provided on request by the corresponding author.

Ethics, consent, permissions
Informed consent was obtained.

Human rights
The manuscript does not report on or involve the use of any animal or human data or tissue. The manuscript does not contain any individual person's data.

References

1. Brown S. Excess mortality of schizophrenia. A meta-analysis. Br J Psychiatry. 1997;171:502–8.
2. Casey DE, Haupt DW, Newcomer JW, Henderson DC, Sernyak MJ, Davidson M, et al. Antipsychotic-induced weight gain and metabolic abnormalities: implications for increased mortality in patients with schizophrenia. J Clin Psychiatry. 2004;65(suppl 7):s4–18.
3. Casey DE. Metabolic issues and cardiovascular disease in patients with psychiatric disorders. Am J Med. 2005;118(suppl 2):s15–22.
4. Osborn DPJ, Levy G, Nazareth I, Petersen I, Islam A, King MB. Relative risk of cardiovascular and cancer mortality in people with severe mental illness from the United Kingdom's general practice research database. Arch Gen Psychiatry. 2007;64:242–9.
5. Gillman MW. Enjoy your fruits and vegetables. BMJ. 1996;313:765–6.
6. Allison DB, Fontaine KR, Heo M, Mentore JL, Cappelleri JC, Chandler LP, et al. The distribution of body mass index among individuals with and without schizophrenia. J Clin Psychiatry. 1999;60:215–20.
7. McCreadie R, Macdonald E, Blacklock C, Tilak-Singh D, Wiles D, Halliday J, et al. Dietary intake of schizophrenic patients in Nithsdale, Scotland: case control study. BMJ. 1998;317:784–5.
8. McCreadie RG. Diet, smoking and cardiovascular risk in people with schizophrenia: descriptive study. Br J Psychiatry. 2003;183:534–9.
9. Holt RI, Abdelrahman T, Hirsch M, Dhesi Z, George T, Blincoe T, et al. The prevalence of undiagnosed metabolic abnormalities in people with serious mental illness. J Psychopharmacol. 2010;24:867–73.
10. McCreadie RG, Kelly C, Connolly M, Williams S, Baxter G, Lean M, et al. Dietary improvement in people with schizophrenia: randomised controlled trial. Br J Psychiatry. 2005;187:346–51.
11. Haddad PM, Sharma SG. Adverse effects of atypical antipsychotics: differential risk and clinical implications. CNS Drugs. 2007;21:911–36.
12. De Hert M, Correll CU, Bobes J, Cetkovich-Bakmas M, Cohen D, Asai I, et al. Physical illness in patients with severe mental disorders. I. Prevalence, impact of medications and disparities in health care. World Psychiatry. 2011;10:52–77.
13. Haddad P. Weight change with atypical antipsychotics in the treatment of schizophrenia. J Psychopharmacol. 2005;19(suppl):s16–27.
14. Heald AH, Sharma R, Anderson SG, Vyas A, Siddals K, Patel J, et al. Dietary intake and the IGF-system: effects of migration in two related populations in India and Britain with markedly different dietary intake. Public Health Nutr. 2005;8:620–7.
15. Alberti KG, Zimmet P, Shaw J. The metabolic syndrome—a new worldwide definition. Lancet. 2005;366:1059–62.
16. World Health Organisation (WHO). Physical status: the use and interpretation of anthropometry. Report of a WHO Expert Committee. WHO. Technical Report Series 854. Geneva: World Health Organization; 1995.
17. World Health Organization: Definition, Diagnosis and Classification of Diabetes Mellitus and its Complications: Report of a WHO Consultation. Part 1: Diagnosis and Classification of Diabetes Mellitus. Geneva: World Health Organisation; 1999.
18. De Hert MA, Van Winkel R, Van Eyck D, Hanssens L, Wampers M, Scheen A, et al. Prevalence of the metabolic syndrome in patients with schizophrenia treated with antipsychotic medication. Schizophr Res. 2006;83:87–93.
19. Martin JL, Lowrie R, McConnachie A, McLean G, Mair F, Mercer SW, et al. Physical health indicators in major mental illness: analysis of QOF data across UK general practice. Br J Gen Pract. 2014;64:e649–56.
20. Heald AH, Montejo AL, Millar H, De Hert M, McCrae J, Correll CU. Management of physical health in patients with schizophrenia: practical recommendations. Eur Psychiatry. 2010;25:S41–5.
21. Galassi A, Reynolds K, He J. Metabolic syndrome and risk of cardiovascular disease: a meta-analysis. Am J Med. 2006;119:812–9.
22. Food Standards Agency (FSA). The balance of good health. London: FSA; 2001.
23. Taylor D, Paton C, Kerwin R. Maudsley prescribing guidelines. 9th ed. London: Informa Healthcare; 1997.
24. Bushe C, Haddad P, Peveler R, Pendlebury J. The role of lifestyle interventions and weight management in schizophrenia. J Psychopharmacol. 2005;19(6 suppl):s28–35.
25. Peet M. Diet, diabetes and schizophrenia: review and hypothesis. Br J Psychiatry. 2004;184(suppl. 47):s102–5.
26. Zino S, Skeaff M, Williams S, Mann J. Randomised controlled trial of effect of fruit vegetable consumption on plasma concentration and antioxidants. BMJ. 1997;314:1787–91.
27. Haddad PM, Wieck A. Antipsychotic-induced hyperprolactinaemia: mechanisms, clinical features and management. Drugs. 2004;64:2291–314.
28. Maguire GA. Prolactin elevation with antipsychotic medication: mechanism of action and clinical consequences. J Clin Psychiatry. 2002;63:56–62.
29. Food Standards Agency (FSA). Low income diet and nutrition survey. London: FSA; 2001.
30. Bodenheimer T, Wagner EH, Grumback K. Improving primary care for patients with chronic illness. JAMA. 2002;288:1775–9.

17

Healthcare professionals' perceptions on the emotional impact of having an inadequate response to antidepressant medications: survey and prospective patient audit

Rajnish Mago[1,5]*, Andrea Fagiolini[2], Emmanuelle Weiller[3] and Catherine Weiss[4]

Abstract

Background: Despite the availability of effective antidepressants, about half of patients with major depressive disorder (MDD) display an inadequate response to their initial treatment. A large patient survey recently reported that 29.8% of MDD patients experiencing an inadequate treatment response felt frustrated about their medication and 19.2% were frustrated with their healthcare provider. This survey and chart audit evaluated healthcare professionals' (HCP) views on the emotional impact of having an inadequate response to antidepressant medication.

Methods: HCPs who frequently treat patients with MDD completed a survey and chart audit of their MDD patients currently experiencing an inadequate response to antidepressant treatment.

Results: 287 HCPs completed 1336 chart audits. HCPs reported that 38% of their patients were trusting/accepting of their MDD medications and 41% of their patients trusted/felt confident with their healthcare provision. Conversely, HCPs reported that 11% of their patients were frustrated with their medication and 5% with their healthcare benefits. HCPs cited impact on daily life (53%) and treatment issues (lack of efficacy and side effects; 50%) as the main drivers for their patients' feelings of frustration. When HCPs recognized patients' feelings of frustration, the top concerns of the HCPs were worsening of symptoms (43%) and non-compliance (41%).

Conclusions: This survey and chart audit highlights the emotional burden associated with inadequate responses to MDD treatment in addition to persistent symptoms. Differences between the views of the HCPs and patients are highlighted and suggest that HCPs may underestimate the full impact that having to try numerous medications has on their patients.

Keywords: Depression, Antidepressant, Frustration, Audit

Background

Despite the availability of many effective antidepressants, in about half of patients, major depressive disorder (MDD) responds inadequately to the initial treatment, leaving patients to cope with persistent symptoms while their medication plan is optimized [1–3]. Persistence of depressive symptoms is known to be associated with various adverse outcomes, including a greater risk of relapse and recurrence [4, 5], a shorter duration between episodes [4], continued impairment in work and relationships [6] and increased overall mortality from comorbid medical disorders [7–10].

We have recently reported the results of a large, international survey of 2096 patients with MDD which was designed to better understand the emotional impact of having an inadequate response to antidepressant

*Correspondence: mago@simpleandpractical.com
5 210 W Rittenhouse Square Suite 404, Philadelphia, PA 19103, USA
Full list of author information is available at the end of the article

medication [11]. The patient survey found that the most frequently reported emotion associated with an inadequate treatment response was 'frustration' (29.8% of respondents). This frustration was directed towards their medication and/or their HCP, and was cited as a cause of patients wanting to stop their medication. To build an effective therapeutic alliance and help patients better engage with their treatment plan, it is essential that HCPs understand the patient's perspective. However, there is often a disconnect between the patient and HCP perceptions of depression management [12]. The aim of this HCP survey and chart audit was to evaluate HCP's views on the emotional impact on the patient of having an inadequate response to antidepressant medication, and to compare these findings with the patient survey.

Methods

This HCP survey and chart audit was conducted in the United States (US), Canada, United Kingdom (UK), Germany, France, and Spain between 14 March and 15 June 2016. No personal identifying information about any patient was requested and the audit was compliant with the European Pharmaceutical Market Research Association (EphMRA) and Association of the British Pharmaceutical Industry (ABPI) Codes of Conduct and all guidelines set forth by the Health Insurance Portability and Accountability Act (HIPAA). In line with the Data Protection Directive 95/46/EC, access to the online audit was secure and all relevant data was kept strictly confidential and anonymous. The authors designed the study and the survey and analyses were conducted by an independent market research agency (Market Strategies International, Livonia, MI, USA funded by Otsuka Pharmaceutical Development & Commercialization, Inc. and H. Lundbeck A/S).

Participants

Respondents were recruited from a database of HCPs who have previously agreed to participate in research. HCP respondents had to be either a board certified/eligible psychiatrist or a primary care physician (PCP; US only) with a 3–35-year history of practicing adult psychiatry in the outpatient setting and currently spending at least 70% of time in direct patient care. All respondents were required to be seeing at least 20 patients with MDD per month. HCPs working in mental health had to be currently initiating prescriptions for MDD (any treatment) including atypical antipsychotics. Primary care physicians were required to be either initiating or refilling prescriptions (any medication) for the treatment of MDD.

Study design

Respondents were blinded to the key study objectives, but were aware that the survey was designed to collect information on current MDD management with the aim of improving patient care. The study was carried out in two distinct parts. The first part was a survey about the HCP's clinical practice, and for the second part, eligible respondents were asked to complete the chart audit for 5 outpatients with MDD who were still experiencing clinically significant depressive symptoms after at least 6 weeks of antidepressant treatment at the recommended dose. It was estimated that it would take 45 min to complete the audits over the course of a week (5–7 min per patient chart, preferably no more than one a day).

Chart audit

To ensure adequate recall, HCP respondents were instructed to complete each patient audit within 8 h of seeing the patient and were encouraged to refer to the patient medical record for accuracy. Full inclusion criteria for suitable patients to be included in the audit are shown in Table 1.

The chart audit included up to 31 items (dependent on responses) and was structured to collect information on: patient characteristics, treatment history, clinical evaluation, HCP perceptions of patient's emotions associated with an inadequate response to treatment and the HCP respondent's perception of whether their patients experience 'frustration' with aspects of their healthcare. As part of the patient characteristics section, HCP respondents were asked to rate their patient's functional ability using the Sheehan Disability Scale (SDS) [13] where a score of 0 represents no impact of symptoms on patient function and 10 represents 'extreme' disruption.

To assess how HCPs recognize patient feelings of frustration and dissatisfaction, respondents were first prompted to indicate how they believed their patients felt

Table 1 Patient criteria for inclusion in audit

Age 18–65 years old

Diagnosed with major depressive disorder (MDD)
Has never had dysthymia
No other comorbid psychiatric conditions (e.g., schizoaffective disorder, etc.)

Being treated in an outpatient setting

Experiencing an MDD episode that required prescription treatment

Treated with an antidepressant at the recommended dose for at least 6 weeks who still experiences clinically significant depressive symptoms

Has been taking prescription medication under your care for at least 3 months for their current episode of MDD and whom you are seeing/ treating in a follow-up visit about their healthcare, choosing from a list of 14 multi-choice answers. Feelings of frustration and dissatisfaction were included as two of the 14 items. The 14 items were: understood, anonymous, frustrated, dissatisfied, neglected, confused, impatient/irritated, apprehensive, hopeless/doubtful, unimportant, ignored, trapped/helpless, none of the above and I am not able to answer this question. If the HCP respondent identified feelings of either frustration or dissatisfaction in their patients, the next set of questions explored which aspects of healthcare they believed the patients were frustrated/dissatisfied with. Further questions included potential sources for frustration/dissatisfaction, and the impact of these feelings.

Data analysis

All HCP responses were coded and analyzed using descriptive statistics (means and frequency of responses).

Results

Sample

A total of 1300 HCPs were screened for inclusion in this survey. Of these, 287 met MDD practice criteria and agreed to the study requirements. Overall, 287 HCPs completed a total of 1336 patient chart audits, and of these 256 HCPs completed all 5 charts. Tables 2 and 3 describe the HCP and patient characteristics, respectively. Overall, 38% of patient charts were from the US, and the rest from the UK, France, Germany, Spain and Canada. Of the 513 US patient charts, half ($n = 254$ or 19% of all charts) were completed by PCPs; all other patient charts were completed by psychiatrists.

Goal setting

Overall, HCPs reported discussing treatment goals with 1189 (89%) of their patients. Of these, most ($n = 1089$; 92%) said their patients agreed with the set goals and only 100 (8%) patients disagreed with the goals. From the HCP perspective, the main goals of treatment were 'improve symptoms of depression' (54.8%), 'improve social functioning' (44%), 'improve symptoms of anxiety' (41%), 'engage in social activities' (39%), 'reach remission and eventually be treatment free' (30%), 'improve sleep problems' (30%), 'improve cognitive symptoms' (28%), 'be able to be productive at work' (27%) and 'be able to better manage home duties' (23%).

Emotions associated with an inadequate response to treatment

Per HCP report, a majority of patients were trusting/accepting (38%) of their medications for MDD and a similar proportion trusted/felt confident (41%) about their healthcare provider. Conversely, HCPs reported that

Table 2 Characteristics of the HCP respondents

Variable	$N = 287$
HCP specialty; n (%)	
Psychiatrist	234 (82%)
US PCP	44 (15%)
Internist/internal medicine	7 (2%)
Nurse practitioner	2 (1%)
Mean years in practice [range]	17.0 years [3–35 years]
Mean percent of time spent in direct patient care	92%
Median estimated numbers of patients seen per month	
MDD	70
Bipolar disorders	30
Schizophrenia	30
Schizoaffective disorder	15
HCP location; n (%)	
US	108 (38%)
Canada	36 (13%)
UK	40 (14%)
Germany	35 (12%)
France	37 (13%)
Spain	31 (11%)
Setting	
Outpatient	251 (88%)
Inpatient	36 (13%)

about one in ten of their patients were frustrated (11%) and/or dissatisfied (9%) with their medication and one in twenty patients were frustrated (5%) and/or dissatisfied with the healthcare provider (Fig. 1).

Further analysis revealed that feelings of frustration and dissatisfaction with medication were identified significantly more frequently by HCPs in patients with a longer history of MDD or who had more antidepressant failures. For example, HCPs identified frustration in 10.7% of patients with a 10-year history of depression ($n = 22$ of 205 patients) compared to 4.5% in patients with a 2-year history ($n = 6$ of 134 patients). Likewise, HCPs identified feelings of frustration with medication in 7.3% of patients who had experienced 3 or more antidepressant treatment failures in the current episode ($n = 48$ of 660 patients) versus 1.8% in patients who had experienced two treatment failures ($n = 7$ of 385 patients) and 2.7% in patients with one treatment failure ($n = 8$ of 291 patients). HCPs were also more likely to identify that their patients were frustrated with healthcare in patients who they had classed (using the SDS scale) as having severe disruption to their daily life (frustration with healthcare was identified in 3.8% of severely affected patients vs. 1.5% of mildly affected patients). Of note, HCPs practicing in Spain and France reported that fewer of their patients were frustrated with medication and/or healthcare (6 and 8%,

Table 3 Patient characteristics per chart audit

Variable	Statistic N = 1336
Setting	
Office	802 (60%)
(US only) Outpatient Community Health Clinic	75 (6%)
(France only) Centre Medical Psychologique	53 (4%)
Hospital Outpatient Clinic	351 (26%)
Telemedicine	12 (1%)
Patient's Home	23 (2%)
Day Clinic	19 (1%)
Other	1 (< 1%)
Length of MDD diagnosis	
< 1 month	88 (7%)
1–3 months	174 (13%)
4–6 months	180 (14%)
7–9 months	65 (5%)
10–12 months	211 (16%)
2–5 years	370 (28%)
6+ years	248 (19%)
Current treatment	
SSRI	800 (60%)
SNRI	320 (24%)
MAOI	7 (< 1%)
TCA	49 (4%)
Other antidepressant	295 (22%)
Anxiolytic	239 (18%)
Antipsychotic	243 (18%)
Hypnotic	76 (6%)
Other treatment for depression	69 (5%)
Mean current ADT duration by treatment class (weeks)	
SSRI	45.4
SNRI	48.7
MAOI	22.0
TCA	106.8
Other antidepressant	38.9
Number of current classes of prescription treatments for depression (this episode); n (%)	
0	6 (< 1%)
1	755 (57%)
2	397 (30%)
3	145 (11%)
4	28 (2%)
5+	5 (< 1%)
Mean number	1.6
Level of functioning (mean SDS scores)	
SDS Mean score	5.1
Work domain	6.0
Social domain	4.7
Home domain	4.5
PHQ-9 score (mean)	6.2

Table 3 (continued)

Variable	Statistic N = 1336
Clinical global impression of change in depression since onset of episode to current visit	
Very much worse	5 (< 1%)
Much worse	63 (5%)
Minimally worse	113 (9%)
No change	248 (19%)
Minimally improved	413 (31%)
Much improved	400 (30%)
Very much improved	94 (7%)

respectively) compared with the USA (15%), Germany (12%), UK (17%) and Canada (17%).

Drivers and consequences of frustration in MDD

When the HCP identified that their patients had feelings of frustration or dissatisfaction with healthcare ($n = 156$ patients), the main drivers of frustration were thought to be: impact on daily life (53%) and treatment issues (i.e., lack of efficacy and side effects; 50%). HCPs considered the medication regimen and having to change treatments as less important (both were considered a driver in 19% of patients) (Fig. 2a). HCPs identified that a wide range of symptoms may be related to frustration with healthcare, the most common being 'feeling down, depressed or hopeless' (38%) and feeling tired or having little energy (28%) (Fig. 2b).

In those patients recognized to be frustrated with their medication ($n = 149$), HCPs indicated that they are most likely to react by asking for a new prescription (37%), to make a new appointment (25%) and/or missing school (23%) (Fig. 3a). Likewise, in those patients believed to be frustrated with overall healthcare (n = 156), HCPs indicated that they were more likely to ask for a new prescription, but also to miss school or work and ask to see the doctor more frequently (Fig. 3b).

When HCPs recognized feelings of frustration in their patient, the top concerns were: worsening of symptoms (43%) and non-compliance (41%) (Fig. 4a). HCPs most commonly suggested non-pharmacological therapies (e.g., cognitive behavioral therapy), adjustment of medication doses, and/or lifestyle changes (Fig. 4b).

Discussion

To the best of our knowledge, this survey is the first to evaluate how HCPs perceive the emotional impact of inadequate response to antidepressant treatment on their patients. Although HCPs reported that a large percentage of their patients experiencing inadequate response to antidepressant treatment had positive feelings about their medication and healthcare, they also identified a range of negative emotions including frustration and dissatisfaction, both with medications and overall healthcare. Such emotions are important to address, as they can directly impact medication adherence. Indeed, noncompliance was one of the top concerns HCPs associated with patient frustration.

The results of this survey indicate that HCPs are aware of the wide range of negative emotions that can potentially be associated with treatment failure and persistent depressive symptoms. No HCP reported that all of their patients included in the audit had only positive feelings towards their medication and/or healthcare. However, comparing the results of this survey to a recent patient survey, it appears that HCPs may significantly underestimate how many of their own patients have negative emotions towards their medication or healthcare, and may not be identifying the full impact of treatment failures on the patient experience. Whereas HCPs identified feelings of frustration with medication in 11% of their patients, the self-reported level of frustration in the patient survey was nearly three times higher (30%). Only half of the HCP respondents recognized frustration in any of their patients. Likewise, whereas HCPs recognized that 12% of their patients are frustrated with their healthcare, the patient survey indicated that a much larger percentage (27%) are frustrated with their overall healthcare, including access to services and medications and experiences with their doctors, nurses and therapists.

Of note, HCPs only considered that 5% their patients are frustrated with their therapeutic relationship compared to 19% of patients in the patient survey. When HCPs did recognize feelings of frustration in their patients, they appeared to be aware of the potential impact of frustration on medication adherence and cited worsening of symptoms and non-adherence as their top concerns associated with frustration. However, it is notable that only 24% of HCPs identified patient frustration in the audit, and these HCPs usually identified it in 2 or 3 of their 5 patient charts. The lack of recognition from the 76% of HCPs likely accounts for the discrepancy between the HCP and patient surveys in the reported prevalence of frustration in this patient population. Recognizing frustration with the therapeutic alliance is vital to address, because 29% of patients in the patient survey reported that they share less information when they are frustrated with their HCP and 27% reported wanting to quit their medication altogether. This insight is supported by the findings of another study based on in-depth interviews which found that MDD patients who had stopped taking their antidepressants had often experienced unsatisfactory interactions with HCPs [14]. Other qualitative studies have identified patient ambiguity and frustration with their medication (including time-frame of treatment, efficacy and tolerability) as key reasons for medication non-adherence [15].

One practical way to improve the therapeutic alliance is to engage the patient in goal setting, so that they have reasonable expectations of their treatment. Moreover, it has been suggested that when patients receive treatment that they perceive as relevant to their individual needs, they are likely to exhibit greater commitment to their treatment regimen [16–18]. This, in turn, may help to significantly decrease discontinuation of treatment, increase

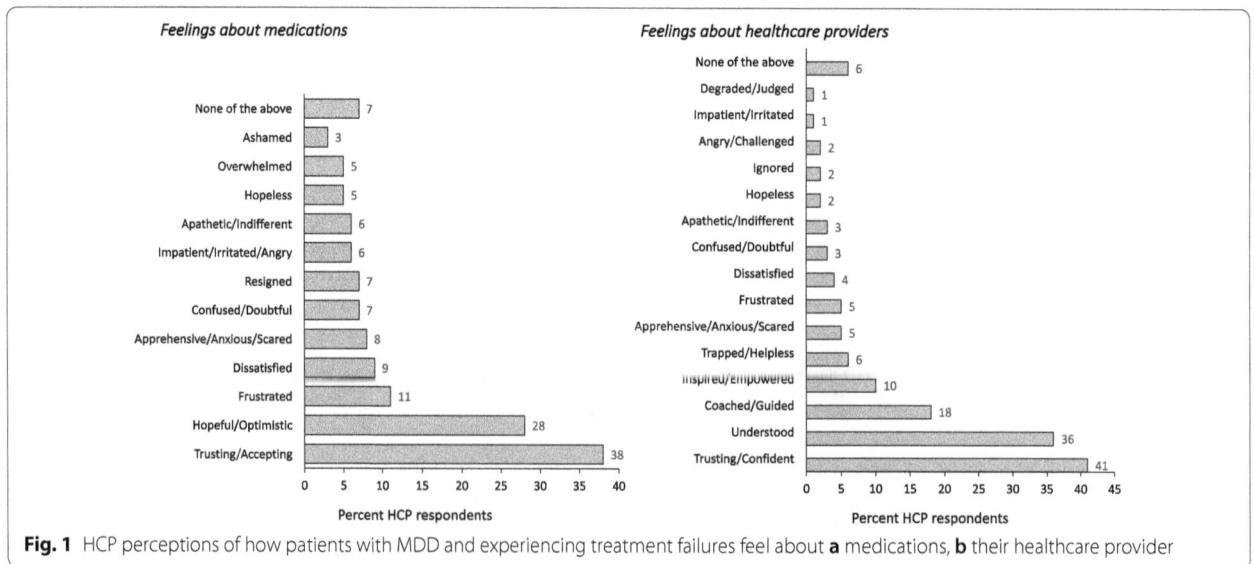

Fig. 1 HCP perceptions of how patients with MDD and experiencing treatment failures feel about **a** medications, **b** their healthcare provider

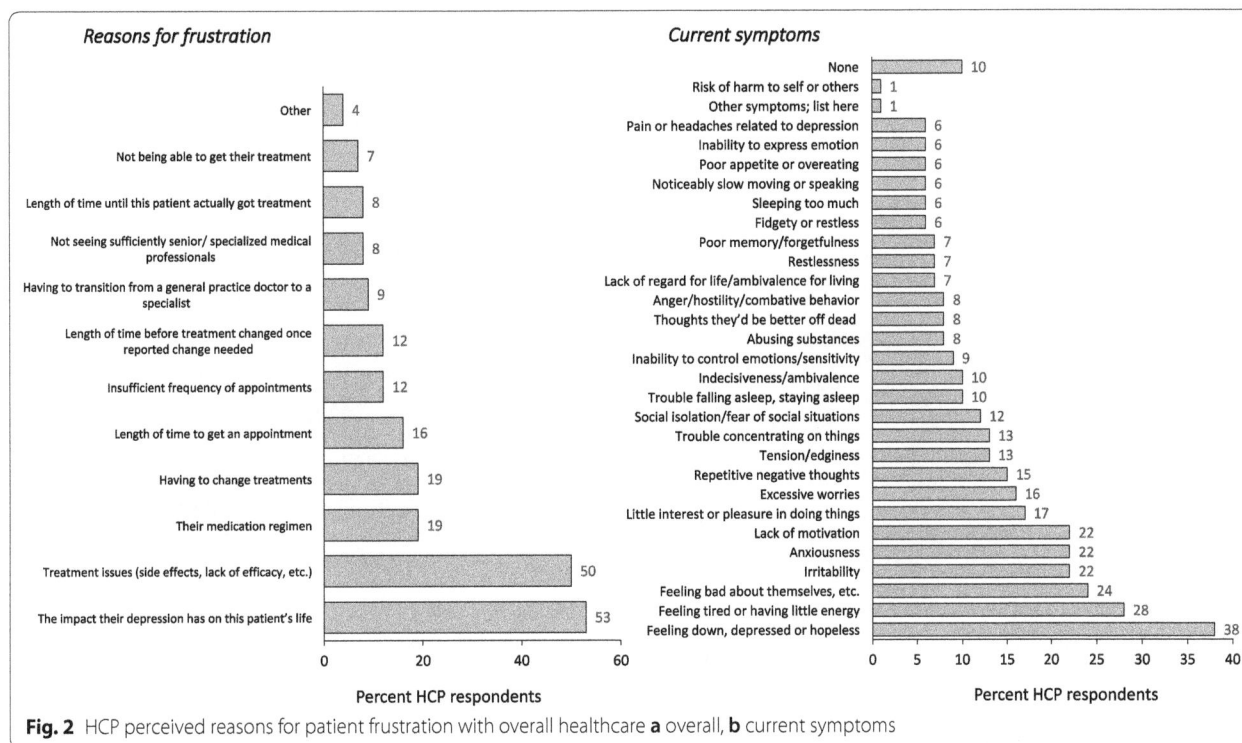

Fig. 2 HCP perceived reasons for patient frustration with overall healthcare **a** overall, **b** current symptoms

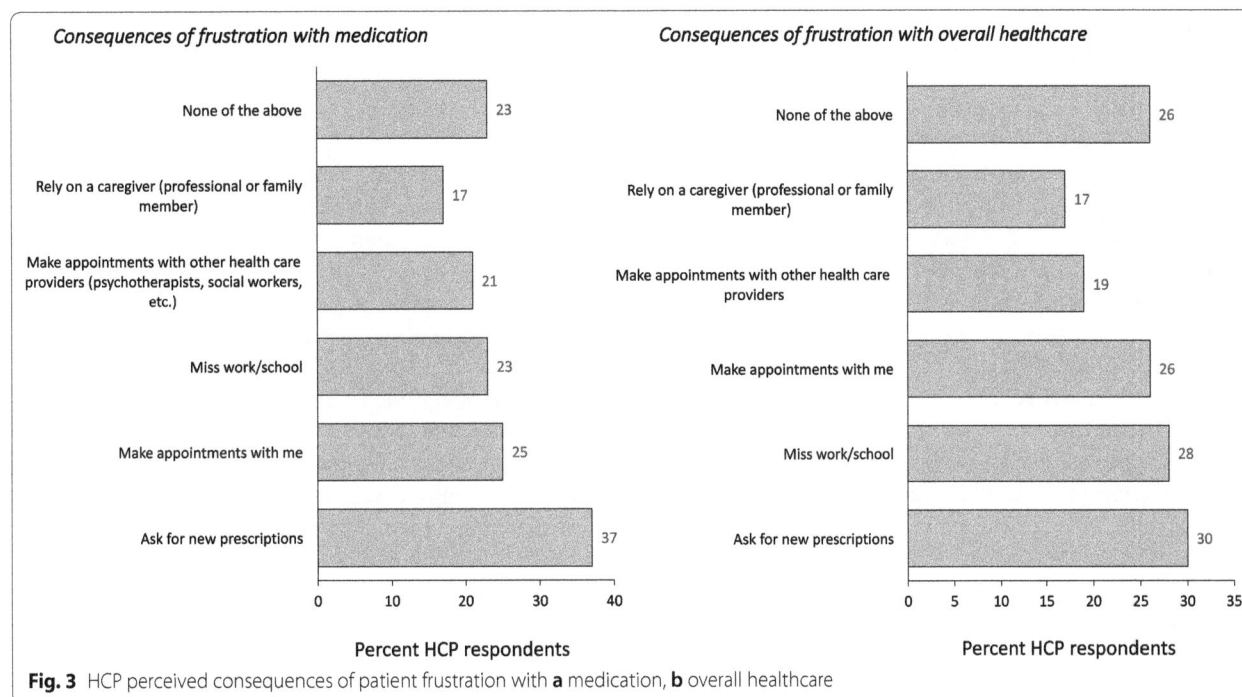

Fig. 3 HCP perceived consequences of patient frustration with **a** medication, **b** overall healthcare

satisfaction, and ultimately improve outcomes. In this survey, HCPs reported that they had discussed treatment goals with 90% of their patients. But in the patient survey, the proportion of patients who said treatment goals had been discussed with their HCPs was smaller (72%).

Effective goal setting requires effective communication between the HCP and patient and it is a therapeutic skill that needs to be learned and practiced [19]. It may also be that some patients in the patient survey did not explicitly realize or remember that their HCP had discussed the

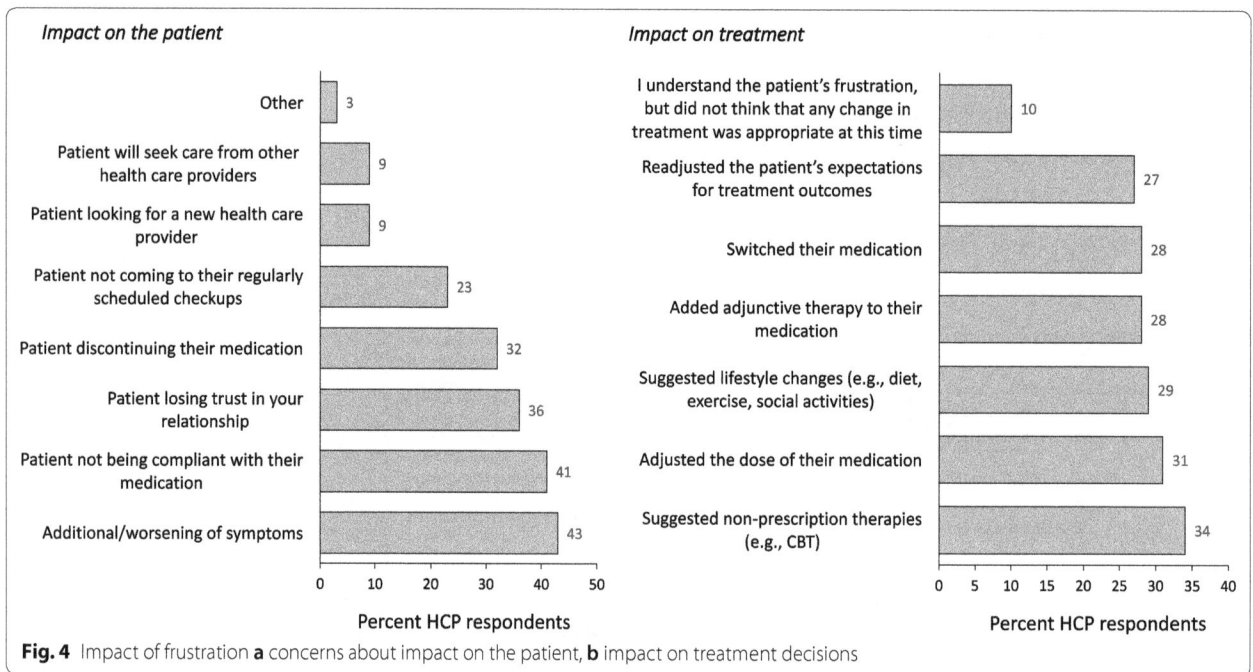

Impact on the patient

Other — 3
Patient will seek care from other health care providers — 9
Patient looking for a new health care provider — 9
Patient not coming to their regularly scheduled checkups — 23
Patient discontinuing their medication — 32
Patient losing trust in your relationship — 36
Patient not being compliant with their medication — 41
Additional/worsening of symptoms — 43

Percent HCP respondents

Impact on treatment

I understand the patient's frustration, but did not think that any change in treatment was appropriate at this time — 10
Readjusted the patient's expectations for treatment outcomes — 27
Switched their medication — 28
Added adjunctive therapy to their medication — 28
Suggested lifestyle changes (e.g., diet, exercise, social activities) — 29
Adjusted the dose of their medication — 31
Suggested non-prescription therapies (e.g., CBT) — 34

Percent HCP respondents

Fig. 4 Impact of frustration **a** concerns about impact on the patient, **b** impact on treatment decisions

goals of treatment. Interestingly, while patients and HCPs both agreed that their top goal for MDD treatment was to address depressive symptoms (55% in the HCP survey and 78% in the patient survey), patients are more inclined to expect improvement in anxiety (61% in patient survey vs. 41% in HCP survey) and sleep issues (51% in patient survey vs. 30% in HCP survey) than HCPs.

Strengths of the study include its international design and the timing of the patient audit where respondents were asked to record the data soon after they had seen the patient (limiting recall bias). Limitations of the survey include all those inherent to survey methodology including the process of recruitment which was limited to a commercial database of HCPs. Although there was consistency of most results across countries, this survey indicated that there may be some national differences in the perception of frustration, with lower levels being reported in Germany and France. This may be because of cultural differences in the patient population and/or in the healthcare system organization for MDD; and indeed, the patient survey found lower levels of patients expressing frustration in France [11]. Studies at the national level may be better able to tease out what aspects of care lead to frustration in each population. In addition, since the patient and HCP surveys were conducted separately, and patients were not matched to the HCP, a limitation of the various comparisons discussed above is that we cannot rule out the possibility that there were inherent differences in the patient populations surveyed. Although both

surveys were conducted in the same countries, the sample size of the HCP survey was smaller than the patient survey ($n = 287$ HCP/1336 patient charts vs. $n = 2096$ patients, respectively), and the relative representation of respondents from each country differed slightly (e.g., 38% of HCP respondents vs. 28.5% patient respondents were from the US). Moreover, it may be that patients experiencing frustration with their healthcare or medication are more likely to participate in a survey as a means to voice their dissatisfaction.

Conclusions

This survey highlights the high prevalence of wide-ranging emotional burden associated with treatment failures in MDD. Although HCPs appear to be aware of some of the problems, the discrepancies between the results of this HCP survey and the patient survey [11] suggest that HCPs may often underestimate the full impact of having to try numerous medications has on their patients. The results can be considered a 'call to action' for clinicians to consider their management approach for patients who show an inadequate response to antidepressant treatment. In particular, HCP awareness of how patients experience 'frustration' appears to be low compared to the self-reported prevalence in patients with MDD. This is important to consider because patients report that feelings of frustration may lead to poor adherence to medication, which will then continue to contribute to poor outcomes in patients.

Abbreviations

ABPI: Association of the British Pharmaceutical Industry; EphMRA: European Pharmaceutical Market Research Association; HCP: healthcare professional; HIPAA: Health Insurance Portability and Accountability Act; MDD: major depressive disorder; PCP: primary care physician.

Authors' contributions

All authors conceptualized the survey and contributed to the interpretation of results and to the final version of the article. EW and CW wrote the first draft of the paper with direction from RM and AF. All authors read and approved the final manuscript.

Author details

[1] Simple and Practical Mental Health, Philadelphia, PA, USA. [2] University of Siena Medical Center, Siena, Italy. [3] H. Lundbeck A/S, Valby, Denmark. [4] Otsuka Pharmaceutical Development & Commercialization, Inc, Princeton, NJ, USA. [5] 210 W Rittenhouse Square Suite 404, Philadelphia, PA 19103, USA.

Acknowledgements

We wish to thank Katy Palmer (Market Strategies International) for help in conducting the study and analyses and Anita Chadha-Patel (ACP Clinical Communications Ltd, funded by Otsuka and H.Lundbeck A/S) for support in the preparation, revisions and editing of this paper. We also thank all the participant HCPs for taking the time to complete the surveys.

Competing interests

RM reports that in the previous 12 months, he received research grants from Alkermes, Allergan, Genomind, Takeda. He has been a consultant for GuidePoint Global, Lundbeck, Neurocrine, and Otsuka. He has developed and delivered educational activities for PsychU, funded by Otsuka Pharmaceuticals. He receives book royalties from On Demand Publishing and Kindle Direct Publishing. AF reports that he is/has been a consultant and/or a speaker and/or has received research grants from Allergen, Angelini, Astra Zeneca, Bristol-Myers Squibb, Boehringer Ingelheim, Pfizer, Eli Lilly, Ferrer, Janssen, Lundbeck, Novartis, Otsuka, and Roche. EW was employed by H.Lundbeck A/S at the time of the study and CW is employed by Otsuka.

Consent for publication

Not applicable.

Funding

This work has been sponsored by Otsuka Pharmaceutical Development & Commercialization, Inc. and H.Lundbeck A/S.

References

1. Rush AJ, Trivedi MH, Wisniewski SR, Stewart JW, Nierenberg AA, Thase ME, Ritz L, Biggs MM, Warden D, Luther JF, et al. Bupropion-SR, sertraline, or venlafaxine-XR after failure of SSRIs for depression. N Engl J Med. 2006;354(12):1231–42.
2. Rush AJ, Trivedi MH, Wisniewski SR, Nierenberg AA, Stewart JW, Warden D, Niederehe G, Thase ME, Lavori PW, Lebowitz BD, et al. Acute and longer-term outcomes in depressed outpatients requiring one or several treatment steps: a STAR*D report. Am J Psychiatry. 2006;163(11):1905–17.
3. Papakostas GI. Managing partial response or nonresponse: switching, augmentation, and combination strategies for major depressive disorder. J Clin Psychiatry. 2009;70(Suppl 6):16–25.
4. Judd LL, Paulus MJ, Schettler PJ, Akiskal HS, Endicott J, Leon AC, Maser JD, Mueller T, Solomon DA, Keller MB. Does incomplete recovery from first lifetime major depressive episode herald a chronic course of illness? Am J Psychiatry. 2000;157(9):1501–4.
5. Paykel ES, Ramana R, Cooper Z, Hayhurst H, Kerr J, Barocka A. Residual symptoms after partial remission: an important outcome in depression. Psychol Med. 1995;25(6):1171–80.
6. Miller IW, Keitner GI, Schatzberg AF, Klein DN, Thase ME, Rush AJ, Markowitz JC, Schlager DS, Kornstein SG, Davis SM, et al. The treatment of chronic depression, part 3: psychosocial functioning before and after treatment with sertraline or imipramine. J Clin Psychiatry. 1998;59(11):608–19.

7. Chang WH, Lee IH, Chen WT, Chen PS, Yang YK, Chen KC. Coexisting geriatric anxiety and depressive disorders may increase the risk of ischemic heart disease mortality—a nationwide longitudinal cohort study. Int J Geriatr Psychiatry. 2017;32(12):e25–33.
8. Ho C, Jin A, Nyunt MS, Feng L, Ng TP. Mortality rates in major and sub-threshold depression: 10-year follow-up of a Singaporean population cohort of older adults. Postgrad Med. 2016;128(7):642–7.
9. Laforest L, Roche N, Devouassoux G, Belhassen M, Chouaid C, Ginoux M, Van Ganse E. Frequency of comorbidities in chronic obstructive pulmonary disease, and impact on all-cause mortality: a population-based cohort study. Respir Med. 2016;117:33–9.
10. Laursen TM, Musliner KL, Benros ME, Vestergaard M, Munk-Olsen T. Mortality and life expectancy in persons with severe unipolar depression. J Affect Disord. 2016;193:203–7.
11. Mago R, Fagiolini A, Weiller E, Weiss C. Understanding the emotions of patients with inadequate response to antidepressant treatments: results of an international online survey in patients with major depressive disorder. BMC Psychiatry. 2018;18(1):33.
12. Lewis L, Hoofnagle L. Patient perspectives on provider competence: a view from the depression and bipolar support alliance. Adm Policy Ment Health. 2005;32(5–6):497–503.
13. Sheehan DV. The Anxiety Disease. New York: Scribner's; 1983.
14. Anderson C, Roy T. Patient experiences of taking antidepressants for depression: a secondary qualitative analysis. Res Social Adm Pharm. 2013;9(6):884–902.
15. Buus N, Johannessen H, Stage KB. Explanatory models of depression and treatment adherence to antidepressant medication: a qualitative interview study. Int J Nurs Stud. 2012;49(10):1220–9.
16. Battle CL, Uebelacker L, Friedman MA, Cardemil EV, Beevers CG, Miller IW. Treatment goals of depressed outpatients: a qualitative investigation of goals identified by participants in a depression treatment trial. J Psychiatr Pract. 2010;16(6):425–30.
17. Dwight-Johnson M, Sherbourne CD, Liao D, Wells KB. Treatment preferences among depressed primary care patients. J Gen Intern Med. 2000;15(8):527–34.
18. Ruggeri M, Salvi G, Bonetto C, Lasalvia A, Allevi L, Parabiaghi A, Bertani M, Tansella M. Outcome of patients dropping out from community-based mental health care: a 6-year multiwave follow-up study. Acta Psychiatr Scand. 2007;437:42–52.
19. Locke EA, Latham GP. Building a practically useful theory of goal setting and task motivation: a 35-year Odyssey. Am Psychol. 2002;57(9):705–17.

18

Fruits and vegetables intake and its subgroups are related to depression

Elham Baharzadeh[1], Fereydoun Siassi[1*], Mostafa Qorbani[2], Fariba Koohdani[3], Neda Pak[4,5] and Gity Sotoudeh[1*]

Abstract

Background: The association of fruits and vegetables (FV) specific subgroups consumption and depression has not been investigated in healthy adult populations. Therefore, the aim of our study was to determine the relationship between intake of FV as well as their subgroups and depression.

Methods: This cross-sectional study was conducted on 400 women attending healthcare centers. The scores of depression, anxiety, and stress were measured using the 21-item depression, anxiety and stress scales questionnaire. The participants' anthropometric and physical activity data were collected and the 147-item semi-quantitative FFQ was used for estimating the FV intake.

Results: After adjustment for confounding variables, the participants in the lower quartiles of total FV, total vegetables, total fruits, citrus, other fruits and green leafy vegetables intake were more likely to experience depression compared to those in the higher quartiles (p trend < 0.03).

Conclusion: Our findings suggest that higher intake of total FV and some of its specific subgroups might be associated with depression.

Keywords: Depression, Diet, Fruits, Vegetables, Women

Background

According to the World Health Organization's (WHO) report, depression is a common mental disorder. Globally, more than 300 million people of all ages suffer from depression. This disease is a major contributor to the overall burden of disease and is the leading cause of disability worldwide. Women are more affected by depression than men [1]. In Iran, the prevalence of mental disorders is 23.4% (27.5% in women and 19.2% in men), with the prevalence of depression being 10.3% (11.4% in women and 9.3% in men) [2]. Several studies have investigated the relationship between fruits and vegetables (FV)

intake and development of depression, but the results are inconsistent. Cross-sectional studies have reported an inverse association between the consumption of FV and depression [3–7]. Some prospective cohort studies have also found that less FV consumption was associated with a higher risk of depression [8, 9]. A meta-analysis study revealed that consumption of FV is inversely related to the risk of depression [10]. Contrary to these results, some cross-sectional studies did not find any relationship between FV consumption and depression [11–13]. Further, in a prospective cohort study, it was found that only vegetables proved to be protective against symptoms of depression, while this effect was not found for fruits [14]. In some cross-sectional studies, an association was found between high consumption of vegetables [15], green leafy vegetables [16], and lower odds of depression, but no relationship was found for fruits [15, 16]. Nevertheless,

---

*Correspondence: siassif@tums.ac.ir; gsotodeh@tums.ac.ir
[1] Department of Community Nutrition, School of Nutritional Sciences and Dietetics, Tehran University of Medical Sciences, Hojatdost Street, Naderi Street, KeshavarzBlv., Tehran, Iran
Full list of author information is available at the end of the article

for vegetable intake, no association was found in other studies [17, 18].

Oxidative stress [19, 20] and inflammation [21] are directly associated with the chance of depression. FV are rich in antioxidants and anti-inflammatory components, which may have beneficial effects in the prevention of depression [17]. Moreover, in FV, there are vitamins, especially folate, B6, C, E, and minerals, including calcium, iron, magnesium, potassium, dietary fiber and phytochemicals especially polyphenols. Vitamin E, C, and polyphenols, which have antioxidant properties, can reduce the oxidative stress. Most of the mentioned nutrients in FV may reduce inflammation, thereby reducing the risk of depression [22, 23]. In addition, FV-rich diets may increase the level of brain-derived neurotrophic factor (BDNF) which is an important protein for neural development and synaptic plasticity. Its low level will result in low mental health including depression [22].

Subgroups of FV have different contents of nutrients, fiber, antioxidants and phytochemicals [24]. Therefore, they may not affect the risk of depression equally. Therefore, it is better to evaluate individual FV or their specific subgroups.

Although the relationship between the intake of FV and depression has been reported in some studies, the specific subgroups of FV and their possible association with depression in apparently healthy population have remained understudied. A cross-sectional study found an inverse relationship between consumption of tomato, as well as tomato products and depression in elderly population [25]. Another cross-sectional study reported that higher consumption of raw FV predicted better mental health. However, this study was only limited to 18–25-year-old subjects [26]. To the best of our knowledge, apart from the mentioned study, no study has investigated the association of intake of FV subgroups and depression in healthy adult populations. Therefore, the aim of our study was to determine the relationship between the consumption of FV, as well as their specific subgroups and depression.

Methods

Subjects

This cross-sectional study was conducted on 400 women attending eight health centers in Khorramabad, Iran from May to October 2017. The inclusion criteria were ages 20–49 years, at least fifth grade elementary education, and body mass index of 18.5–34.9 kg/m^2. On the other hand, the exclusion criteria were pregnancy and lactation, diagnosis of depression by a psychiatrist within a year prior to the start of the study, currently taking an antidepressant medication or in the past year, and use of tobacco or alcohol at least once a week. Women with

diagnoses such as diabetes, cardiovascular disease, cancer, hypertension, kidney and liver disease, hyperthyroidism, epilepsy and MS, regular use of any medication or following special diet were excluded from the study. The objective and protocol of the study were explained to the participants, and informed consent was obtained from them before the study. The Ethics Committee of Tehran University of Medical Sciences approved the protocol of this study.

Assessment of depression status

The Depression, Anxiety, Stress Scales (DASS, 21-items) questionnaire was used to measure the score of depression. This questionnaire was provided by Lovibond in 1995, which was validated by Afzali et al. for Iran [27, 28]. In the short form of the DASS questionnaire, for each subscale of depression, anxiety and stress, 7 questions have been presented. Individuals responded to each question based on to what extent that item applied to them during the last week (from 0 to 3: not at all, to some degree, to a considerable degree and very much, respectively). The scores on the DASS-21 were multiplied by 2 to calculate the final score. Based on the total score of depression, the subjects were divided into five groups of normal (0–9), mild (10–13), moderate (14–20), severe (21–27), and very severe (> 27) depression. However, due to the limited number of cases in some groups, they were simply divided into two groups of normal (< 10) and depressed (≥ 10) [29].

Anthropometric and physical activity assessment

Weight was measured with minimal clothing and without shoes by a digital scale (Seca 813, Germany) with a measurement accuracy of 100 g. Their height was measured without shoes to the nearest 0.5 cm with a gauge. To calculate the body mass index (BMI), the weight was divided by the square of height (kg/m^2). The International Physical Activity Questionnaire (IPAQ)—short form— was used to assess the physical activity of the participants [30]. Inquiries were made regarding vigorous and moderate activity and walking for at least 10 min/day during the previous 7 days. To calculate the activity, the duration and frequency of activity days were multiplied by the metabolic equivalent task value of the activity. The sum of the scores was calculated as the total physical activity per week.

Dietary assessment

The usual dietary intake during the past year was assessed using a validated semi-quantitative food frequency questionnaire (FFQ) which included 147 food items [31]. In addition, some questions related to local spices and vegetables were added to the questionnaire. Finally, the number of questions reached 161 questions. The participants were asked to report their frequency of consumption of each food item during the previous year on a daily, weekly, or monthly basis. For estimating the daily food intake, the information of the FFQ was converted to g/day. The food items were analyzed for their energy and nutrients content using the Nutritionist IV software (First Databank, San Bruno, CA), modified for Iranian foods. The software database is drawn from United States Department of Agriculture (USDA) [32] food composition tables [33].

FV was divided into specific groups including cruciferous vegetables, green leafy vegetables, other vegetables, berries, citrus fruits, and other fruits based on previous studies [34, 35]. The Healthy Eating Index (HEI-2015) score [36] summarizes the consumption of 13 foods or nutrients including total fruits, whole fruits, total vegetables, greens and beans, whole grains, dairy products,

total protein foods, seafood and plant proteins, fatty acids, refined grains, sodium, added sugars, and saturated fats. Each component was scored on a scale of 0–5 or 0–10. Similar to another study [24], we excluded FV when calculating the HEI score.

Statistical analysis

Data analysis was performed using the SPSS version 16 (SPSS Inc.). The Kolmogorov–Smirnov test was used to evaluate the data normality. The data with an abnormal distribution were logarithmically transformed for statistical analyses. The geometric mean (standard error of mean) was calculated for the transformed data. The independent t test was employed to compare the quantitative variables between the two groups (depressed and healthy subjects). The mean values of the quantitative variables across the FV quartiles were then compared using the ANOVA test. Further, the ANCOVA test

Table 1 Characteristic of study participants according to quartiles of total vegetables and fruits intake

	Quartiles of total vegetables and fruits intake				
	1 (n = 100)	2 (n = 100)	3 (n = 100)	4 (n = 100)	p-trend[a]
g/day (median)	233.9	332.1	378.3	451.6	
Age (years)	33.3 ± 7	34.0 ± 7.7	34.2 ± 7.5	34.1 ± 7.1	0.4
Education (years)	12.1 ± 3.4	12.8 ± 3.1	12.5 ± 3.1	12.4 ± 3.8	0.6
BMI (kg/m²)	25.7 ± 3	26.2 ± 3.36	26.3 ± 2.6	25.5 ± 3	0.7
Physical activity (MET/h/week)	487.4 ± 275.6	473.1 ± 292.5	546.7 ± 247.9	500.7 ± 340.5	0.3
Height (cm)	161.6 ± 4.7	161.5 ± 4.7	161.8 ± 4.1	161.9 ± 4.7	0.5
Weight (kg)	66.8 ± 7.9	67.9 ± 9.6	68.8 ± 7.3	66.4 ± 7.7	0.9
Family size (n)	4.3 ± 1.3	4.5 ± 1.1	4.4 ± 1.3	4.4 ± 1.4	0.7
Dietary supplement use (%)	45 (45%)	49 (49%)	47 (47%)	53 (53%)	0.5[b]
Energy intake (kcal)	1579.6 ± 288.5[c]	1614.5 ± 266	1629.4 ± 289.6	1752.1 ± 355.6	< 0.001
Protein intake (g)	56 ± 9.5[c]	58.7 ± 10.1	59.5 ± 9.7	64.8 ± 11.5	< 0.001
Carbohydrate intake (g)	218.5 ± 47.1[c]	237 ± 44.5	240.1 ± 48.6	261 ± 57.4	< 0.001
Fat intake (g)	52.8 ± 13.7[c]	48 ± 11.3	48 ± 13.1	50.8 ± 15.2	0.003[d]
Energy of protein (%)	14.2 ± 1.2	14.6 ± 1.4	14.6 ± 1.3	14.8 ± 1.4	0.001
Energy of carbohydrate (%)	55.6 ± 5.3	58.9 ± 4.3	59.2 ± 5.2	59.7 ± 4.4	< 0.001[d]
Energy of fat (%)	30.6 ± 5.7	27.1 ± 4.6	27 ± 5.2	26.4 ± 4.5	< 0.001[d]
Total fiber intake (g)	38.9 ± 18.2[c]	42.8 ± 14.4	40.5 ± 16.8	46.8 ± 18.7	< 0.001[d]
Healthy eating index score	46.6 ± 5.3[e]	47 ± 4.8	48.3 ± 6.1	50.4 ± 7.6	< 0.001[d]

Values are means (standard deviations) or percentages unless stated otherwise

Vegetables include white cabbage, red cabbage, broccoli, cauliflower, spinach, lettuce, vegetable greens, carrot, yellow squash, cucumber, tomato, green squash, eggplant, celery, green peas, green beans, garlic, onion, bell peppers, turnip, mushroom, green peppers, olive, corn, leek and artichoke

Fruits include strawberry, blackberry, mulberry, orange, tangerine, sweet lemon, sour lemon, dried berries, grapefruit, cantaloupe, melon, pears, apricot, cherry, apple, plum, peach, persimmon, nectarine, greengage, figs, kiwi fruit, pomegranate, date, plum, sour cherry, banana, apple juice, cantaloupe juice, grapes, raisin, dry peach and apricot, fruit juice

[a] ANOVA

[b] Chi-square test

[c] Geometric mean ± SEM

[d] Kruskal–Wallis test

[e] Median ± interquartile range

was utilized to compare the mean FV intake in the two groups after adjusting for potential confounders including BMI, energy intake, and HEI score. Variables with p value < 0.05 in ANOVA test were selected for adjustment. In addition, based on evidence from the literature, we selected age and physical activity as potential confounders [37]. Total vegetables and total fruits intake were mutually adjusted. For all of the vegetables and fruits sub-groups, FV intake was adjusted.

The relationship between FV intake and odds of depression was analyzed by simple logistic regression. In addition to the unadjusted analysis (Model 1), we used multivariable models to assess the relationship between FV intake and depression (Model 2). In Model 2, we adjusted for age, BMI, physical activity, energy intake, and HEI. Total vegetables and total fruits intake were mutually adjusted. For all of the vegetables and fruits subgroups, other subgroups of FV intake were also adjusted. Tests for trend were performed by introducing the categorical variables as continuous parameters

in the models. p values less than 0.05 were considered significant.

Results

The prevalence of mild, moderate, severe, and very severe depression was 10%, 8.5%, 5.8%, and 1%, respectively. The characteristics of the participants according to the quartiles of intake of total vegetables and fruits are presented in Tables 1, 2, and 3. With elevation of the total FV (Table 1), total vegetables (Table 2) and total fruits (Table 3) quartiles, the subjects had higher intake of energy, protein, carbohydrate, total fiber, percentage of energy from carbohydrate (p trend < 0.04), and lower intake of fat and percentage of energy from fat (p trend < 0.005). Upon increasing the total FV and total vegetables, the subjects had a higher percentage of energy from protein (p-trend < 0.002). In addition, with an elevation of the total FV and total fruits quartiles, the subjects had a higher HEI score (p-trend < 0.001).

Table 2 Characteristic of study participants according to quartiles of total vegetables intake

	Quartiles of total vegetables intake				
	1 (n = 100)	2 (n = 100)	3 (n = 100)	4 (n = 100)	p-trend[a]
g/day (median)	119.6	170.6	200.6	251.7	
Age (years)	34.3 ± 7.5	32.7 ± 7.1	34.3 ± 7.4	34.3 ± 7.1	0.5
Education (years)	12 ± 3.6	13 ± 3	12.7 ± 3.4	12.2 ± 3.4	0.8
BMI (kg/m²)	25.9 ± 3.2	25.6 ± 2.6	25.9 ± 3.1	26.4 ± 3.1	0.1
Physical activity (MET/h/week)	497 ± 292.4	510 ± 273.2	473 ± 256.8	527.8 ± 338.1	0.6
Height (cm)	161.4 ± 4.7	161.7 ± 4.9	162 ± 4.3	161.8 ± 4.4	0.4
Weight (kg)	66.7 ± 7.4	66.9 ± 8	68 ± 9	68.3 ± 8.5	0.1
Family size (n)	4.5 ± 1.2	4.3 ± 1.3	4.4 ± 1.3	4.4 ± 1.2	0.8
Dietary supplement use (%)	50 (50%)	46 (46%)	57 (57%)	41 (41%)	0.5[b]
Energy intake (kcal)	1600.3 ± 276.5[c]	1606.6 ± 289.7	1632.7 ± 274.5	1734.4 ± 366.0	0.001
Protein intake (g)	56.9 ± 9.1[c]	58.0 ± 10.5	59.6 ± 8.9	64.5 ± 12.2	< 0.001
Carbohydrate intake (g)	224.6 ± 50.7[c]	238.4 ± 47.1	240.6 ± 50.1	251.9 ± 56.1	< 0.001
Fat intake (g)	51.7 ± 13.3[c]	47.0 ± 11.5	48.4 ± 11.4	52.7 ± 16.5	0.004[d]
Energy of protein (%)	14.2 ± 1.4	14.5 ± 1.2	14.6 ± 1.2	14.9 ± 1.4	< 0.001
Energy of carbohydrate (%)	56.4 ± 6	59.5 ± 4.2	59.1 ± 4.7	58.3 ± 4.7	< 0.001[d]
Energy of fat (%)	29.7 ± 6.1	26.6 ± 4.3	27.1 ± 5	27.7 ± 5	< 0.001[d]
Total fiber intake (g)	40.8 ± 18.4[c]	42.3 ± 16.8	40.9 ± 17.0	44.7 ± 16.9	0.034[d]
Healthy eating index score	46.9 ± 5.6[e]	48.7 ± 6.6	47.6 ± 4.5	49 ± 7.5	0.06[d]

Values are means (standard deviations) or percentages unless stated otherwise

Total vegetables are defined as in Table 1

[a] ANOVA

[b] Chi-square test

[c] Geometric mean ± SEM

[d] Kruskal–wallis test

[e] Median ± interquartile range

Table 3 Characteristic of study participants according to quartiles of total fruits intake

	Quartiles of total fruits intake				
	1 (*n* = 100)	2 (*n* = 100)	3 (*n* = 100)	4 (*n* = 100)	*p*-trend[b]
g/day (median)	103.7	177.8	229.6	229.6	
Age (years)	34 ± 7.3	33.4 ± 7.7	34.8 ± 6.8	33.4 ± 7.3	0.8
Education (years)	12.1 ± 3.5	12.8 ± 3.1	12.2 ± 3.3	12.7 ± 3.6	0.3
BMI (kg/m²)	26.3 ± 3	25.8 ± 3.1	26 ± 2.7	25.6 ± 3.1	0.1
Physical activity (MET/h/week)	474.7 ± 287.9	495.5 ± 235.7	515.9 ± 282.7	521.8 ± 349.6	0.2
Height (cm)	161.8 ± 4.6	162.1 ± 4.4	161 ± 4.3	161.9 ± 4.9	0.6
Weight (kg)	68.5 ± 8.8	67.6 ± 9	67.1 ± 6.9	66.7 ± 8.1	0.1
Family size (n)	4.3 ± 1.3	4.3 ± 1.2	4.6 ± 1.1	1.4 ± 4.3	0.7
Dietary supplement use (%)	37 (37%)	56 (56%)	42 (42%)	59 (59%)	0.5[c]
Energy intake (kcal)	1603 ± 273.3[d]	1561.3 ± 254.6	1689.6 ± 350.8	1721.8 ± 319.2	0.001
Protein intake (g)	57.0 ± 9.9[d]	57.0 ± 9.6	62.2 ± 11.5	62.8 ± 10.3	0.001
Carbohydrate intake (g)	218.2 ± 45.3[d]	227.9 ± 42.9	250.7 ± 51.2	260.3 ± 55.6	0.001
Fat intake (g)	56.8 ± 12.6[d]	48.2 ± 10.5	50.9 ± 16.4	49.6 ± 12.6	< 0.001[e]
Energy of protein (%)	14.3 ± 1.4	14.6 ± 1.3	14.7 ± 1.1	14.6 ± 1.4	0.051
Energy of carbohydrate (%)	54.7 ± 5	58.5 ± 4.2	59.5 ± 4.5	60.6 ± 4.5	< 0.001[e]
Energy of fat (%)	31.6 ± 5.6	27.5 ± 4.5	26.4 ± 4.5	25.6 ± 4.4	< 0.001[e]
Total fiber intake (g)	42.7 ± 16.4[d]	43.5 ± 15.7	45.6 ± 16.3	50.6 ± 19.6	< 0.001[e]
Healthy eating index score	47.1 ± 5.3[f]	46.6 ± 4.7	47.4 ± 6.9	50.4 ± 6.0	< 0.001[e]

Values are means (standard deviations) or percentages unless stated otherwise

Total fruits were defined as in Table 1

[a] ANOVA

[b] Chi square test

[c] Geometric mean ± SEM

[d] Kruskal–Wallis test

[e] Median ± interquartile range

The comparison of FV intake between depressed and healthy subjects is presented in Table 4. The intake of total FV and all of their subgroups were significantly lower in depressed subjects as compared to their healthy counterparts (*p* < 0.02). After adjustment for confounding variables, these differences remained significant for total FV, total vegetables, cruciferous vegetables, other vegetables, total fruits, citrus fruits, and other fruits (*p* < 0.02).

The odds ratio (OR) of depression across quartiles of FV intake, before and after adjustment for confounding factors, is presented in two different models in Table 5. Before adjusting the confounders, the subjects in the lowest quartile of total FV intake and its all subgroups had a higher OR of depression compared with those in the highest quartile (*p* trend < 0.04). After adjusting for confounders, the participants in the lowest quartile of total FV, total vegetables, total fruits, citrus, other fruits and green leafy vegetables had a higher OR of depression compared with those in the highest quartile

(*p*-trend < 0.03). Finally, the participants in the first quartile of berries (*p* = 0.01) had a higher OR compared with those in the highest quartile. However, no dose–response relationship was observed.

Discussion

This study examined the relationship between the intake of various FV and depression among apparently healthy women. The results of this study suggested that a high intake of total FV, total vegetables, total fruits, citrus, other fruits and green leafy vegetables was independently related to a lower OR of depression. In addition, berries were inversely associated with depression, although no clear dose–response relationship was found.

Studies conducted to investigate the relationship between specific subgroups of FV and depression are very limited and there is no study in healthy adult populations. Our study provided evidence supporting benefits

Table 4 Fruits and vegetables intake across depressed and healthy subjects

Daily intake (g)	Depressed (n = 101) Mean ± SD	Healthy (n = 299) Mean ± SD	p^a	p^b	p^c
Total vegetables and fruits	289.1 ± 104.7	373.2 ± 76.4	< 0.001	< 0.001	< 0.001
Total vegetables	160.2 ± 69.1	197.1 ± 54.9	< 0.001[d]	< 0.001	< 0.001
Cruciferous vegetables	4.0 ± 5.0	6.5 ± 6.5	< 0.001[d]	< 0.001	0.005
Green leafy vegetables	16.3 ± 13.9[e]	23.9 ± 12.6	< 0.001	< 0.001	0.06
Dark yellow vegetables	5.1 ± 4.1	6.2 ± 4.5	0.01	0.011	0.1
Other vegetables	130.6 ± 55.2	157.9 ± 45.4	< 0.001[d]	< 0.001	0.016
Total fruits	118.5 ± 53.7[e]	170.6 ± 48.6	< 0.001	< 0.001	< 0.001
Berries fruits	0.5 ± 0.5	0.8 ± 0.6	< 0.001[d]	< 0.001	0.1
Citrus fruits	25.3 ± 12.5	35.2 ± 10.9	< 0.001[d]	< 0.001	< 0.001
Other fruits	93.8 ± 45.9[e]	134.4 ± 44.5	< 0.001	< 0.001	< 0.001

Total vegetables and fruits are defined as in Table 1

Cruciferous vegetables include white cabbage, red cabbage, broccoli, cauliflower

Green leafy vegetables include spinach, lettuce, and green vegetables such as basil, parsley, cress, leek, spearmint, origany, coriander and scallion

Dark yellow vegetables include carrot, yellow squash

Other vegetables include cucumber, tomato, zucchini, eggplant, celery, green pea, green bean, garlic, onion, green pepper, bell peppers, turnip, mushroom, olive, corn and artichoke

Berries fruits include strawberry, white mulberry black mulberry and dried berries

Citrus fruits include orange, tangerine, grapefruits, sweet lemon, sour lemon, orange juice

Other fruits include cantaloupe, melon, pear, apricot, cherry, apple, peach, nectarine, greengage, fig, kiwi fruit, persimmon, pomegranate, date, plum, sour cherry, banana, pineapple, grapes, dry peach and apricot, raisin and fruit juice

Values are means (standard deviations)

[a] Unadjusted, Student t test

[b] Adjusted for energy intake; ANCOVA test

[c] Adjusted for age, body mass index, physical activity, energy intake and healthy eating index score. Total vegetables and total fruits intake were mutually adjusted. For each vegetables and fruits sub-groups, total fruits and vegetables intake was adjusted; ANCOVA test

[d] Mann–Withney test

[e] Geometric mean ± SEM

of consuming citrus, other fruits, green leafy vegetables and to a lesser extent berries.

Our findings are consistent with the results of other studies, suggesting an inverse relationship between FV consumption and depression. Cross-sectional studies [3–5, 7] and some prospective cohort studies [8, 9] have suggested that lower FV consumption was associated with a higher risk of depression. In addition, the inverse relationship between depression and fruits [9, 17, 18, 38] or vegetables [9, 15, 39, 40] consumptions has been separately indicated. A meta-analysis study indicated that intakes of both fruits and vegetables were inversely related to the risk of depression [10]. In subgroup analysis by the study design, higher fruits intake was associated to lower risk of depression in both cross-sectional and cohort studies. However, the association between higher vegetable intake and lower risk of depression was found in only cohort studies [11]. Contrary to these studies, the association between depression and FV intake or fruits and vegetables individually was not shown in other studies [3, 12–15, 17, 18, 32, 41, 42].

In some cross-sectional studies in elderly subjects, there was an association between high consumption of green leafy vegetables [16] as well as tomato and tomato products [25] and lower odds of depression. A case–control study which compared consumptions of food groups between depressed and healthy women revealed that subjects with more intake of citrus, berries, melons, other fruits, green leafy vegetables, yellow vegetables, and other vegetables had a lower chance of developing depression [43]. Since these are findings from a case–control study, the possibility that depression may influence the FV intake of subjects cannot be ruled out. In addition, other dietary components have not been controlled either.

Relevant data from clinical trials are scarce. Dietary improvements including increasing fruits and vegetables intake in patients with depression reduced the symptoms of depression [44]. However, in some other studies, higher intake of FV [45], concord grape juice [46] and blueberry juice [45] supplementation did not improve depression.

Table 5 Odds ratio (95% CI) of depression according to quartiles (Q) of fruits and vegetables intake

Daily intake	Q1	Q2	Q3	Q4	p-trend*
Total vegetables and fruits g/day (median)	233.9	332.1	378.3	451.6	
Cases of depressed	55	19	17	10	
Model 1 p	11 (5.12–23.59) <0.001	2.1 (0.92–4.8) 0.07	1.84 (0.79–4.25) 0.1	1	<0.001
Model 2 p	18.83 (7.96–44.51) <0.001	2.98 (1.23–7.2) 0.01	2.47 (1.02–5.96) 0.04	1	<0.001
Total vegetables g/day (median)	125.4	176.6	203.2	245.8	
Cases of depressed	54	16	14	17	
Model 1 p	5.73 (2.98–11.01) <0.001	0.93 (0.44–1.96) 0.8	0.79 (0.36–1.71) 0.5	1	<0.001
Model 2 p	4.43 (2.06–9.51) <0.001	1.14 (0.50–2.59) 0.7	1.07 (0.46–2.5) 0.8	1	0.001
Cruciferous vegetables g/day (median)	2.5	3.1	6.2	6.2	
Cases of depressed	44	24	22	11	
Model 1 p	4.92 (2.33–10.42) <0.001	1.79 (0.82–3.91) 0.1	1.53 (0.69–3.37) 0.2	1	0.001
Model 2 p	1.6 (0.57–4.48) 0.3	0.94 (0.34–2.55) 0.9	1.29 (0.52–3.21) 0.5	1	0.6
Green leafy vegetables g/day (median)	14.3	21.6	24.8	31.6	
Cases of depressed	49	17	15	20	
Model 1 p	3.84 (2.05–7.19) <0.001	0.81 (0.4–1.67) 0.5	0.7 (0.33–1.47) 0.3	1	<0.001
Model 2 p	1.61 (0.64–4.02) 0.3	0.55 (0.22–1.35) 0.1	0.58 (0.24–1.4) 0.2	1	0.02
Dark yellow vegetables g/day (median)	2.1	4.3	5.7	7.7	
Cases of depressed	34	25	20	22	
Model 1 p	1.82 (0.97–3.42) 0.06	1.18 (0.61–2.27) 0.6	0.88 (0.44–1.57) 0.7	1	0.03
Model 2 P	0.45 (0.18–1.09) 0.07	0.61 (0.26–1.41) 0.2	0.68 (0.3–1.53) 0.3	1	0.2
Other vegetables g/day (median)	102.7	144.6	166.2	190.3	
Cases of depressed	49	24	9	19	
Model 1 p	4.09 (2.17–7.73) <0.001	1.34 (0.68–2.65) 0.3	0.42 (0.18–0.98) 0.04	1	<0.001
Model 2 p	2.05 (0.88–4.79) 0.09	1.43 (0.64–3.23) 0.3	0.5 (0.19–1.33) 0.1	1	0.07
Total fruits g/day (median)	108.3	155.6	180	209.2	
Cases of depressed	58	17	14	12	
Model 1 p	10.12 (4.91–20.85) <0.001	1.5 (0.67–3.33) 0.3	1.19 (0.52–2.72) 0.6	1	<0.001
Model 2 p	11.08 (4.96–24.75) <0.001	2.12 (0.90–5.01) 0.08	1.27 (0.54–2.99) 0.5	1	<0.001
Berries fruits g/day (median)	0.4	0.5	0.3	0.6	
Cases of depressed	53	20	12	16	
Model 1 p	5.72 (2.95–11.11) <0.001	1.33 (0.64–2.75) 0.4	0.69 (0.30–1.54) 0.3	1	0.001
Model 2 p	2.77 (1.24–6.18) 0.01	0.81 (0.34–1.91) 0.6	0.68 (0.27–1.68) 0.4	1	0.3

Table 5 (continued)

Daily intake	Q1	Q2	Q3	Q4	p-trend*
Citrus fruits g/day (median)	24.7	34.3	36.4	37.6	
Cases of depressed	55	22	12	12	
Model 1 p	8.96 (4.36–18.42) <0.001	2.06 (0.96–4.45) 0.06	1 (0.42–2.34) 1	1	<0.001
Model 2 p	3.14 (1.34–7.38) 0.008	1.27 (0.53–3.04) 0.5	0.68 (0.27–1.74) 0.4	1	0.004
Other fruits g/day (median)	85.1	121.1	141	167.4	
Cases of depressed	55	19	14	13	
Model 1 p	8.17 (4.04–16.52) <0.001	1.57 (0.72–3.38) 0.2	1.08 (0.48–2.45) 0.8	1	<0.001
Model 2 p	4.93 (1.97–12.31) 0.001	1.61 (0.67–3.89) 0.2	1.03 (0.43–2.51) 0.9	1	<0.001

Model 1: unadjusted

Model 2: adjusted for age, body mass index, physical activity, energy intake and healthy eating index. Total vegetables and total fruits intake were mutually adjusted. For each vegetables and fruits sub-groups, other sub-groups of fruits and vegetables intake was adjusted

Fruits and vegetables are defined as in Tables 1 and 4

* Tests for trend were performed by entering the categorical variables as continuous parameters in the models

The biological mechanisms for the inverse association of FV intake and depression are not clear.

However, this association may be due to the large amount of bioactive compounds present in FV [24]. FV have a high content of micronutrients and phytochemicals including antioxidants and anti-inflammatory components which have detrimental effects on depression [17]. Antioxidants such as carotenoids, vitamin C, and vitamin E might prevent depressive symptoms [42]. High intake of B vitamins such as folic acid have been associated with lower risk of depression [47]. FV also supplies dietary fiber whose role in improving mood has been suggested [48]. Green leafy vegetables are good sources of folate and magnesium which are important in the prevention of depression. Folate is involved in the metabolism of monoamines such as serotonin in the brain [42]. Reduced synthesis of serotonin results to depressed mood [49]. In magnesium deficiency, high levels of calcium and glutamate reduce synaptic function and lead to depression [50]. In addition, lower levels of C-reactive protein, a marker of low-grade inflammation, has been reported in magnesium sufficiency [22]. In a study on rats, it was found that tomato juice inhibited monoamine oxidase (MAO) enzyme. This result suggested the anti-depressant properties of tomato [51]. In addition, Aronia melanocarpa berry juice with the highest polyphenol contents among fruits could yield an antidepressant effect in rats [52]. A study found that heptamethoxy flavone (HMF), a citrus flavonoid, increases the expression of BDNF in the hippocampus in rats, thereby exerting anti-depressant effects [53].

Women who were included in the present study were not informed of their depression status, which is one of the strengths of this study. When subjects are aware of their depression disorder, they might change their food intake. Another strength of our study was the adjustment for many confounding variables, especially the overall quality of diet. However, this study was limited in some aspects. First, there is a probability of error in answering FFQ questions. The reliability and validity of the utilized FFQ were not assessed for this population. Second, although we adjusted for many confounding variables, there may still be residual confounding variables which would affect our results. In addition, as with all cross-sectional studies, the present study reveals the existence or the absence of a relationship, while it does not specify causality. Further, FV-rich diets have been accompanied by a healthy lifestyle which may have not been adjusted in our analysis. Finally, our findings may not be generalized to other populations.

Conclusions

In conclusion, we found that higher consumption of total FV, total vegetables, total fruits, citrus, other fruits, green leafy vegetables and berries might be associated with a lower OR of depression. The findings from this study support encouragement of FV consumption as part of a healthy diet and highlight the importance of FV consumption and a number of their subgroups in mitigating the chance of depression. Further studies focusing specifically on FV subgroups are required to confirm these findings.

Abbreviations
FV: fruits and vegetables; BDNF: brain-derived neurotrophic factor; BMI: body mass index; DASS: Depression Anxiety Stress Scale; FFQ: food frequency questionnaire; WHO: World Health Organization; IPAQ: international physical activity questionnaire; HEI: healthy eating index; OR: odds ratio; MAO: monoamine oxidase; HMF: heptamethoxy flavone.

Authors' contributions
The authors' contributions are as follows: FS and GS conceived and developed the idea for the paper and revised the manuscript; EB contributed to data collection and wrote numerous drafts; MQ, FK and NP contributed to data analysis and interpretation of the data. All authors read and approved the final manuscript.

Author details
[1] Department of Community Nutrition, School of Nutritional Sciences and Dietetics, Tehran University of Medical Sciences, Hojatdost Street, Naderi Street, KeshavarzBlv., Tehran, Iran. [2] Non-communicable Diseases Research Center, Alborz University of Medical Sciences, Karaj, Iran. [3] Department of Cellular, Molecular Nutrition, School of Nutritional Sciences and Dietetics, Tehran University of Medical Sciences, Tehran, Iran. [4] Shariati Hospital, School of Medicine, Tehran University of Medical Sciences, Tehran, Iran. [5] Children Hospital of Excellence, School of Medicine, Tehran University of Medical Sciences, Tehran, Iran.

Acknowledgements
The authors thank the support of Lorestan University of Medical Sciences (LUMS).

Competing interests
The authors declare that they have no competing interests.

Consent for publication
Not applicable.

Funding
This research project was supported by Tehran University of Medical Sciences (TUMS) (Grant No. 96-450-18).

References
1. WHO (The World Health Organization). Depression. http://www.who.int/mediacentre/factsheets/fs369/en/. Accessed Jun 2017.
2. Noorbala AA, Faghihzadeh S, Kamali K, Bagheri Yazdi SA, Hajebi A, Mousavi MT, Akhondzadeh S, Faghihzadeh E, Nouri B. Mental Health Survey of the Iranian Adult Population in 2015. Arch Iran Med (AIM). 2017;20:3.
3. McMartin SE, Jacka FN, Colman I. The association between fruit and vegetable consumption and mental health disorders: evidence from five waves of a national survey of Canadians. Prev Med. 2013;56(3):225–30.
4. Poorrezaeian M, Siassi F, Milajerdi A, Qorbani M, Karimi J, Sohrabi-Kabi R, Pak N, Sotoudeh G. Depression is related to dietary diversity score in women: a cross-sectional study from a developing country. Ann Gen Psychiatry. 2017;16(1):39.
5. Payne ME, Steck SE, George RR, Steffens DC. Fruit, vegetable, and antioxidant intakes are lower in older adults with depression. J Acad Nutr Diet. 2012;112(12):2022–7.
6. Bishwajit G, O'Leary DP, Ghosh S, Sanni Y, Shangfeng T, Zhanchun F. Association between depression and fruit and vegetable consumption among adults in South Asia. BMC Psychiatry. 2017;17(1):15.
7. Saghafian F, Malmir H, Saneei P, Keshteli AH, Hosseinzadeh-Attar MJ, Afshar H, Siassi F, Esmaillzadeh A, Adibi P. Consumption of fruit and vegetables in relation with psychological disorders in Iranian adults. Eur J Nutr. 2018;57(6):2295–306.
8. Lai JS, Hure AJ, Oldmeadow C, McEvoy M, Byles J, Attia J. Prospective study on the association between diet quality and depression in mid-aged women over 9 years. Eur J Nutr. 2017;56(1):273–81.
9. Gangwisch JE, Hale L, Garcia L, Malaspina D, Opler MG, Payne ME, Rossom RC, Lane D. High glycemic index diet as a risk factor for depression: analyses from the Women's Health Initiative. Am J Clin Nutr. 2015. https://doi.org/10.3945/ajcn103846
10. Liu X, Yan Y, Li F, Zhang D. Fruit and vegetable consumption and the risk of depression: a meta-analysis. Nutrition. 2016;32(3):296–302.
11. Fulkerson JA, Sherwood NE, Perry CL, Neumark-Sztainer D, Story M. Depressive symptoms and adolescent eating and health behaviors: a multifaceted view in a population-based sample. Prev Med. 2004;38(6):865–75.
12. Mistry R, McCarthy WJ, Yancey AK, Lu Y, Patel M. Resilience and patterns of health risk behaviors in California adolescents. Prev Med. 2009;48(3):291–7.
13. Meegan AP, Perry IJ, Phillips CM. The association between dietary quality and dietary guideline adherence with mental health outcomes in adults: a cross-sectional analysis. Nutrients. 2017;9(3):238.
14. Tsai AC, Chang T-L, Chi S-H. Frequent consumption of vegetables predicts lower risk of depression in older Taiwanese–results of a prospective population-based study. Public Health Nutr. 2012;15(6):1087–92.
15. Woo J, Lynn H, Lau W, Leung J, Lau E, Wong S, Kwok T. Nutrient intake and psychological health in an elderly Chinese population. Int J Geriatr Psychiatry. 2006;21(11):1036–43.
16. Mamplekou E, Bountziouka V, Psaltopoulou T, Zeimbekis A, Tsakoundakis N, Papaerakleous N, Gotsis E, Metallinos G, Pounis G, Polychronopoulos E. Urban environment, physical inactivity and unhealthy dietary habits correlate to depression among elderly living in eastern Mediterranean islands: the MEDIS (MEDiterranean ISlands Elderly) study. J Nutr Health Aging. 2010;14(6):449–55.
17. Mihrshahi S, Dobson A, Mishra G. Fruit and vegetable consumption and prevalence and incidence of depressive symptoms in mid-age women: results from the Australian longitudinal study on women's health. Eur J Clin Nutr. 2015;69(5):585–91.
18. Sánchez-Villegas A, Delgado-Rodríguez M, Alonso A, Schlatter J, Lahortiga F, Majem LS, Martínez-González MA. Association of the Mediterranean dietary pattern with the incidence of depression: the Seguimiento Universidad de Navarra/University of Navarra follow-up (SUN) cohort. Arch Gen Psychiatry. 2009;66(10):1090–8.
19. Perez-Cornago A, Lopez-Legarrea P, de la Iglesia R, Lahortiga F, Martinez JA, Zulet MA. Longitudinal relationship of diet and oxidative stress with depressive symptoms in patients with metabolic syndrome after following a weight loss treatment: the RESMENA project. Clin Nutr. 2014;33(6):1061–7.
20. Black C, Penninx B, Bot M, Odegaard A, Gross M, Matthews K, Jacobs D. Oxidative stress, anti-oxidants and the cross-sectional and longitudinal association with depressive symptoms: results from the CARDIA study. Transl Psychiatry. 2016;6(2):e743.
21. Howren MB, Lamkin DM, Suls J. Associations of depression with C-reactive protein, IL-1, and IL-6: a meta-analysis. Psychosom Med. 2009;71(2):171–86.
22. Rooney C, McKinley MC, Woodside JV. The potential role of fruit and vegetables in aspects of psychological well-being: a review of the literature and future directions. Pro Nutr Soc. 2013;72(4):420–32.
23. Black CN, Bot M, Scheffer PG, Cuijpers P, Penninx BWJH. Is depression associated with increased oxidative stress? A systematic review and meta-analysis. Psychoneuroendocrinology. 2015;51:164–75.
24. Muraki I, Imamura F, Manson JE, Hu FB, Willett WC, van Dam RM, Sun Q. Fruit consumption and risk of type 2 diabetes: results from three prospective longitudinal cohort studies. Br Med J. 2013;347:f5001.
25. Niu K, Guo H, Kakizaki M, Cui Y, Ohmori-Matsuda K, Guan L, Hozawa A, Kuriyama S, Tsuboya T, Ohrui T. A tomato-rich diet is related to depressive symptoms among an elderly population aged 70 years and over: a population-based, cross-sectional analysis. J Affect Disord. 2013;144(1):165–70.
26. Brookie KL, Best GI, Conner TS. Intake of raw fruits and vegetables is associated with better mental health than intake of processed fruits and vegetables. Front Psychol. 2018;9:487.
27. Afzali A, Delavar A, Borjali A, Mirzamani M. Psychometric properties of DASS 42 as assessed in a sample of Kermanshah High School students. J Res Behav Sci. 2007;5(2):81–92.
28. Lovibond S, Lovibond P. Manual for the Depression Anxiety Stress Scale. Sydney: Psychological Foundation of Australia; 1995.
29. UNSW. Depression Anxiety and Stress Scale (DASS). http://www.psy.unsw.edu.au/groups. Accessed Dec 2017.
30. Committee IR. Guidelines for data processing and analysis of the International Physical Activity Questionnaire (IPAQ)–short and long forms. Retrieved September 2005, 17: 2008.

31. Esfahani FH, Asghari G, Mirmiran P, Azizi F. Reproducibility and relative validity of food group intake in a food frequency questionnaire developed for the Tehran Lipid and Glucose Study. J Epidemiol. 2010;20(2):150–8.

32. National Nutrient Database for Standard Reference. United States Department of Agricultural. 2015. https://ndb.nal.usda.gov/ndb/. Accessed Dec 2017.

33. Sánchez-Villegas A, Verberne L, De Irala J, Ruíz-Canela M, Toledo E, Serra-Majem L, Martínez-González MA. Dietary fat intake and the risk of depression: the SUN Project. PLoS ONE. 2011;6(1):e16268.

34. Liu S, Manson JE, Lee IM, Cole SR, Hennekens CH, Willett WC, Buring JE. Fruit and vegetable intake and risk of cardiovascular disease: the Women's Health Study. Am J Clin Nutr. 2000;72(4):922–8.

35. Liu S, Serdula M, Janket S-J, Cook NR, Sesso HD, Willett WC, Manson JE, Buring JE. A prospective study of fruit and vegetable intake and the risk of type 2 diabetes in women. Diabetes Care. 2004;27(12):2993–6.

36. Overview & Background of The Healthy Eating Index. National Cancer Institute. 2015. https://epi.grants.cancer.gov/hei/. Accessed Dec 2017.

37. Nooyens AC, Bueno-de-Mesquita HB, van Boxtel MP, van Gelder BM, Verhagen H, Verschuren WM. Fruit and vegetable intake and cognitive decline in middle-aged men and women: the Doetinchem Cohort Study. Br J Nutr. 2011;106(5):752–61.

38. Liu C, Xie B, Chou C-P, Koprowski C, Zhou D, Palmer P, Sun P, Guo Q, Duan L, Sun X. Perceived stress, depression and food consumption frequency in the college students of China Seven Cities. Physiol Behav. 2007;92(4):748–54.

39. Shahar S, Hassan J, Sundar VV, Kong AYW, Chin SP, Ahmad SA, Lee LK. Determinants of depression and insomnia among institutionalized elderly people in Malaysia. Asian J Psychiatry. 2011;4(3):188–95.

40. Ribeiro SM, Malmstrom TK, Morley JE, Miller DK. Fruit and vegetable intake, physical activity, and depressive symptoms in the African American Health (AAH) study. J Affect Disord. 2017;220:31–7.

41. Hintikka J, Tolmunen T, Honkalampi K, Haatainen K, Koivumaa-Honkanen H, Tanskanen A, Viinamäki H. Daily tea drinking is associated with a low level of depressive symptoms in the Finnish general population. Eur J Epidemiol. 2005;20(4):359–63.

42. Chi SH, Wang JY, Tsai AC. Combined association of leisure-time physical activity and fruit and vegetable consumption with depressive symptoms in older Taiwanese: results of a national cohort study. Geriatr gerontol Int. 2016;16(2):244–51.

43. Kargarnovin Z, Pourghassem Gargari B, Ranjbar F, Rashidkhani B, Zareiy S, Hosein Poor S, Nasiri Z. The association of food groups with major depression in adult women resident in tabriz. Urmia Med J. 2014;24(11):872–82.

44. Jacka FN, O'Neil A, Opie R, Itsiopoulos C, Cotton S, Mohebbi M, Castle D, Dash S, Mihalopoulos C, Chatterton ML. A randomised controlled trial of dietary improvement for adults with major depression (the 'SMILES' trial). BMC Med. 2017;15(1):23.

45. Krikorian R, Shidler MD, Nash TA, Kalt W, Vinqvist-Tymchuk MR, Shukitt-Hale B, Joseph JA. Blueberry supplementation improves memory in older adults. J Agric Food Chem. 2010;58(7):3996–4000.

46. Krikorian R, Nash TA, Shidler MD, Shukitt-Hale B, Joseph JA. Concord grape juice supplementation improves memory function in older adults with mild cognitive impairment. Br J Nutr. 2010;103(5):730–4.

47. Skarupski KA, Tangney C, Li H, Ouyang B, Evans DA, Morris MC. Longitudinal association of vitamin B-6, folate, and vitamin B-12 with depressive symptoms among older adults over time. Am J Clin Nutr. 2010;92(2):330–5.

48. Kaczmarczyk MM, Miller MJ, Freund GG. The health benefits of dietary fiber: beyond the usual suspects of type 2 diabetes mellitus, cardiovascular disease and colon cancer. Metabolism. 2012;61(8):1058–66.

49. Mayeux R, Stern Y, Cote L, Williams JB. Altered serotonin metabolism in depressed patients with Parkinson's disease. Neurology. 1984;34(5):642.

50. Tarleton EK, Littenberg B, MacLean CD, Kennedy AG, Daley C. Role of magnesium supplementation in the treatment of depression: a randomized clinical trial. PLoS ONE. 2017;12(6):e0180067.

51. Milind P, Suman M. Eat tomato a day to keep depression at bay. Asian J Biol Sci. 2009;4(2):258–62.

52. Tomić M, Ignjatović Đ, Tovilović-Kovačević G, Krstić-Milošević D, Ranković S, Popović T, Glibetić M. Reduction of anxiety-like and depression-like behaviors in rats after one month of drinking Aronia melanocarpa berry juice. Food Funct. 2016;7(7):3111–20.

53. Sawamoto A, Okuyama S, Yamamoto K, Amakura Y, Yoshimura M, Nakajima M, Furukawa Y. 3,5,6,7,8,3',4'-heptamethoxyflavone, a citrus flavonoid, ameliorates corticosterone-induced depression-like behavior and restores brain-derived neurotrophic factor expression, neurogenesis, and neuroplasticity in the hippocampus. Molecules (Basel, Switzerland). 2016;21(4):541.

19

The relation between immunologic variables and symptom factors in patients with major depressive disorder

Yang-Whan Jeon, Sang-Ick Han and E. Jin Park*[ID]

Abstract

Background: The associations between depression and immunity were investigated by measuring the scores of Hamilton Rating Scale for Depression (HRSD) and peripheral lymphocyte parameters in patients with major depressive disorder (MDD).

Methods: Forty-nine patients with MDD were recruited and their clinical symptoms are evaluated with 17-item HRSD which was factorized using the confirmatory factor analysis (i.e., depression factor, insomnia factor, and anxiety factor). Basic immunologic variables such as CD4, CD8, and CD56-positive cell numbers were measured by flow cytometry. Natural killer cell activity (NKCA) was also assessed by ELISA method using K-562 cells as target cells. All patients were treated for 4 weeks with selective serotonin reuptake inhibitors. Immunologic and clinical variables were measured both at baseline and after medication.

Results: CD8-positive cell number was increased ($p < .05$) and CD4/CD8 ratio was decreased ($p < .01$) after medication. NKCA showed a significant positive correlation with anxiety factor scores of HRSD ($p < .05$) at baseline. However, except NKCA, there was no correlation between other immunologic measures and symptom factors.

Conclusion: These results suggest that immunologic measure such as NKCA may be an important variable for symptom of MDD such as anxiety during acute depressive state.

Keywords: Major depressive disorder, Immunologic variables, Anxiety, Selective serotonin reuptake inhibitor

Introduction

Major depressive disorder (MDD) is one of the most common mental disorders. 10–25% of women and 5–10% of men may become susceptible to the condition once or more in their life [1]. Patients with MDD have a mortality rate over twice higher than normal and MDD is also known as a risk factor that can increase the morbidity of various medical diseases [2, 3]. Many researchers have demonstrated that changes of immune functions may play an important role in increasing mortality and morbidity among patients with MDD [4, 5].

However, there were controversial reports on immune functions in patients with MDD: immunosuppression or activation of the immune system [6, 7]. Several methods had been used to measure lymphocytes, determine how the lymphocytes function, and assess markers of immune activity in patients with MDD. There were different reports on the number of lymphocytes: the number of lymphocytes or natural killer (NK) cells has increased, decreased, or unchanged [8–12]. The functions of lymphocytes have been assessed on the basis of lymphocyte proliferation by mitogen stimulation, NK cell activity (NKCA), and the cytokine secretion. Many researchers have reported that lymphocyte proliferation by mitogen was decreased and a consistent decrease in NKCA in patients with MDD [9, 13]. However, no consistent report has been made on the number of lymphocytes in patients

*Correspondence: zahir@catholic.ac.kr
Department of Psychiatry, College of Medicine, Incheon St. Mary's Hospital, The Catholic University of Korea, 56 Dongsu-ro, Bupyeong-gu, Incheon 21431, South Korea

with MDD and limited research has been conducted on their immune functions in Korea.

These controversial results are probably due to inter-relationship with the immune system and heterogeneity among patients with MDD. The patients with MDD diagnosed according to the criteria in the fourth edition of the diagnostic and statistical manual of mental disorders (DSM-IV) are not identical to one another but show quite different clinical symptoms [14]. For this reason, many researchers have tried to categorize MDD according to the aspect of melancholy or the subtype of accompanying symptoms in examining the immune system [15, 16]. It is, therefore, necessary to classify a diversity of clinical symptoms of MDD in valid way. This study employed the 17-item Hamilton Rating Scale for Depression (HRSD), which has been widely used in clinical practice and research, to examine immune functions in patients with MDD in terms of those symptom factors divided by confirmational factor analysis [17]. Many studies have examined the factor structure of the HDRS, with the original 17-item version of the scale being the most studied. Though some evidence of a relatively stable factor has been provided, not all studies of the 17-item scale factor support this finding [17–23].

As the literature review found that fluoxetine, a selective serotonin reuptake inhibitor (SSRI), was effective in restoring T cells negatively affected by stress and that NK cells became more active as depressive symptoms improved, an attempt was made to investigate immunologic variables before and after medication in patients with MDD [24–26].

This study aimed to examine immunologic changes by SSRI in patients with MDD and determine correlation between the symptom factors in HRSD and the immunologic variables. We hypothesized that immunologic variables would change after medication and some symptom factors would be correlated with immunologic variables.

Methods

Subjects and symptom assessment

This study was conducted in 49 outpatients diagnosed with MDD at the department of psychiatry, Incheon St. Mary's Hospital in the Catholic University of Korea. Diagnosis of MDD was confirmed by structured clinical interview for DSM-IV by two psychiatrists (EJP and SIH) [27]. The subjects were treated with SSRIs and doses of SSRIs varied depending on patients' symptom improvement and side effects. Those who were at high risk of committing suicide or had psychotic symptoms, who had history of bipolar disorder, drug or alcohol dependence, schizophrenia, or other psychotic disorders, and who had a history of taking medication on a current episode of MDD within a month were excluded. Patients

with abnormal findings in a battery of clinical laboratory test (including urine analysis, complete blood count, renal and liver function test, mineral panel, thyroid indices, chest X-ray, and electrocardiogram) were excluded. Those who had suffered from an immunologic disease or a malignant tumor were also excluded. In addition, those who had taken any other medicine during the 4 week period of treatment or who were found to have suffered from a cold or symptoms of inflammation by medical history or physical examinations were excluded. 17-item HRSD was used to assess the symptoms of MDD in the subjects at baseline and after 4 week treatment. HRSD was applied by trained psychiatric residents. EJP had trained the residents for interrater reliability using video recordings of ten cases of patients with MDD. This study was conducted with the approval of the Institutional Review Board of Incheon St. Mary's Hospital, the Catholic University of Korea (IRB number OCMC07MI002) and all the participants were given a full explanation of its purpose before they made a written consent. The participants signed the consent form accepting to participate and also for permission to published.

Flow cytometry

A peripheral blood sample was taken from each subject at baseline and after 4 week treatment. The peripheral blood was treated with EDTA for flow cytometric analysis. All the tests were performed within 4 h after sampling and each sample was stored at room temperature (18–20 °C) before the analysis. To examine the immune status of the subjects, CD4-positive (helper T cell), CD8-positive (suppressor T cell), and CD56-positive cells (NK cell) were counted in the following way: 50 μL of the whole blood sample treated with EDTA was mixed with 5 μL of an antibody to each antigen (PE-CY5 conjugated mouse anti-human CD3, FITC conjugated mouse anti-human CD4, PE conjugated mouse anti-human CD8, and PE conjugated mouse anti-human CD56) (Immunotech, Marseille, France); then, each mixture was incubated in a darkroom for 30 min. Erythrocytes were then lysed by incubation in 2 mL of lysing solution (Immunotech, Marseille, France) and the sediments were washed in phosphate-buffered saline. Fluorescence was analyzed by flow cytometry (FACScan, Becton–Dickinson, CA, USA). Staining of CD3, CD4, and CD8 was performed by triple stain, and each positive population of CD4 and CD8 was separated from the gating cells with CD3-positive lymphocytes. CD56 were stained with a single preparation. Isotype controls (Immunotech, Marseille, France) were stained as the negative control, and the percentage of positive signal group in the gated lymphocytes was calculated.

Assessment of natural killer cell activity

To determine the cytotoxic activity of NK cells on the K-562 tumor cell line (ATCC, Rockville, MD, USA), we used a modified lactate dehydrogenase (LDH) release assay. Mononuclear cells as effector cells, at a concentration of $8 \times 10^5/100$ mL in a 200 μL culture medium, were mixed with K-562 cells, as target cells, at a concentration of $1 \times 10^4/100$ mL. The assay was performed in 96-well U-bottom culture plates (Corning Glass Works, Corning, NY, USA) and incubated for 4 h at 37 °C in a 5% CO_2 humid atmosphere. After the reaction, we sampled a 100 μL medium and used ELISA (Roche Diagnostics, Roche, Mannheim, Germany) to measure the amount of LDH isolated from K-562 cells as follows: we transferred the medium to a flat-bottom microplate (Molecular Devices Co., Sunnyvale, CA, USA) and added the same dose of a reagent (LDH substrate mixture) to it, and let it react at room temperature (15–25 °C) with light blocked out for 30 min, and measured absorbance at 490 nm wavelength. Culture media was used for the spontaneous LDH assay, and Triton X-100 solution was added to the media to determine the maximum amount of LDH isolated from K-562 cells, so that the cells could be lysed completely. On the basis of the absorbance in each condition, the following equation was used to assess activity of NK cells (% cytotoxicity):

$$\text{Natural killer cell activity} (\% \text{ cytotoxicity})$$
$$= \frac{\text{LDH}_{\text{experimental}} - \text{LDH}_{\text{effector cells}} - \text{LDH}_{\text{spontaneous}}}{\text{LDH}_{\text{maxiaml}} - \text{LDH}_{\text{spontaneous}}}$$
$$\times 100$$

$\text{LDH}_{\text{experimental}}$ is the value obtained by culturing both NK cells and K-562 cells, $\text{LDH}_{\text{effector cells}}$ is the value obtained by culturing NK cells separately, $\text{LDH}_{\text{spontaneous}}$ is the value obtained by culturing K-562 cells separately, and $\text{LDH}_{\text{maximal}}$ is the value obtained from K-562 cells cultured with triton X-100 added.

Statistical analyses

The factor analysis divided the 17-item HRSD into depression factors (Fd), insomnia factors (Fi), and anxiety factors (Fa) by confirmational factor analysis. Fd included item 1 (depressed mood), item 2 (feeling of guilt), item 7 (work and activities), item 8 (retardation: psychomotor), and item 13 (somatic symptoms general); Fi included item 4 (insomnia early), item 5 (insomnia middle), and item 6 (insomnia late); and Fa included item 9 (agitation), item 10 (anxiety: psychological), item 11 (anxiety: somatic), item 15 (hypochondriasis), and item 16 (loss of weight). T test and one-way analysis of variances were used to compare the immunologic variables

in terms of the demographic data and the clinical characteristics. Bonferroni test was applied for age group. To determine if immunologic variables differed across age and whether other demographic data impacted immunologic variables, we conducted a series of multivariable linear regression analysis. In these models, we included age and recent episode. Paired T test was used to compare the total scores of HRSD, the scores for three symptom factors, the number of lymphocyte subtypes, and the number and activity of NK cells at baseline and after medication. To determine the correlation between the number of lymphocyte subtypes, the number and activity of NK cells, and the three symptom factors of HRSD, we used Pearson's method and compared r and p values at baseline and after treatment after controlling age and recent episode. The significance level for all the statistics was set at .05. Statistical processing was performed using Statistica (version 12.0)

Results

Demographics and clinical characteristics

Forty-nine patients with MDD were included. Table 1 presents the demographic and clinical characteristics. Subjects were treated with escitalopram ($N=27$; mean daily dose, 12.8 mg; range, 5–20 mg/day), paroxetine ($N=12$; mean daily dose, 50 mg; range, 25–50 mg/day), and sertraline ($N=10$; mean daily dose, 75 mg; range, 50–100 mg/day). Response to treatment was defined as $\geq 50\%$ reduction of the baseline HAM-D score after 4 week treatment.

Table 1 Demographic and clinical characteristics of the subjects at baseline

Variables	Number (%)
Age (years)	50.9 ± 13.6
20–39	11 (22.4)
40–59	24 (49.0)
60≦	14 (28.6)
Sex	
Males	7 (14.3)
Females	42 (85.7)
Onset age (years)	48.1 ± 15.5
Recent episode	
Single	26 (53.1)
Recurrent	23 (46.9)
Duration of current episode (months)	2.0 ± 2.2
Response	
Responders	23 (46.9)
Non-responders	26 (53.1)

Immunologic variable and HRSD scores

For the number of lymphocyte subtypes and the number and activity of NK cells by the demographic and clinical characteristics of the subjects at baseline, there were significant differences in CD4/CD8 ratio ($p=.04$) and NKCA ($p=.01$) among age groups. In addition, single episode group had significantly greater NKCA ($p=.01$) (Table 2).

Figure 1 presents plots of immunologic variables and HRSD scores at baseline and after 4 week treatment. After controlling for age and recent episode, there were significant increase CD8-positive cells ($p=.03$) and decrease CD4/CD8 ratio ($p=.02$) after medication. After 4 week treatment, both total score of HRSD and the scores of Fd, Fa, and Fi were significantly lower (Table 3).

Table 2 Descriptive statistics of lymphocyte subsets and NKCA at baseline by the characteristics of the subjects

Variables	CD3, %	CD4, %	CD8, %	CD4/CD8, %	CD56, %	NKCA, %
Age (years)						
20–39	66.0±9.0	38.7±6.1	27.2±4.3	1.4±.2	16.8±6.7	9.8±7.6
40–59	64.1±8.4	40.8±6.1	23.3±5.7	1.9±.6*	18.4±6.6	17.1±11.1
60≦	61.1±9.9	39.3±5.6	21.8±6.1	1.9±.5	21.2±8.8	22.6±11.2[†]
Sex						
Males	63.1±11.3	40.0±7.9	23.2±6.3	1.8±.5	21.2±9.3	17.1±7.6
Females	63.7±8.7	39.9±5.7	23.8±6.0	1.8±.5	18.4±7.0	17.0±11.8
Recent episode						
Single	62.4±8.3	38.9±6.1	23.4±5.6	1.8±.5	20.5±8.1	20.3±12.3
Recurrent	65.1±9.7	41.0±5.7	24.1±6.1	1.8±.5	17.0±6.1	13.4±8.8*
Response						
Responders	62.8±8.7	40.0±5.5	22.8±5.2	1.8±.5	20.8±7.9	17.0±9.7
Non-responders	64.4±9.4	40.0±6.4	24.6±6.2	1.7±.6	17.1±6.5	17.1±12.6

* $p<.05$, a significant difference between 20 and 39 years and 40–59 years by Bonferroni test

[†] $p<.05$, a significant difference between 20 and 39 years and 60≦ years by Bonferroni test

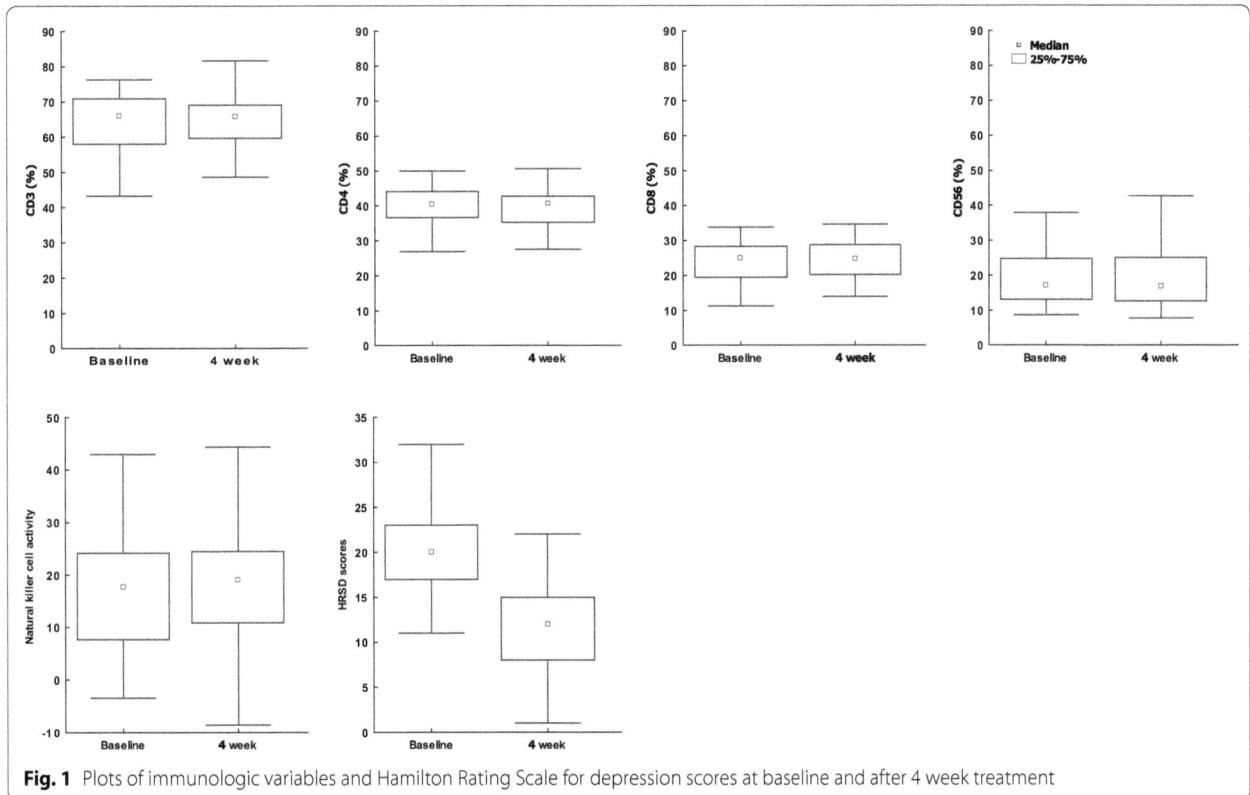

Fig. 1 Plots of immunologic variables and Hamilton Rating Scale for depression scores at baseline and after 4 week treatment

Table 3 Immunologic variables and symptom factor scores in patients with major depressive disorder at baseline and after 4 week treatment

Variables	At baseline	After treatment	t value	p
CD3 (%)	63.6 ± 9.0	64.7 ± 8.9	− 1.1	N.S.
CD4 (%)	39.9 ± 5.9	39.9 ± 6.0	.0	N.S.
CD8 (%)	23.8 ± 5.8	24.8 ± 5.4	− 2.2	.03.
CD4/CD8	1.8 ± .5	1.7 ± .4	3.3	.002.
CD56 (%)	18.8 ± 7.3	19.6 ± 8.7	− 1.1	N.S.
NKCA (%)	17.0 ± 11.2	18.5 ± 11.6	− 1.0	N.S.
HRSD, total	20.3 ± 5.5	11.4 ± 5.2	9.1	< .001
Fd	7.3 ± 2.3	4.3 ± 2.3	8.4	< .001
Fi	3.4 ± 1.5	1.3 ± 1.5	7.8	< .001
Fa	4.1 ± 1.7	2.5 ± 1.4	6.0	< .001

Partial correlation between immunologic variables and HRSD scores

At baseline, NKCA was positively correlated with Fa ($r = .35$, $p = .02$). After treatment, Fi was positively correlated with CD4/CD8 ($r = .33$, $p = .03$) (Table 4).

Discussion

The patients with MDD in this study were significantly increased in the number of CD8-positive cells and, consequently, a significant decrease in the CD4/CD8 ratio after medication. Severe depression was associated with lower CD8-positive cells in a large-scale meta-analysis among medically healthy persons, and as severity of depression may decrease after medication, CD4/CD8 ratio is correlated with the severity of depression [9, 28].

Medication made no change in NKCA in this study. Frank et al. reported that the responders to medication shown increased NKCA after the medication, whereas the non-responders shown decreased; others found that the decrease in NKCA lasted for 6 months during which medication was given [26]. No change in NKCA by medication in this study is inconsistent with the previous findings probably because of the differences in subjects' demographic variables. In this study, 47% of subjects responded and 53% made no response after 4 week treatment. The ratio of responders seems to be relatively low, given that about 67% of patients with MDD are usually expected to respond to medication. Further research needs to execute long-term follow-up of NKCA in patients with MDD, since some non-responders are likely to respond to the medication 6–8 weeks later [29].

Our model contained three symptom factors of HRSD: Fd, Fi, and Fa. Correlation between these factors and the immunologic variables was assessed at baseline and after treatment. NKCA was significantly positively correlated with anxiety factors in HRSD at baseline. More than half of individuals with a lifetime history of MDD report a lifetime history of one or more anxiety disorder, with the anxiety disorders predating the onset of MDD in the majority of cases and that depression disorder is accompanied by anxiety symptoms in most cases and immunologic research concerning anxiety has found that depressed patients with panic disorder may have a larger number of T cells and mitogen stimulation make greater lymphocyte proliferation than those without panic disorder and NKCA positively correlated with the score for Taylor's manifest anxiety in cancer patients [30–35].

Table 4 Partial correlation between immunologic variables and symptom factor scores in patients with major depressive disorder before and 4 weeks after the treatment after controlling age and recent episode

Variables	Before treatment				After treatment			
	HRSD (total)	Fd	Fi	Fa	HRSD (total)	Fd	Fi	Fa
CD3	r = .11	r = .13	r = .10	r = .07	r = .11	r = .13	r = − .01	r = .14
	p = .47	p = .40	p = .51	p = .65	p = .79	p = .39	p = .97	p = .36
CD4	r = .02	r = − .02	r = .09	r = − .03	r = .13	r = .04	r = .17	r = .11
	p = .87	p = .88	p = .54	p = .82	p = .84	p = .80	p = .25	P = .48
CD8	r = .15	r = .23	r = .06	r = .25	r = .03	r = .16	r = − .21	r = .10
	p = .32	p = .11	p = .69	p = .32	p = .84	p = .27	p = .16	p = .51
CD4/CD8	r = − .14	r = − .21	r = − .03	r = − .13	r = .03	r = − .18	r = .33	r = − .02
	p = .37	p = .15	p = .85	p = .37	p = .82	p = .23	p = .03*	p = .87
CD56	r = − .03	r = .00	r = .03	r = − .08	r = − .13	r = − .01	r = − .08	r = − .25
	p = .84	p = .99	p = .84	p = .61	p = .39	p = .94	p = .58	p = .09
NKCA	r = .13	r = .23	r = − .23	r = .35	r = − .05	r = .00	r = − .09	r = − .01
	p = .38	p = .12	p = .12	p = .02*	p = .76	p = .98	p = .53	p = .97

* p < .05

From these findings, the result that symptoms of anxiety were correlated with the immunologic variables in patients with MDD may provide a clue to the immunologic changes observed among patients with MDD.

We analyzed by controlling two demographic variables, which showed difference in immunologic measures at baseline and after medication. (1) Age. The age group from 40 to 59 years accounted for 49% and older patients had significantly greater NKCA. The early reports suggested that NK cell numbers and activity were unchanged with aging, but more recent investigators have generally described an increase in the proportion of CD56^{dim} (mature) NK cells, a decrease in the number, and/or activity of NK cells, with a decreased affinity for target cells [36–39]. A recent study reported that psychosocial resources correlate with the expression of the cell surface maker CD57 (a marker of terminal maturation and senescence) on NK cells. These findings provide support that the sense that one has substantial resources may retard age-associated aspects of the microenvironment in which NK cells develop and mature, independent of effects on distress [40]. (2) Recurrence of MDD. The patients with single episode had significantly greater NKCA at baseline than those with recurrent episode. Recurrence of depression may contribute to immunologic decrease such as NKCA.

At present, major depressive disorders are diagnosed through patient interviews, symptom checklists based on diagnostic criteria of DSM-IV or DSM-5, self-reported scales, and scales by clinicians. However, there is a controversy over the objectivity of the assessment based on these symptoms and limitations on the establishment of an individualized treatment plan [41–43].

Biomarkers are indicators of normal biological processes, pathogenic processes, or pharmacological responses to a therapeutic intervention that can be measured and evaluated objectively [44]. However, the biomarker study of depression is difficult because of the heterogeneity of the disorder.

From the results, we carefully suggest that NKCA could be the possibility of being a diagnostic biomarker of anxiety-dominant depression subtype. CD+8 may also be an objective indicator of the severity and change of depression.

Results of this study in a limited small population could not be generalized to the patients with MDD. To overcome such a limitation, it is necessary to include normal control in the population and conduct in-depth, more systematic, wide-ranging research by assessing immune responses to antibodies and immune mediators, such as cytokine, as well as by counting immunocytes and by measuring their activity. An additional limitation to absent a healthy control sample is that it is difficult to determine whether immunological changes over time are related to technical changes in two assays or to experimental conditions unrelated to symptomatic changes in subjects.

It has been reported that a decrease of cell-mediated and innate immune responses is correlated with vulnerability to infectious diseases among patients with depression and that depression is correlated with immunologic activity among patients with cardiovascular diseases or inflammatory diseases, such as rheumatoid arthritis [5, 45–47]. These results imply that changes of immune functions among patients with MDD may depend on their age and chronicity of the condition, and such changes can also affect physical health of the patients.

Our research has provided new perspectives on the contribution of cellular immunity to major depression disorders and antidepressant treatment response as a potential biomarker.

Conclusion

This study aimed to examine the immunologic changes by medication in patients with MDD, assess correlation between immunologic variables and symptom factors, and determine association between depression disorder and immune functions. Fifty-one patients with MDD who had no history of taking psychotropic drugs during the period of MDD episodes and had no major physical disease participated in this study. The 17-item Hamilton Rating Scale for Depression (HRSD) was used to assess the symptoms among the subjects, and the items in HRSD were divided into depression, insomnia, and anxiety factors by confirmational factor analysis. To assess the immune functions in the subjects, we used flow cytometry to count NK cells and lymphocytes in peripheral blood, employed ELISA using K-562 to assess activity of NK cells, and provided 4 week treatment with a selective serotonin inhibitor to observe changes of symptoms. We also counted NK cells and lymphocytes in peripheral blood, assessed their activity, and determined correlation between these variables and the three factors in HRSD. After treatment, the number of CD8-positive cells increased significantly ($p<.05$) and the CD4/CD8 ratio dropped significantly ($p<.01$). Positive correlation was found between the anxiety factors and NKCA at baseline ($r=.36$, $p=.01$); however, no correlation was found after treatment. As medication improved the symptoms of MDD, immune functions changed. The symptoms of anxiety, which accompanied MDD, were found to have a principal impact on such immunologic variables as NKCA.

Authors' contributions
EJP and SIH contributed to the major building of the manuscript, and JYW participated with other authors in the interpretation of the data. EJP drafted the manuscript and all authors revised it critically. All authors read and approved the final manuscript.

Acknowledgements
Not applicable.

Competing interests
The authors declare that they have no competing interests.

Consent for publication
The participants signed the consent form accepting to participate and also for permission to published.

Funding
The study was part of the corresponding author's doctor of philosophy in medical science/psychiatry program and all the costs were borne by her.

References

1. Kessler RC, Berglund P, Demler O, Jin R, Koretz D, Merikangas KR, Rush AJ, Walters EE, Wang PS. The epidemiology of major depressive disorder: results from the national comorbidity survey replication (NCS-R). JAMA. 2003;289:3095–105.
2. Penninx BW, Geerlings SW, Deeg DJ, van Eijk JT, van Tilburg W, Beekman AT. Minor and major depression and the risk of death in older persons. Arch Gen Psychiatry. 1999;56:889–95.
3. Rudisch B, NemeroV CB. Epidemiology of comorbid coronary artery disease and depression. Biol Psychiatry. 2003;54:227–40.
4. Evans DL, Ten Have TR, Douglas SD, Gettes DR, Morrison M, Chiappini MS, Brinker-Spence P, Job C, Mercer DE, Wang YL, Cruess D, Dube B, Dalen EA, Brown T, Bauer R, Petitto JM. Association of depression with viral load, CD8 T lymphocytes, and natural killer cells in women with HIV infection. Am J Psychiatry. 2002;159:752–9.
5. Zautra AJ, Yocum DC, Villanueva I, Smith B, Davis MC, Attrep J, Irwin M. Immune activation and depression in women with rheumatoid arthritis. J Rheumatol. 2004;31:457–63.
6. Irwin MR, Miller AH. Depressive disorders and immunity: 20 years of progress and discovery. Brain Behav Immun. 2007;21:374–83.
7. Sluzewska A. Indicators of immune activation in depressed patients. Adv Exp Med Biol. 1999;461:59–73.
8. Evans DL, Folds JD, Petitto JM, Golden RN, Pedersen CA, Corrigan M, Gilmore JH, Silva SG, Quade D, Ozer H. Circulating natural killer cell phenotypes in men and women with major depression. Arch Gen Psychiatry. 1992;49:388–95.
9. Herbert TB, Cohen S. Depression and immunity—a meta-analytic review. Psychol Bull. 1993;113:472–86.
10. Maes M, Lambrechts J, Bossman E, Jacobs J, Suy E, Vandervost C, DeJonekheere C, Mihner B, Raus J. Evidence for a systemic immune activation during depression: results of leukocyte enumeration by flow cytometry in conjunction with monoclonal antibody staining. Psychol Med. 1992;22:45–53.
11. Ravindran A, Griffith J, Merali Z, Anisman H. Circulating lymphocyte subsets in obsessive compulsive disorder, major depression and normal controls. J Affect Disord. 1999;52:1–10.
12. Farid Hosseini R, Jabbari Azad F, Talaee A, Miri S, Mokhber N, Farid Hosseini F, Esmaeili H, Mahmoudi M, Rafatpanah H, Mohammadi M. Assessment of the immune system activity in Iranian patients with major depression disorder (MDD). Iran J Immunol. 2007;4(1):38–43.
13. Zorrilla EP, Luborsky L, McKay JR, Rosenthal R, Houldin A, Tax A, Mccorkle R, Selgman DA, Schmidt K. The relationship of depression and stressors to immunological assays: a meta- analytic review. Brain Behav Immun. 2001;15:199–226.
14. American Psychiatric Association. Diagnostic and statistical manual of mental disorders. 4th ed. Washington, D.C: American Psychiatric Press; 2000.
15. Maes M, Stevens W, Peeters D, DeClerck L, Scharpe S, Bridts C, Schotte C, Cosyns P. A study on the blunted natural killer cell activity in severely depressed patients. Life Sci. 1992;50:505–13.
16. Grosse L, Carvalho LA, Birkenhager TK, Hoogendijk WJ, Kushner SA, Drexhage HA, Bergink V. Circulating cytotoxic T cells and natural killer cells as potential predictors for antidepressant response in melancholic depression. Restoration of T regulatory cell populations after antidepressant therapy. Psychopharmacology (Berl). 2016;233(9):1679–88.
17. Hamilton M. A rating scale for depression. J Neurol Neurosurg Psychiatry. 1960;23:56–62.
18. O'Brien KP, Glaudin V. Factorial structure and factor reliability of the Hamilton Rating Scale for Depression. Acta Psychiatr Scand. 1988;78:113–20.
19. Hamilton M. Development of a rating scale for primary depressive illness. Br J Soc Clin Psychol. 1967;6:278–96.
20. Zheng YP, Zhao JP, Phillips M, Liu JB, Cai MF, Sun SQ, Huang MF. Validity and reliability of the Chinese Hamilton Depression Rating Scale. Br J Psychiatry. 1988;152:660–4.
21. Marcos T, Salamero M. Factor study of the Hamilton Rating Scale for Depression and the Bech Melancholia Scale. Acta Psychiatr Scand. 1990;82:178–81.
22. Fleck MP, Poirier-Littre MF, Guelfi JD, Bourdel MC, Loo H. Factorial structure of the 17-item Hamilton Depression Rating Scale. Acta Psychiatr Scand. 1995;92:168–72.
23. Bech P, Stage KB, Nair NP, Larsen JK, Kragh-Sørensen P, Gjerris A. The Major Depression Rating Scale (MDS). Inter-rater reliability and validity across different settings in randomized moclobemide trials. Danish University Antidepressant Group. J Affect Disord. 1997;42:39–48.
24. Freire-Garabal M, Nunez MJ, Losada C, Pereiro D, Riveiro MP, González-Patiño E, Mayán JM, Rey-Mendez M. Effects of fluoxetine on the immunosuppressive response to stress in mice. Life Sci. 1997;60:403–13.
25. Hernandez ME, Martinez-Fong D, Perez-Tapia M, Estrada-Garcia I, Estrada-Parra S, Pavón L. Evaluation of the effect of selective serotonin-reuptake inhibitors on lymphocyte subsets in patients with a major depressive disorder. Eur Neuropsychopharmacol. 2010;20:88–95.
26. Evans DL, Lynch KG, Benton T, Dubé B, Gettes DR, Tustin NB, Lai JP, Metzger D, Douglas SD. Selective serotonin reuptake inhibitor and substance P antagonist enhancement of natural killer cell innate immunity in human immunodeficiency virus/acquired immunodeficiency syndrome. Biol Psychiatry. 2008;63:899–905.
27. First MB, Spitzer RL, Gibbon M, Williams JBW. Structured clinical interview for DSM-IV axis I disorders. Seoul: Hana; 2000 (**Korean translation**).
28. Schleifer S, Keller S, Bartlett J. Depression and immunity: clinical factors and therapeutic course. Psychiatry Res. 1999;85:63–9.
29. Frank MG, Hendricks SE, Burke WJ, Johnson DR. Clinical response augments NK cell activity independent of treatment modality: a randomized double-blind placebo controlled antidepressant trial. Psychol Med. 2004;34:491–8.
30. Kessler RC, Nelson CB, McGonagle KA, Liu J, Swartz M, Blazer DG. Comorbidity of DSM-III-R major depressive disorder in the general population: results from the US National Comorbidity Survey. Br J Psychiatry suppl. 1996;168:17–30.
31. Fava M, Rankin MA, Wright EC, Alpert JE, Nierenberg AA, Pava J, Rosenbaum JF. Anxiety disorders in major depression. Compr Psychiatry. 2000;41:97–102.
32. Philip TN, Joseph B. Symptomatic and syndromal anxiety and depression. Depress Anxiety. 2001;14:79–85.
33. Nemeroff CB. Comorbidity of mood and anxiety disorders: the rule, not the exception? Am J Psychiatry. 2002;159:3–4.
34. Andreoli A, Keller SE, Rabaeus M, Zaugg L, Garrone G, Taban C. Immunity, major depression, and panic disorder comorbidity. Biol Psychiatry. 1992;31:896–908.
35. Tashiro M, Itoh M, Kubota K, Kumano H, Masud MM, Moser E, Arai H, Sasaki H. Relationship between trait anxiety and natural killer cell activity in cancer patients: a preliminary PET study. Psychooncology. 2001;10:541–6.
36. Fiatarone MA, Morley JE, Bloom ET, Benton D, Solomon GF, Makinodan T. The effect of exercise on natural killer cell activity in young and old subjects. J Gerontol. 1989;44:37–45.
37. Grubeck-Loebenstein B, Della Bella S, Iorio AM, Michel JP, Pawelec G, Solana R. Immunosenescence and vaccine failure in the elderly. Aging Clin Exp Res. 2009;21:201–9.
38. Miyaji C, Watanabe H, Minagawa M, Toma H, Kawamura T, Nohara Y, Nozaki H, Sato Y, Abo T. Numerical and functional characteristics of lymphocyte subsets in centenarians. J Clin Immunol. 1997;17:420–9.

39. Rukavina D, Laskarin G, Rubesa G, Strbo N, Bedenicki I, Manestar D, Glavas M, Christmas SE, Podack ER. Age-related decline of perforin expression in human cytotoxic T lymphocytes and natural killer cells. Blood. 1998;92:2410–20.

40. Segerstrom SC, Al-Attar A, Lutz CT. Psychosocial resources, aging, and natural killer cell terminal maturity. Psychol Aging. 2012;27:892–902.

41. Hilsenroth MJ, Baity MW, Mooney MA, Meyer GJ. DSM-IV major depressive episode criteria: an evaluation of reliability and validity across three different ratingmethods. Int J Psychiatr Clin Pract. 2004;8(1):3–10.

42. Phillips J, Frances A, Cerullo MA, Chardavoyne J, Decker HS, First MB, Ghaemi N, Greenberg G, Hinderliter AC, Kinghorn WA, LoBello SG, Martin EB, Mishara AL, Paris J, Pierre JM, Pies RW, Pincus HA, Porter D, Pouncey C, Schwartz MA, Szasz T, Wakefield JC, Waterman GS, Whooley O, Zachar P. The six most essential questions in psychiatric diagnosis: a pluralogue part 1: conceptual and definitional issues in psychiatric diagnosis. Philos Ethics Humanit Med. 2012;7:3.

43. Stein DJ, Phillips KA, Bolton D, Fulford KW, Sadler JZ, Kendler KS. What is a mental/psychiatric disorder? From DSM-IV to DSM-V. Psychol Med. 2010;40(11):1759–65.

44. Biomarkers Definitions Working Group. Biomarkers and surrogate endpoints: preferred definitions and conceptual framework. Clin Pharmacol Ther. 2001;69(3):89–95.

45. Cohen S, Miller G. Stress, immunity and susceptibility to upper respiratory infection. In: Ader R, Felten D, Cohen N, editors. Psychoneuroimmunology. San Diego: Academic Press; 2000. p. 499–509.

46. Lesperance F, Frasure-Smith N, Theroux P, Irwin M. The association between major depression and levels of soluble intercellular adhesion molecule 1, interleukin-6, and C-reactive protein in patients with recent acute coronary syndromes. Am J Psychiatry. 2004;161:271–7.

47. Miller GE, Stetler CA, Carney RM, Freedland KE, Banks WA. Clinical depression and inflammatory risk markers for coronary heart disease. Am J Cardiol. 2002;90:1279–83.

20

A comparison of three-factor structure models using WISC-III in Greek children with learning disabilities

Anna Adam[1*], Grigoris Kiosseoglou[2], Grigoris Abatzoglou[1] and Zaira Papaligoura[2]

Abstract

Background: Children with learning disabilities are a heterogeneous group of children with a common characteristic discrepancy on the progress and development of their individual learning abilities. A few statistical analyses have been published regarding the factor analysis of the Greek Edition of Wechsler Intelligence Scale for Children-III. The aim of the research is the emergence of a new factorial model which describes the General Intelligence (g) of children and adolescents with learning disabilities, and that differs from the already existing intelligence models. This study aims to compare three-factor structure models of WISC-III in children with learning disabilities in the Greek population.

Methods: A sample of 50 children were selected on the basis of research criteria from a total of 122 children who evaluated in a child psychiatric service in a general hospital, in a residential area in Greece. The Wechsler Intelligence Scale for Children—Third Edition was used to assess children's cognitive function. Using multi-factor analysis, three alternative factor models were compared.

Results: Analysis of factor structure models suggests a new bi-factorial model that more appropriately describes the areas of cognitive development of children with learning disabilities. The first factor includes Comprehension, Picture Arrangement, Coding, Block Design, and Object Assembly, whereas the second one combines Information, Similarities, Arithmetic, Vocabulary, and Picture Arrangement.

Conclusions: The present study shows the existence of a factorial model with two factors: one aggregating the Comprehension verbal subtest with four performance subtests and the other the Picture Arrangement performance subtest with four verbal subtests. This two-factor model includes the loadings in two factors that relate to sequencing abilities and verbal reasoning abilities of children. These findings assert the clinical utility of the intelligence evaluation in the specific population.

Keywords: WISC-III, Factor structure, Learning disabilities, Comprehension, Picture arrangement

Background

The Wechsler Intelligence Scale for Children-Third Edition (WISC-III) is a widely used tool to measure intelligence that is systematically used for assessing children and adolescents with learning disabilities [1]. Children's performance on the intelligence test guides the

*Correspondence: adaann@auth.gr; infoadamanna@gmail.com
[1] School of Medicine, Service of Child and Adolescent Psychiatry, AHEPA Hospital, Third Psychiatric Clinic, Aristotle University of Thessaloniki, Thessaloniki, Greece
Full list of author information is available at the end of the article

educational placement and determines the cognitive strengths and weaknesses of children.

The WISC-III factor structure of a group of children with special educational needs has been adequately studied and the data corroborate both the existence of a major factor for general intelligence and a two-factor model with verbal and performance factors [2]. The model proposed by Wechsler based on multiple-factor analysis is a model with four factors: (a) verbal comprehension, (b) freedom of distractibility, (c) perceptual organization, and (d) processing speed. According to researchers [3, 4], this model adequately describes the cognitive abilities of children with special educational needs. Wechsler also indicated that the four-factor model provides the best fit for multiple groups, such as a clinical sample of children with learning disabilities, reading disorders, or attention-deficit disorders [5].

The use of factor analysis models is a key tool in evaluating specific populations. Similar studies use special education samples, such as children with learning disabilities or other academic difficulties identifying four- and five-factor structure models on the WISC-III [4, 6–9]. Burton et al. [10] reported that the five-factor model concludes verbal comprehension, constructional praxis, visual reasoning, freedom from distractibility, and processing speed in a mixed clinical sample of 318 children. However, these factor models were contingent on the administration of the supplemental subtests.

Researches that examine WISC-III results in Greek special populations, such as children with mental retardation, organic disabilities, psychiatric disorders, or learning disabilities, are limited [11, 12]. The adaptation of the Greek scale is based on the British version of the WISC-III [5] and any modification made with the particularities of the Greek language and culture. Based on the analysis of the factor structure in WISC-III in the Greek weighting population, a three-factor model emerges, similar, to four-factor model proposed by Wechsler [13]. The Freedom from Distractibility Factor is not found, as well as in the Belgian–French Edition [14].

The present study aims to examine the factor structure of WISC-III and to compare three alternative factor models that best describe the intelligence of children and adolescents with learning disabilities in the Greek population. Because index scores are used for the interpretation of the test, it is critical to validate the factor structure of the WISC-III in the specific population. This study is an effort, for the first time in the Greek field, to detect the factor structure of the test in a clinical population. It is part of a wider research that scrutinizes the interaction of individual, family, social, and school factors in the performance of WISC-III in children with learning disabilities. The study of the scale's factor structure in the particular population is an attempt to visualize the factor model that more precisely describes the areas of cognitive development.

Methods
Aim and study design
According to the above, we investigate: (a) the existence of a single-factor model which includes a major factor (g) for intelligence; (b) validation of the expected model on which the subtests information, similarities, arithmetic,

vocabulary, and comprehension load on the verbal factor and the subscale picture completion, coding, picture arrangement, block design, and object assembly load on the performance factor; (c) the existence of a new modified factor model that fits better than the single or the expected factor model the data of the Greek sample studied.

The main objectives of the present study are expressed by the following research questions: Is there a strong structural factor that represents intelligence? Is the expected model verified? Multi-factor analyses are applied to children's performances in WISC-III to point out the aggregation of the ten core subscales in individual meaningful factors.

Participants
The total number of children and adolescents evaluated for their educational disabilities is 122. Out of the total of 122 children, 50 children were selected who met the following research criteria: (1) the initial referral was to evaluate the learning problem or the school failure of the child, (2) reported learning difficulties that met diagnostic criteria for learning disabilities, (3) a 3-year interval between two evaluations of the child with the WISC-III that meets the criteria for the high reliability of the scale in children with learning disabilities [15], and (4) the sample included children with severe psychopathology (pervasive developmental disorders, mental retardation, etc.) or organic diseases (neurological, endocrinological disorders, chronic diseases, etc.) who attend the service for evaluating their educational difficulties. The remaining 72 children did not meet the entry criteria, as there was insufficient evidence to perform a comprehensive psychometric assessment by administering the WISC-III.

The sample consisted of 50 children and adolescents (30 males and 20 females), who received comprehensive psychological evaluations for their learning disabilities. Their ages ranged from 7 to 15 years, and the average age of the participants was $M = 11.5$ years (SD = 2.05). From the total sample, 52% were elementary school students and 48% junior high and high school students. Of the participants, 74% attended schools in the urban area of Thessaloniki, 20% in suburban areas, and 6% attended schools in rural areas.

From the total sample, 58% of the children were diagnosed according to the criteria of the ICD-10 Classification of Mental and Behavioral Disorders [16] concerning Pervasive and Specific Developmental Disorders (F80–F89), and more specifically, the Phonological disorders, the Specific developmental disorders of scholastic skills, and the Pervasive developmental disorders. The rest of the children were diagnosed with Behavioral and

Emotional Disorders (F90–F98), as well as the Intellectual Disabilities (F70–F79). From the total sample of children, 10% were students with high performance in school, 62% exhibited average performance, and 28% were children with school failure.

Data collection

The study is part of a larger research that was carried out in the Child and Adolescent Service of the Third Psychiatric Clinic of the AHEPA University Hospital of Thessaloniki in Greece, from October 2010 to June 2016. The intelligence quotients of school aged children and adolescents were measured by the Greek version of the Wechsler Intelligence Scale for Children, Third Edition (WISC-III) [17]. The test was performed individually by an educational psychologist, and its duration was about 60–90 min. The scale consists of 13 subscales that assess the intellectual abilities; five core verbal, five core performance scales, two supplemental, and one optional subscale ($M = 10$; SD$=3$). The first ten subscales deduce the Full Scale (FSIQ), verbal (VIQ), and performance (PIQ) intelligence indexes ($M = 100$; SD$=15$). For research purposes, only the first ten mandatory subscales were administered to participants.

Statistical analyses

Scaled scores of the ten WISC-III subscales were analyzed using exploratory and confirmatory factor analysis. Exploratory factor analysis (EFA) was applied first to identify an initial factor structure for the underlying subtests. Then, confirmatory factor analysis (CFA) was used to validate specific patterns that have been revealed initially from EFA and to relate the observable scores of WISC-III subtests to factors. The goal of the multifactorial exploratory and confirmatory analyses was to find the model that most efficiently describes the data structure.

EFA was applied using maximum-likelihood as extraction method that is considered the best one if data are relatively normally distributed [18]. We also used oblique rotation that allows the extracted factors to correlate. The sample size $n = 50$ of this research is considered marginally sufficient to yield a recognizable factor pattern [19, 20]. In addition, the subjects-to-variables ratio $50/10 = 5$ meets the minimum requirement for EFA, because it is no lower than 5 [21]. Three well-known criteria were used to determine the number of factors to retain: Kaiser's eigenvalue > 1 [22], Cattell's scree test [23], and Horn's parallel analysis [24]. All EFAs were performed using IBM SPSS Statistics 24 program.

Concerning CFA, the recent simulation studies showed that sample sizes of $n = 50$ participants are associated with satisfactory fit and reliable parameter estimates [25],

especially in models with large factor loadings and high factor intercorrelations [26].

To evaluate the fit of the CFA models, we followed Hu and Bentler [27] guidelines for acceptable model fit: CFI and TLI values close to .95 or greater, SRMR values close to .08 or below, and RMSEA values close to .06 or below.

Finally, to compare the fit of non-nested CFA models, we calculated differences in BIC (Bayesian information criterion) values between models [28], while a Chi-square difference test was computed to compare nested models [29].

All CFAs were conducted using Mplus 5.0 program [30] based on maximum-likelihood estimation of parameters. It must be noted that Pearson correlation coefficient was used to calculate correlations among the WISC-III subtests.

Results

Table 1 shows Pearson correlations among ten subtest scores as well as the values of skewness and kurtosis. As expected, all correlations are positive and significant ($p < .01$). We also observe that all values of skewness and kurtosis are between -1 and $+1$, so we can conclude that the distribution of subtest scores fits the normal shape almost adequately.

EFA was applied first to explore the factor structure for the underlying WISC-III core subtests. The Kaiser–Meyer–Olkin measure of sampling adequacy (KMO) was .89, indicating that EFA was appropriate for this sample. The results from Kaiser's and Cattell's criteria pointed to the presence of one dominant factor and another one, secondary and less important, while parallel analysis suggested a one-factor solution. We also considered the Chi-square goodness-of-fit test, produced from EFA. For the one-factor solution, it was found that $\chi^2(35) = 56.33$, $p = .013$, which means that there is additional significant amount of covariance among the subtest scores after one factor has been extracted. In contrary, for the two-factor solution, the test was not significant ($\chi^2(26) = 24.34$, $p = .556$), indicating that the sample data are likely to have arisen from two correlated factors. Thus, we decided to adopt, as initial factor structure of the ten subtests, the two-factor solution. The pattern matrix presented in Table 2 displays the rotated factor loadings of the ten subtests for one- and two-factor solution. After inspecting the pattern of loadings for the two-factor solution, and setting the cutoff at .41, it was found that the first factor was mainly defined by the performance subtests except "Picture Arrangement" which had higher loading on the second factor, while the second factor was loaded mainly by the verbal subtests except "Comprehension" which had higher loading on the first factor.

Table 1 Measures of shape and Pearson correlations among WISC-III subtests

	S	K	IN	SI	AR	VO	CO	PC	CD	PA	BD
IN	.07	.36	–								
SI	.02	−.07	.69	–							
AR	−.40	−.01	.55	.69	–						
VO	−.10	−.09	.68	.75	.62	–					
CO	−.38	−.59	.54	.59	.65	.66	–				
PC	−.44	−.28	.39	.47	.62	.43	.56	–			
CD	−.39	−.56	.39	.39	.50	.51	.51	.51	–		
PA	−.58	−.45	.52	.58	.64	.59	.48	.45	.57	–	
BD	−.67	−.24	.45	.47	.65	.47	.56	.61	.49	.55	–
OA	−.67	−.19	.52	.49	.53	.49	.67	.60	.54	.51	.76

S skewness, K kurtosis, IN information, SI similarities, AR arithmetic, VO vocabulary, CO comprehension, PC picture completion, CD coding, PA picture arrangement, BD block design, OA object assembly

All correlations are significant ($p < .01$)

Table 2 Exploratory factor analysis

	One factor	Two rotated factors	
		Factor 1	Factor 2
Information	.71	.03	−.75
Similarities	.78	−.06	−.92
Arithmetic	.82	.38	−.50
Vocabulary	.79	−.03	−.89
Comprehension	.79	.44	−.41
Picture completion	.68	.69	−.05
Coding	.64	.50	−.19
Picture arrangement	.73	.33	−.45
Block design	.74	.93	.10
Object assembly	.75	.87	.03
Eigenvalue	5.99	5.99	1.01
Variance (%)	59.89	59.89	10.09

Maximum-likelihood–direct oblimin factor loadings for one- and two-factor solution

Loadings > |.41| highlighted in italic

Next, to validate the pattern of two-factor loadings proposed by EFA, CFA was conducted in the following way: first, a CFA was used to test the fit of the model with two correlated factors (M2) resulting from EFA. Then, a one-factor model (M1) in which all subtests loaded on a single factor was considered, and a Chi-square difference test for nested models was computed to compare M1 and M2 models to decide whether the one fitted significantly better or worse than the other. Finally, a third CFA was conducted to test the fit of the expected two-factor model (M3) in which all five performance subtests load on a factor (performance factor), while all five verbal subtests load on another one (verbal). The two non-nested models M3 and M2 were compared via Bayesian information criterion, BIC index. The model with the smallest BIC value is considered to be the best model.

After inspection of modification indices given by Mplus program, we allowed a correlation between the errors terms of Block Design and Object Assembly subtests for the three models. Table 3 contains fit indices for the three alternative models. We observe that model M2, corresponding to the two correlated factor solution proposed by EFA fits the data very well: $\chi^2 = 38.39$, $df = 33$, $p = .24$, CFI = .98, TLI = .98, RMSEA = .057, and SRMR = .050. The correlation between factors was $r = .85$, $p < .001$. Standardized loadings (Table 4) range from .66 to .85 supporting an internally consistent solution, and are all significant ($p < .001$).

For the one-factor model M1, we observe (Table 3) that it fits the data well but worse than model M2: $\chi^2 = 49.94$, $df = 34$, $p = .038$, CFI = .95, TLI = .93, RMSEA = .097, and SRMR = .059. Furthermore, according to the Chi-square difference in the fit between the nested models M1 and M2: $\Delta\chi^2 = \chi^2(M1) - \chi^2(M2) = 11.55$, $\Delta df = df(M1) - df(M2) = 1$, $p < .001$, it was found that model M1 fits the data significantly worse than model M2.

Finally, model M3 fits the data satisfactory (Table 3) but slightly worse than model M2: $\chi^2 = 41.58$, $df = 33$, $p = .15$, CFI = .97, TLI = .96, RMSEA = .072, and SRMR = .053. To compare the non-nested models M2 and M3, we calculated the difference in BIC values between the two models: BIC(M3)–BIC(M2) = 2460.7–2457.5 = 3.2. According to Kass and Raftery [28], difference in BIC of 2–6 points is considered as positive evidence in favor of the model with the smaller BIC. Hence, we can conclude that model M2 fits the observed data better than model M3.

Table 3 Summary of fit indices for three alternative CFA models

Models	χ^2	df	p	CFI	TLI	RMSEA	SRMR	BIC
Single-factor (M1)	49.94	34	.038	.95	.93	.097	.059	2465.1
Correlated two-factor (M2)[a]	38.39	33	.238	.98	.98	.057	.050	2457.5
Correlated two-factor (M3)[b]	41.58	33	.145	.97	.96	.072	.053	2460.7

[a] M2: factor 1 is loaded by performance subtests except "Picture Arrangement" which loads on the second factor; factor 2 is loaded by verbal subtests except "Comprehension" which loads on the first one

[b] M3: factor 1 is loaded by performance subtests; factor 2 is loaded by verbal subtests

Table 4 Confirmatory factor analysis

Subtests	Factor 1	Factor 2	R^2
Comprehension	.81		.66
Picture completion	.73		.53
Coding	.66		.44
Block design	.75		.56
Object assembly	.79		.63
Information		.76	.58
Similarities		.85	.73
Arithmetic		.81	.65
Vocabulary		.84	.70
Picture arrangement		.72	.52

Correlated two-factor model; standardized loadings

All loadings are significant ($p < .001$)

Discussion

Findings from this study demonstrated that the (g) factor reflecting General Intelligence, as emerged from a single-factor model, remains a major factor for children with learning disabilities. These findings are consistent with the previous surveys. According to Poulson and Scardapane, the scale's factor structure in a population of individuals with special educational needs has confirmed the existence of a powerful factor for General Intelligence and partial two-factor models, the Verbal and Performance Intelligence Scale [2].

However, adopting a single-factor model does not allow us to better understand the cognitive abilities of the children while taking into account individual variations in their performance on each of the two scales. Even though the single-factor model provides information on children's cognitive potential, it does not allow researchers to deepen their intrapersonal profile. These findings are in agreement with Konold et al. [3] and Grice et al. [4] which conclude in models with more than one factor.

The expected model has been validated as a sufficiently good illustrative model, as anticipated, however, a new alternative model emerges that outweighs it and better fulfills the statistical criteria. The new proposed two-factor model better adapts to General Intelligence of children with learning disabilities. This model consists of two new factors. The first factor that relates to the sequencing abilities of children consists of four performance subtests and one verbal subtest: picture completion, coding, block design, object assembly, and comprehension. The second factor, which relates to the verbal reasoning abilities of children, consists of four verbal and one performance subtests: information, similarities, arithmetic, vocabulary, and picture arrangement. This new two-factor model fits more adequately than both the single-factor model and the expected model.

This finding could be particularly noteworthy, as it is different from any similar research, probably due to the correlation observed between comprehension (verbal subtest) and picture arrangement (practical subtest). Krippner [31], Brannigan [32], and Beebe et al. [33] point out that these two subtests are indicators of measuring social competence and social maturity. In addition, Rapaport et al. [34] emphasize that Comprehension and Picture Arrangement can be considered complementary, voicing common abilities in relation to social understanding.

At the same time, Sattler [35] reported that Comprehension measures the child's social knowledge and the level of social maturation and Picture Arrangement evaluates the child's ability to comprehend and evaluate social situations. The correlation of these two connotations led to their association as a measurement of "social intelligence" [36]. The relevance of the two subtests may partially explain this new model. In addition, there is no absolute agreement between researchers about linking these two abstracts to the measurement of "social intelligence" [37]. This discrepancy is related to the variety in the definition of social competence and maturity [33].

One possible explanation might be that even though Picture Arrangement is a performance subtest, it can also measure the ability for verbal sequencing in children that have well-developed verbal skills [5]. This finding is asseverated by the clinical practice, as well as the children who understand and tell the story correctly in picture arrangement subtest to achieve better results than the children who fail in understanding the content of the stories. This hypothesis, however, needs further investigation.

Giannitsas and Mylonas [13] conducted factor analyses in the weighting Greek sample and resulted in three factors, verbal comprehension, perceptual organization, and processing speed. These results are not validated in the present study; however, the majority of surveys measure children's performance in 13 WISC-III subtests (primary and complementary), while our study is based on the ten core endorsements. A key advantage is that it is the first study that examines the factor structure of WISC-III in a clinical population in children of Greece.

However, there are certain limitations, concerning the heterogeneous nature of the sample, which consisted of children with a variety of diagnoses. In addition, a larger sample would allow for separate factor analyses across different clinical populations to determine if the findings of this study are replicable. Although the sample of the survey fulfills the research's criteria, a larger sample would allow the conclusions to be strengthened. For example, individual diagnostic categories in the group of children with learning disabilities could be evaluated. In addition, the factor structure of the scale could be examined in different age and sex groups.

Conclusions

The new proposed model follows the widely used model of two individual factors (VIQ and PIQ); however, it has some significant differences, as Performance and Verbal subscales cannot be allocated equally to the two factors, but they cross each other. This study provides evidence that the first factor relates to the sequence abilities of children, the ability to think with logical sequences, rationally, and to perceive the elements in a specific order. These skills are very important in comprehension, and written and oral language. The second factor related to verbal reasoning abilities focuses on the ability of children to think in a structured way and to comprehend concepts composed by words. These skills are an essential element of the learning process.

These results may provide useful information to psycho-educational assessments and improve educational planning and therapeutic interventions in children with learning disabilities in the Greek population. Nevertheless, it is critical to further investigate the meaning and interpretation of these factors in clinical populations.

Authors' contributions
All authors contributed toward data analysis, drafting, and critically revising the paper, and agree to be accountable for all aspects of the work. All authors read and approved the final manuscript.

Author details
[1] School of Medicine, Service of Child and Adolescent Psychiatry, AHEPA Hospital, Third Psychiatric Clinic, Aristotle University of Thessaloniki, Thessaloniki, Greece. [2] School of Psychology, Aristotle University of Thessaloniki, Thessaloniki, Greece.

Acknowledgements
Not applicable.

Competing interests
The authors declare that they have no competing interests.

Consent for publication
Not applicable.

Funding
This research did not receive any specific grant from funding agencies in the public, commercial, or not-for-profit sectors.

References
1. Nicholson C, Alcorn C. Interpretation of the WISC-III and Its Subtests, Paper presented at the 25th Annual Meeting of the National Association of School Psychologists. Washington DC;1993:1–16.
2. Poulson MK, Scardapane JR. The factor structure of the WISC-III for unclassified, learning disabled, and high-IQ groups. Arch Clin Neuropsychol. 1997;12:388.
3. Konold TR, Kush JC, Canivez GL. Factor replication of the WISC-III in three independent samples of children receiving special education. J Psychoeduc Assess. 1997;15:123–37.
4. Grice JW, Krohn EJ, Logerquist S. Cross-validation of the WISC-III factor structure in two samples of children with learning disabilities. J Psychoeduc Assess. 1999;17:236–48.
5. Wechsler D. Wechsler intelligence scale for children: third edition manual. San Antonio: The Psychological Corporation; 1991.
6. Donders J, Warschausky S. A structural equation analysis of the WISC-III in children with traumatic head injury. Child Neuropsychol. 1996;2:185–92.
7. Watkins MW, Kush JC. Confirmatory factor analysis of the WISC-III for students with learning disabilities. J Psychoeduc Assess. 2002;20(1):4–19.
8. Cockshott FC, Marsh NV, Hine DW. Confirmatory factor analysis of the Wechsler Intelligence Scale for Children-third edition in an Australian clinical sample. Psychol Assess. 2006;18(3):353–7.
9. Kush JC, Watkins MW. Structural validity of the WISC-III for a national sample of Native American students. Can J Sch Psychol. 2007;22(2):235–48.
10. Burton DB, Sepehri A, Hecht F, VandenBroek A, Ryan JJ, Drabman R. A confirmatory factor analysis of the WISC-III in a clinical sample with cross-validation in the standardization sample. Child Neuropsychol. 2001;7(2):104–16.
11. Filippatou D, Livaniou L. Comorbidity and WISC-III profiles of Greek children with attention deficit, hyperactivity disorder, learning disabilities and language disorders. Psychol Rep. 2005;97:485–504.
12. Rotsika V, Vlassopoulos M, Legaki L, Sini A, Rogakou E, Sakellariou K, et al. The WISC-III profile in Greek children with learning disabilities: different language, similar difficulties. Int J Test. 2009;9:271–82.
13. Giannitsas ND, Mylonas C. Factor analysis for the Hellenic WISC-III: domains of cognitive development. Psychology (HJP). 2004;11(3):422–43.
14. Grégoire J. Factor structure of the French adaptation of the WISC-III: three or four factors. Int J Test. 2001;1:271–81.
15. Ganivez G, Watkins M. Long term stability of the Wechsler Intelligence Scale for Children-Third Edition among students with disabilities. School Psych Rev. 2001;30:438–53.
16. World Health Organization. International statistical classification of diseases and related health problems 10Th revision (ICD-10); 2008.
17. Georgas J, Paraskevopoulos IN, Besevegis E, Giannitsas ND. The Hellenic WISC-III. Athens: Psychometric Laboratory. University of Athens; 1997.
18. Fabrigar LR, Wegener DT, MacCallum RC, Strahan EJ. Evaluating the use of exploratory factor analysis in psychological research. Psychol Methods. 1999;4:272–99.
19. Arrindell WA, van der Ende J. An empirical test of the utility of the observations-to-variables ratio in factor and components analysis. Appl Psychol Meas. 1985;9:165–78.
20. De Winter JCF, Dodou D, Wieringa PA. Exploratory factor analysis with small sample sizes. Multivariate Behav Res. 2009;44:147–81.
21. Bryant FB, Yarnold PR. Principal components analysis and exploratory and confirmatory factor analysis. In: Grimm LG, Yarnold PR, editors. Reading and understanding multivariate statistics. Washington DC: American Psychological Association; 1995. p. 99–136.

22. Kaiser HF. The application of electronic computers to factor analysis. Educ Psychol Meas. 1960;20:141–51.

23. Cattell RB. The scree test for the number of factors. Multivariate Behav Res. 1966;1:245–76.

24. Horn JL. A rationale and test for the number of factors in factor analysis. Psychometrika. 1965;30:179–85.

25. Sideridis G, Simos P, Papanicolaou A, Fletcher J. Using structural equation modeling to assess functional connectivity in the brain. Educ Psychol Meas. 2014;74:733–58.

26. Wolf EJ, Harrington KM, Clark SL, Miller MW. Sample size requirements for structural equation models. Educ Psychol Meas. 2013;73:913–34.

27. Hu L, Bentler PM. Cutoff criteria for fit indexes in covariance structure analysis: conventional criteria versus new alternatives. Struct Equ Model. 1999;6:1–55.

28. Kass RE, Raftery AE. Bayes factors. J Am Stat Assoc. 1995;90:773–95.

29. Steiger JH, Shapiro A, Browne MW. On the multivariate asymptotic distribution of sequential Chi square statistics. Psychometrika. 1985;50:253–63.

30. Muthén LK, Muthén BO. Mplus User's Guide. 5th ed. Los Angeles: Muthén & Muthén; 2007.

31. Krippner S. WISC comprehension and picture arrangement subtests as measures of social competence. J Clin Psychol. 1964;20(3):366–7.

32. Brannigan G. Scoring difficulties on the Wechsler intelligence scales. Psychol Sch. 1975;12(3):313–4.

33. Beebe DW, Pfiffner LJ, McBurnett K. Evaluation of the validity of the Wechsler Intelligence Scale for Children-Third edition comprehension and picture arrangement subtests as measures of social intelligence. Psychol Assess. 2000;12(1):97–101.

34. Rapaport D, Gill MM, Schafer R. Diagnostic psychological testing. New York: International Universities Press; 1968.

35. Sattler J. Assessment of children. 3rd ed. San Diego CA: JM Sattler; 1992.

36. Ott SL, Spinelli S, Rock D, Roberts S, Amminger G, Erlenmeyer-Kimling L. The New York high-risk project: social and general intelligence in children at risk for schizophrenia. Schizophr Res. 1998;31(1):1–11.

37. Lipsitz JD, Dworkin RD, Erlenmeyer-Kimling L. Wechsler comprehension and picture arrangement subtests and social adjustment. Psychol Assess. 1993;5(4):430–7.

21

Analysis of global research output on diabetes depression and suicide

Waleed M. Sweileh[*]

Abstract

Background: Diabetic patients, during the course of the disease, are most likely to experience depressive symptoms that might ultimately lead to suicidal ideation or suicide. The size of literature in diabetes depression/suicide is a good indicator of national and international efforts to address psychological co-morbidities associated with diabetes mellitus (DM). Therefore, the objective of this study was to give a comprehensive analysis, both quantitative and qualitative, of scientific literature in diabetes depression/suicide.

Methods: SciVerse Scopus was used to retrieve relevant literature up to 2016.

Results: In total, 1664 journal documents were retrieved with an average of 26.9 citations per article and an h-index of 98. Publications started in 1949 but showed a steep and noticeable increase after 2001. Retrieved articles were published in 641 different journals with *Diabetes Care* journal being the top productive one with a total of 130 (7.8%) articles. Researchers from 83 different countries participated in retrieved publications. Researchers from the United States of America participated in publishing 685 articles. There was a strong and positive correlation between research output and Gross Domestic Product ($r = 0.083$; $p < 0.001$) but not with prevalence or mortality caused by DM. Researchers from 4870 different institutions/organizations participated in publishing retrieved articles. Publications from the *University of Washington, Seattle, USA* had the highest h-index (38), while "*VA medical centers*" had the highest number of publications (75; 4.5%). In total, 5715 authors appeared in retrieved articles giving an average of 3.4 authors per article. Top cited articles focused on prevalence, impact of depression on glycemic control, and potential risk of diabetic complications. The total number of publications in depression/suicide in diabetic patients was lesser than that in cardiac (1938) or in cancer (1828) patients. However, publications in diabetes depression/suicide exceeded those in cardiac and cancer in the last 2 years of the study period.

Conclusion: The current study showed a noticeable growth of publications indicative of the importance of this topic. Research focusing on the psychiatric component of diabetes mellitus needs to be strengthened and encouraged. At the practical level, screening for depression/suicide among patients attending primary healthcare clinics is needed to optimize health and quality of life of diabetic patients.

Keywords: Diabetes mellitus, Depression, Suicide, Research output, Bibliometric analysis

Background

Diabetes mellitus (DM) is a chronic metabolic disease that requires careful changes in life style that can be demanding and difficult to implement by some diabetic patients [1]. According to World Health Organization's (WHO) recent report, the number of people diagnosed with diabetes mellitus (DM) has risen from 108 million in 1980 to 422 million in 2014 [2]. In 2012, an estimated 1.5 million deaths were directly caused by diabetes and another 2.2 million deaths were attributable to high blood glucose [2]. Diabetes mellitus is considered as a national and global health burden. It is estimated that at least 10% of healthcare expenditures in many countries is invested in preventing and combating DM complications [3]. Diabetes mellitus is not only a health and economic

*Correspondence: waleedsweileh@yahoo.com
Department of Physiology and Pharmacology/Toxicology, College of Medicine and Health Sciences, Nablus, Palestine

burden but also a social and psychological challenge that could ultimately lead to chronic depression.

Depression is a common mental disorder and according to the WHO, more than 300 million people worldwide had depression. Depression is a serious illness and if not properly addressed, it can affect the normal function of affected people and might sometimes lead to suicide [4]. Globally, there is an increased trend of suicide [5]. According to the WHO, close to 800,000 deaths occur annually due to suicide and the majority (78%) of these cases occur in low- and middle-income countries (LMIC) [6]. Psychiatric disorders are known to impair the control of chronic diseases such as DM and behavioral interventions in such conditions might have more pronounced effects than medications [7].

Diabetic patients, and during the course of the disease, are most likely to experience depressive symptoms that might ultimately lead to suicidal ideation or suicide. Published studies showed that individuals with diabetes have an increased incidence of major depression when compared to the general population [8–10]. The high prevalence of depression among diabetic patients had led to the term "diapression" [11]. Vascular changes due to DM could be the biological basis for the development of depression among diabetic patients [12]. The relationship between diabetes and depression could be bidirectional with one disease leading to the increased risk of having the other disease [13]. Regardless of the directionality of the disease, the presence of depression in diabetes mellitus could worsen self-care, poor medication adherence, increased healthcare cost, poor glycemic control, potential risk of diabetic micro- and macro-vascular complications, and poor QOL [14–16]. The presence of depression in diabetic patients could lead to suicide ideation and suicide attempts. Studies have shown that diabetic patients, particularly type 1 DM, have higher risk of suicide ideation and suicidal attempts than non-diabetic patients [17, 18].

In light of increasing incidence of diabetes mellitus and in light of geographical and social differences in healthcare services and health literacy in diabetes, the need to assess the growth of research on diabetes depression/suicide becomes very important. Quantitative and qualitative analysis of publications in a particular area is usually called bibliometrics or scientometrics in which statistical methods are applied on a set of retrieved publications [19]. Bibliometric analysis is a growing field of information science which had been applied to various scientific disciplines [20–24]. Bibliometric analysis is a key element in establishing baseline data for future comparison in any scientific subject. Bibliometric analysis in diabetes depression/suicide could help to establish strategies for improving the volume and quality of research in this

field and the results could help to identify research gaps that future studies could focus on. The size of literature and research productivity in diabetes depression/suicide are good indicators of national and international efforts to decrease the health and economic burden of DM and the national and international efforts to address psychological co-morbidities associated with diabetes that could affect the QOL and glycemic control in diabetic patients.

To date, no studies have been published to summarize global research efforts, research trends, and geographical distribution of research output in diabetes depression/suicide, despite that several bibliometric analyses in diabetes research activity had been published [21, 25–28]. Therefore, the objective of this study was to give a comprehensive analysis, both quantitative and qualitative, of scientific literature in diabetes depression/suicide.

Methods

Bibliographic database

For the purpose of this study, only peer-reviewed articles published in scientific journals indexed in SciVerse Scopus were retrieved. Gray literature such as governmental and non-governmental reports, brochures, dissertations, theses, and newsletters were not included because some of the gray literature especially thesis and dissertation might have been published as research articles in peer-reviewed journals and therefore, they will create false-positive results due to overlap. The choice of Scopus database was based on the understanding of the author that it is larger than Web of Science and includes 100% of Medline [29]. Furthermore, Scopus has many analytic functions that facilitate bibliometric investigations of retrieved literature and therefore, it had been used in many previously published articles in the medical field.

Research strategy and keywords

To achieve the goal of the study, a set of related keywords pertaining or indicative of diabetes along with keywords related to depression or suicide were used. Keywords used in the search strategy were obtained from available systematic reviews [30–35]. The search strategy and keywords used along with the number of documents retrieved in each step are shown in Additional file 1: Appendix S1. To avoid any misinterpretation, we excluded publications in gestational diabetes mellitus and in experimental animals. The search strategy was based on searching for specific keywords in title of articles and not in abstract or author keywords. Actually, search for keywords in abstract and/or keywords yielded too many false-positive results that could negatively affect the validity of the study.

Validity check

The validity of research strategy was checked by manual review of top 20 cited articles to guarantee the absence of false-positive results. Furthermore, visualized author keywords were used to check for any irrelevant terms or false-positive results. For example, it was noticed that some keywords such as neuropathic pain, diabetes insipidus were present in retrieved articles and therefore, such keywords were excluded. Finally, research productivity of top active authors was retrieved manually and compared with those obtained using the current search strategy. The correlation between the manually obtained results and those obtained by search strategy was high with an interclass correlation of 96.8% indicative of high validity of the results and very low percentage of false negative.

Bibliometric indicators

Retrieved documents were refined, analyzed, and mapped to show research contribution and research trends. The time span of the study was set from 1997 to 2016. The Hirsch index (h-index) was used to assess the quality of published literature, while impact factor (IF) obtained from Journal Citation Report (2016) was used to assess the strength of publishing journals. Analysis of growth of publications with time was presented graphically using Statistical Package for Social Sciences (SPSS 21). For mapping keywords as well as international research collaboration, VOSviewer software was used [36]. In VOSviewer, the extent of collaboration is assessed by the thickness of a line connecting any two items such as countries or authors. For research productivity, the larger circle size or font size presenting a country or author, the greater the research productivity or citations of the listed author or country [36]. For geographical distribution of publications, ArcMap 10.1 software was used. Active institutions/organizations as well as most preferred journals for publishing articles in DSM were presented as top ten ones.

Results

The total number of retrieved articles was 1664. Research articles constituted the majority (1311; 78.8%) of retrieved documents followed by review articles (160; 9.6%) (Table 1). The main language in retrieved articles was English (1497; 90.0%) followed by German (67; 4.0%) and Spanish (30; 1.8%). Retrieved documents had an h-index of 98 and the highest number of citations recorded was 2060 for a meta-analysis study published in 2001 about the prevalence of depression among diabetic patients [37]. Retrieved documents received a total number of citations of 44,775, an average of 26.9 citations per article. The vast majority of retrieved articles was about diabetes depression, while

Table 1 Types of retrieved documents

Document type	Frequency	% ($N = 1664$)
Article	1311	78.8
Review	160	9.6
Letter	63	3.8
Note	57	3.4
Conference paper	22	1.3
Editorial	19	1.1
Short Survey	18	1.1
Article in Press	14	0.8

Table 2 Subject areas of retrieved documents

Document type	Frequency	% ($N = 1664$)[a]
Medicine (General and Internal)	765	46.0
Biochemistry, Genetics and immunology, Biology, and Molecular Biology	311	18.7
Psychology	227	13.6
Nursing	220	13.2
Neuroscience	80	4.8
Social Sciences and Humanities	92	5.5
Pharmacology, Toxicology and Pharmaceutics	47	2.8
Health Professions	41	2.5
Multidisciplinary and Miscellaneous	17	1.0

[a] Total percentage exceeds 100% due to overlap in certain subject areas

46 (2.8%) articles were about diabetes suicide and suicidal ideation.

Of retrieved articles, 765 (46%) were in the subject area of "Medicine", 311 (18.7%) were in the subject area of "Biochemistry, genetics, immunology, and molecular biology", while 227 (13.6%) were in the subject area of "psychology". Various subject areas of retrieved articles are shown in Table 2.

Growth of publications in diabetes depression/suicide started in 1949 with an article published in *The New England Journal of Medicine* about the effects of a large dose of insulin taken for suicidal attempt [38]. The number of publications in diabetes depression/suicide started in 1949, but remained very low until 2001. After 2001, the number of publications showed a steep and noticeable increase. Figure 1 shows the annual growth of publications in diabetes depression/suicide. Approximately, 92% of retrieved articles were published during the period from 2001 to 2016. The remaining 8% were published from 1949 to 2001. The highest number of publications recorded was 200 publications obtained in 2015.

Growth of publications was compared with that in other chronic diseases, particularly cancer and cardiac diseases. The total number of publications in diabetes depression/suicide (1664) was lesser than that in cardiac diseases depression/suicide (1938) and lesser than that in cancer depression/suicide (1828). However, the growth of publications in the three diseases showed that the ones in diabetes depression/suicide exceeded the other two in the last 2 years of the study period. Figure 2 showed the growth of publications in the three diseases with focus on the past three decades to facilitate comparison of growth of publications.

Retrieved articles were published in 641 different journals. Names of journals that published at least 10 documents are shown in Table 3 along with their most recent IF. The active list included a total of 18 journals with *Diabetes Care* being the top productive one with a total of 130 (7.8%) articles. More than half (10; 55.6%) of top active journals were in the field of diabetes and six were in the field of psychiatry/psychology (6; 33.3%), one (*Plos One*) was multidisciplinary, and one was in internal medicine. Seventeen journals in the active list had an official IF and two had an IF above five.

Researchers from 83 different countries participated in publishing retrieved articles. Countries with a minimum productivity of 10 documents are listed in Table 4 along with the reported prevalence of DM in each country. No significant correlation existed between prevalence of DM and research productivity in diabetes depression/suicide. The most productive country was the United States of America (USA) with a total productivity of 685 documents followed by the United Kingdom (UK) with a total productivity of 125 documents. No significant correlation was found between research output and prevalence of DM or mortality caused by DM per 100,000 population. However, there was a strong and positive correlation between research output and GDP ($r = 0.083$; $p < 0.001$). Despite that there was no significant correlation between research output and mortality rate caused by DM, there was a general trend of increased mortality caused by DM with low research output. This trend was obvious in countries such as Oman, Bahrain, Jordan, Morocco, South Africa, and Mexico (data not shown). Geographical distribution of publications showed that Africa, East Europe, and South America had poor research output in the field of diabetes depression/suicide. Figure 3 is a world map for geographical distribution of publications.

Researchers from 4870 different institutions/organizations participated in publishing retrieved articles. Institutions/organizations with a minimum productivity of 10

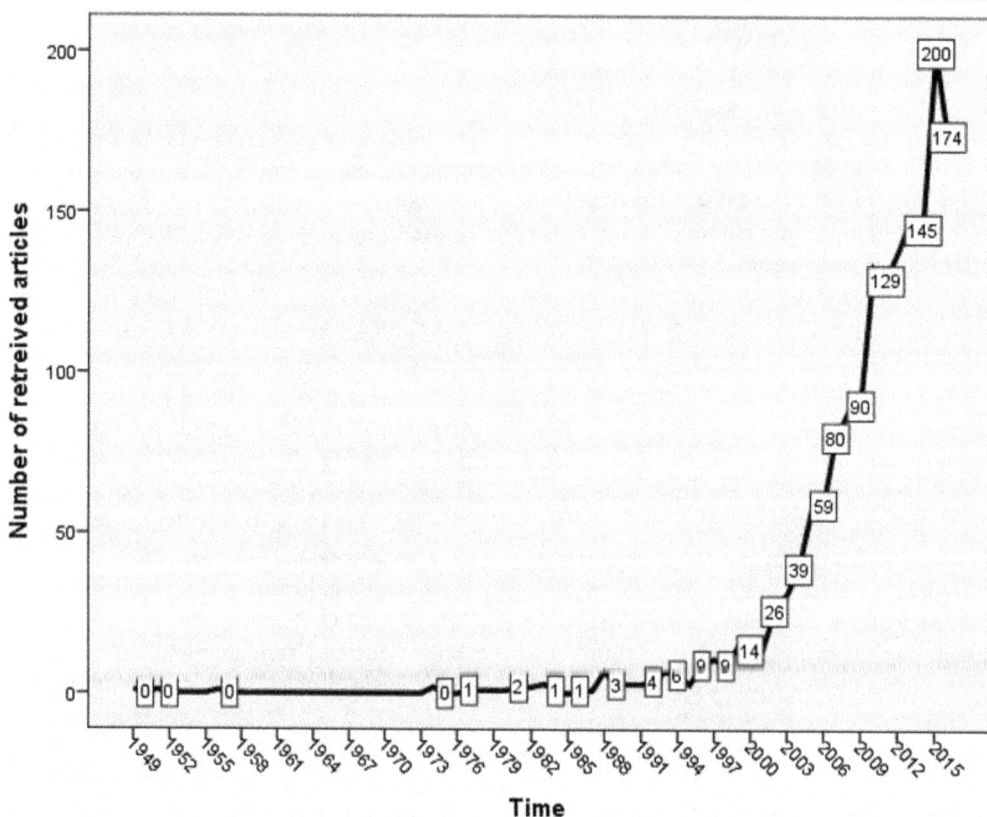

Fig. 1 Growth of publications in diabetes depression/suicide

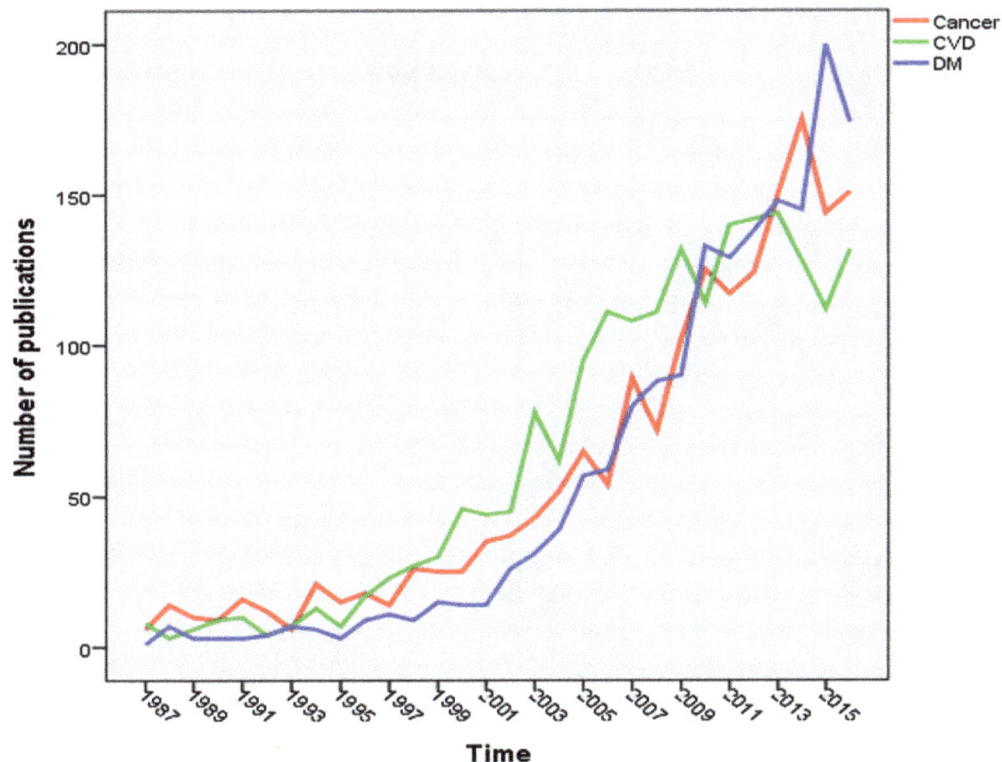

Fig. 2 Comparison of growth of publications in diabetes depression/suicide with that in cardiac diseases and in cancer (1986–2016). DM, diabetes mellitus; CVD, cardiovascular diseases

Table 3 List of journals with a minimum of 10 publications in diabetes depression/suicide

Journal	Frequency	% (N = 1664)	IF	Publisher
Diabetes Care	130	7.8	11.9	ADA
Diabetic Medicine	69	4.1	3.054	Wiley
Diabetes Research and Clinical Practice	39	2.3	3.693	Elsevier
General Hospital Psychiatry	29	1.7	2.279	Elsevier
Journal of Affective Disorders	28	1.7	3.432	Elsevier
Journal of Psychosomatic Research	26	1.6	2.809	Elsevier
Psychosomatic Medicine	25	1.5	3.863	LWW
Diabetologia	24	1.4	6.080	Springer Berlin Heidelberg
Diabetologe	23	1.4	0.072	Springer Medizin
Plos One	22	1.3	2.806	Public Library of Science
Journal of Diabetes and Its Complications	21	1.3	2.734	Elsevier
Diabetes Educator	17	1.0	1.811	Sage
Psychosomatics	17	1.0	1.436	Elsevier
BMC Psychiatry	16	1.0	2.613	BioMed Central
Journal of General Internal Medicine	13	0.8	3.701	Springer US
Journal of The Japan Diabetes Society	11	0.7	N/A	Japan Diabetes Society
Current Diabetes Reports	10	0.6	3.387	Current Medicine Group
Diabetes Spectrum	10	0.6	N/A	ADA

IF, impact factor; ADA, American Diabetes Association

Table 4 List of countries with minimum participation of 10 articles in diabetes depression/suicide based on country affiliation of authors

Country	Frequency	% (N = 1664)	Prevalence of DM [93]	Mortality per 100,000 population caused by DM [94]	GDP (trillions)
United States	674	40.5	9.1%	14.78	18.04
United Kingdom	125	7.5	7.7%	4.91	2.86
Germany	121	7.3	7.4%	11.43	3.36
Netherlands	100	6.0	6.1%	8.99	0.75
Australia	77	4.6	7.3%	11.05	1.2
Canada	71	4.3	7.2%	11.01	1.55
China	57	3.4	9.4%	14.8	11.06
India	41	2.5	7.8%	25.4	2.1
Japan	37	2.2	10.1%	4.37	4.38
Brazil	35	2.1	8.1%	39.74	1.8
Italy	31	1.9	8.5%	13.13	1.82
Poland	31	1.9	9.5%	10.07	0.477
Iran	25	1.5	10.3%	16.34	0.425
Mexico	23	1.4	10.4%	89.56	1.14
Turkey	23	1.4	13.2%	12.61	0.717
France	21	1.3	8.0%	8.78	2.42
Taiwan	21	1.3	–	–	1.177
Norway	19	1.1	6.6%	8.64	0.387
Spain	19	1.1	9.4%	9.86	1.19
Finland	17	1.0	7.7%	4.66	0.232
South Korea	15	0.9	9.5%	16.01	1.378
Sweden	14	0.8	6.9%	9.68	0.496
Austria	13	0.8	6.0%	15.84	0.377
Switzerland	13	0.8	5.6%	7.67	0.671
Saudi Arabia	12	0.7	14.4%	35.61	0.646
Croatia	11	0.7	9.9%	14.04	0.049
Hong Kong	11	0.7	–	–	0.309
Nigeria	11	0.7	4.3%	42.95	0.877
Belgium	10	0.6	6.4%	8.03	0.455
Pakistan	10	0.6	9.8%	39.65	0.271

documents were shown in Table 5. The active top 10 list included seven institutions in the USA, two in Netherlands and one in Canada. Publications from the *University of Washington, Seattle, USA* had the highest *h*-index (38) while "VA medical centers" had the highest number of publications (75; 4.5%).

In total, 5715 authors participated in publishing the retrieved documents giving an average of 3.4 authors per article. Authors with a minimum productivity of 10 documents and belong to a network of authors are visualized in Fig. 4. Visualization map of active authors included 36 authors grouped into six clusters. The largest cluster (red cluster) included 14 authors forming a network of collaboration. The size of the circle in the map reflects the size of the productivity, while the lines connecting the circles reflect the extent of author collaboration. Authors with the highest productivity include Katon W.J., Pouwer F., and Lustman P.J.

Top 20 cited articles are listed in Table 6. Top cited articles discussed issues related to epidemiology, impact of depression on glycemic control, diabetic complications/mortality, medication adherence, and quality of life. Four articles in top 20 cited articles discussed depression as a risk factor for diabetes and the bidirectional relationship between diabetes and depression. Analysis of author keywords using VOSviewer mapping showed that the following author keywords were most frequently encountered: "quality of life", epidemiology, prevalence, complications, screening, "primary care", adherence, self-management, mortality,

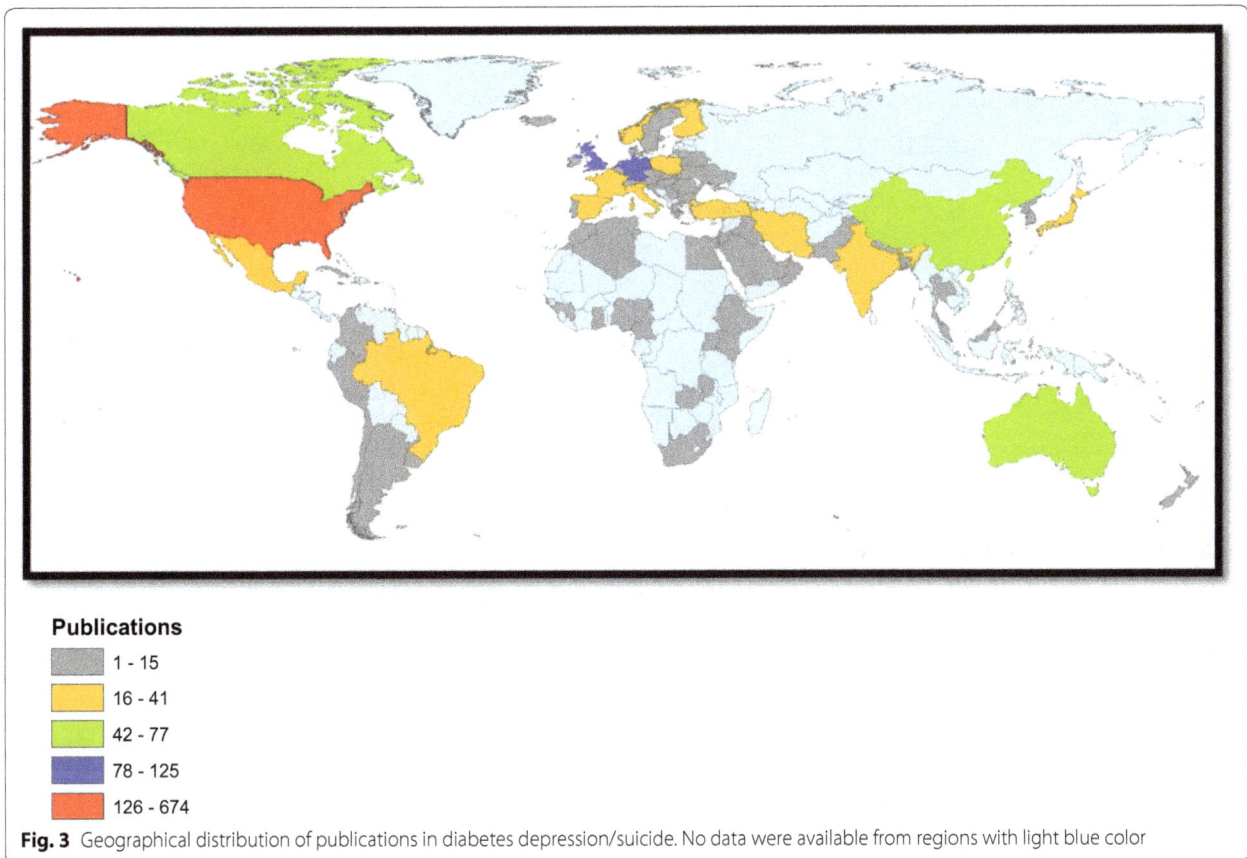

Publications

	1 - 15
	16 - 41
	42 - 77
	78 - 125
	126 - 674

Fig. 3 Geographical distribution of publications in diabetes depression/suicide. No data were available from regions with light blue color

Table 5 List of top active institutions/organizations

Institution/Organization	Frequency	% (N = 1664)	h-index of the publications	Country
VA Medical Center	75	4.5	31	USA
University of Washington, Seattle	73	4.4	38	USA
Tilburg University	51	3.1	22	Netherlands
VU University Medical Center	43	2.6	22	Netherlands
Johns Hopkins University	39	2.3	23	USA
Washington University in St. Louis, School of Medicine	37	2.2	26	USA
University Michigan Ann Arbor	34	2.0	15	USA
McGill University	31	1.9	8	Canada
Harvard Medical School	31	1.9	16	USA
University of California, Los Angeles	30	1.8	14	USA

women, "African–Americans", Hispanics, and other related terms (Fig. 5).

Discussion

The purpose of this study was to assess and analyze global research output and research trends on diabetes depression/suicide. The current study was conducted based on the assumption that diabetes mellitus is a potential risk factor for depressive symptoms which could lead to suicidal ideation and death [39–41]. The current study showed that keywords such as screening and "primary healthcare" were most commonly encountered indicating that screening for depression primary healthcare centers is strongly advocated by researchers.

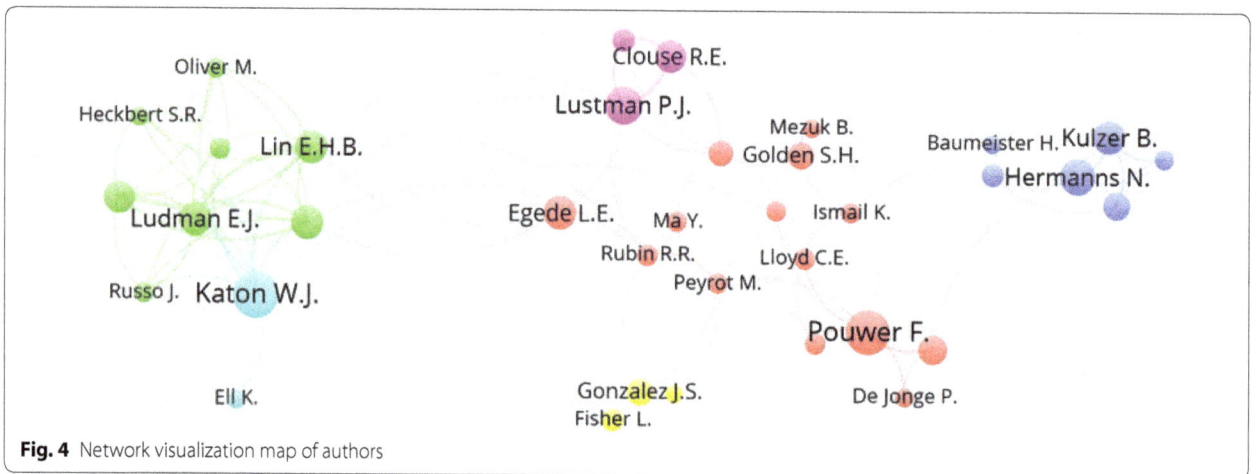

Fig. 4 Network visualization map of authors

Table 6 Top 20 cited articles in diabetes depression/suicide

Title	References	Year	Source title	Cited by
The prevalence of comorbid depression in adults with diabetes: a meta-analysis	[37]	2001	Diabetes Care	2056
Depression and poor glycemic control: a meta-analytic review of the literature	[95]	2000	Diabetes Care	1047
Association of depression and diabetes complications: a meta-analysis	[96]	2001	Psychosomatic Medicine	987
Depression and diabetes: impact of depressive symptoms on adherence, function, and costs	[97]	2000	Archives of Internal Medicine	935
Depression and type 2 diabetes over the lifespan: a meta-analysis	[40]	2008	Diabetes Care	572
The prevalence of co-morbid depression in adults with Type 2 diabetes: a systematic review and meta-analysis	[39]	2006	Diabetic Medicine	537
Relationship of depression and diabetes self-care, medication adherence, and preventive care	[98]	2004	Diabetes Care	528
Prevalence of depression in adults with diabetes: an epidemiological evaluation	[99]	1993	Diabetes Care	480
The pathways study: a randomized trial of collaborative care in patients with diabetes and depression	[100]	2004	Archives of General Psychiatry	475
Depression as a risk factor for the onset of type 2 diabetes mellitus. a meta-analysis	[101]	2006	Diabetologia	441
Examining a bidirectional association between depressive symptoms and diabetes	[102]	2008	JAMA—Journal of the American Medical Association	432
Comorbid depression is associated with increased health care use and expenditures in individuals with diabetes	[103]	2002	Diabetes Care	426
Depression and risk for onset of type ii diabetes: a prospective population-based study	[104]	1996	Diabetes Care	417
Relationship of depression to diabetes types 1 and 2: epidemiology, biology, and treatment	[105]	2003	Biological Psychiatry	412
Cognitive behavior therapy for depression in type 2 diabetes mellitus. A randomized, controlled trial	[106]	1998	Annals of Internal Medicine	395
The association of comorbid depression with mortality in patients with type 2 diabetes	[107]	2005	Diabetes Care	371
Depression and diabetes treatment nonadherence: a meta-analysis	[108]	2008	Diabetes Care	347
Depression predicts increased incidence of adverse health outcomes in older Mexican Americans with type 2 diabetes	[109]	2003	Diabetes Care	338
Levels and risks of depression and anxiety symptomatology among diabetic adults	[110]	1997	Diabetes Care	321
Diabetes, depression, and quality of life: a population study	[111]	2004	Diabetes Care	314

Subject areas of the retrieved literature

The current study showed that approximately 20% of publication in diabetes depression/suicide was within biochemistry/genetics/molecular biology subject area indicating that there was intensive research in the biological relationship between diabetes and depression. The hypothalamic–pituitary–adrenal (HPA) axis, cortisol, increased catecholamine, and proinflammatory cytokine

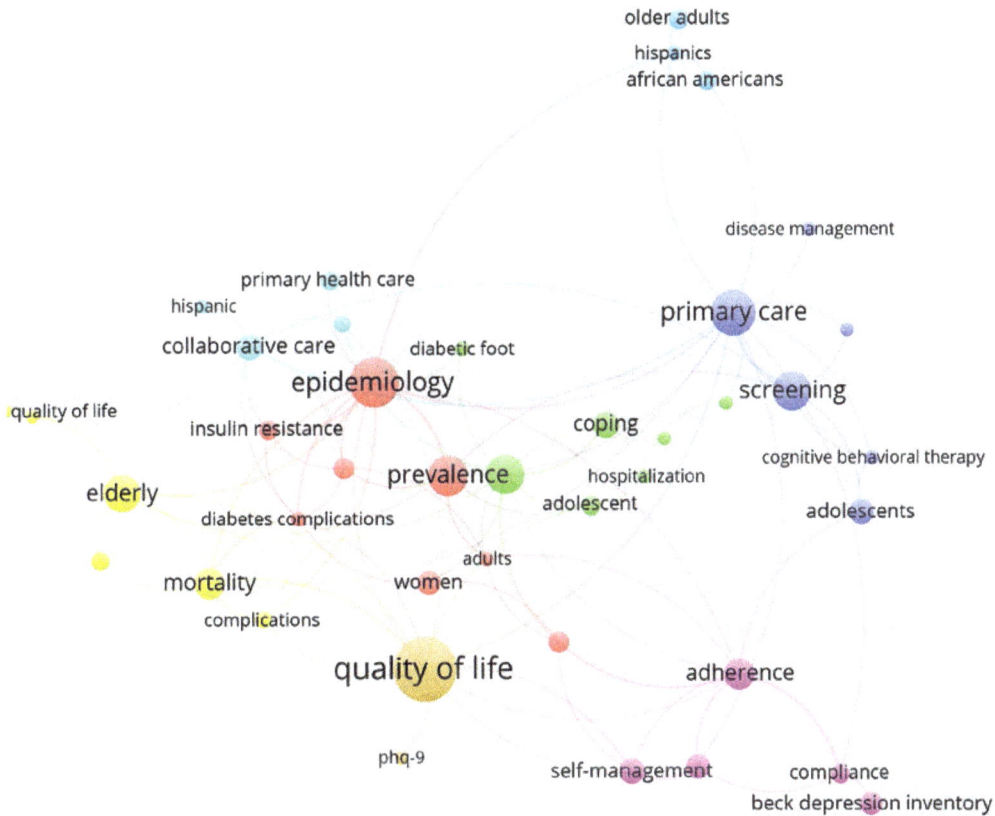

Fig. 5 Network visualization map of relevant author keywords

levels play a key role in development of insulin resistance [12, 42, 43]. The current study also showed that approximately 14% of retrieved documents were within the subject area of psychology. This was unsurprising given that coping behaviors and social support for diabetic patients might be different among different cultures and ethnicities [44–54].

Growth of publications
Research in diabetes depression/suicide started more than six decades ago, but the number of publications accelerated and showed a dramatic increase in the past decade. The growth of publication could be due to several factors. The overall increase in number of scholars, institutions, peer-reviewed journals, and global research output in the field of medicine positively affected the number of publications in diabetes depression/suicide. Second, certain findings regarding the scientific link between depression and poor glycemic control have triggered more research in this field. A third potential reason for the growth of publications was the debate about the bidirectional relationship between diabetes and depression and the role of depression as a potential risk factor

for diabetes [13, 55–59]. The growth of publications is of great relevance to mental health practitioners and should argue in favor of routine depression screening in diabetic patients in primary healthcare facilities [60–68].

Comparison with other diseases
The current study showed that the growth of research on diabetes depression showed a steeper increase than that on cardiac or cancer-depression research. Actually, in the last 3 years of the study period, the number of publications in diabetes depression/suicide exceeded that of cardiac or cancer publications indicating a global interest in this field. Furthermore, h-index of publications related to diabetes depression was very close to that of cardiac and cancer suggesting that depression in all chronic diseases is a serious problem that is of interest to scholars.

Geographical distribution of publications
The current study showed that geographical distribution of publications was skewed toward developed countries, particularly USA, Canada, Australia, Germany, Netherlands, and UK. Other countries such as Brazil, India, and China were among top active countries. In 2000, India had the highest number of

people with diabetes mellitus followed by China and the United States. It is predicted that by 2030 diabetes mellitus may afflict up to 79.4 million, 42.3 million, and 30.3 million individuals in India, China, and the USA, respectively, in 2030 [69–71]. Unfortunately, diabetes has been rising more rapidly in MLIC which necessitates more rigorous research in these countries to minimize diabetic complications and mortality [2]. Previously published studies also showed that contribution of LMIC to diabetes research did not match the health and economic burden of diabetes in these countries [21, 25, 27, 28, 72–74]. Not only diabetes research but also mental health research in LMIC was reported to be scarce [75–77]. The low research productivity from LMIC was also reflected in top 10 active institutions in diabetes depression/suicide research where no institution from LMIC showed up in the list.

Highly cited documents

An important aspect discussed in the top cited documents was the impact of depression on medication adherence and the potential risk of poor glycemic control. Studies showed that co-morbid diabetes and depression decreased the likelihood of adherence to lifestyle changes, specifically, diet, medication adherence, and physical activity resulting in elevated HbA1c and consequently poor self-care/self-management with increased risk of retinopathy, nephropathy, cardiac dysfunction, and mortality [78–84]. It had been found that depressive disorders decrease the desire to seek treatment making depression as an initial step of poor diabetes outcomes [85].

Limitations

The current study, like other bibliometric studies, has limitations that are inherent to bibliometric methodology and nature the database used [86–92]. Scopus database is not 100% comprehensive of literature, and therefore, some literature was missed particularly the ones published in un-indexed journals from developing countries. Second, the potential presence of false-negative results is a possibility due to the use of title search strategy. However, the title research strategy was used to minimize the false-positive results.

Conclusion

The current study showed an increasing interest of researchers in the psychiatric aspects of diabetes. This increasing interest is believed to promote the health of diabetic patients through initial screening of depression and through psychological and pharmacological treatment of the diseases. As a chronic disease with increasing global health burden, researchers need to get involved in all aspects that can alleviate the future complications of the disease to minimize health and economic burden of the disease. Future studies should focus on both epidemiological aspects in various cultures in developing countries and on the biological basis of depression in diabetic patients.

Abbreviation
DM: diabetes mellitus; WHO: World Health Organization.

Author contributions
WS: concept, data extraction, analysis and presentation, manuscript preparation, and manuscript submission and follow-up. The author read and approved the final manuscript.

Acknowledgements
None.

Competing interests
The author declares no competing interests.

Consent for publication
Not applicable.

Funding
None.

References
1. Armstrong C. Ada updates standards of medical care for patients with diabetes mellitus. Am Fam Physician. 2017;95(1):40–3.
2. World Health Organization: Global Report on Diabetes: World Health Organization; 2016.
3. Roglic G, Unwin N, Bennett PH, Mathers C, Tuomilehto J, Nag S, Connolly V, King H. The burden of mortality attributable to diabetes: realistic estimates for the year 2000. Diabetes Care. 2005;28(9):2130–5.
4. World Health Organization; Depression (Fact Sheet) http://www.who.int/mediacentre/factsheets/fs369/en/. Accessed 29 Jan 2018.
5. Bertolote JM, Fleischmann A. A global perspective in the epidemiology of suicide. Suicidologi. 2015;7(2):6–8.
6. World Health Organization; Suicide (Fact Sheet). http://www.who.int/mediacentre/factsheets/fs398/en. Accessed 04 July 2017.
7. Cezaretto A, Siqueira-Catania A, de Barros CR, Salvador EP, Ferreira SRG. Benefits on quality of life concomitant to metabolic improvement in intervention program for prevention of diabetes mellitus. Qual Life Res. 2012;21(1):105–13.
8. Poulsen K, Pachana NA. Depression and anxiety in older and middle-aged adults with diabetes. Aust Psychol. 2012;47(2):90–7.
9. Rubin RR, Peyrot M. Psychological issues and treatments for people with diabetes. J Clin Psychol. 2001;57(4):457–78.
10. Huang C-J, Lin C-H, Lee M-H, Chang K-P, Chiu H-C. Prevalence and incidence of diagnosed depression disorders in patients with diabetes: a National Population-Based Cohort Study. Gen Hosp Psychiatry. 2012;34(3):242–8.
11. Ciechanowski P. Diapression: an integrated model for understanding the experience of individuals with co-occurring diabetes and depression. Clin Diabetes. 2011;29(2):43–9.
12. Champaneri S, Wand GS, Malhotra SS, Casagrande SS, Golden SH. Biological basis of depression in adults with diabetes. Curr Diab Rep. 2010;10(6):396–405.

13. Pan A, Lucas M, Sun Q, Van Dam RM, Franco OH, Manson JE, Willett WC, Ascherio A, Hu FB. Bidirectional association between depression and type 2 diabetes mellitus in women. Arch Intern Med. 2010;170(21):1884–91.

14. Egede LE, Osborn CY. Role of motivation in the relationship between depression, self-care, and glycemic control in adults with type 2 diabetes. Diab Educator. 2010;36(2):276–83.

15. Fisher L, Glasgow RE, Strycker LA. The Relationship between diabetes distress and clinical depression with glycemic control among patients with type 2 diabetes. Diabetes Care. 2010;33(5):1034–6.

16. Egede LE, Ellis C. Diabetes and depression: global perspectives. Diab Res Clin Pract. 2010;87(3):302–12.

17. Pompili M, Lester D, Innamorati M, De Pisa E, Amore M, Ferrara C, Tatarelli R, Girardi P. Quality of life and suicide risk in patients with diabetes mellitus. Psychosomatics. 2009;50(1):16–23.

18. Pompili M, Forte A, Lester D, Erbuto D, Rovedi F, Innamorati M, Amore M, Girardi P. Suicide risk in type 1 diabetes mellitus: a systematic review. J Psychosom Res. 2014;76(5):352–60.

19. Thompson DF, Walker CK. A descriptive and historical review of bibliometrics with applications to medical sciences. Pharmacotherapy. 2015;35(6):551–9.

20. Dalton J, Garvey J, Samia LW. Evaluation of a Diabetes Disease Management Home Care Program. Home Health Care Manag Pract. 2006;18(4):272–85.

21. Sweileh WM, Zyoud SH, Al-Jabi SW, Sawalha AF. Bibliometric analysis of diabetes mellitus research output from middle eastern arab countries during the period (1996–2012). Scientometrics. 2014;101(1):819–32.

22. Sweileh WM, Al-Jabi SW, Sawalha AF, AbuTaha AS, Zyoud SH. Bibliometric analysis of medicine-related publications on poverty (2005–2015). SpringerPlus. 2016;5(1):1888.

23. Sweileh WM, Al-Jabi SW, Sawalha AF, Zyoud SH. Bibliometric profile of the global scientific research on autism spectrum disorders. SpringerPlus. 2016;5(1):1480.

24. Zyoud SH, Waring WS, Al-Jabi SW, Sweileh WM. Global cocaine intoxication research trends during 1975–2015: a bibliometric analysis of web of science publications. Subst Abuse. 2017;12(1):6.

25. Liu L, Jiao JH, Chen L. Bibliometric study of diabetic retinopathy during 2000–2010 by Isi. Int J Ophthalmol. 2011;4(4):333–6.

26. Peykari N, Djalalinia S, Kasaeian A, Naderimagham S, Hasannia T, Larijani B, Farzadfar F. Diabetes research in middle east countries; a scientometrics study from 1990 to 2012. J Res Med Sci. 2015;20(3):253–62.

27. Somogyi A, Schubert A. Correlation between National Bibliometric and Health Indicators: the Case of Diabetes. Scientometrics. 2005;62(2):285–92.

28. Yan B, Xiao H. Bibliometric analysis of diabetes literatures published in recent ten years. Acad J Sec Milit Med Univ. 2006;27(6):652–5.

29. Falagas ME, Pitsouni EI, Malietzis GA, Pappas G. Comparison of pubmed, scopus, web of science, and google scholar: strengths and weaknesses. FASEB J. 2008;22(2):338–42.

30. Werfalli M, Raubenheimer P, Engel M, Peer N, Kalula S, Kengne AP, Levitt NS. Effectiveness of community-based peer-led diabetes self-management programmes (Comp-Dsmp) for improving clinical outcomes and quality of life of adults with diabetes in primary care settings in low and middle-income countries (Lmic): a systematic review and meta-analysis. BMJ Open. 2015;5(7):e007635.

31. Teljeur C, Moran PS, Walshe S, Smith SM, Cianci F, Murphy L, Harrington P, Ryan M. Economic evaluation of chronic disease self-management for people with diabetes: a systematic review. Diabetic Med. 2016;34(8):1040–9.

32. Ahmad Sharoni SK, Minhat HS, Mohd Zulkefli NA, Baharom A. Health education programmes to improve foot self-care practices and foot problems among older people with diabetes: a systematic review. Int J Older People Nurs. 2016;11(3):214–39.

33. Lau Y, Htun TP, Wong SN, Tam WSW, Klainin-Yobas P. Efficacy of internet-based self-monitoring interventions on maternal and neonatal outcomes in perinatal diabetic women: a systematic review and meta-analysis. J Med Internet Res. 2016;18(8):e220.

34. Chrvala CA, Sherr D, Lipman RD. Diabetes self-management education for adults with type 2 diabetes mellitus: a systematic review of the effect on glycemic control. Patient Educ Couns. 2016;99(6):926–43.

35. Cui M, Wu X, Mao J, Wang X, Nie M. T2dm Self-management via smartphone applications: a systematic review and meta-analysis. PLoS ONE. 2016;11(11):e0166718.

36. van Eck NJ, Waltman L: Vosviewer Manual. In: Leiden: Univeristeit Leiden. vol. 1; 2013.

37. Anderson RJ, Freedland KE, Clouse RE, Lustman PJ. The prevalence of comorbid depression in adults with diabetes: a meta-analysis. Diabetes Care. 2001;24(6):1069–78.

38. Vogl A, Youngwirth SH. The Effects of a single dose of 2000 units of protamine zinc insulin taken by a diabetic patient with suicidal intent. N Engl J Med. 1949;241(16):606–9.

39. Ali S, Stone MA, Peters JL, Davies MJ, Khunti K. The prevalence of co-morbid depression in adults with type 2 diabetes: a systematic review and meta-analysis. Diabet Med. 2006;23(11):1165–73.

40. Mezuk B, Eaton WW, Albrecht S, Golden SH. Depression and type 2 diabetes over the lifespan: a meta-analysis. Diabetes Care. 2008;31(12):2383–90.

41. Nouwen A, Winkley K, Twisk J, Lloyd CE, Peyrot M, Ismail K, Pouwer F. Type 2 diabetes mellitus as a risk factor for the onset of depression: a systematic review and meta-analysis. Diabetologia. 2010;53(12):2480–6.

42. Jacobson AM, Samson JA, Weinger K, Ryan CM. Diabetes, the brain, and behavior: is there a biological mechanism underlying the association between diabetes and depression? Int Rev Neurobiol. 2002;51:455–79.

43. Musselman DL, Betan E, Larsen H, Phillips LS. Relationship of depression to diabetes types 1 and 2: epidemiology, biology, and treatment. Biol Psychiaty. 2003;54(3):317–29.

44. Black SA. Increased health burden associated with comorbid depression in older diabetic mexican Americans: results from the hispanic established population for the epidemiologic study of the elderly survey. Diabetes Care. 1999;22(1):56–64.

45. Chlebowy DO, Coty MB, Fu L, Hines-Martin V. Comorbid Diabetes and Depression in African Americans: Implications for the Health Care Provider. J Racial Ethnic Health Dispar. 2017;5:1–6.

46. De Groot M, Auslander W, Williams JH, Sherraden M, Haire-Joshu D. Depression and poverty among african american women at risk for type 2 diabetes. Ann Behav Med. 2003;25(3):172–81.

47. De Groot M, Lustman PJ. Depression among African-Americans with diabetes: a dearth of studies [2]. Diabetes Care. 2001;24(2):407–8.

48. Egede LE. Beliefs and attitudes of african americans with type 2 diabetes toward depression. Diab Educator. 2002;28(2):258–68.

49. Gary TL, Crum RM, Cooper-Patrick L, Ford D, Brancati FL. Depressive symptoms and metabolic control in African-Americans with Type 2 Diabetes. Diabetes Care. 2000;23(1):23–9.

50. Hernandez R, Ruggiero L, Prohaska TR, Chavez N, Boughton SW, Peacock N, Zhao W, Nouwen A. A Cross-Sectional Study of depressive symptoms and diabetes self-care in African Americans and Hispanics/Latinos with diabetes: the role of self-efficacy. Diab Educator. 2016;42(4):452–61.

51. Husaini BA, Hull PC, Sherkat DE, Emerson JS, Overton MT, Craun C, Cain VA, Levine RS. Diabetes, depression, and healthcare utilization among African Americans in primary care. J Natl Med Assoc. 2004;96(4):476–84.

52. Kim MT, Kim KB, Ko J, Jang Y, Levine D, Lee HB. Role of depression in diabetes management in an ethnic minority population: a case of Korean Americans with type 2 diabetes. BMJ Open Diab Res Care. 2017;5(1):e000337.

53. Rehman SU, Shakaib A, Rashid S. Regarding depressive symptoms and metabolic control in African-Americans with type 2 diabetes [5] (multiple letters). Diabetes Care. 2000;23(10):1596–7.

54. Shah ZC, Huffman FG. Depression among hispanic women with type 2 diabetes. Ethn Dis. 2005;15(4):685–90.

55. Chen PC, Chan YT, Chen HF, Ko MC, Li CY. Population-based cohort analyses of the bidirectional relationship between type 2 diabetes and depression. Diabetes Care. 2013;36(2):376–82.

56. Golden SH, Lazo M, Carnethon M, Bertoni AG, Schreiner PJ, Diez Roux AV, Lee HB, Lyketsos C. Examining a bidirectional association between depressive symptoms and diabetes. JAMA. 2008;299(23):2751–9.

57. Jaser SS, Holl MG, Jefferson V, Grey M. Correlates of depressive symptoms in urban youth at risk for type 2 diabetes mellitus. J Sch Health. 2009;79(6):286–92.

58. Renn BN, Feliciano L, Segal DL. The bidirectional relationship of depression and diabetes: a systematic review. Clin Psychol Rev. 2011;31(8):1239–46.

59. Yu M, Zhang X, Lu F, Fang L. Depression and risk for diabetes: a meta-analysis. Can J Diab. 2015;39(4):266–72.

60. Burton C, Simpson C, Anderson N. Diagnosis and treatment of depression following routine screening in patients with coronary heart disease or diabetes: a database cohort study. Psychol Med. 2013;43(3):529–37.

61. Corathers SD, Kichler J, Jones NHY, Houchen A, Jolly M, Morwessel N, Crawford P, Dolan LM, Hood KK. Improving depression screening for adolescents with type 1 diabetes. Pediatrics. 2013;132(5):e1395–402.

62. Fleer J, Tovote KA, Keers JC, Links TP, Sanderman R, Coyne JC, Schroevers MJ. Screening for depression and diabetes-related distress in a diabetes outpatient clinic. Diabet Med. 2013;30(1):88–94.

63. Hermanns N, Caputo S, Dzida G, Khunti K, Meneghini LF, Snoek F. Screening, evaluation and management of depression in people with diabetes in primary care. Prim Care Diab. 2013;7(1):1–10.

64. Holt RG, van der Feltz-Cornelis CM. Key concepts in screening for depression in people with diabetes. J Affec Disorders. 2012;142:S72–9.

65. Monaghan M, Singh C, Streisand R, Cogen FR. Screening and identification of children and adolescents at risk for depression during a diabetes clinic visit. Diabetes Spectr. 2010;23(1):25–31.

66. Roy T, Lloyd CE, Pouwer F, Holt RIG, Sartorius N. Screening tools used for measuring depression among people with type 1 and type 2 diabetes: a systematic review. Diab Med. 2012;29(2):164–75.

67. Silverstein J, Cheng P, Ruedy KJ, Kollman C, Beck RW, Klingensmith GJ, Wood JR, Willi S, Bacha F, Lee J, et al. Depressive symptoms in youth with type 1 or type 2 diabetes: results of the pediatric diabetes consortium screening assessment of depression in diabetes study. Diabetes Care. 2015;38(12):2341–3.

68. Van Steenbergen-Weijenburg KM, De Vroege L, Ploeger RR, Brals JW, Vloedbeld MG, Veneman TF, Hakkaart-Van Roijen L, Rutten FF, Beekman AT, Van Der Feltz-Cornelis CM. Validation of the Phq-9 as a screening instrument for depression in diabetes patients in specialized outpatient clinics. BMC Health Serv Res. 2010;10:235.

69. Wild S, Roglic G, Green A, Sicree R, King H. Global prevalence of diabetes: estimates for the year 2000 and projections for 2030. Diabetes Care. 2004;27(5):1047–53.

70. Whiting DR, Guariguata L, Weil C, Shaw J. Idf diabetes atlas: global estimates of the prevalence of diabetes for 2011 and 2030. Diabetes Res Clin Pract. 2011;94(3):311–21.

71. Kaveeshwar SA, Cornwall J. The current state of diabetes mellitus in India. Australas Med J. 2014;7(1):45.

72. De Lusignan S. Bibliometric analysis of primary care research, childhood obesity, the importance of understanding small area data and diabetes. Inform Prim Care. 2011;18(4):217–8.

73. Caglar C, Demir E, Kucukler FK, Durmus M. A bibliometric analysis of academic publication on diabetic retinopathy disease trends during 1980–2014: a global and medical view. Int J Ophthalmol. 2016;9(11):1663–8.

74. Nolan CK, Spiess KE, Meyr AJ. Where art thou diabetic foot disease literature? A bibliometric inquiry into publication patterns. J Foot Ankle Surg. 2015;54(3):295–7.

75. Razzouk D, Sharan P, Gallo C, Gureje O, Lamberte EE, de Jesus Mari J, Mazzotti G, Patel V, Swartz L, Olifson S. Scarcity and inequity of mental health research resources in low-and-middle income countries: a global survey. Health Policy. 2010;94(3):211–20.

76. Siriwardhana C, Sumathipala A, Siribaddana S, Samaraweera S, Abeysinghe N, Prince M, Hotopf M. Reducing the scarcity in mental health research from low and middle income countries: a success story from Sri Lanka. Int Rev Psychiatry. 2011;23(1):77–83.

77. Lund C. Poverty, inequality and mental health in low-and middle-income countries: time to expand the research and policy agendas. Epidemiol Psychiatr Sci. 2015;24(2):97.

78. Coelho CR, Zantut-Wittmann DE, Parisi MCR. A cross-sectional study of depression and self-care in patients with type 2 diabetes with and without foot ulcers. Ostomy Wound Manag. 2014;60(2):46–51.

79. Gaitonde P, Shaya FT. Relationship between depression, self-care behaviors, and treatment success among older medicare beneficiaries with type 2 diabetes. J Pharm Health Serv Res. 2016;7(4):241–5.

80. Kokoszka A. Treatment adherence in patients with type 2 diabetes mellitus correlates with different coping styles, low perception of self-influence on disease, and depressive symptoms. Patient Preference Adherence. 2017;11:587–95.

81. Matsunaga S, Tanaka S, Fujihara K, Horikawa C, Iimuro S, Kitaoka M, Sato A, Nakamura J, Haneda M, Shimano H, et al. Association between all-cause mortality and severity of depressive symptoms in patients with type 2 diabetes: analysis from the japan diabetes complications study (jdcs). J Psychosom Res. 2017;99:34–9.

82. Rees G, Xie J, Fenwick EK, Sturrock BA, Finger R, Rogers SL, Lim L, Lamoureux EL. Association between diabetes-related eye complications and symptoms of anxiety and depression. JAMA Ophthalmol. 2016;134(9):1007–14.

83. Shin N, Hill-Briggs F, Langan S, Payne JL, Lyketsos C, Golden SH. The association of minor and major depression with health problem-solving and diabetes self-care activities in a clinic-based population of adults with type 2 diabetes mellitus. J Diabetes Complications. 2017;31(5):880–5.

84. Sumlin LL, Garcia TJ, Brown SA, Winter MA, García AA, Brown A, Cuevas HE. Depression and adherence to lifestyle changes in type 2 diabetes: a systematic review. Diab Educator. 2014;40(6):731–44.

85. Egede LE. Effect of depression on self-management behaviors and health outcomes in adults with type 2 diabetes. Curr Diab Rev. 2005;1(3):235–43.

86. Sweileh WM, Wickramage K, Pottie K, Hui C, Roberts B, Sawalha AF, Zyoud SH. Bibliometric analysis of global migration health research in peer-reviewed literature (2000–2016). BMC Public Health. 2018;18(1):777.

87. Sweileh WM. Bibliometric analysis of literature in aids-related stigma and discrimination. Transl Behav Med. 2018. https://doi.org/10.1093/tbm/iby072.

88. Sweileh WM. Bibliometric analysis of medicine—related publications on refugees, asylum-seekers, and internally displaced people: 2000–2015. BMC Int Health Hum Rights. 2017;17(1):7.

89. Sweileh WM. Bibliometric analysis of peer-reviewed literature in transgender health (1900–2017). BMC Int Health Hum Rights. 2018;18(1):16.

90. Sweileh WM. Global output of research on epidermal parasitic skin diseases from 1967 to 2017. Infect Dis Poverty. 2018;7(1):74.

91. Sweileh WM. Global research output in the health of international arab migrants (1988–2017). BMC Public Health. 2018;18(1):755.

92. Sweileh WM. Global research trends of World Health Organization's top eight emerging pathogens. Global Health. 2017;13(1):9.

93. World Health Organization (WHO). Diabetes Country Profile. http://www.who.int/diabetes/country-profiles/en/. Accessed 29 Jan 2018.

94. World Health Rankings: Diabets mellitus death rate per 100,000 age standardized. 2016.

95. Lustman PJ, Anderson RJ, Freedland KE, de Groot M, Carney RM, Clouse RE. Depression and poor glycemic control: a meta-analytic review of the literature. Diabetes Care. 2000;23(7):934–42.

96. de Groot M, Anderson R, Freedland KE, Clouse RE, Lustman PJ. Association of depression and diabetes complications: a meta-analysis. Psychosom Med. 2001;63(4):619–30.

97. Ciechanowski PS, Katon WJ, Russo JE. Depression and diabetes: impact of depressive symptoms on adherence, function, and costs. Arch Intern Med. 2000;160(21):3278–85.

98. Lin EH, Katon W, Von Korff M, Rutter C, Simon GE, Oliver M, Ciechanowski P, Ludman EJ, Bush T, Young B. Relationship of depression and diabetes self-care, medication adherence, and preventive care. Diabetes Care. 2004;27(9):2154–60.

99. Gavard JA, Lustman PJ, Clouse RE. Prevalence of depression in adults with diabetes: an epidemiological evaluation. Diabetes Care. 1993;16(8):1167–78.

100. Katon WJ, Von Korff M, Lin EH, Simon G, Ludman E, Russo J, Ciechanowski P, Walker E, Bush T. The pathways study: a randomized trial of collaborative care in patients with diabetes and depression. Arch Gen Psychiatry. 2004;61(10):1042–9.

101. Knol MJ, Twisk JW, Beekman AT, Heine RJ, Snoek FJ, Pouwer F. Depression as a risk factor for the onset of type 2 diabetes mellitus. A meta-analysis. Diabetologia. 2006;49(5):837–45.

102. Golden SH, Lazo M, Carnethon M, Bertoni AG, Schreiner PJ, Diez Roux AV, Lee HB, Lyketsos C. Examining a bidirectional association between depressive symptoms and diabetes. JAMA. 2008;299(23):2751–9.

103. Egede LE, Zheng D, Simpson K. Comorbid depression is associated with increased health care use and expenditures in individuals with diabetes. Diabetes Care. 2002;25(3):464–70.

104. Eaton WW, Armenian H, Gallo J, Pratt L, Ford DE. Depression and risk for onset of type ii diabetes. A prospective population-based study. Diabetes Care. 1996;19(10):1097–102.

105. Musselman DL, Betan E, Larsen H, Phillips LS. Relationship of depression to diabetes types 1 and 2: epidemiology, biology, and treatment. Biol Psychiatry. 2003;54(3):317–29.

106. Lustman PJ, Griffith LS, Freedland KE, Kissel SS, Clouse RE. Cognitive behavior therapy for depression in type 2 diabetes mellitus. A randomized, controlled trial. Ann Intern Med. 1998;129(8):613–21.

107. Katon WJ, Rutter C, Simon G, Lin EH, Ludman E, Ciechanowski P, Kinder L, Young B, Von Korff M. The association of comorbid depression with mortality in patients with type 2 diabetes. Diabetes Care. 2005;28(11):2668–72.

108. Gonzalez JS, Peyrot M, McCarl LA, Collins EM, Serpa L, Mimiaga MJ, Safren SA. Depression and diabetes treatment nonadherence: a meta-analysis. Diabetes Care. 2008;31(12):2398–403.

109. Black SA, Markides KS, Ray LA. Depression predicts increased incidence of adverse health outcomes in older Mexican Americans with type 2 diabetes. Diabetes Care. 2003;26(10):2822–8.

110. Peyrot M, Rubin RR. Levels and Risks of Depression and Anxiety Symptomatology among Diabetic Adults. Diabetes Care. 1997;20(4):585–90.

111. Goldney RD, Phillips PJ, Fisher LJ, Wilson DH. Diabetes, depression, and quality of life: a population study. Diabetes Care. 2004;27(5):1066–70.

22

Determinants of depression among people with epilepsy in Central Ethiopia

Asrat Chaka[1], Tadesse Awoke[2], Zegeye Yohannis[1], Getinet Ayano[1], Minale Tareke[3*], Andargie Abate[3] and Mulugeta Nega[4]

Abstract

Background: Depression is the most frequently and highly occurring mental disorders in epilepsy patients. When depression is comorbid with epilepsy, it leads to low employment and poor quality of life. Thus, the aim of this study was to assess the prevalence and associated factors of depression among people living with epilepsy in Central Ethiopia.

Methods: Institution-based cross-sectional study was conducted from April to May 2015 at Amanuel Mental Specialized and TikurAnbesa Hospitals, Addis Ababa, Ethiopia. Samples of 422 epilepsy patients were selected, and data on depression were collected using validated questionnaire using face-to-face interview technique. Logistic regression analysis was performed to assess predictors of depression.

Results: The study indicated that the prevalence of depression among people with epilepsy was 43.8%. Factors associated with depression were being female (AOR 2.48; 95% CI, 1.61.3.81), being single (AOR 2.23; 95% CI 1.38–3.60), perceived stigma (AOR 2.47; 95% CI 1.59–3.83), medication adherence (AOR 2.85; 95% CI 1.64–4.96), and current substance use (AOR 2.10; 95% CI 1.34–3.30).

Conclusion: There is a high prevalence of depression among epilepsy patients. Early detection and prompt management of depressive symptoms are critically important in reducing depression burden among people living with epilepsy.

Keywords: Comorbidity, Depression, Epilepsy

Introduction

Epilepsy is a disease of the brain defined by at least two unprovoked (or reflex) Seizures occurring within > 24 h apart; one unprovoked (or reflex) seizure and a probability of further seizures similar to the general recurrence risk (at least 60%) after two unprovoked seizures, occurring over the next 10 years [1]. It is a common neurological condition characterized by recurrent seizures and abnormal electrical activity in the brain that causes an involuntary change in body movement or function, sensation, awareness, or behavior [2]. More than 80% of people with epilepsy live in developing countries, and a

majority of them do not have recourse to any effective treatment [3].

Depression is highly prevalent in the patient with epilepsy and is the most frequent comorbid psychiatric problem [4]. According to Diagnostic and Statistical Manual of Mental Disorders, Fifth Edition (DSM-5), depressive disorder is defined as at least one of the symptoms, either depressed mood or loss of interest or pleasure for at least 2 weeks, and includes at least other four symptoms from a list of criteria items, which are severe enough to cause severe distress or impairment in executing important functional roles [5].

Data from population-based studies have revealed a more complex, bidirectional relation between the two disorders, whereby not only are people with epilepsy at greater risk of developing depression but also people with depression are at greater risk of developing epilepsy. The

*Correspondence: minale23@gmail.com
[3] College of Medicine and Health Science, Bahir Dar University, Bahir Dar, Ethiopia
Full list of author information is available at the end of the article

existing common neurobiological pathogenic mechanisms shared by depressive disorders and epilepsy include neurotransmitter disturbances in the central nervous system such as serotonin, norepinephrine, dopamine, glutamate, and gamma-aminobutyric acid (GABA); endocrine disturbances such as hyperactive hypothalamic pituitary–adrenal axis, resulting in high serum concentrations of cortisol; and inflammatory mechanisms (in particular, interleukin-1β has been found to play a pathogenic role in patients with mood disorders) [6].

Depression is the most frequent psychiatric comorbidity in people with epilepsy with a prevalence rate ranging from 9.5 to 63% [7–12]. It leads to underemployment, lower rates of marriage, and a greater chance of social isolation when compared to counterparts [13, 14]. The high magnitude of depression among people living with epilepsy negatively influences their quality of life and increases suicidal tendency [15, 16]. Factors such as side effects of antiepileptic drugs, perceived stigma, fear of seizures, discrimination, joblessness, lack of social support, increased seizure frequency, and nonadherence to their medication have contributed to inducing depression among epilepsy patients [17, 18].

Despite this burden and consequences, there is a limited literature on the magnitude of depression and associated factors in people with epilepsy in the study area. Therefore, this study was intended to fill the gaps by assessing the prevalence and associated factors of depression among people living with epilepsy. It also helps to integrate mental health service in primary healthcare unit by early diagnosis and timely treatment of comorbid cases.

Methods

Study settings and population

Institution-based cross-sectional study was conducted from April to May 2015 at Amanuel Mental Specialized and TikurAnbesa Hospitals neurology clinics, located in Addis Ababa (capital city of Ethiopia). Amanuel Mental Specialized Hospital (AMSH) and TkurAnbesa Hospital (TAH) are the largest referral centers for people in Ethiopia as well as served as being medical teaching institutions. The AMSH and TAH have three and two neurologic outpatient clinics, respectively. Both hospitals provide medical and neurologic care.

The study populations comprised all epilepsy patients who were receiving treatments in their respective hospitals. All patients aged 18 years and above who have been diagnosed with epilepsy and provided with treatment in the outpatient epilepsy clinics in both hospitals were included in the study. Patients unable to communicate and seriously ill were excluded from the study.

Sample size and Sampling procedures

The sample size was calculated using a single population proportion formula $[n_o = (Z\alpha_{/2})^2 \times (P - q))/d^2$, where n_o is the minimum sample size, Z the standardized normal distribution value at $\alpha/2$, P the proportion of depression, and d is the margin of error]. By taking the proportion of depression at 49.3% [19], $Z\alpha_{/2}$ at 95% CI (1.96), and tolerable margin of error at (0.05), the minimum sample size was 384. By adding 10% for nonresponse rate, 423 participants were involved in the study.

Sampling interval was determined by dividing the total study population who had followed up during one month before data collection period (1600) by total sample size (422). Sampling fraction is $1600/422 \approx 4$. Hence, the sample interval is 4. The first study population was selected by lottery method, and the next study participants were chosen at regular intervals (every 4th), and the selected respondents were interviewed by data collectors.

Data collection and quality assurance

Data were collected using instruments that measure depression, perceived stigma, Medication Adherence Scale, and social support-related questionnaires. The Patient Health Questionnaire (PHQ)-9 is the nine-item depression scale which is a powerful tool for clinicians to screen depression and monitor treatment response. The tool is based directly on the nine diagnostic criteria for major depressive disorder among epilepsy patients [20]. PHQ-9 is validated and extensively used in Ethiopia [21, 22]. The score of greater than or equal to 5 was considered to indicate probable depression in patients in this study. Patient medication adherence was measured using self-reported questions.

Perceived stigma was assessed via a three-item stigma scale with an overall possible score ranging from 0 (no felt stigma) to 3 (maximally felt stigma) [23]. Social support was measured by the three Oslo scale of social support measurement [24].

The questionnaire was designed and modified appropriately and translated into local language (Amharic) to be understood by all participants and translated back to English again to ensure its consistency. Training was given for four data collectors (psychiatry nurses) and one supervisor (BSc Nursing) for 2 days. The pretest was done at TikurAnbesa hospital 2 weeks before the day of actual data collection. The data collectors were supervised daily, and the filled questionnaires were checked properly by the supervisor and the principal investigator.

Data management and processing

The coded data were checked, cleaned, and entered into epi.info version 3.5 and then exported into Statistical Package for the Social Sciences (SPSS) window version 20 for analysis. Descriptive statistic was used to explain the study participants in relation to study variable. Bivariate and multivariate logistic regression analyses were conducted to identify associated factors of depression among people with epilepsy. The strength of the association was interpreted by odds ratio with 95% CI, and the p-value less than 0.05 was considered as statistically significant.

Ethical consideration

Ethical clearance was obtained after approval from the Institutional Review Board (IRB) of the College of Medicine and Health Sciences, the University of Gondar and from Amanuel Mental Specialized Hospital. The data collectors have clearly explained the aims of the study to the study participants. Information was collected after obtaining written consent from each participant. The right to exercise refusal was given to the study participants as well as their discontinuation from participation at any point in time. Confidentiality was maintained throughout the study. Those study participants suffering from recurrent severe suicidal thought was treated by communicating with psychiatry case team.

Result

Sociodemographic characteristics

The mean age of respondents was 31.57 ($\pm$ SD 9.91). Nearly one-third (33.9%) of the respondents were between 25- and 34-aged groups and almost half of them were single (50. 2%) by marital status. A majority of them were living in the urban area (88.2%) (Table 1).

Clinical- and medication-related characteristics

The majority (86%) of them had no family history of mental illness. Among the study respondents, nearly one-third (36%) had more than 10 years of duration of illness. Most (66.4%) of the study respondents were taking more than one antiepileptic drugs, had social support (85.3%), and had felt no stigma (62.3%) (Table 2).

Substance related factors of the respondents

Most (67.8%) of the study participants had no history of substance use; however, the remaining (32.2%) used the substance. Among the total study participants who had used the substance, 79 (18.7%) were reported drinking alcohol (Fig. 1).

Table 1 Sociodemographic distribution of epilepsy patients on follow up at AMSH and TAH, 2015

Variables	Numbers	Percent (%)
Sex		
Male	249	59.0
Female	173	41
Age		
18–24	105	24.9
25–34	143	33.9
35–44	113	26.8
45–54	48	11.4
≥55	13	3.1
Ethnicity		
Amhara	138	32.7
Oromo	126	29.9
Tigre	24	5.7
Gurage	119	28.2
Others	15	3.6
Marital status		
Single	212	50.2
Divorce	58	13.7
Widowed	9	2.1
Married	143	33.9
Religion		
Orthodox	270	64.0
Muslim	98	23.0
Protestant	54	12.6
Residence		
Urban	372	88.2
Rural	50	11.8
Education		
Unable to read and write	24	5.7
Primary (1–8)	145	34.4
Secondary (9–12)	172	40.8
Diploma and degree	81	19.2
Occupation		
Not employed	41	9.7
Employed	381	90.3
With whom living now		
Family	396	93.8
Alone	14	3.3
Relative/friend	12	2.8

Prevalence of depression among epilepsy patients

The distribution of PHQ-9 among respondents showed a mean score and standard deviation of 4.83 $\pm$ 4.68. Using cutoff point of five and above, 43.8% of the respondents had depression with 95% confidence interval (38.9%, 48. 8%). More females (52.4%) were affected by depression than males (47.6%) (Table 3).

Table 2 Description of clinical and psychosocial factors of patients with epilepsy at AMSH and TAH, 2015

Variables	Frequency	Numbers	Percent (%)
Family history of mental illness	Yes	59	14
	No	363	86
Seizure frequency per month	No seizure	243	57.6
	1–3	173	41.0
	4 and above	6	1.4
Duration of epilepsy illness	<1 year	19	4.5
	1–5 years	115	27.3
	6–10 years	136	32.2
	>10 years	152	36
Types of epilepsy diagnosed	Grandmal	251	59.5
	Petimal	108	25.6
	Other	63	14.9
Type of antiepileptic drug	Mono therapy	142	33.6
	Polytherapy	280	66.4
Medication adherence	Adherence	330	78.2
	Poor adherence	92	21.8
Social support	Yes	360	85.3
	No	62	14.7
Perceived stigma	No felt stigma	263	62.3
	Felt stigma	159	37.7

Table 3 Factors associated with depression among epilepsy patients at under follow up at AMSH and TASH, 2015

Variables	Depression		COR (95% CI)	AOR (95% CI)
	Yes	No		
Sex				
Female	97	76	2.36 (1.56–3.47)	2.62 (1.68–4.09)*
Male	88	161	1.00	1.00
Marital status				
Single	110	102	2.35 (1.51–3.66)	2.04 (1.25–3.34)*
Divorced/separated	27	31	1.89 (1.01–3.54)	
Widowed	3	6	1.089 (0.26–4.55)	
Married	45	98	1.00	1.00
Medication adherence				
Yes	162	168	1.00	1.00
No	23	69	2.89 (1.72–4.86)	2.65 (1.52–4.65)*
Perceived stigma				
No	94	169	1.00	1.00
Yes	91	68	2.40 (1.60–3.60)	2.65 (1.65–4.07)*
Current substance use (alcohol, chat, cigarette)				
Yes	77	59	2.15 (1.42–3.26)	2.14 (1.34–3.39)*
No	108	178	1.00	1.00

*p < 0.05; 1.00 = Reference; COR crude odds ratio, AOR adjusted odds ratio

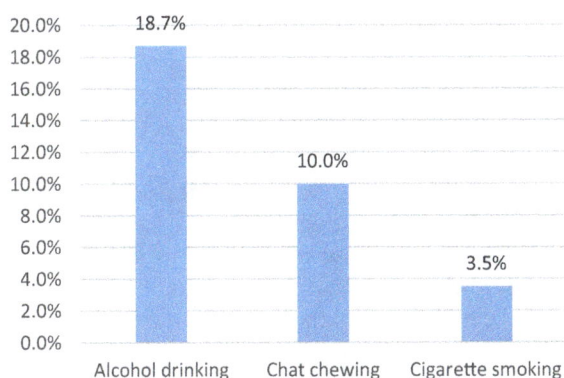

Fig. 1 Bar graph showing the distribution of current substance use among epilepsy patients at AMSH and TAH, 2015

Factors associated with depression among epilepsy patients

The associations of all potential explanatory variables and depression were checked using logistic regression model. However, only being female, single, perceived stigma, poor medication adherence, and current use of substance were significantly associated with depression in bivariate and multivariate logistic regression ($p < 0.05$).

Being female was 2.6 times more likely to have depression when compared to males (AOR 2.62, 95% CI 1.68–4.09). Similarly, being single was around twice more likely to have depression compared to married participants (AOR 2.04, 95% CI 1.25–3.34).

Moreover, those who have poor medication adherence and having perceived stigma had close to three odds of having depression compared to their counterparts (AOR 2.65, 95% CI 1.52–4.65; AOR 2.65, 95% CI 1.65–4.07, respectively). In addition, current substance use (alcohol drinking, Khat chewing, and cigarette smoking) were significantly associated with depression. Depression was two times more likely among current substance users (AOR 2.14, 95% CI 1.34–3.39) (Table 3).

Discussion

In this study, the prevalence rate of depression among epilepsy patients was 43.8% (38.9, 48.8%). It is consistent with the study done at the University of Gondar Hospital (45.2%) [25] and Sudan (45.5%) [26].

This finding was lower than the result from the study conducted at the Jimma University Specialized Hospital (49.3%) [19]. Other studies conducted in Nigeria and Gaza stated that depression had been prevalent among 85.5 and 63% of participants, respectively [9, 27] which are very high compared with the current study, and they were almost three times higher in magnitude than that reported in a study done in Canada [11]. This difference might be due to the sociocultural variation and instrument, since those authors used BDI which has items similar to somatic complaints, and this might have led to overestimating the prevalence.

However, the current study's finding regarding prevalence rate is higher than the report described in Amanuel Mental Specialized Hospital (33.3%) [28], Kenya (16.5%) [29], Iran (9.5%) [8], Thailand (20%) [30], and Greek (22.5%) [31]. These discrepancies might be due to the difference in study participants, method, culture, time, and settings.

In this study, the researchers found a high prevalence of depression among female compared to male respondents which are consistent with the study done in Gaza [9]. However, the study in Nigeria and Ethiopia [19, 27] revealed that no significant relationship between gender and depression in people with epilepsy. The difference is most likely due to diverse methodological approaches, cultural variation, and different instruments they used to measure depression. In general, females faced difficulty in performing normal activities of daily living, and they might face several risks or hardships with regard to reproductive activity and pregnancy. Furthermore, women with epilepsy face difficulty in decision-making with regard to important major life events such as marriage or bearing children. Thus, these consequences might increase depression among females.

With regard to marital status in this study, those who were married were less likely to be depressed compared to those with single status, and having another marital status. This finding was consistent with the previous study in Jimma Ethiopia [19] but inconsistent with other studies in which the authors found no significant difference among different marital statuses [27, 28]. This might be due to marriage-related change of lifestyles because of some kind of guardian-like protective effect of the marital status where adherence to healthy activities is greatly increased—and behaviors leading to health risks are reduced. Moreover, married people also have higher levels of emotional support.

The study has also shown that patients who were not adherent to their medication had depression compared to those who were adherent. This hypothesis is supported by previous studies [19, 25]. The high rates of poor adherence demonstrated in this study are causing concerns, given the consequences of antiepileptic discontinuation. It might be assumed that patients who discontinue medication will be more likely to relapse and have very poor and less control over the disease than those who continue medications.

Moreover, in this study, stigma was associated with depression which is supported by different studies [19, 28]. The previous study conducted in Ethiopia among epilepsy among patients found perceived stigma to be a common problem among people living with epilepsy [32]. This is because people with epilepsy might be overprotected and restricted from doing many activities by their family members, friends, or teachers. Overprotection arising from stigmatization can have severe consequences. Eventually, this stigma shatters a person's hope and self-esteem leading to negative outcomes related to recovery including depressive symptoms, social avoidance, and a preference for adopting avoidance of coping strategies.

In this particular study, current substance use has a significant association with depression. This result is supported by Epilepsy Action Australia report [33]. Substance use among people taking antiepileptic medications is likely to be more sensitive to the effects of substances. The substance can interfere with the metabolism of these medications and therefore increase the chance of seizures. Some medications can enhance the toxic effects of alcohol, and people can feel severely intoxicated after drinking only a small amount. Skipping a dose, taking extra medication, or altering the time of taking regular antiepileptic medications before drinking will not alter this reaction but may cause additional adverse effects or seizures [33].

In general, the implication of this finding indicates that people living with epilepsy need strong counseling in terms of adherence, by way of creating awareness in the community and addressing misperception issues attached to epilepsy. Collaborative efforts among different stakeholders and clinicians are recommended to bring effective management strategies to neurologic clinics. In addition, generating additional evidence through further research is required.

A limitation of this study was that it was not possible to clarify the cause–effect relationship between depression and epilepsy due to the cross-sectional nature of the study. A prospective study could help to establish clearly whether epilepsy predisposes to depression or a consequence of depression predispose to epilepsy. Another limitation includes recall bias—regarding the duration of illness and substance-use-related factor—which was not assessed by a standard tool.

Conclusion

The finding showed that there is a high prevalence of comorbid depression (43.8%) among epilepsy patients at the AMSH and TAH. The epilepsy-related sociodemographic variables like being female, single, and clinical-related factors including poor medication adherence, current substance use, and perceived stigma were significantly associated with depression. Early recognition of depression symptoms in people with epilepsy should be of great concern for healthcare providers to help them provide appropriate counseling regarding adherence and substance use.

Author details

[1] Department of Psychiatry, Amanuel Mental Specialized Hospital, Addis Ababa, Ethiopia. [2] Department of Epidemiology and Biostatistics, University of Gondar, Gondar, Ethiopia. [3] College of Medicine and Health Science, Bahir Dar University, Bahir Dar, Ethiopia. [4] College of Medicine and Health Science, Haramaya University, Harer, Ethiopia.

Acknowledgements

The authors would like to thank the University of Gondar and AMSH. The authors are also grateful to data collectors, supervisors, and study participants, and their important contribution for this study is duly acknowledged.

Authors' contributions

All authors contributed toward data analysis, drafting, and critically revising the paper, and agree to be accountable for all aspects of the work. All authors read and approved the final manuscript.

Competing interests

The authors have declared that there are no conflicts of interest in this work.

Consent for publication

Not applicable.

Funding

This research work is funded by the University of Gondar and Amanuel Mental Specialized Hospital.

References

1. Mathern G, Nehlig A. ILAE Adopts an operational definition of epilepsy intended to be used clinically. Flower Mound: International League Against Epilepsy; 2014.
2. Fisher RS, Acevedo C, Arzimanoglou A, Bogacz A, Cross JH, Elger CE, Engel J Jr, Forsgren L, French JA, Glynn M, et al. ILAE Official Report: a practical clinical definition of epilepsy. Epilepsia. 2014;55(4):475–82.
3. De Boer HM, Mula M, Sander JW. The global burden and stigma of epilepsy. Epilepsy Behav. 2008;12(4):540–6.
4. Gilliam FG, Barry JJ, Hermann BP, Meador KJ, Vahle V, Kanner AM. Rapid detection of major depression in epilepsy: a multicentre study. Lancet Neurol. 2006;5(5):399–405.
5. American Psychiatric Association, Mula M. Diagnostic and statistical manual of mental disorders. 5th ed. Washington, DC: American Psychiatric Association; 2013.
6. Mula M. Neuropsychiatric symptoms of epilepsy. Cham: Springer; 2016.
7. Kanner AM, Schachter SC, Barry JJ, Hersdorffer DC, Mula M, Trimble M, Hermann B, Ettinger AE, Dunn D, Caplan R. Depression and epilepsy: epidemiologic and neurobiologic perspectives that may explain their high comorbid occurrence. Epilepsy Behav. 2012;24(2):156–68.
8. Asadi-Pooya A, Sperling M. Depression and anxiety in patients with epilepsy, with or without other chronic disorders. Iran Red Crescent Med J. 2011;13(2):112–6.
9. Sheer AA: Depression among epileptic patients in Governmental Community Mental Health Centers in Gaza Strip. Gaza: The Islamic University – Gaza; 2012.
10. Todorova K, Arnaoudova M. Depressive disorders in epilepsy. J IMAB Annu Proc (Sci Pap.). 2010;16:3.
11. Wong ST, Manca D, Barber D, Morkem R, Khan S, Kotecha J, Williamson T, Birtwhistle R, Patten S. The diagnosis of depression and its treatment in Canadian primary care practices: an epidemiological study. CMAJ Open. 2014;2(4):E337.
12. Nidhinandana S, Chinvarun Y, Sithinamsuwan P, Udommongkol C, Suwantamee J, Wongmek W, Suphakasem S. Prevalence of depression among epileptic patients at Phramongkutklao Hospital. J Med Assoc Thai. 2007;90(1):32.
13. Baker GA. The psychosocial burden of epilepsy. Epilepsia. 2002;43(s6):26–30.
14. Nabukenya AM, Matovu JK, Wabwire-Mangen F, Wanyenze RK, Makumbi F. Health-related quality of life in epilepsy patients receiving anti-epileptic drugs at National Referral Hospitals in Uganda: a cross-sectional study. Health Qual Life Outcomes. 2014;12(1):1.
15. Gabb MG, Barry JJ. The link between mood disorders and epilepsy. J Adv Med. 2005;5(6):S572–8.
16. Kralj-Hans I, Goldstein LH, Noble AJ, Landau S, Magill N, McCrone P, Baker G, Morgan M, Richardson A, Taylor S. Self-management education for adults with poorly controlled epILEpsy [SMILE (UK)]: a randomised controlled trial protocol. BMC Neurol. 2014;14:69.
17. Grabowska-Grzyb A, Jędrzejczak J, Nagańska E, Fiszer U. Risk factors for depression in patients with epilepsy. Epilepsy Behav. 2006;8(2):411–7.
18. Jones R, Butler J, Thomas V, Peveler R, Prevett M. Adherence to treatment in patients with epilepsy: associations with seizure control and illness beliefs. Seizure. 2006;15(7):504–8.
19. Tsegabrhan H, Negash A, Tesfay K, Abera M. Co-morbidity of depression and epilepsy in Jimma University specialized hospital, Southwest Ethiopia. Neurol India. 2014;62(6):649.
20. Kroenke K, Spitzer R, Williams J. The PHQ-9: validity of a brief depression severity measure. J Gen Intern Med. 2001;16(9):606–13.
21. Gelaye B, Williams MA, Lemma S, Deyessa N, Bahretibeb Y, Shibre T, Wondimagegn D, Lemenhe A, Fann JR, Vander Stoep A. Validity of the patient health questionnaire-9 for depression screening and diagnosis in East Africa. Psychiatry Res. 2013;210(2):653–61.
22. W/giorgis T, Wordofa B. Prevalence of depression and associated factors among adult diabetic patients attending outpatient department, at Felege Hiwot Referral Hospital, Bahir Dar, Northwest Ethiopia. Int J Health Sci Res (IJHSR). 2016;6(9): 264–276.
23. Pungrassami P, Kipp AM, Stewart PW, Chongsuvivatwong V, Strauss R, Van Rie A. Tuberculosis and AIDS stigma among patients who delay seeking care for tuberculosis symptoms. Int J Tuberc Lung Dis. 2010;14(2):181–7.
24. Bøen H. Characteristics of senior centre users–and the impact of a group programme on social support and late-life depression. Norsk Epidemiol. 2012;22(2):261–9.
25. Bifftu BB, Dachew BA, Tiruneh BT, Birhan Tebeje N. Depression among people with epilepsy in Northwest Ethiopia: a cross-sectional institution based study. BMC Res Notes. 2015;8:585.
26. Saadalla A, Elbadwi A. Depression among Sudanese epileptic patients. Indian J Basic Appl Med Res. 2016;5(4):808–11.
27. Onwuekwe IO, Ekenze OS, Bzeala-Adikaibe, Ejekwu J. Depression in patients with epilepsy: a study from Enugu, South East Nigeria. Ann Med Health Sci Res. 2012;2(1):10–3.
28. Tegegne MT, Mossie TB, Awoke AA, Assaye AM, Gebrie BT, Eshetu DA. Depression and anxiety disorder among epileptic people at Amanuel Specialized Mental Hospital, Addis Ababa, Ethiopia. BMC Psychiatry. 2015;15:210.
29. Kiko N. Prevalence and factors associated with depression among patients with epilepsy in a Kenyan tertiary care hospital. Nairobi: Aga Khan University; 2013.
30. Phabphal K, Sattawatcharawanich S, Sathirapunya P, Limapichart K. Anxiety and depression in Thai epileptic patients. Med J Med Assoc Thai. 2007;90(10):2010.
31. Zis P, Yfanti P, Siatouni A, Tavernarakis A, Gatzonis S. Determinants of depression among patients with epilepsy in Athens, Greece. Epilepsy Behavior. 2014;33:106–9.
32. Tegegne MT, Awoke AA. Perception of stigma and associated factors in people with epilepsy at Amanuel Specialized Mental Hospital, Addis Ababa, Ethiopia. Int J Psychiatry Clin Pract. 2016;21(1):58–63.
33. Epilepsy Action Australia. Seizure smart: Alcohol and Epilepsy. 2011. Accessed 17 Jan 2017.

23

Resting-state brain activity in Chinese boys with low functioning autism spectrum disorder

Gaizhi Li[1,3], Kathryn Rossbach[2], Wenqing Jiang[3] and Yasong Du[3*]

Abstract

Background: This study aimed to explore the resting-state fMRI changes in Chinese boys with low functioning autism spectrum disorder (LFASD) and the correlation with clinical symptoms.

Methods: The current study acquired resting-state fMRI data from 15 Chinese boys with LFASD and 15 typically developing (TD) boys to examine the local brain activity using the regional homogeneity (ReHo) and amplitude of low-frequency fluctuation (ALFF) indexes; the researchers also examined these measures and their possible relationships with clinical symptoms using the autism behavior checklist.

Results: Results indicated that boys with LFASD exhibited increased ReHo in the right precuneus and inferior parietal gyrus (IPG), increased ALFF in right middle temporal gyrus, angular gyrus and IPG. However, no correlation was found between the ALFF/ReHo score and clinical symptoms in the LFASD group.

Conclusions: Some of the brain regions had ReHo/ALFF values that were higher in the boys with LFASD than the TD group and these differentiated brain areas in boys with LFASD were all on the right cerebrum, which supported 'atypical rightward asymmetry' in boys with LFASD.

Keywords: Low functioning autism spectrum disorder, Resting-state functional magnetic resonance imaging, Regional homogeneity, Amplitude of low-frequency fluctuation, Autism behavior checklist

Introduction

Autism spectrum disorders (ASDs) are increasingly prevalent neurodevelopmental disorders characterized by impaired social interaction and repetitive behaviors [1]. Long distance under-connectivity and local over-connectivity in individuals with autism have been reported by many studies [2, 3]. Research indicates that the regional connectivity differences found between samples with ASD and typically developing (TD) control groups should be examined carefully as high variability among ASD subjects may be contributing to these apparent differences.

Resting-state fMRI is a method of functional brain imaging that can be used to evaluate regional interactions that occur when a subject is not performing an explicit task [4]. Resting-state data obtained through the scans can be analyzed using a variety of methods. ReHo and ALFF are two methods widely used for characterizing local spontaneous activity of RS-fMRI data. ReHo measures the local synchronization of the time series of neighboring voxels, whereas ALFF/fALFF measures the amplitude of time series fluctuations at each voxel [5–7].

Many studies have been completed examining psychiatric disorders using ReHo and ALFF [8, 9], some of which studied ASD. Using the ReHo, both increases and decreases of ReHo value were observed in resting-state fMRI studies of individuals with ASD, but with poor replication across studies. For example, Paakki et al. [10] used the ReHo approach to study adolescents with ASD and found that compared with the controls,

*Correspondence: yasongdu@163.com
[3] Department of Child & Adolescent Psychiatry, Shanghai Mental Health Center, Shanghai Jiao Tong University School of Medicine, No 600 Wanping Nan Road, Xuhui, Shanghai 200030, China
Full list of author information is available at the end of the article

the subjects with ASD had significantly decreased ReHo in the right superior temporal sulcus region, right inferior and middle frontal gyri, right insula and right postcentral gyrus. Further, significantly increased ReHo was shown in the left inferior frontal and anterior subcallosal gyrus [10]. While Shukla et al. [11] found that ReHo was lower in the ASD than the TD group in the superior parietal and anterior prefrontal regions, higher ReHo was detected in lateral and medial temporal regions, predominantly in the right hemisphere in the ASD group, thus they proposed that ReHo is a sensitive measure for detecting cortical abnormalities in ASD. With regard to ALFF/fALFF, Itahashi et al. [12] reported that patients with High Functioning ASD showed significantly decreased fALFF values in a large cluster, including the right LING (lingual gyri), middle occipital gyrus (MOG), FG (fusiform gyri), and cerebellum. Di Martino et al. [13] used ReHo, ALFF, voxel mirrored homotopic connectivity (VMHC) and degree centrality (DC) in their research, and reported that two clusters exhibited ASD-related abnormalities in three measures, one from the left posterior insula to the central and parietal operculum (which exhibited ASD-related decreases in VMHC, ReHo and DC), and the other cluster was located in right dorsal superior frontal cortex (which exhibited ASD-related increases in fALFF, ReHo and DC).

These studies focused on high functioning autism spectrum disorder or Asperger syndrome, even though one-third of individuals with ASD are on the lower functioning end of the autism spectrum according to the latest CDC reports [14]. To our knowledge, no report of the correlation between clinical symptoms and ALFF/ReHo value has been examined in Chinese children with LFASD.

ASD is about four times more common among boys than among girls [14]; thus, it is more difficult to recruit girls for a study of this nature simply due to the lack of girls with ASD. Further, researchers proposed that the neurobiological mechanism for boys and girls may differ [15]. Therefore, results may be biased or inaccurate if a study was to include both boys and girls.

In the current research study, we aimed to explore the difference between the boys with LFASD and TD using Reho and ALFF, and examined the correlation between ReHo/ALFF and clinical symptoms. We hypothesized that (1) the ReHo, ALFF of resting-state brain activity would be different between boys with LFASD and typically developing controls in brain areas shown to display functional alterations in previous studies; (2) the differentiated brain areas may be correlated with the clinical symptoms.

Methods

Participants

Participants in the LFASD sample included a clinically referred sample of consecutive cases of children with an ASD diagnosis within the Shanghai Mental Health Center, Shanghai Jiao Tong University School of Medicine between April 2015 and April 2017. Diagnoses were based on DSM-5 (American Psychiatric Association, 2013) criteria and determined by an MD-level clinician, under the supervision of an MD/Ph.D. Professor (Dr. Du, the corresponding author). All participants also completed the WISC-IV Chinese version.

The children in the typically developing control group (TD group) were recruited from primary and middle schools in Shanghai. Children were excluded if they had any type of psychiatric disorder based on the Kiddie-SADS-present and lifetime version [16], which was conducted by an MD-level clinician, under the supervision of an MD/Ph.D. Professor (Dr. Du).

Parents of all the children completed the autism behavior checklist (ABC) after receiving instructions from the psychological professionals working in Shanghai Mental Health Center, Shanghai Jiao Tong University School of Medicine, and questionnaires were scored and interpreted by an MD-level clinician working in the Shanghai Mental Health Center, Shanghai Jiao Tong University School of Medicine. The ABC was used to rule out the presence of ASD-related symptoms in the TD group. No children in the control group had elevated scores on the ABC.

This study was approved by the Shanghai Mental Health Center Ethics Committee. Parents provided written informed consent for their children. Children who were verbal and could write their name, and also judged to be capable of providing assent, signed their name on this form too.

Measures

WISC-IV Chinese version

The WISC-IV Chinese version is an individually administered instrument designed to measure intelligence [17]. The WISC-IV Chinese version contains 10 core subtests and five additional subtests. These are combined into four index scores [Verbal Comprehension Index (VCI), Perceptual Reasoning Index (PRI), Processing Speed Index (PSI), Working Memory Index (WMI)] and one full scale intelligence (FSIQ) score, which ranges from 40 to 160.

Autism behavior checklist

The autism behavior checklist includes 57 items and five domains, including the sensory, relating, body concept, language and social self-help domain [18]. It was introduced into China by Yang et al. and has been widely used in clinical and scientific research [19, 20]. It can be used with individuals aged from 18 months to 35 years, as a screening tool for ASD.

MRI data acquisition

All MRI data were acquired using a 3.0 T MRI system (Siemens MAGNETOM Trio Tim) with a phased array whole-head coil. The functional images were acquired using a gradient echo-planar imaging sequence (repetition time (TR) 2000 ms, echo time (TE) 30 ms, flip angle 77°, slice thickness 3 mm, matrix size 74*74). Two-hundred and forty volumes were acquired in a single run.

During the scan, each of the participants was instructed to remain relaxed in the scanner, lying as still as possible, with his or her eyes closed, but to stay awake while in the dim scanner room. In addition, a high-resolution T1-weighted spoiled gradient recalled (SPGR) 3D MRI image was acquired (TR 2530 ms, TE 3.25 ms, 1-mm-slice thickness, matrix size 256*256).

Data preprocessing

Preprocessing was performed in MATLAB R2010b (Mathworks, Natick, MA) using data processing assistant for resting-state fMRI (DPARSF advanced edition) software [21]. DPARSF pipeline analysis was used to do the preprocessing. The first step was to remove the first ten time points for signal equilibrium and to allow the participants' adaptation to the scanning noise, slice timing and realign, then a report of head motion was created based on the realign parameters estimated by SPM (as shown in "ExcludeSubjects.txt" in the "Realign Parameter" directory). According to the report, three participants with ASD and three TD participants were excluded due to excessive motion ($\geq \pm 2.5$ mm translation and $\geq \pm 2.5$ rotation from the first volume in any axis). For inter-subject comparison to be feasible, the individual brain was transformed or spatially normalized into a standardized template using unified segmentation on a T1 image. The whole-brain signal, six motion parameters, the cerebrospinal fluid (CSF), and the white matter signals were also removed as nuisance variables to reduce the effects of head motion and non-neuronal BOLD fluctuations in a regression analysis. A Gaussian filter (a 4 mm FWHM) was used to smooth the fMRI data (for ReHo, this step was performed after ReHo calculation). Removing the systematic drift or trend using a linear model was the last step.

Statistical analysis

Resting-state fMRI data analysis toolkit (REST 1.8) was used to perform the data analysis [22]. To explore the between-group patterns, two-sample t tests were performed on the ALFF and ReHo, respectively, with age/FSIQ as covariates. Partial correlation analysis was applied to analyze the correlation between ALFF/ReHo and clinical symptoms using age/FSIQ as covariates in REST. A correction for multiple comparisons was performed using Monte Carlo simulation with a corrected threshold of $P < 0.005$ (two-tailed).

Results
Demographic data

Nineteen boys with LFASD participated in our study. One of them could not cooperate in the WISC-IV administration, so only 18 boys with LFASD completed the WISC-IV Chinese version, and three boys were excluded due to excessive head motion. The mean age of the LFASD group was 8.87 ± 3.11. Eighteen typically developing boys were included, three of whom were excluded due to excessive head motion; all the boys in the control group completed the WISC-IV Chinese version, and the mean age of the TD group was 10.53 ± 2.61. No significant difference was observed when it came to age between the two groups (t = -1.588, $P = 0.124$). The mean FSIQ score was 50.47 ± 11.25 for the LFASD group and 127.27 ± 13.84 for the TD group, and the difference between the groups was statistically significant ($P < 0.001$). The clinical data of the LFASD group were assessed using the ABC and the total score is 66.50 ± 23.61; the subscale data are shown in Table 1.

Group difference

In the current research study, using ReHo values, the boys with LFASD had statistically significantly higher scores than the TD children when it came to the Precuneus (BA 23) and Inferior Parietal Gyrus, IPG (BA 40) (See Fig. 1 and Table 2). At the same time, using ALFF values, the boys with LFASD had statistically significantly higher scores when it came to the Right Middle Temporal Gyrus MTG (BA 21), Angular gyrus (BA 39) and IPG (BA 40) (see Fig. 2 and Table 2).

Correlation analysis

When examining the LFASD group, based on the correlation analysis between the ReHo value and the ABC subscale and total scores, no significant correlation was observed. In addition, there was no significant correlation observed between the ALFF score and ABC scores (see Table 3).

Discussion

ASD is a neurodevelopmental disorder with an unknown biological basis. Many studies have confirmed the morphological difference between children with ASD and

Table 1 Demographic data of the LFASD and TD groups

	LFASD group ($n = 15$)	TD group ($n = 15$)	t	P
Age	8.87 ± 3.11	10.53 ± 2.61	− 1.588	0.124
FSIQ	50.47 ± 11.25	127.27 ± 13.84	− 16.679	< 0.001
ABC				
Sensory	12.94 ± 6.86	–		
Relating	12.81 ± 9.10	–		
Body concept	11.88 ± 6.84	–		
Language	15.94 ± 7.49	–		
Social self-help	12.94 ± 4.81	–		
Total ABC score	66.50 ± 23.61	–		

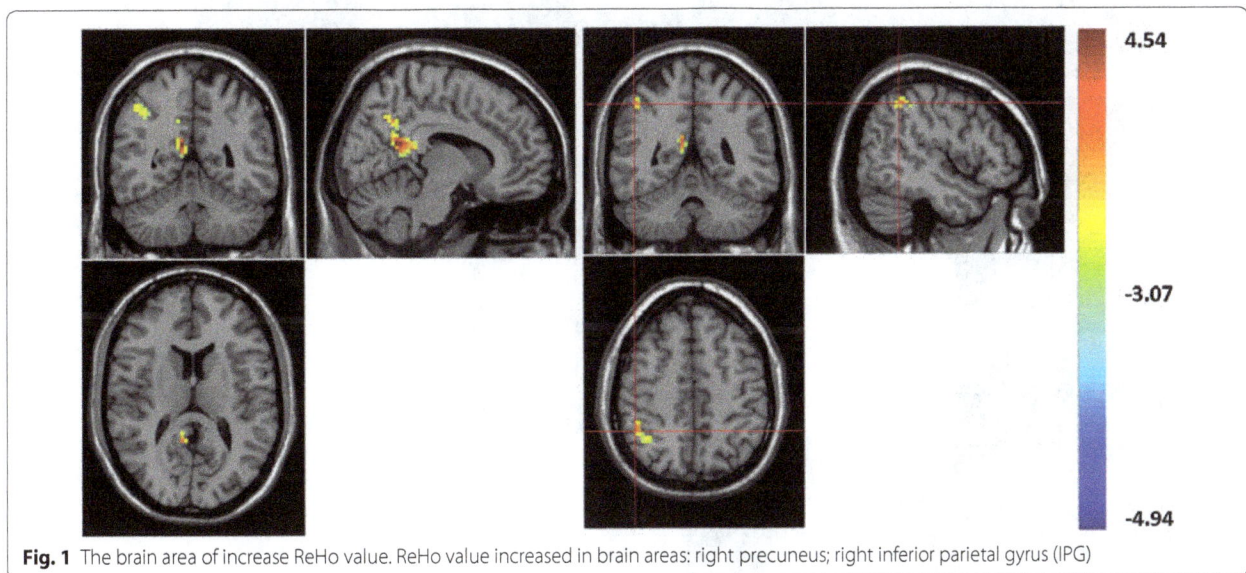

Fig. 1 The brain area of increase ReHo value. ReHo value increased in brain areas: right precuneus; right inferior parietal gyrus (IPG)

TD children [23–26]. As a part of a functional MRI study, resting-state data, especially the ReHo and ALFF, are two important methods widely used for characterizing local spontaneous brain activity of children with ASD. Up until now, evidence has been limited for children with low functioning ASD. In the current study, we explored the difference between Chinese boys with LFASD and TD boys using ReHo and ALFF. We also examined whether any relationship existed between abnormal spontaneous brain activity and clinical manifestation by looking at the pattern of relationships between regional brain measures and clinical symptoms in the LFASD group.

Unfortunately, excessive motion and floor task performance are issues that hinder successful scanning of young children and account for significant data loss [27] and, in our study, seven participants' data had to be discarded due to head motion and lack of cooperation.

With respect to the group difference, our findings show that all the differentiated brain areas are on the right side of the cerebrum. These results within the right cerebrum are the same as reports from Shukla et al. [11] as they also found that higher ReHo were predominantly in the right hemisphere in the ASD group. Atypical rightward asymmetry was also reported to be a feature in ASD in another study [28].

According to our findings, there are four regions: precuneus (BA 23), IPG (BA 40), MTG (BA 21) and angular gyrus (BA 39) that significantly differ from typically developed children. MTG (BA 21) which is a part of temporal lobe has been regarded as an important brain area mainly engaged in the face recognition. Interestingly, the impairment of face recognition in individuals with ASD is frequently reported [29]. Cheng et al. [30] used rs-fMRI in a large sample to explore the functional connectivity of subjects with autism and controls. They identified two key systems, the first one in the middle temporal gyrus/superior temporal sulcus region that has reduced cortical functional connectivity (and increased

Table 2 The brain regions of ALFF/ReHo score between the LFASD and TD groups

	Voxels	L/R	Brain regions	BA	x	y	z	Peak
ALFF	22	R	MTG	21	51	−30	−9	4.4535
	36	R	Angular	39	42	−63	45	4.0839
	22	R	IPG	40	54	−36	51	4.5399
ReHo	59	R	Precuneus	23	9	−51	18	4.4852
	35	R	IPG	40	48	−48	48	3.8732

MTG middle temporal gyrus, *IPG* inferior parietal gyrus

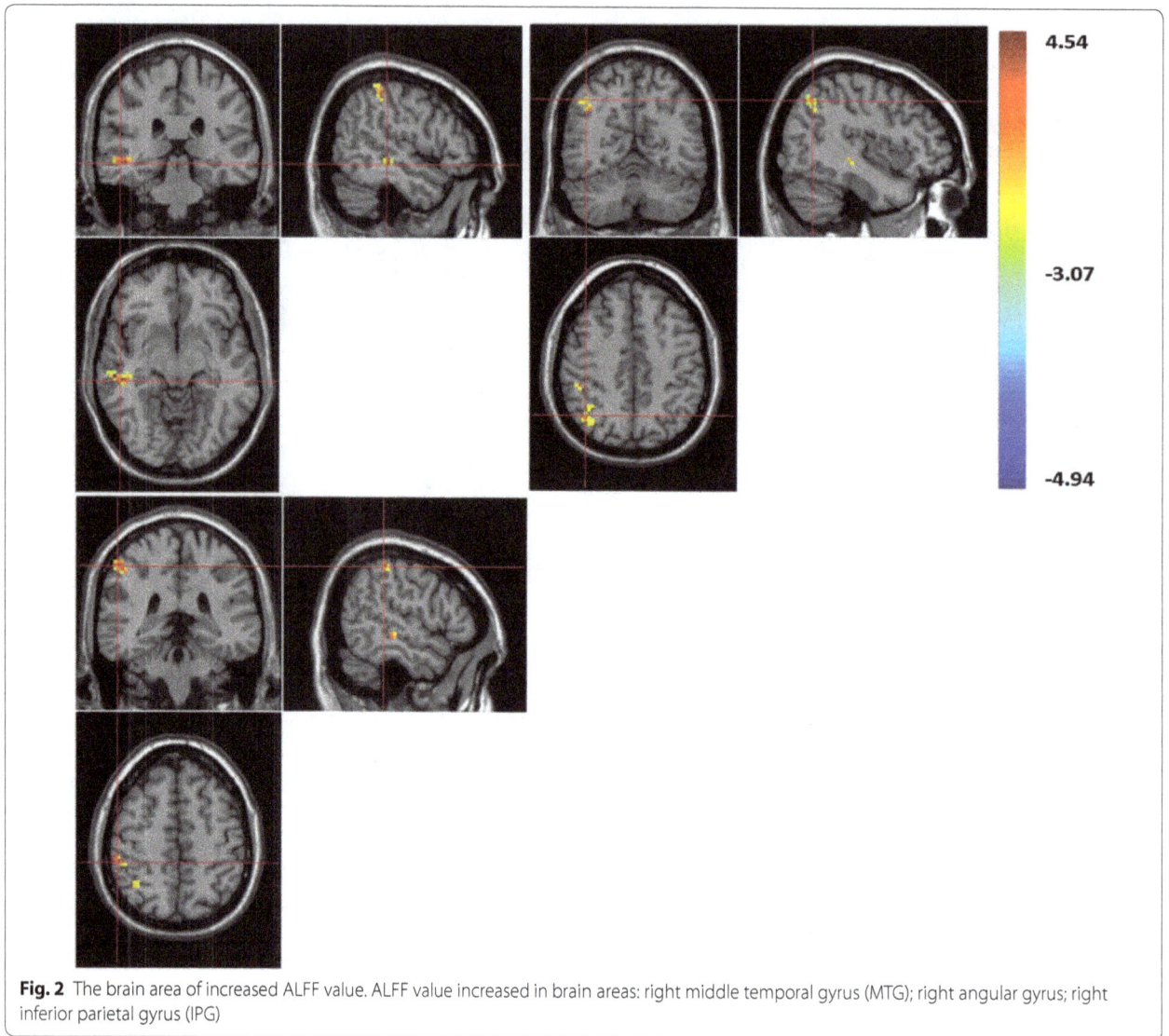

Fig. 2 The brain area of increased ALFF value. ALFF value increased in brain areas: right middle temporal gyrus (MTG); right angular gyrus; right inferior parietal gyrus (IPG)

with the medial thalamus). This area is implicated in face expression processing involved in social behavior. The middle temporal gyrus system is also implicated in theory of mind processing. A second key system is in the precuneus/superior parietal lobule region with reduced functional connectivity, which is implicated in spatial functions including of oneself and of the spatial environment. Our finding regarding the different resting state in boys with LFASD is partly consistent with Cheng's study, as the precuneus/superior parietal lobule regions

Table 3 Correlation between ALFF/ReHo score and behavioral scores (ABC)

	Brian areas	Sensory	Social	Language	Body concept	Self-care	Total score
ALFF	Right MTG						
	r	−0.049	0.244	0.392	0.252	0.404	0.320
	P	0.875	0.421	0.185	0.406	0.171	0.286
	Right angular						
	r	−0.434	0.049	0.173	0.121	0.082	−0.003
	P	0.139	0.874	0.572	0.693	0.790	0.992
	Right IPG						
	r	−0.338	0.057	−0.267	0.150	0.288	−0.052
	P	0.258	0.852	0.378	0.624	0.341	0.865
ReHo	Right precuneus						
	r	−0.375	−0.359	−0.259	−0.060	0.309	−0.254
	P	0.207	0.229	0.393	0.846	0.304	0.403
	Right IPG						
	r	−0.024	0.005	−0.412	−0.158	0.014	−0.160
	P	0.939	0.987	0.162	0.607	0.965	0.602

MTG middle temporal gyrus, *IPG* inferior parietal gyrus

were both reported; however, the Angular gyrus was not observed in his study.

The precuneus (BA 23), IPG (BA 40) and angular gyrus (BA 39) are part of the occipital lobe. The precuneus (BA 23) is reported to be correlated with the reflective, self-related processing, awareness and conscious information processing, episodic memory, and visuospatial processing [31]. IPG (BA 40) has been involved in the perception of emotions in facial stimuli and interpretation of sensory information. The inferior parietal lobule is concerned with language, mathematical operations, and body image, particularly the supramarginal gyrus and the angular gyrus. The angular gyrus (BA 39) is engaged in transferring visual information to Wernicke's area, in order to make meaning out of visually perceived words. It is also involved in a number of processes related to language, number processing and spatial cognition, memory retrieval, attention, and theory of mind [32].

Nonetheless, in the current study, no significant correlations were found for the ALFF/ReHo values and clinical symptoms. In past studies, facial recognition, spatial cognition and theory of mind were the basic impairments in resting time of children with ASD, but these neuro-psychological features were not assessed in the current study. This may be the reason that no relationship has been found between spontaneous brain activity and clinical manifestation. Therefore, the increased ALFF/ReHo may not be the neurological bases for clinical symptoms in the boys with LFASD. Thus, we suggest that the local connectivity of LFASD was higher than the TD group, but future larger samples will be needed to clarify this question.

The current results indicate that the resting-state activity is impaired mainly in the right hemisphere of the boys with LFASD, which is important for clinical practice. If results are able to be replicated, when boys with LFASD are being treated, the focus could be surrounding the right hemisphere. Additionally, this research could help support locating a more specific deficit in brain function related to ASD which could eventually aid in earlier detection and better treatment overall.

Limitations

There are some limitations in our study. The first is that since we studied Chinese boys with LFASD, the sample size was relatively small. By only using boys in the study we cannot generalize our studies across genders. In addition, this is a cross-sectional study, thus we cannot conclude the developmental-related changes, even though age was as covariate when analyzed. Additionally, the typical developing group had a fairly high FSIQ; this was simply a result of the sample used, but may have impacted the study since the difference in IQ was so large between the two groups. Future longitudinal studies are needed to characterize the brain-clinical associations in Chinese boys with LFASD.

Conclusion

In the present study, we used the measures of ReHo/ALFF to study the relationship between local connectivity and clinical symptoms in Chinese boys with LFASD. Some of the brain regions had ReHo/ALFF values that were higher in the boys with LFASD than the TD group. According to our study, all the resting-state differentiated brain areas in boys with LFASD were on the right cerebrum, which supported 'atypical rightward asymmetry' in boys with LFASD.

Abbreviations
ABC: autism behavior checklist; ALFF: amplitude of low-frequency fluctuation; ASD: autism spectrum disorder; BA: Brodmann area; BOLD: blood oxygenation level dependent; CARS: Childhood Autism Rating Scale; DSM-5: diagnostic and statistical manual of mental disorders (5th ed); FC: functional connectivity; FOV: field of view; FSIQ: full scale IQ; FWHM: full width half maximum; HFASD: high functioning autism spectrum disorder; IPG: inferior parietal gyrus; IQ: intelligence quotient; K-SADS-PL: Kiddie schedule for affective disorders and schizophrenia-present and lifetime version; LFASD: low functioning autism spectrum disorder; MNI: monireal neurological institute; MTG: middle temporal gyrus; NVIQ: nonverbal IQ; PRI: Perceptual Reasoning Index; PSI: Processing Speed Index; ReHo: regional homogeneity; ROI: region of interest; SNR: signal to noise ratio; TD: typically developing; TR/TE: repetition time/echo time; VCI: Verbal Comprehension Index; VIQ: verbal IQ; WISC-IV: Wechsler Intelligence Scale for children, the fourth edition; WMI: Working Memory Index.

Authors' contributions
GL and YS designed the study, GL analyzed the MRI data and wrote this manuscript, YD is funded by the foundations and is the corresponding author. WJ collected the MRI data and clinical data. KR revised our manuscript. All authors read and approved the final manuscript.

Author details
[1] Shanxi Medical University, The First Hospital of Shanxi Medical University, Taiyuan, China. [2] NCSP, Greater Atlanta area, Atlanta, USA. [3] Department of Child & Adolescent Psychiatry, Shanghai Mental Health Center, Shanghai Jiao Tong University School of Medicine, No 600 Wanping Nan Road, Xuhui, Shanghai 200030, China.

Acknowledgements
We thank all the volunteers who participated in this study.

Competing interests
The authors declare that they have no competing interests.

Consent for publication
The parents signed the informed consent including consent for publication.

Funding
The current study was funded by the following foundations: the National Natural Science Foundation of China (No. 81771477), the doctoral foundation of Shanxi Medical University (BS201706), the doctoral foundation of Shanxi Province, and the Postdoctoral Foundation of Shanxi Medical University.

References
1. American Psychiatric Association. Diagnostic and statistical manual of mental disorders. 5th ed. Washington, DC: American Psychiatric Association; 2013.
2. Supekar K, Uddin LQ, Khouzam A, Phillips J, Gaillard WD, Kenworthy LE, et al. Brain hyperconnectivity in children with autism and its links to social deficits. Cell Rep. 2013;5(3):738–47.
3. Hahamy A, Behrmann M, Malach R. The idiosyncratic brain: distortion of spontaneous connectivity patterns in autism spectrum disorder. Nat Neurosci. 2015;18(2):302–9.
4. Biswal BB. Resting state fMRI: a personal history. Neuroimage. 2012;62(2):938–44.
5. Zang Y, Jiang T, Lu Y, He Y, Tian L. Regional homogeneity approach to fMRI data analysis. Neuroimage. 2004;22(1):394–400.
6. Kendall M, Gibbons JDR. Correlation methods. Oxford: Oxford University Press; 1990. p. 35–8.
7. Zou QH, Zhu CZ, Yang Y, Zuo XN, Long XY, Cao QJ, et al. An improved approach to detection of amplitude of low-frequency fluctuation (ALFF) for resting-state fMRI: fractional ALFF. J Neurosci Methods. 2008;172(1):137–41.
8. Zang YF, He Y, Zhu CZ, Cao QJ, Sui MQ, Liang M, et al. Altered baseline brain activity in children with ADHD revealed by resting-state functional MRI. Brain Dev. 2007;29(2):83–91.
9. Zang YF, Zuo XN, Milham M, Hallett M. Toward a meta-analytic synthesis of the resting-state fMRI literature for clinical populations. BioMed Res Int. 2015. https://doi.org/10.1155/2015/435265.
10. Paakki JJ, Rahko J, Long X, Moilanen I, Tervonen O, Nikkinen J, et al. Alterations in regional homogeneity of resting-state brain activity in autism spectrum disorders. Brain Res. 2010;1321:169–79.
11. Shukla DK, Keehn B, Müller RA. Regional homogeneity of fMRI time series in autism spectrum disorders. Neurosci Lett. 2010;476(1):46–51.
12. Itahashi T, Yamada T, Watanabe H, Nakamura M, Ohta H, Kanai C, et al. Alterations of local spontaneous brain activity and connectivity in adults with high-functioning autism spectrum disorder. Mol Autism. 2015;6(1):1.
13. Di Martino A, Yan CG, Li Q, Denio E, Castellanos FX, Alaerts K, et al. The autism brain imaging data exchange: towards a large-scale evaluation of the intrinsic brain architecture in autism. Mol Psychiatry. 2014;19:659–67.
14. Christensen DL, Baio J, Braun KV, et al. Prevalence and characteristics of autism spectrum disorder among children aged 8 years—autism and developmental disabilities monitoring network, 11 sites, United States, 2012. MMWR Surveill Summ. 2016;65:1–23.
15. Ecker C, Andrews DS, Gudbrandsen CM, Marquand AF, Ginestet CE, Daly EM, et al. Association between the probability of autism spectrum disorder and normative sex-related phenotypic diversity in brain structure. JAMA Psychiatry. 2007;74(4):329–38.
16. Kaufman J, Birmaher B, Brent D, Rao U, Flynn C, Moreci P, et al. Schedule for affective disorders and schizophrenia for school-age children-present and lifetime version (K-SADS-PL): initial reliability and validity data. J Am Acad Child Adolesc Psychiatry. 1997;36:980–8.
17. Zhang HC. The revision of WISC-IV Chinese version. Psychol Sci. 2009;32(5):1177–9.
18. Krug DA, Arick J, Almond P. Behavior checklist for identifying severely handicapped individuals with high levels of autistic behavior. J Child Psychol Psychiatry. 1980;21(3):221–9.
19. Yang XL, Huang YQ, Jia MX, Chen SK. Test report of autism behavior checklist. Chin Mental Health J. 1993;7(6):279–80.
20. Jiang LX, Li GZ, Du YS. Comparison of screening tools for ASD. Chin J Nerv Mental Dis. 2015;41(3):189–92.
21. Yan CG, Zang YF. DPARSF: a MATLAB toolbox for "pipeline" data analysis of resting-state fMRI. Front Syst Neurosci. 2011;4:13.
22. Song XW, Dong ZY, Long XY, Li SF, Zuo XN, Zhu CZ, et al. REST: a toolkit for resting-state functional magnetic resonance imaging data processing. PloS ONE. 2011;6(9):e25031.
23. Amaral DG, Schumann CM, Nordahl CW. Neuroanatomy of autism. Trends Neurosci. 2008;31:137–45.
24. Balardin JB, Sato JR, Vieira G, Feng Y, Daly E, Murphy C, et al. Relationship between surface-based brain morphometric measures and intelligence in autism spectrum disorders: influence of history of language delay. Autism Res. 2015;8(5):556–66.
25. Maximo JO, Keown CL, Nair A, Müller RA. Approaches to local connectivity in autism using resting state functional connectivity MRI. Front Hum Neurosci. 2013;7:605.
26. Wass S. Distortions and disconnections: disrupted brain connectivity in autism. Brain Cognit. 2011;75:18–28.
27. Yerys BE, Jankowski KF, Shook D, Rosenberger LR, Barnes KA, Berl MM, et al. The fMRI success rate of children and adolescents: typical development, epilepsy, attention deficit/hyperactivity disorder, and autism spectrum disorders. Hum Brain Mapp. 2009;30(10):3426–35.
28. Joseph RM, Tanaka J. Holistic and part-based face recognition in children with autism. J Child Psychol Psychiatry. 2003;44(4):529–42.
29. Åsberg Johnels J, Hovey D, Zürcher N, Hippolyte L, Lemonnier E, Gillberg C, et al. Autism and emotional face-viewing. Autism Res. 2017;10(5):901–10.
30. Cheng W, Rolls ET, Gu H, Zhang J, Feng J. Autism: reduced connectivity between cortical areas involved in face expression, theory of mind, and the sense of self. Brain. 2015;138(Pt 5):1382–93.
31. Zhang S, Li CR. Functional connectivity mapping of the human precuneus by resting state fMRI. Neuroimage. 2012;59(4):3548–62.
32. Seghier ML. The angular gyrus. Neuroscientist. 2013;19(1):43–61.

24

Perceived stigma among non-professional caregivers of people with severe mental illness, Bahir Dar, northwest Ethiopia

Temesgen Ergetie[1*], Zegeye Yohanes[2], Biksegn Asrat[3], Wubit Demeke[2], Andargie Abate[4] and Minale Tareke[1]

Abstract

Background: The stigmatization of mental illness is currently considered to be one of the most important issues facing caregivers of severely mentally ill individuals. There is a dearth of information about the prevalence and associated factors of perceived stigma among caregivers of people with severe mental illness in the study area.

Objective: To assess the prevalence and associated factors of perceived stigma among non-professional caregivers of people with severe mental illness, Bahir Dar, northwest Ethiopia.

Method: Institutional based cross-sectional study was conducted from May to June, 2016 at Felege Hiwot Referral Hospital among 495 caregivers of people with the severe mental illness. Pre-tested structured family interview schedule questionnaire was used. Binary logistic regression was applied to identify factors associated with perceived stigma and interpreted using odds ratio with 95% confidence interval. Statistical significance was considered at p value < 0.05.

Result: The overall prevalence of perceived stigma was found to be 89.3%. Being female, rural residency, lack of social support, long duration of relationship with the patient and currently not married were found significantly associated with the perceived stigma of caregivers.

Conclusion: Prevalence of perceived stigma is very high in the current study. Thus, stigma reduction program and expanding of strong social support should better be implemented by different stakeholders for caregivers of people with severe mental illness.

Keywords: Caregivers, Perceived stigma, Severe mental illness

Introduction

The burden of mental health problems is increasing globally [1]. Mental illness accounted for 13% of world's disease burden and this figure will be increased to 15% by the year 2020 [2, 3]. Studies showed that approximately 450 million persons affected by mental illness and their devastating effects at personal and national levels are quite significant [1, 2, 4]. Due to different reasons, in low- and middle-income countries, about third quarter of people who need mental health service do not get any kind of intervention [5]. Stigma is one of the barriers that can prevent patients with mental illnesses from getting appropriate treatment or care [6].

Stigma is a social process, practiced or expected and characterized by separation, rejection, and blame or discredit about an individual or groups [7]. Stigma occurs at three levels, namely, organizational, public and personal level. Organizational stigma refers to the stigma that exists at system level which is defined as the rules, policies, and procedures of private and governmental entities in positions of power that restrict the rights and chances of people with disabling conditions [8]. Public stigma occurs at the group level and can be defined as the trends of massive social groups endorsing stereotype behavior and acting against a stigmatized group [9]. Personal level stigma is the stigma existing at the individual level. Perceived stigma existing at the

*Correspondence: Tomtemesgen@gmail.com
[1] Department of Psychiatry, College of Medicine and Health Sciences, Bahir Dar University, Po box 79, Bahir Dar, Ethiopia
Full list of author information is available at the end of the article

personal level which is respondent's beliefs in which those people with mental illness are generally stigmatized [10].

Facing stigmatization of mentally ill individual is one of the most important issues in mental health field until now [11]. It involves an isolation of person labeled as different from "us" who are believed to possess negative traits, resulting in negative feelings, discrimination, and status loss for the marginalized persons [12].

Feeling of stigmatization was not the only problem of people with severe mental illness, but also their family members who help care for them report feeling stigmatized as a result of their relationship with the loved one with mental illness [13–16]. Practically, 43–92% of the care providers of people with mental illness reported the feeling of being stigmatized [17]. In the United States, a study revealed that 43% of caregivers of people with mental illness perceived that they were stigmatized by others because of having a mentally ill individual within their relatives [15]. In Morocco, caregivers of schizophrenia patients reported high level of perceived stigma and faced serious impacts on their family members [18]. A community-based study conducted in Ethiopia showed that perceived stigma was 75% among caregivers of people with severe mental illness (SMI) [19]. Perceived stigma has affected caregivers of people with SMI in several ways including emotional, relationship, financial, health, and time stressors. They also described the feeling of being separated, ignored, blamed and criticized by peers, neighbors, coworkers and even mental health professionals [20]. Caregivers of people with mental illness are exposed to shame, low self-worth, and social isolation as a result of perceived stigma. Caregivers' expectation of devaluation and discrimination from others leads them to adopt harmful coping mechanisms such as secrecy or withdrawal. As a result, caregivers hide patients, and patients may not get proper treatment or will be noncompliance [13].

A study revealed that perceived stigma of caregivers is associated with higher education, living with the patient in an urbanized area, being female, and a patient who had early age onset of illness, multiple admission and longer duration of the illness [14].

Even though studies around the globe demonstrated the high magnitude of perceived stigma, in Ethiopia, there are few previous studies that reported on perceived stigma specifically among non-professional caregivers of people with SMI.

Therefore, this study was proposed to determine the magnitude of perceived stigma and predictive factors among non-professional caregivers of people with SMI in the study area.

Methods

Study design and period

The facility-based cross-sectional study was conducted from May to June 2016 at Felege-Hiwot Referral Hospital (FHRH). The Hospital is found in the capital city of Amhara Regional state which is located 553 km far from the capital city of Ethiopia, Addis Ababa. It was established in 1963 as district hospital and changed into referral hospital in 2002. Psychiatry unit was established in 1990 and currently, there are five psychiatry outpatient units which provide services for about 70–90 patients per day.

Sample size determination and sampling procedure

Sample size and Sampling procedures

The sample size was determined using single-population proportion formula $[n = ((z\alpha/2)2p(1 - p))/d2]$ with the following assumptions: 95% confidence interval (CI) ($Z\alpha/2 = 1.96$) and the proportion (p) of perceived stigma of caregivers to be 75% from previous study at Buta Jira [19], marginal error 4%. By adding 10% non-response rate, a total of 495 study populations were involved.

The study participants were selected using systematic random sampling technique. The numbers of patients with SMI who had monthly regular follow-up estimated were 1482; of these, 526 people with schizophrenia, major depressive disorder (MDD) (600) and bipolar disorders (356). The total sample size was allocated proportionally to each SMI patient caregivers. Sampling fraction was 3 (i.e. $1482/495 \approx 3$) for all samples. Lottery method was used to get the first participant who arrived at outpatient settings for each type of severely mentally ill patients' caregivers. Then after, ever 3rd caregivers were interviewed according to their arrival in outpatient settings for each type of caregivers independently. A caregiver who provides more care was interviewed when the patient had more than one caregiver.

Operational definitions

Caregiver

Someone who provided more than 6 months of care and regularly responsible for taking care of patients more than other immediate or non-immediate family relative rather than by a health professional.

Immediate family relative

Father/mother, son/daughter and brother/sister.

Non-immediate family relative
Other relatives and friends.

Severe mental illness
Mental illness that includes schizophrenia, major depressive and bipolar disorders.

Data-collection instruments and procedures
Data were collected using standardized Family Interview Schedule (FIS) questionnaire, which was developed as part of a world health organization study on the course and outcome of schizophrenia [21]. FIS questionnaire was 14-item questions regarding stigma that might affect families. Each stigma item was rated on a four-point scale, not at all (0), sometimes (1), often (2) and a lot (3) with respect to stigma. To assess the distribution of stigma responses between groups, a stigma sum score was computed by summarizing all positive responses (≥ 1) for each of the 14 items. The presence of just one positive answer on the stigma questionnaire was enough to represent a form of perceived stigma [19].

Social support was measured using the Oslo-3 Social Support Scale (OSS-3) with three questions. We used the sum score scale ranging from 3 to 14, which has three broad categories: "poor support" 3–8, "moderate support" 9–11 and "strong support" 12–14 [22].

A semi-structured questionnaire was used to collect socio-demographic, relationship and clinical factors. Data were collected using pre-tested structured questionnaires using face to face interview. Five data collectors (BSc nurses) and one MSc in mental health supervisor were recruited to conduct face to face interview of the caregivers for a month duration.

Data quality management
Data quality control issue is ensured by conducting pre-test among 25 caregivers in the study area 1 week before the actual data-collection periods. One-day training was given for data collectors and supervisors on how to use the questionnaires, how to approach the participants of the study and about the purpose of the study. In addition to this, English questionnaires were translated to local language respondents' Amharic language. Supervisor and principal investigator were closely followed the whole period of data-collection process. Supervision was held regularly during the data-collection period. Collected data were checked on a daily basis for its completeness.

Data processing and analysis
Data were checked, coded, cleaned and entered into Epi-Info version 7 and exported to SPSS version 20 for analysis. Frequency, percentage, mean, standard deviation, tables, and charts were used to report the results of the data. Bivariate logistic regression analysis used to examine the association between dependent and independent variables. All variables with $p < 0.2$ in bivariate analysis were fitted into the multivariate logistic regression model to identify factors associated with perceived stigma. The association was interpreted using odds ratio and 95% confidence interval. $p < 0.05$ was considered statistically significant in this study.

Ethical consideration
Ethical clearance obtained from University of Gondar ethical review board committee before data-collection period. The official letter was obtained and given for Amhara regional health bureau and Felege-Hiwot Referral Hospital. The study participants were informed about the purpose of the study. Written informed consent was obtained from participants during data-collection period, and they were informed that participation was on the voluntary basis and had full right to withdraw at any time during the interview process. They were also informed that refusal to participate had no negative consequences on the patients' care, and participation had no financial benefit. Confidentiality was maintained throughout the study.

Results
Socio-demographic characteristics
Out of 495 recruited caregivers, 478 participated in the study yielding a response rate of 96.56%. The mean age of caregivers was 37.08 (± 13.4 SD) years. Nearly half of caregivers were females 244 (51%) and rural residents 262 (54.8%). Majority of respondents were Amhara by ethnicity 469 (98.1%), Orthodox religion follower 384 (80.3%) and currently not married 374 (78.2%) (Table 1).

Psychosocial factors
Nearly half of the caregivers had poor social support 260 (54.4%), others had moderate social supports 136 (28.5%), and strong social supports 82 (17.1%).

Relationship factors
Caregivers who have the duration of relationship with the patient for about 20–39 years were 238 (49.8%) and not live together with the patient 279 (58.4%) (Table 2).

Clinical factors
Almost half of patient's illness onset was below the ages of 20 years 262 (54.8%) and 307 (64.2%) had history of admission (Table 3).

Table 1 Socio-demographic characteristics of caregivers at Felege-Hiwot Referral Hospital, Bahir Dar, northwest Ethiopia, July, 2016 ($n = 478$)

Variables	Categories	Frequency	Percent
Age	18–24	89	18.6
	25–34	138	28.9
	35–44	108	22.6
	44–54	81	16.9
	≥ 55	62	13
Sex	Male	234	49
	Female	244	51
Residence	Urban	216	45.2
	Rural	262	54.8
Ethnicity	Amhara	469	98.1
	Others[a]	9	1.9
Religion	Orthodox	384	80.3
	Muslim	88	18.4
	Others[b]	6	1.3
Marital status	Currently not married	374	78.2
	Currently married	104	21.8
Educational status	Unable to read and write	121	25.3
	Primary	115	24.1
	Secondary	90	18.8
	Diploma and above	152	31.8
Job	Government employee	73	15.3
	Private employee	72	15.1
	Merchant	65	13.6
	Farmer	143	29.9
	House wife	71	14.9
	Student	54	11.3

Others[a] = Tigrie, Oromo and Guragie; Others[b] = Protestant and Catholic

Table 2 Relationship factors of caregivers of people with SMI at Felege-Hiwot Referral Hospital, Bahir Dar, northwest Ethiopia, July, 2016 ($n = 478$)

Variables	Categories	Frequency	Percent
Type of relationship	Mother	64	13.4
	Father	113	23.6
	Spouse	98	20.5
	Child	75	15.7
	Brother/sister	83	17.4
	Other relatives/friends	45	9.4
Duration of relationship with the patient (years)	0–19	181	37.9
	20–39	238	49.8
	40–59	59	12.3
Do you live together with patients	Yes	199	41.6
	No	279	58.4

Table 3 Clinical factors of caregivers of people with SMI at Felege-Hiwot Referral Hospital, Bahir Dar, northwest Ethiopia, July, 2016 ($n = 478$)

Variables	Categories	Frequency	Percent
Types of diagnosis	Schizophrenia	175	36.6
	Bipolar disorders	115	24.1
	MDD	188	39.3
Age of illness onset (years)	≤ 20	262	54.8
	21–40	135	28.2
	≥ 40	81	16.9
Duration patient's Illness (years)	≤ 1	111	23.2
	> 1	367	76.8
Duration of treatment of patients (years)	≤ 1	205	42.9
	2–5	178	37.2
	6–10	75	15.7
	≥ 11	20	4.2
Admission	No	171	35.8
	Yes	307	64.2

Prevalence of perceived stigma

The prevalence of perceived stigma in our study was 89.3% (95%, CI 84.6, 91.9). The mean and standard deviation of FIS scale was 7.6 and 8.1 respectively and its minimum and maximum value ranges from 0 to 34. Regarding the proportion of perceived stigma toward each item, three quarters (75.2%) of the caregivers agreed with the item "Felt grief or depression because of it", followed by "Helping other people to understand what it is like to have a family member with psychiatric problem' '(43.9%). The least frequently endorsed item was 'felt that somehow it might be your fault' (14.6%) (Table 4).

Associated factors with perceived stigma

In the bivariate logistic regression analysis, sex, residence, social support, age of onset of illness, patient's duration of treatment, marital status, care giver's educational level, patient's numbers of hospital admission and duration of relationship with the patient were significantly associated with previewed stigma at p value < 0.2 level and entered for further analysis into multivariate logistic regression to control confounding factors. On the other hand, ethnicity, religion, types of diagnosis, duration of illness, the age of respondents, job, types of the relationship of caregivers with the patient and living together or not living together were not statistically significant. In the logistic regression,

Table 4 Proportion of perceived stigma response of caregivers to each item at Felege-Hiwot Referral Hospital, Bahir Dar, northwest Ethiopia, July, 2016 ($n = 478$)

S. no	Items	Negative responses	Any positive response			
		Not at all total (%)	Some times	Often	A lot	Total (%)
1	Worried about being treated differently	365 (76.4%)	58	14	41	113 (23.6%)
2	Worried people would know about it	352 (73.7%)	46	27	53	126 (26.3%)
3	Felt the need to hide this fact	356 (74.4%)	52	21	49	122 (25.6%)
4	Helping other people to understand what it is like to have a family member with psychiatric problem	268 (56.1%)	134	33	43	210 (43.9%)
5	Making an effort to keep this fact a secret	349 (73%)	57	23	49	129 (27%)
6	Worried about being avoided	381 (80%)	46	24	27	97 (20%)
7	Explaining to others that (name) isn't like their picture of "crazy" people	341 (71.3%)	85	25	27	137 (28.7%)
8	Worried that people would blame you for his or her problems	401 (83.9%)	44	18	15	77 (16.1%)
9	Worried that a person looking to marry would be reluctant to marry into your family	352 (73.6%)	54	20	52	126 (26.4%)
10	Worried about taking him or her out	359 (75.1%)	48	17	54	126 (24.9%)
11	Felt ashamed or embarrassed about it	335 (70.1%)	125	17	1	143 (29.9)
12	Sought out people who also have a family member who has had psychiatric problem	301 (63%)	79	20	78	177 (37%)
13	Felt grief or depression because of it	119 (24.9%)	140	61	158	359 (75.1%)
14	Felt that somehow it might be your fault	408 (85.4%)	50	12	8	70 (14.6%)

after controlling confounding factors, sex, residency, social support, marital statuses, and numbers of admission and duration of relationship with the patient were found statistically significant.

Female caregivers were three times more likely to have perceived stigma compared to male caregivers (AOR = 3.02, 95% CI 1.30, 7.11), not currently married were three times more likely to have perceived stigma compared to currently married caregivers (AOR = 3.20, 95% CI 1.48, 6.91) and caregivers who lived in rural were three times more likely to have perceived stigma compared to who lived in urban areas (AOR = 2.80, 95% CI 1.20, 6.54). Caregivers who had poor social support were five times more likely to have perceived stigma compared to caregivers who have strong social support (AOR = 5.06, 95% CI 1.96, 13.13).

Caregivers who gave care for patients for 20–39-year duration were five times more likely to have perceived stigma compared to those who gave care for 6 months–19 years of duration (AOR = 4.92, 95% CI 1.30, 18.67). In addition to this, caregivers who cared for the patient who had the history of admission were 77% less likely to have perceived stigma compared those who gave no history of admission (AOR = 0.23, 95% CI = 0.10, 0.51) (Table 5).

Discussion

The increment in the prevalence of perceived stigma globally needs a better understanding of the local burden and most common influencing factors. In the current study, the overall prevalence of perceived stigma among caregivers of people with SMI was found to be 89.3% which was in line with the study done in Morocco which was 86.7% [18].

However, the prevalence in this study was higher than the prevalence reported in the United States (43%), Belgium (86%) and Butajira, Ethiopia (75%) [15, 19, 23]. The difference might be due to variation in sample size, instruments they used, cultural, socio-demographic characteristics of participants and study population. In addition to this, perceived stigma in our study might be due to a misperception about mental illness and most of the time people believed that mental illness is happened as a result of supernatural punishment. Furthermore, the sample size in Butajira was 178 and conducted at the community level, however, the current study was done at health institution among 478 caregivers of people with SMI. There was also an educational status difference.

In this study, perceived stigma among female caregivers was higher than male caregivers, which was in line with the previous studies done in China and American [14, 24]. This might be due to the reason in which the role of caring and social burden for the female is more burdensome increasing their vulnerability to perceived stigma.

Table 5 Factors associated with perceived stigma among caregivers of people with SMI attending at Felege-Hiwot Referral Hospital, Bahir Dar, northwest Ethiopia, July, 2016 ($n = 478$)

Explanatory variables	Category	Perceived stigma		COR (95% CI)	AOR (95% CI)
		Yes	No		
Sex	Male	199	35	1.0	1.0
	Female	228	16	2.51 (1.35, 4.67)	3.03 (1.29, 7.11)[a]
Residency	Urban	187	29	1.0	1.0
	Rural	240	22	1.70 (0.94, 3.304)	2.80 (1.20, 6.54)[a]
Social support	Poor	244	16	5.59 (2.77, 11.30)	5.06 (1.96, 13.13)[a]
	Moderate	123	13	3.47 (1.64, 7.36)	2.43 (0.91, 6.45)
	Strong	60	22	1.0	1.0
Age onset of illness (years)	≤ 20	254	8	1.0	1.0
	21–39	100	35	0.09 (0.04, 0.20)	0.47 (0.75, 8.12)
	≥ 40	73	8	0.29 (0.10, 0.79)	0.40 (0.14, 1.13)
Duration of treatment (years)	< 1	191	14	1.0	1.0
	2–5	159	19	0.61 (0.30, 1.26)	0.22 (0.64, 16.22)
	6–10	64	11	0.43 (0.18, 0.99)	0.14 (0.62, 15.85)
	≥ 11	13	7	0.14 (0.05, 0.40)	0.12 (0.39, 11.64)
Marital status	Currently not married	350	24	5.11 (2.80, 9.34)	3.20 (1.48, 6.91)[a]
	Currently married	77	27	1.0	1.0
Educational level	Unable to read and write	102	19	0.46 (0.21, 0.99)	1.00 (0.35, 2.86)
	Primary	106	9	1.01 (.41, 0.2.48)	1.45 (0.49, 4.26)
	Secondary	79	11	0.62 (0.26, 1.46)	0.74 (0.26, 2.06)
	Diploma and above	140	12	1.0	1.0
History of admission	No	146	25	1.0	1.0
	Yes	281	26	1.85 (1.03, 3.32)	0.23 (0.10, 0.51)[a]
Duration of care for the patient	6 moths–19 years	149	32	1.0	1.0
	20–39 years	227	11	4.43 (2.17, 9.10)	4.92 (1.30, 18.67)[a]
	≥ 40 years	51	8	1.37 (0.060, 3.16)	3.80 (1.20, 11.98)[a]

COR crude odds ratio, *AOR* adjusted odds ratio

[a] Statistically significant at *p* value < 0.05

Caregivers who were currently not married and lived in the rural area were three times more likely to have perceived stigma compared to those who were currently married and lived in the urban area. This result has concurred with the findings documented in India and China [25, 26]. This might be due to lack of intimate social support to share stressful feelings, having low self-esteem and poor coping mechanism which are common among not married people exposing them to have perceived stigma. This thought is supported by the current study stating that poor social support increased the level of perceived stigma. In addition, caregivers who lived in the rural area experienced the high level of perceived stigma. These could be due to rural residents' lack of awareness and cultural belief about the causes of mental illness such as spiritual possessions, the result of a sinful act or punishment from God [27].

Caregivers who had poor social support were five times more likely to have perceived stigma compared to those with strong social support. This result is in line with the data from a study conducted in China [26]. The possible reason could be the assumptions that caregivers who had a mentally ill person with family members might isolate themselves from the societies and cannot share different roles, responsibilities and their feelings.

Regarding duration of patient care, those who gave care for longer duration were more likely to have perceived stigma than those who gave care for a relatively shorter duration which is in line with the previous result in China [14]. Perception of stigma may be increased when the duration of caring increased. Because caring for people with severe mental illness causes a burden for caregivers in every aspect of life including economic, social, financial, physical and psychological consequences.

Admitted patient caregivers had a lower level of perceived stigma compared to caregivers who had no SMI family members with a history of admission. The current finding is inconsistent with the previous institution-based study was done in China [14]. The difference might be due to the difference in study design (follow-up study), measurement tool (Camberwell Family Interview) and study population (schizophrenia caregivers) in China. Moreover, the information might create awareness since they exchange information about mental illness with different health professionals and other peoples who cared people with several mental illnesses during their hospital stay.

Limitation of the study

Since the study was conducted only using quantitative design, it might not explore well the perception of caregivers' perceived stigma. In addition, a way of using an interpretation tool may exaggerate the presence of perceived stigma. Most comparison parts of discussions are not culturally matched.

Conclusion

This study finding showed a high prevalence of perceived stigma among caregivers of people with severe mental illness at Felege-Hiwot Referral Hospital, Bahir Dar. Being female, rural residency, poor social support, currently not being married and long duration of caring for patient were found to be significantly associated with the perceived stigma of caregivers of people with the severe mental illness. Therefore, it is very important to increase strong social support towards caregivers of people with mental illness by collaborating with different stakeholders and link them to support groups such as nongovernmental organizations and social workers, and to formulate certain interventions that focus on reduction of perceived stigma among caregivers.

Authors' contributions
TE conceived and designed the study. TE organized the data-collection process. TE, ZY, WD, BA, AA, and MT analyzed the data. TE and MT prepared the manuscript. All authors read and approved the final manuscript.

Author details
[1] Department of Psychiatry, College of Medicine and Health Sciences, Bahir Dar University, Po box 79, Bahir Dar, Ethiopia. [2] Amanuel Specialized Mental Hospital, Addis Ababa, Ethiopia. [3] Department of Psychiatry, College of Medicine and Health Sciences, Gondar University, Gondar, Ethiopia. [4] College of Medicine and Health Sciences, Bahir Dar University, Po box 79, Bahir Dar, Ethiopia.

Acknowledgements
The authors would like to thank the data collectors, supervisor, study participants and Felege-Hiwot Referral Hospital psychiatry clinic staffs for their genuine cooperation during the study period.

Competing interests
The authors declare that they have no competing interests.

Consent for publication
Not applicable.

Funding
The research is funded by the University of Gondar.

References
1. Organization WH. The world health report 2001: mental health: new understanding, new hope. Geneva: World Health Organization; 2001.
2. Desjarlais R. World mental health: problems and priorities in low-income countries. Oxford: Oxford University Press; 1995.
3. Murray CJ, Lopez AD. Global burden of disease. Cambridge: Harvard University Press; 1996.
4. Rafiyah I. burden on family caregivers caring for patients with schizophrenia and its related factors. Nurs Media J Nurs. 2011;1(1):29–41.
5. Andrews L. Non-specialist health worker interventions for the care of mental, neurological, and substance-abuse disorders in low-and middle-income countries. Issues Ment Health Nurs. 2016;37(2):131–2.
6. Cooper AE, Corrigan PW, Watson AC. Mental illness stigma and care seeking. J Nerv Ment Dis. 2003;191(5):339–41.
7. Goffman E. Stigma: notes on the management of spoiled identity. New York: Simon and Schuster; 2009.
8. Corrigan PW, Kerr A, Knudsen L. The stigma of mental illness: explanatory models and methods for change. Appl Prev Psychol. 2005;11(3):179–90.
9. Werner P, Aviv A, Barak Y. Self-stigma, self-esteem and age in persons with schizophrenia. Int Psychogeriatr. 2008;20(1):174–87.
10. Griffiths KM, Christensen H, Jorm AF, Evans K, Groves C. Effect of web-based depression literacy and cognitive–behavioural therapy interventions on stigmatising attitudes to depression. Br J Psychiatry. 2004;185(4):342–9.
11. Crisp R. A qualitative study of the perceptions of individuals with disabilities concerning health and rehabilitation professionals. Disabil Soc. 2000;15(2):355–67.
12. Link BG, Yang LH, Phelan JC, Collins PY. Measuring mental illness stigma. Schizophr Bull. 2004;30(3):511–41.
13. Phelan JC, Bromet EJ, Link BG. Psychiatric illness and family stigma. Schizophr Bull. 1998;24(1):115–26.
14. Phillips MR, Pearson V, Li F, Xu M, Yang L. Stigma and expressed emotion: a study of people with schizophrenia and their family members in China. Br J Psychiatry. 2002;181(6):488–93.
15. Struening EL, Perlick DA, Link BG, Hellman F, Herman D, Sirey JA. Stigma as a barrier to recovery: the extent to which caregivers believe most people devalue consumers and their families. Psychiatric Serv. 2001;52(12):1633–8.
16. Thara R, Srinivasan T. How stigmatising is schizophrenia in India? Int J Soc Psychiatry. 2000;46(2):135–41.
17. Van Brakel WH. Measuring health-related stigma—a literature review. Psychology Health Med. 2006;11(3):307–34.
18. Kadri N, Manoudi F, Berrada S, Moussaoui D. Stigma impact on Moroccan families of patients with schizophrenia. Can J Psychiatry. 2004;49(9):625–9.
19. Shibre T, Negash A, Kullgren G, Kebede D, Alem A, Fekadu A, Fekadu D, Medhin G, Jacobsson L. Perception of stigma among family members of individuals with schizophrenia and major affective disorders in rural Ethiopia. Soc Psychiatry Psychiatr Epidemiol. 2001;36(6):299–303.
20. Joanne Riebschleger PhDM, Maureen Mickus PhDM, Christine Liszewski MD, Eaton M. How are the experiences and needs of families of individuals with mental illness reflected in medical education guidelines? Acad Psychiatry. 2008;32(2):119.
21. Sartorius N, Janca A. Psychiatric assessment instruments developed by the World Health Organization. Soc Psychiatry Psychiatr Epidemiol. 1996;31(2):55–69.
22. Dalgard OS, Dowrick C, Lehtinen V, Vazquez-Barquero JL, Casey P, Wilkinson G, Ayuso-Mateos JL, Page H, Dunn G. Negative life events, social support and gender difference in depression. Soc Psychiatry Psychiatr Epidemiol. 2006;41(6):444–51.
23. Catthoor K, Schrijvers D, Hutsebaut J, Feenstra D, Persoons P, De Hert M, Peuskens J, Sabbe B. Associative stigma in family members of psychotic patients in Flanders: an exploratory study. World J Psychiatry. 2015;5(1):118.

24. Gonzalez JM, Perlick DA, Miklowitz DJ, Kaczynski R, Hernandez M, Rosen-heck RA, Culver JL, Ostacher MJ, Bowden CL. Factors associated with stigma among caregivers of patients with bipolar disorder in the STEP-BD study. Psychiatric Serv. 2007;58(1):41–8.

25. Yannawar PB, Gajendragad JM, Gotewal S, Singh SB. Comparative study of perception of stigma among caregivers of persons with Bipolar affective disorder and Schizophrenia.

26. Yin Y, Zhang W, Hu Z, Jia F, Li Y, Xu H, Zhao S, Guo J, Tian D, Qu Z. Experiences of stigma and discrimination among caregivers of persons with schizophrenia in China: a field survey. PLoS ONE. 2014;9(9):e108527.

27. Tilahun D, Hanlon C, Fekadu A, Tekola B, Baheretibeb Y, Hoekstra RA. Stigma, explanatory models and unmet needs of caregivers of children with developmental disorders in a low-income African country: a cross-sectional facility-based survey. BMC Health Serv Res. 2016;16(1):152.

25

The effect of training interventions of stigma associated with mental illness on family caregivers

Farshid Shamsaei[1], Fatemeh Nazari[2] and Efat Sadeghian[3*]

Abstract

Background: Stigma is one of the most destructive features of mental illnesses that may affect the family caregivers. This study aimed to analyze the effect of training interventions of stigma on family caregivers of the mental illness patients.

Materials and methods: This quasi-experimental pre- and post-test study was performed on a single group of 43 family caregivers of mental illness patients in Hamadan Psychiatric Hospital, Iran, in 2015. The samples were taken through convenience sampling method and the data collection tool was a stigma questionnaire made by the researchers. The questionnaires were filled by the participants within pre-intervention and 1-month post-intervention. All the data were analyzed by SPSS version 16, and the mean and standard deviation by paired t test and Wilcoxon test.

Results: Findings of this study demonstrated that women included 60% of the family caregivers. The average age of caregivers and the duration of caregiving were 41.67 ± 11.62 years and 66.28 ± 7.99 months, respectively. The mean and standard deviation for pre-intervention stigma score were 82.47 ± 12.23 indicating that the family caregivers suffered from some problems arisen from living with mental patients. They include not getting married, unable to find a job, embarrassment, humiliation by others, disgrace, and shame. Our results revealed that the mean and standard deviation of stigma score decreased to 29.28 ± 7.52 after training, and this difference was statistically significant ($P < 0.001$).

Conclusions: According to the results of present study, training interventions reduce the issues caused by stigma and help the family members of mental patients to face and cope with the problem.

Keywords: Family caregivers, Mental illness, Stigma, Training

Introduction

Family caregivers play the most prominent role in caregiving for mental illnesses patients, and there is a growing body of literature on the family burden and stigma, lack of caregiver support, and equivocal success, with interventions aiming at alleviating the care-giving burden [1, 2].

Family caregivers have to bear the negative effects caused by prejudice and stigmatization in addition to support of the patients both emotionally and physically. Stigma is one of the most destructive features of mental illnesses that may affect the family caregivers, patients' families, and the patients themselves [3, 4]. In other words, many authorities in the field of psychological health believe that the most important obstacle to the mental patients treatment is "mental illness stigma" rather than the medication shortage, specialists, or facilities [5].

The stigma arisen from taking care of mental patients leads the prejudice, losing social status, preventive

*Correspondence: sadeghianefat@gmail.com
[3] Chronic Diseases (Home Care) Research Centre, School of Nursing and Midwifery, Hamadan University of Medical Sciences, Hamadan, Iran
Full list of author information is available at the end of the article

behavior strategies such as withdrawal, decreased life quality, disease intensity, drug abuse, failing to take the medications and to pursue the treatments, and confusion in the family [6]. Link and Phelan [6] announced that stigma includes five elements of labeling, stereotyping, cognitive isolation, emotional reactions, and prejudice so that a person in the society is labeled for any special characteristic which is different from the formalities of society and placed in minority [7, 8].

The stigma results the feeling of embarrassment in many family caregivers of mental patients. It should be noted that a low percentage of these members undergoes education and sufficient information considering the mental illnesses, signs and symptoms, correct approaches for facing the patients, and stereotyping [9–11].

Limited and mistaken information about psychological health and tendency for hiding the family member illness in family caregivers leads a remarkable augmentation in being stigmatized [12]. One of the effective approaches in reducing the stigma and omitting the negative attitude of society to these patients is to help the family caregivers understand the illness, encourage to accept pharmaceutical therapy, identify the early symptoms of relapse, and assure the rapid omission of disease attacks. The mentioned practices may result in better recovery of the patient and reduced social and personal disabilities. In addition, they might lead the family caregivers to better play their supportive and therapeutic roles [13].

In spite of various research projects on stigma reduction programs, few studies have examined how to overcome stigma toward family caregivers of mental illness patients [14, 15]. It seems that the stigma reduction strategies vary according to the contextual factors including politics, socioeconomic status, culture, religion and media. Iran is a Middle-East Islamic country with an approximately 79-million population [15] in which religious culture is dominant. In Iran, families play the key role in taking care of the mental illness patients, and social variables as well as the misbeliefs of people pose them some problems such as stigma. Therefore, this study was performed to analyze the effect of training stigma interventions associated with mental illness on family caregivers.

Materials and methods

This quasi-experimental pre- and post-test study was conducted on a group of patients in Hamadan Psychiatric Hospital, Iran, in 2015. The sample included 43 mental patients family members who had the most prominent role in taking care of the mental patients and were selected through convenience sampling method. Sample size was measured according to a similar study [16] with

reliability level of 95% and statistical power of 80% using the following equation:

$$n = \frac{(Z1-\alpha/2 + Z1 - /2)^2 S^2}{d^2} = \frac{(1.96 + 0.84)^2 (4.64)^2}{(2)^2} = 43$$

The study inclusion criteria: (1) mental illness of one of the family members (e.g., schizophrenia, schizoaffective, bipolar disorders type I, major depressive disorder, etc.) diagnosed by the psychiatrist based on the diagnostic criteria of the 5th edition of the Diagnostic and Statistical Manual of Mental Disorders (DSM-5), (2) at least 1-year experience in taking care of the mental patient, (3) the patient is an adult, and 4) lack of mental retardation, chronic diseases, and drug addiction history in the family. The exclusion criteria included absence in more than two sessions of the trainings during the study and incidence of unpredicted stressors in the family.

To design the questionnaire as the data collection means, a full literature review was performed using different databases including *PsycINFO*, SID, Prequest, Up-to-date, Scopus, Pub med and Ovid. Therefore, the stigma evaluation questionnaire was designed for the family caregivers of the patients with chronic mental disorders. Afterwards, face and content validity in both quantitative and qualitative aspects, construct validity in addition to the internal consistency were all assessed. The primary tool consisting of 38 items was analyzed regarding the face and content validity based on the qualitative and quantitative features (CVR and CVI). In this stage, some items were omitted and merged, reducing to 33 items. The construct validity was examined through exploratory *factor analysis* and sample size of 356 which led the final remaining 30 items. The results of Cronbach's alpha (0.83) and retest (0.87) were indicative of a high internal consistency and reliability of the tool.

Each item was answered as a Likert scale with five choices (i.e., never, rarely, sometimes, often, and always). The scores of zero, one, two, three, and four were attributed to the answers never, rarely, sometimes, often, and always, respectively. Therefore, the minimum score for the questionnaire was determined as zero and the maximum 120. Overall, the score ranges of 0–29, 30–59, 60–89, and 90–120 were interpreted as weak, moderate, severe, and strongly severe stigma, respectively, categorized into four groups of 25%.

Intervention

Mental Illness Stigma Reduction Programs: a large number of programs and initiatives have attempted to reduce mental illness stigma. They can be roughly divided into two categories: training interventions that involve in-person communication between an educator/speaker and a small moderate-sized group, and mass media campaigns and broad multifaceted interventions. Some initiatives include both of these components [16, 17]. Training interventions typically involve an educational component in which information about the causes of mental illness, mental health treatment, and the experiences of people with mental health problems are provided to counteract the stereotypes and prejudice, and promote attitudes affirmation to the people with mental illness [18].

In this study, we used training interventions that involve in-person communication between an educator/speaker and a small group.

The content of the intervention sessions:

1. Providing information about the research and family's experience of stigma.

   The purpose of this session was to meet the family caregivers, to provide them with information about the research objective and to determine the time and place of the education to be given. In addition, in this session, basics of psychological health were explained and the participants were asked to share and discuss their experiences about stigma if any.
2. Providing information about the mental illness.

   Aim of the second session was an introduction to mental illnesses and their reasons, treatments, and taking care of the mental patients. These aims were achieved by giving presentations and delivering pamphlets.
3. Providing information about roles of family in taking care of mental illness.

   The third session was held to clarify the importance and roles of the family in treatment and care for the mental patients. Therefore, the roles of family members in treatment and interactions with the patients were discussed in groups.
4. How to know stigma and teach skills for coping with stigma.

   In the fourth session, the purpose of stigma analysis is the effective factors on causing it, effects of accepting the stigma on treatment protocols, problems due to the stigma in families, confronting the stigma, and beliefs in the mental illnesses.

When participants were selected, they were divided into 9 groups (Each consisting of 4–5 people). Pretest was done before intervention. The education program included four sessions that lasted 60–75 min. We used a different day in the same week for each group. Sessions started with an evaluation of the past session. All participants completed the education program.

Education program was presented by a psychiatric nurse in cooperation with an associate professor of nursing. Post-test occurred 1 week after intervention.

Statistical analysis

Data were analyzed using SPSS 16 packet program. The descriptive analysis included absolute and relative frequency distribution, mean, and standard deviation. Moreover, comparison of the mean scores, paired t test, and Wilcoxon test were utilized for the analytical statistics. The significance was set at $\alpha = 0.05$.

Results

According to the findings of our study, the average age of participants was 41.2 years, mostly consisting of women (60.5%). The average duration of taking care of the patients was 66.3 months and average duration of taking care during a week was 71 h (Table 1). The most common disorders among the patients were bipolar disorders type

Table 1 Socio-demographic characteristics of caregivers

Characteristics	N	%
Sex		
Male	26	60.5
Female	17	39.5
Ages (years)		
>30	6	13.9
30–39	12	27.9
40–49	21	48.8
≤50	4	9.3
Marital status		
Single	11	25.6
Married	27	62.8
Divorced	3	7
Widowed	2	4.6
Educational level		
Primary school	9	20.9
High school	27	62.8
University	7	16.3
Employment status		
Employed	10	23.2
Unemployed	3	7
Retired	2	4.6
Business	11	23.6
Agricultural worker	9	20.9
Housework	8	18.6
Relationship with patient		
Spouses	10	28.3
Parents	21	40.6
Children	7	12.9
Siblings	5	18.2

I (44.2%), obsessive–compulsive disorders 26.4%, Major depressive disorder 21% and schizophrenia 9.3%.

The mean stigma score pre-intervention was 82.47 ± 12.23, which declined to 29.28 ± 7 post-intervention. The difference of stigma questionnaire score between two pre- and post-intervention times was statistically significant ($P < 0.001$) (Table 2). The latter finding demonstrates that short-term training programs can also reduce the stigma in family caregivers of mental patients.

Discussion

Results of the current study indicate that the mean stigma score is high in family caregivers of the mental illness patients before the training intervention. In other words, stigma is one of the problems arisen from caregiving and living with a mental patient as mentioned in the literature [19–22].

The present study aimed to investigate the effects of training on encountering the stigma in family caregivers of the mental illness patients. Our results showed that education could be effective on reducing the stigma score among the family caregivers.

The studies performed by Uchino and Cuhadar demonstrated that training could diminish the stigma in family caregivers of the patients with schizophrenia and mood disorder, which are compliant with the findings of this study [23, 24]. On the other hand, Kiropoulos et al. showed in Australia that training had no influence on stigma, which is not in line with our results [25].

The inconsistency between the current study and the study conducted by Kiropoulos et al. might be due to two major reasons [25]. The first reason is that training in the present study was face-to-face and direct contact with the caregivers. Corrigan et al. also emphasizes the positive and remarkable impact of direct training [5], while Kiropoulos et al. performed their training intervention via internet. Furthermore, their study population included several different cultures, such as Greeks, English-speaking people, and Italians. However, all the participants of the present study were familiar with Persian language and almost enjoy the similar culture [25].

Moreover, results of the studies performed by Bernhard et al. and Yang et al. indicated that training, knowledge, and attitude of the caregivers may improve the mental illness [11, 16]. In addition, Cuhadar et al. and Cook et al. also reached the conclusion that the hiding rate by the caregivers significantly declined post-intervention [24, 26].

Moreover, the findings of current study revealed that the preventive behaviors of the caregivers diminished, and their social interactions increased after training, as they are compliant with the results of Uchino et al. [23, 24, 26].

It was observed in the present research that the parents of mental patients did not blame themselves anymore after the training sessions, and they have mainly solved their ideas toward this problem. Accordingly, Yin et al. and Cuhadar and Cam mentioned in their studies that parents considerably blamed themselves less after the trainings [20, 24].

One of the limitations of the current study was the short period of training program, as it seems that long-term trainings and continuous follow-ups improve the efficacy of interventions. Moreover, the sample size could be considered as another limitation, and a more comprehensive study with larger sample size will enhance the generalizability of the results. In addition, applying a research-made questionnaire was also among the limitations of this study. Another limitation is related to sampling method. The data were collected by convincing sampling. This method may represent the views of a specific group rather than the entire population.

Despite the aforementioned limitations, findings of this study provide crucial empirical evidence regarding the effects of stigma confrontation training on family caregivers of people with mental illness in the Iran.

Conclusions

This study demonstrated that stigma is one of the problems and challenges of mental patients' family caregivers, and insufficient knowledge regarding the stigma phenomenon might exacerbate the problem. Therefore, the current research provided an evidence for the short-term efficacy of the training program in improving stigma-related knowledge of family caregivers of mental illness people.

Table 2 Comparison of mean scores of stigma before and after intervention

Stigma score	Before intervention N (%)	After intervention N (%)	P
Mild	0	24 (55.8)	< 0.001*
Moderate	1 (2.3)	19 (44.2)	
Severe	30 (69.8)	0	
Strongly severe	12 (27.9)	0	
Mean ± SD	82.47 ± 12.23	29.28 ± 7.52	< 0.001**

* Wilcoxon signed rank test

** Paired sample *t* test

Abbreviations

CVI: content validity index; CVR: content validity ratio; DSM 5: diagnostic and statistical manual of mental disorders 5th edition; *PsycINFO*: *psychological information*; Pub med; pub medline; SID: scientific information database; SPSS: statistical package for the social sciences.

Authors' contributions

FSH and FN conceived the study, prepared the protocol and developed the training programs. ES and FN developed the analysis plan and performed the statistical analyses. FSH and ES were major contributors in writing the manuscript. All authors read and approved the final manuscript.

Author details
[1] Behavioural Disorders and Substance Abuse Research Centre, Hamadan University of Medical Sciences, Hamadan, Iran. [2] Department of Nursing and Midwifery, Hamadan University of Medical Sciences, Hamadan, Iran. [3] Chronic Diseases (Home Care) Research Centre, School of Nursing and Midwifery, Hamadan University of Medical Sciences, Hamadan, Iran.

Acknowledgements
This study is funded by the Behavioural disorders and substance abuse research centre, Hamadan University of Medical sciences in Iran. Researchers would like to thank families for taking part in the study and project staff for their valuable contribution.

Competing interests
The authors declare that they have no competing interests.

Consent for publication
Not applicable.

Funding
This work was supported by Hamadan University of Medical sciences, Hamadan, Iran (No. 9406313526).

References

1. Shamsaei F, Cheraghi F, Esmaeilli R. The family challenge of caring for the chronically mentally ill: a phenomenological study, Iran. J Psychiatry Behav Sci. 2015;9(3):e1898.
2. Ergetie T, Yohanes Z, Asrat B, Demeke W, Abate A, Tareke M. Perceived stigma among non-professional caregivers of people with severe mental illness, Bahir Dar, northwest Ethiopia. Ann Gen Psychiatry. 2018;17:42.
3. Shamsaei F, Kermanshahi SM, Vanaki Z, Holtforth MG. Family care giving in bipolar disorder: experiences of stigma. Iran J Psychiatry. 2013;8(4):188–94.
4. Stuart H. Reducing the stigma of mental illness. Glob Ment Health. 2016;3:e17.
5. Corrigan PW, Morris SB, Michaels PJ, Rafacz JD, Rüsch N. Challenging the public stigma of mental illness: a meta-analysis of outcome studies. Psychiatr Serv. 2012;63(10):963–73.
6. Link BG, Phelan JC. Conceptualizing stigma. Annu Rev Sociol. 2001;27:363–85.
7. Hatzenbuehler ML, Phelan JC, Link BG. Stigma as a fundamental cause of population health inequalities. Am J Public Health. 2013;103(5):813–21.
8. Zegwaard MI, Aartsen MJ, Cuijpers P, Grypdonck MH. Review: a conceptual model of perceived burden of informal caregivers for older persons with a severe functional psychiatric syndrome and concomitant problematic behaviour. J Clin Nurs. 2011;20(15–16):2233–58.
9. Hadlaczky G, Hökby S, Mkrtchian A, Carli V, Wasserman D. Mental health first aid is an effective public health intervention for improving knowledge, attitudes, and behaviour: a meta-analysis. Int Rev Psychiatry. 2014;26(4):467–75.
10. Dixon LB, Lucksted A, Medoff DR, Burland J, Stewart B, Lehman AF, et al. Outcomes of a randomized study of a peer-taught family-to-family education program for mental illness. Psychiatr Serv. 2011;62(6):591–7.
11. Yang LH, Lai GY, Tu M, Luo M, Wonpat-Borja A, Jackson VW, et al. A brief anti-stigma intervention for Chinese immigrant caregivers of individuals with psychosis: adaptation and initial findings. Trans Cult Psychiatry. 2014;51(2):139–57.
12. Shamsaei F, Kermanshahi SM, Vanaki Z, Hajizadeh E, Hayatbakhsh MR. Experiences of family caregivers of patients with bipolar disorder. Asia Pac. Psychiatry. 2010;2(4):201–7.
13. Bejerholm U, Eklund M. Occupational engagement in persons with schizophrenia: relationships to self-related variables, psychopathology, and quality of life. Am J Occup Ther. 2007;61(1):21–32.
14. Chan Jemma WW, Law LS. Combining education and video-based contact to reduce stigma of mental illness: "The Same or Not the Same" anti-stigma program for secondary schools in Hong Kong. Soc Sci Med. 2009;68(8):1521–6.
15. Taghva A, Farsi Z, Javanmard Y, Atashi A, Hajebi A, Noorbala AA. Strategies to reduce the stigma toward people with mental disorders in Iran: stakeholders' perspectives. BMC Psychiatry. 2017;17:17.
16. Bernhard B, Schaub A, Kummler P, Dittmann S, Severus E, Seemuller F, et al. Impact of cognitive psychoeducational interventions in bipolar patients and their relatives. Eur Psychiatry. 2006;21(7):81–6.
17. Corrigan P, Gelb B. Three programs that use mass approaches to challenge the stigma of mental illness. Psychiatr Serv. 2006;57(3):3393–8.
18. Brown SA, Evans Y, Espenschade K, O'Connor M. An examination of two brief stigma reduction strategies: filmed personal contact and hallucination simulations. Community Ment Health J. 2010;64(5):494–9.
19. Pitman JO, Noh S, Colema D. Evaluating the effectiveness of a consumer delivered anti-stigma program: replication with graduate-level helping professionals. Psychiatr Rehabil J. 2010;33(3):3236–8.
20. Yin Y, Zhang W, Hu Z, Jia F, Li Y, Xu H, et al. Experiences of stigma and discrimination among caregivers of persons with schizophrenia in China: a field survey. PLoS ONE. 2014;9(9):108–52.
21. Kenneth A, Korley D, Kwaku Poku A, Seth O. Experiences of caregivers of people living with serious mental disorders. Glob Health Action. 2015;8:1–9.
22. Zachary S, Claire M, Iranpour C, Chey T, Jackson J, Vikram P, et al. Global prevalence of common mental disorders: a systematic review and meta-analysis 1980–2013. Int J Epidemiol. 2014;43(2):476–93.
23. Uchino T, Maeda M, Uchimura N. Psychoeducation may reduce self-stigma of people with schizophrenia and schizoaffective disorder. Kurume Med J. 2012;59(1, 2):25–35.
24. Cuhadar D, Cam O. Effectiveness of psycheducation in reducing internalized stigmatization in patients with bipolar disorder. Arch Psychiatr Nurs. 2014;28(1):62–6.
25. Kiropoulos L, Griffiths K, Blashki G. Effects of a multilingual information website intervention on the levels of depression literacy and depression-related stigma in Greek-Born and Italian-Born immigrants living in Australia: a randomized controlled trial. J Med Internet Res. 2011;13(2):1–25.
26. Cook JE, Vaughns VP, Meyer IH, Busch JTA. Intervening within and across levels: a multilevel approach to stigma and public health. Soc Sci Med. 2014;103:101–9.

26

Validity of the PHQ-9 and PHQ-2 to screen for depression in nationwide primary care population in Latvia

Elmars Rancans[1], Marcis Trapencieris[2], Rolands Ivanovs[1] and Jelena Vrublevska[1*] ⓘ

Abstract

Background: Depression is highly underdiagnosed in primary care settings in Latvia. Screening for depression in primary care is potentially an efficient way to find undetected case s and improve diagnostics. We aimed to validate both a nine-item and two-item Patient Health Questionnaire (PHQ-9 and PHQ-2) in the Latvian and Russian languages in primary care settings using a representative sample in Latvia.

Materials and methods: The study was carried out within the framework of the National Research Program BIO-MEDICINE to assess the prevalence of mental disorders at 24 primary care facilities. During a 1-week period, all consecutive adult patients were invited to complete the PHQ-9 and PHQ-2. Criterion validity was assessed against the Mini International Neuropsychiatric Interview (MINI).

Results: There were 1467 patients who completed the PHQ-9 and the MINI. Overall, the PHQ-9 items showed good internal reliability (Cronbach's alpha 0.81 for Latvian version and 0.79 for Russian version of the PHQ-9). A cut-off score of 8 or greater was established for the PHQ-9 (sensitivity 0.75 and 0.79, specificity 0.84 and 0.80 for Latvian and Russian languages, respectively). For the PHQ-2, a score of 2 or higher (sensitivity 0.79 and 0.79, specificity 0.65 and 0.67 for Latvian and Russian languages) detected more cases of depression than a score of 3 or higher.

Conclusions: We suggest GPs ask patients to respond to the first 2 questions of the PHQ-9. If their score is positive, the patients should then complete the PHQ-9.

Keywords: Depression, Primary care, General practitioners, Validation

Background

Depression is a common psychiatric condition that has widespread consequences both at the individual and societal level. It is among the leading non-fatal diseases globally [1]. Long term consequences of depression include reduced quality of life, risk of suicide, increased rates of hospital admission, increased risk for chronical medical conditions and stigmatization [2–5].

The WHO study on psychological problems in general health care across 14 countries found that 14% of individuals suffered from major depression [6]. Despite the fact that most care for depression is delivered by general practitioners, under-recognition of depression has been extensively described [7]. Depression is often under-detected in primary care: approximately 50% of GPs correctly identify depression cases, and even fewer, 34%, record it in their notes [8].

Despite rich data from studies of depression in primary care in Western Europe [9, 10], there still is a need for studies from Eastern Europe [11]. The best available data suggest that under-diagnosis of depression is particularly salient for Latvia, where the 12-month prevalence of depression has been estimated at 7.8%, but according to the data from the Latvian National Health Service, only 4423 unique patients have been diagnosed with a mood disorder by general practitioners (GPs) [12, 13].

*Correspondence: vrublevskaja@inbox.lv
[1] Department of Psychiatry and Narcology, Riga Stradins University, Tvaika Street 2, Riga 1005, Latvia
Full list of author information is available at the end of the article

Because of large estimates of underdiagnosed and undertreated depression in primary care, improved screening could reduce the burden of depression. Routine primary care screening can facilitate improvement of the diagnosis rates of adult depression and has been recommended by the US Preventive Services Task Force [14, 15]. However, it is notable that some national guidelines doubt the effectiveness of screening for depression [16].

It is essential that depression screening tools are reliable and valid to ensure that the results they generate are clinically correct [17]. There are numerous studies assessing the reliability and validity of depression screening tools, but there is currently no consensus on one particular screening tool to be used for depression screening across primary healthcare settings [18]. Moreover, to be acceptable in practice, it is essential that instruments are easy and quick to use [19].

The Patient Health Questionnaire-9 (PHQ-9) was developed as a depression screener for depression in primary care. The PHQ-9 is a self-rating instrument for depression developed in the late 1990s from the Primary Care Evaluation of Mental Disorders (PRIME-MD) [20] and based on the Diagnostic and Statistical Manual of Mental Disorders, Fourth Edition (DSM-IV) criteria for MDD [21]. This tool consisting of 9 items is known for its ease of completion for the patient, ease of scoring and interpretation, and public availability. It is used among racially and ethnically diverse populations. Respondents rate the scale items from 0 to 3 according to the frequency of their experience over the previous 2-week period (not at all, several days, more than half the days, or nearly every day). A cut-off score of ≥ 10 has been recommended for detecting cases of major depressive disorder (MDE) [21, 22]. Over 100 studies have examined the PHQ-9 in primary care [22]. Moreover, the PHQ-9 has been validated in medical populations [23–25], general populations [26–29] and psychiatric samples [30–34].

Of recent interest has been the use of fewer screening questions from the PHQ–9 [35, 36]. The PHQ-2 was developed for depression screening, with some evidence for a role in diagnosing depression [35, 37, 38]. These 2 questions, collectively known as the PHQ-2, ask about the frequency of the symptoms of depressed mood and anhedonia, scoring each as 0 (not at all) to 3 (nearly every day). The validation study of the PHQ-2 by Kroenke et al. included a sample of 580 primary care patients [35].

A valid depression screener in Latvian and Russian is important for Latvia because 61.8% of the population is Latvian, with the remainder being people from Russian language-speaking nations (Russia, Belarus, and Ukraine) [39, 40].

The aim of our study was to validate the PHQ-9 and PHQ-2 in Latvian and Russian languages using the Mini International Neuropsychiatric Interview (MINI) as the reference standard in a representative primary care sample.

Materials and methods

The current study was carried out in 2015 within the framework of the National Research Program, BIOMEDICINE 2014–2017, a cross-sectional study to assess the prevalence of mental disorders in primary care settings in Latvia. The study recruited patients from 24 primary care facilities all over the country that covered all regions of Latvia. The survey was conducted in the two most commonly spoken languages in Latvia (Latvian and Russian). The programme was financed by the Latvian Ministry of Education and Science. The main aim of this programme is to develop new prevention, treatment, and diagnostic methods and practices, as well as biomedical technologies to improve public health in Latvia. The programme has existed since 2007 and comprises certain areas: cardiovascular and metabolic diseases, oncological diseases, and childhood and infectious diseases. Mental health was included in the programme for the first time.

During a 1-week period in each GP's facility, all consecutive patients aged 18 years or older visiting a primary care physician with any health concerns were invited to participate in the study. Those who visited their GP for any administrative reasons were not included in the sample. No further restrictions on patient selection were implemented.

All consecutive patients were invited to complete the paper-and-pencil form of the PHQ-9 in the preferred language (Latvian or Russian) before seeing the GP, followed by interview with a structured socio-demographic questionnaire. All uncertainties and questions raised were explained by a psychiatrist. Both versions of the PHQ-9 in Latvia have been previously adapted and used in a nationwide general population study [41]. However, at that time, no cut-off score for Latvia was established, and a cut-off score ≥ 10 has been applied as recommended by Kroenke et al. [21]. In 2014, within the pilot project of the National Research Programme, BIOMEDICINE, that was conducted at 6 primary care facilities, the cut-off score of the PHQ-9 of ≥ 10 for both languages was established [42]. However, that study included validation of the PHQ-9 and not the PHQ-2 and had considerable limitations such as a small sample size that was not representative of the primary care population nationwide.

No more than 2 weeks after completing the PHQ-9, four psychiatrists who were blind to the PHQ-9 scores interviewed the respondents over the phone with the Mini International Neuropsychiatric Interview (MINI), Version 6.0.0. The MINI is a structured diagnostic interview that was validated by convergence with the

Structured Clinical Interview for the DSM-III-R Patient Version (SCID-P) and the Composite International Diagnostic Interview (CIDI) and by expert professional opinion [43]. The good psychometric characteristics of the MINI, its ability to be administered rapidly, and its acceptability to patients made it a good choice for research purposes [44]. The MINI has been translated and adapted for both Latvian and Russian languages by the authorship holders and previously has been used in population-based study [13]. The MINI was used as the standard to determine the presence of major depressive episodes and was conducted over the telephone. Administering the MINI over the telephone is acceptable and was applied in other studies [45, 46]. In this study, all modules of the MINI were used. Participants diagnosed with depression or suicide ideations or attempt were referred for appropriate care.

This study was approved by the Ethics Committee of the Riga Stradins University, Riga, Latvia. The project was conducted in accordance with the Declaration of Helsinki and its subsequent amendments. All patients were enrolled after providing written informed consent. Neither participating family practices nor patients were compensated for their participation.

Statistical analysis

The internal reliability of the PHQ-9 was assessed by Cronbach's alpha coefficient. The criterion validity of the PHQ-9 and the PHQ-2 was assessed by receiver operating characteristic (ROC) analysis. The criterion validity of the PHQ-9 and the PHQ-2 was analysed in terms of sensitivity, specificity, and positive and negative predictive values for different cut-off scores. The Latvian and Russian versions of the MINI, which is used to diagnose major depressive disorder, were used as the criterion standard. Data analyses were performed in Stata version 14 (Stata Corp). A separate analysis was conducted for the Latvian and Russian languages.

Results

In total, 1604 patients were invited to complete the PHQ-9 scale, and 1585 of them completed the PHQ-9. From those who completed the PHQ-9, 100 patients did not answer a telephone call three times and were excluded, and 1485 patients were interviewed with the MINI over the telephone. In the final analysis, 1467 patients (448 men and 1019 women) were included. The questionnaires of 18 patients had to be dropped out due to insufficient data quality.

The main characteristics of those who were included in the analysis are shown in Table 1. For both languages, a separate analysis was applied. According to the MINI, 10.2% (95% CI 8.7–11.8) of the whole population had

Table 1 Characteristics of the total sample (*n* = 1467)

	Latvian % (*n*)	Russian % (*n*)
Total	100 (912)	100 (555)
Lifetime depression	27.6 (252)	28.7 (159)
Past only depression	19.0 (173)	16.4 (91)
Current depression	8.7 (79)	12.3 (68)
Gender		
Male	30.7 (280)	30.3 (168)
Female	69.3 (632)	69.7 (387)
Age groups		
18–34	17.7 (161)	8.7 (48)
35–54	30.6 (279)	31.7 (176)
55–64	22.3 (203)	26.3 (146)
65+	29.5 (269)	33.3 (185)
Education		
Primary or less	16.2 (148)	15.4 (78)
Secondary	53.4 (487)	54.3 (310)
Higher than secondary	29.8 (272)	29.7 (164)
No answer	0.6 (5)	0.6 (3)
Socioeconomic status		
Above average	5.2 (47)	4.3 (24)
Average	71.3 (650)	60.9 (338)
Below average	23.5 (214)	34.8 (193)
No answer	0.1 (1)	0.0 (0)

current depression and 28.1% (95% CI 25.9–30.4) had experienced at least one depressive episode in the past. Current depression was found in 8.7% of those who completed the PHQ-9 in Latvian and 12.3% in Russian. The reliability (Cronbach's alpha) for the Latvian version of the PHQ-9 scale was 0.82 and 0.79 for the Russian version.

The performance of the PHQ-9 was compared against the diagnosis of major depression as determined by the MINI, a reliable standard. The sensitivity, specificity, and likelihood ratio are presented separately for the Latvian and Russian languages in Tables 2 and 3, respectively. At a cut-off score of 8 or above, the sensitivity of the Latvian version of the PHQ-9 was 0.75, and the specificity was 0.84. For the Russian version of the PHQ-9, they were 0.79 and 0.80, respectively. The positive likelihood ratio was 4.57 for the Latvian version and 4.0 for the Russian version at this cut-off score. A cut-off score of 10 for the PHQ-9 Latvian language decreased sensitivity to 60.8% and increased specificity to 91.1%. A cut-off score of 10 for the PHQ-9 Russian language decreased sensitivity to 67.7% and increased specificity to 89.7%. The cut-offs chosen in the ROC curve analysis where the ones closer is to the upper left corner. ROC curve analysis (Figs. 1, 2) supported the criterion validity of the PHQ-9 in

Table 2 Sensitivity, specificity, and likelihood ratios at various cut-off points of the Latvian version of the PHQ-9

PHQ-9 score	Sensitivity (%)	Specificity (%)	Classified (%)	LR+	LR−
≥ 6	82.3	69.6	70.7	2.71	0.25
≥ 7	77.2	77.3	77.3	3.40	0.29
≥ 8	74.7	83.7	82.9	4.57	0.30
≥ 9	70.9	87.9	86.4	5.84	0.33
≥ 10	60.8	91.1	88.5	6.84	0.43
≥ 11	55.7	94.1	90.8	9.47	0.47
≥ 12	49.4	95.8	91.8	11.75	0.53
≥ 13	44.3	97.4	92.8	16.78	0.57
≥ 14	36.7	98.2	92.9	20.39	0.64

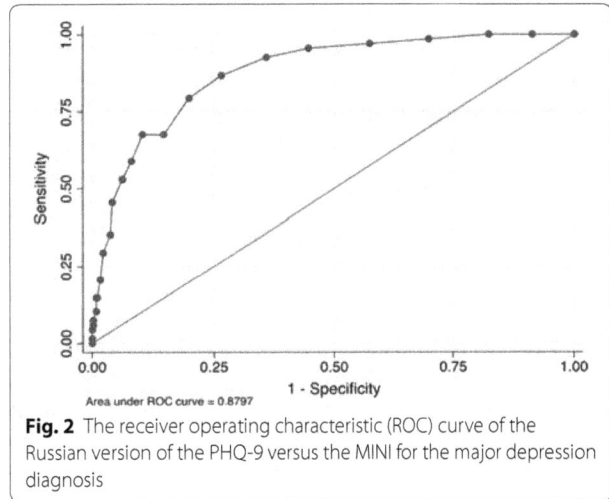

Fig. 2 The receiver operating characteristic (ROC) curve of the Russian version of the PHQ-9 versus the MINI for the major depression diagnosis

Table 3 Sensitivity, specificity, and likelihood ratios at various cut-off points of the Russian version of the PHQ-9

PHQ-9 score	Sensitivity (%)	Specificity (%)	Classified (%)	LR+	LR−
≥ 6	92.7	64.2	67.8	2.59	0.11
≥ 7	86.8	73.5	75.1	3.28	0.18
≥ 8	79.4	80.1	80.0	4.00	0.26
≥ 9	67.7	85.4	83.2	4.64	0.38
≥ 10	67.7	89.7	87.0	6.59	0.36
≥ 11	58.8	92.0	87.9	7.34	0.45
≥ 12	52.9	93.8	88.8	8.59	0.50
≥ 13	45.6	95.9	89.7	11.10	0.57
≥ 14	35.2	96.3	88.8	9.55	0.67

Table 4 Sensitivity, specificity, and likelihood ratios at various cut-off points of the Latvian version of the PHQ-2

PHQ-2 score	Sensitivity (%)	Specificity (%)	Classified (%)	LR+	LR−
≥ 1	89.9	40.7	45.0	1.52	0.25
≥ 2	78.5	64.6	65.8	2.22	0.33
≥ 3	55.7	89.9	87.0	5.52	0.49
≥ 4	36.00	94.2	89.4	6.59	0.66
≥ 5	22.8	98.0	91.5	11.16	0.79
≥ 6	15.2	98.4	91.2	9.73	0.86

Table 5 Sensitivity, specificity, and likelihood ratios at various cut-off points of the Russian version of the PHQ-2

PHQ-2 score	Sensitivity (%)	Specificity (%)	Classified (%)	LR+	LR−
≥ 1	94.1	38.2	45.1	1.52	0.15
≥ 2	79.4	66.5	68.1	2.37	0.31
≥ 3	58.8	87.7	84.1	4.77	0.47
≥ 4	45.6	92.8	87.0	6.34	0.59
≥ 5	27.9	96.3	87.9	7.56	0.75
≥ 6	19.1	98.2	88.5	10.34	0.82

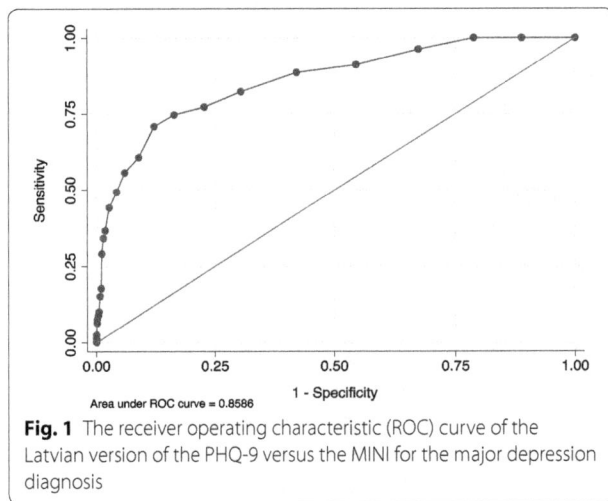

Fig. 1 The receiver operating characteristic (ROC) curve of the Latvian version of the PHQ-9 versus the MINI for the major depression diagnosis

differentiating between patients with and without major depression (AUC=0.86 for Latvian version and 0.88 for Russian version).

We also performed validity analysis for both languages of the PHQ-2 against the MINI The sensitivity, specificity, LR+ and LR− for all possible PHQ-2 thresholds for both Latvian and Russian languages are presented in Tables 4 and 5. At the threshold ≥ 2, the PHQ-2 Latvian version correctly identified 78.5% of MINI cases (sensitivity) and 64.6% of non-cases of depression (specificity).

The PHQ-2 Russian version correctly identified 79.4% of cases and 66.5% of non-cases. The positive likelihood ratio was 2.21 and 2.37 at this cut-off score for the Latvian and Russian languages, respectively. The PHQ-2 demonstrated moderate overall accuracy relative to the MINI for discriminating between cases and non-cases of depression, with an AUC of 0.79 for the Latvian version and AUC of 0.80 for the Russian version.

Discussion

The main aim of this study was to assess the validity of the PHQ-9 and the PHQ-2 and to establish a cut-off score to identify depression in the nationwide sample of patients attributable to Latvia visiting their GP because of health concerns. The screener was primarily developed for use in primary care settings and is the only questionnaire that has been tested in a primary care sample in Latvia.

Instruments that can be used in both screening and scaling modes have a particular advantage in that their weaknesses can be compensated by each other [47].

Within 18 studies performed with the PHQ-9, the prevalence of depression, as diagnosed by the gold-standard tests, ranged from 2.5 to 37.5% [48]. In our study, the point prevalence of depression was estimated at 10.2%, which is consistent with the findings from the other studies.

Despite the fact that the brief PHQ-9 is commonly used to screen for depression with 10 often recommended as a cut-off score, we found that a cut-off score of ≥ 8 on the PHQ-9 was the best at detecting depression in primary care patients in Latvia. Interestingly, the optimal cut-off points for major depression fall in the severity range of 5–9, as described by Kroenke et al. [21] for the category of patients with mild depressive symptoms. In the meta-analysis by Manea et al. [48], the PHQ-9 was found to have acceptable diagnostic properties for detecting depression for cut-off scores between 8 and 11. Its validity was supported by the AUC value that suggests a moderate accuracy of the questionnaire.

The pooled estimates of sensitivity and specificity for a cut-off score of 8 reported by Manea et al. [48] were 0.82 (95% CI 0.66–0.92) and 0.83 (95% CI 0.69–0.92), respectively. In our study, the rates of sensitivity and specificity for the Latvian language version were 0.75 and 0.83 and for the Russian language version were 0.79 and 0.80, respectively. In a study with primary care elderly patients, in which the criterion validity was evaluated by administering both the PHQ-9 and the MINI, the reported optimal cut-off score for major depressive disorder with the best validity characteristics was ≥ 7 (sensitivity 0.92, specificity 0.78) [49]. Our study showed lower sensitivity, but higher specificity. Although, we have also studied

primary care populations, the comparison of the studies cannot be made easily. In our study, we included all patients who visit their GP because of medical concerns, but in the study by Lamers et al. [49], only the patients 60 years or older diagnosed with certain chronic medical disorders were included.

The sensitivity of screening instruments is considered good when their range is 0.79–0.97 and when their specificity is 0.63–0.86 [50]. Both languages of the PHQ-9 had relatively low sensitivity and acceptable specificity. The moderate specificity of the PHQ-9 for diagnosing major depression can be explained because it is possible to diagnose the disorder without having either of the two cardinal symptoms of major depression. As such, the summed score does not match perfectly with the MINI, which is a structured diagnostic interview based on DSM-IV criteria [51].

The internal consistency (alpha coefficient) of the PHQ-9 in this study was 0.82 for the Latvian version and 0.79 for the Russian version. For a self-report instrument to be reliable, it is suggested that Cronbach's alpha be at least 0.70 [52]. However, it was lower than that from studies in the US (alpha coefficient = 0.79–0.89) [53, 54].

Recently, the PHQ-9 validation study in six primary care settings in Latvia was performed with a total sample size of 293 patients [42]. The estimated cut-off score was ≥ 10 with sensitivity 86.49% and specificity 89.36% for both languages. In the pilot project of the PHQ-9 validation, the PHQ-9 validity parameters were better than in this study. It is notable that the pilot study had considerable limitations. First, there was a small number of subjects. Second, not all Latvian regions were covered; therefore, the results cannot be representative. Third, the study was conducted by one interviewer. This study was conducted with a larger sample of patients and covered all Latvian regions and was performed by four mental health professionals who specialize in psychiatry and who were blind to the PHQ-9 and PHQ-2 results.

Our findings support the fact that an estimated cut-off score of 10 cannot be generalized across countries and populations.

The 2-question screener was sensitive for diagnosis of major depression when compared with the MINI with sensitivities of 0.90 and 0.94 for Latvian and Russian versions for thresholds of 1 or greater. Sensitivities for threshold 2 or greater comprised 0.79 for both language versions of the PHQ-2, and these sensitivities were acceptable. However, the specificities for threshold 1 or greater were not acceptable, but for threshold 2 or greater they were modest for both language versions of the PHQ-2: 0.65 for the Latvian version and 0.67 for the Russian version. At the most commonly used threshold ≥ 3 [35], the sensitivity for the Latvian and Russian versions was 0.56 and 0.59 and the specificity was 0.90 and 0.88, respectively. The finding that the score ≥ 2 was more successful at detecting depression is in accordance with similar finding reported by previous studies [55]. Another study to include a primary care sample (but not exclusively) reported a sensitivity of 0.83 and a specificity of 0.92 when the PHQ-2 (threshold score of 3 or higher) was compared with a health professional interview in 580 patients [35]. The patients who received the reference standard interview had to be contacted within 48 h of the screening interview. In our study, the reference standard was provided by the telephone within 2 weeks after the screening phase, which may have introduced bias into the results. A study conducted in older patients using the DSM-IV as a reference standard reported a sensitivity of 1.0 and a specificity of 0.77 for the PHQ-2 [56]. However, in this study, construct validity cut-off points were not reported. A study conducted in an outpatient clinic in Germany reported sensitivity and specificity was 78 and 79%, respectively, for major depression determined by a PHQ-2 score of 3 or more [37]. At a threshold score of 3 or higher and using a recognized reference standard, our sensitivity results for the PHQ-2 are generally not as high as those of other studies. This outcome can be explained as the result of a truly consecutive sample of patients in primary care, a reference standard that was administered not immediately but within 2 weeks after screening or even simply chance. Another of the limitations is its cross-sectional design; longitudinal studies are needed to establish the sensitivity to change. Inclusion of currently diagnosed and treated patients may increase bias in studies by inflating estimates of screening accuracy [57].

The strengths of this study are that all the patients were from primary care and they all received the MINI reference standard assessment. Our study included a large sample size, covered all Latvian regions and was conducted in urban and rural settlements and is representative to primary care in Latvia. Respondents were interviewed by four psychiatrists who were blind to the PHQ-9 estimates.

Conclusion and implications for practice

In summary, the Latvian and Russian versions of the PHQ-9 and PHQ-2 have moderate psychometric properties for screening for major depression in general practice with a recommended cut-off score of 8 or greater for the PHQ-9 and 2 or greater for the PHQ-2. For GPs who wish to screen their patients for depression, we suggest they ask patients to respond to the first 2 questions of the PHQ-9 (i.e., the PHQ-2); if their score is positive (if they score 2 or more), the patients should then complete the PHQ-9.

In a study on the 12-month prevalence of depression and healthcare utilization in the general population of Latvia, certain risk factors for depression were identified [13], and these factors could be useful for GPs to identify the target population and initiate screening with the PHQ-2 and PHQ-9.

In this study, established cut-off points of the PHQ-9 and PHQ-2 together with the established risk factors for having depression in the study conducted in the general population [13] have been used within the framework of the National Research Programme, BIO-MEDICINE, to develop diagnostic and treatment algorithms for depression in primary care in Latvia.

Abbreviations
AUC: the area under curve; GP: general practitioner; LR+, LR–: likelihood ratio for positive and negative results; MINI: The Mini International Neuropsychiatric Interview; PHQ-9: The Patient Health Questionnaire-9; PHQ-2: The Patient Health Questionnaire-2; ROC: a receiver operating characteristic; US: The United States; WHO: The World Health Organization.

Authors' contributions
ER conceived the presented idea and study design. ER, MT, JV worked on the technical details. ER, MT, RI. JV analysed the data. MT performed statistical analysis. JV wrote the manuscript in consultation with ER. All authors discussed the results and contributed to the final manuscript. All authors read and approved the final manuscript.

Author details
[1] Department of Psychiatry and Narcology, Riga Stradins University, Tvaika Street 2, Riga 1005, Latvia. [2] Institute of Philosophy and Sociology, University of Latvia, Kalpaka bulv. 4, Riga, Latvia.

Acknowledgements
None.

Competing interests
The authors declare that they have no competing interests.

Consent for publication
Not applicable.

Funding
The study was supported by The National Research Programme BIOMEDICINE 2014–2017 (Nr. 5.8.1.).

References
1. Whiteford HA, Degenhardt L, Rehm J, Baxter AJ, Ferrari AJ, Erskine HE, et al. Global burden of disease attributable to mental and substance use disorders: findings from the Global Burden of Disease Study 2010. Lancet. 2013;382(9904):1575–86.
2. Scott KM, Von Korff M, Angermeyer MC, Benjet C, Bruffaerts R, de

Girolamo G, et al. Association of childhood adversities and early-onset mental disorders with adult-onset chronic physical conditions. Arch Gen Psychiatry. 2011;68(8):838–44.

3. Holmstrand C, Bogren M, Mattisson C, Brådvik L. Long-term suicide risk in no, one or more mental disorders: the Lundby Study 1947–1997. Acta Psychiatr Scand. 2015;132(6):459–69.

4. Guthrie EA, Dickens C, Blakemore A, Watson J, Chew-Graham C, Lovell K, et al. Depression predicts future emergency hospital admissions in primary care patients with chronic physical illness. J Psychosom Res. 2016;82:54–61.

5. Parcesepe AM, Cabassa LJ. Public stigma of mental illness in the United States: a systematic literature review. Adm Policy Ment Health. 2013;40(5):384–99.

6. Ustun TB, Korff VM. Mental illness in general health care: an international study. In: Ustun TB, Sartorius N, editors. Mental illness in general health care: an international study. Chichester: Wiley; 1995. p. 347–60.

7. Hirschfeld RM, Keller MB, Panico S, Arons BS, Barlow D, Davidoff F, et al. The National Depressive and Manic-Depressive Association consensus statement on the undertreatment of depression. JAMA. 1997;277(4):333–40.

8. Mitchell AJ, Vaze A, Rao S. Clinical diagnosis of depression in primary care: a meta-analysis. Lancet. 2009;374(9690):609–19.

9. Katon W, Schulberg H. Epidemiology of depression in primary care. Gen Hosp Psychiatry. 1992;14(4):237–47.

10. King M, Nazareth I, Levy G, Walker C, Morris R, Weich S, et al. Prevalence of common mental disorders in general practice attendees across Europe. Br J Psychiatry. 2008;192(5):362–7.

11. Winkler P, Krupchanka D, Roberts T, Kondratova L, Machů V, Höschl C, et al. A blind spot on the global mental health map: a scoping review of 25 years' development of mental health care for people with severe mental illnesses in central and eastern Europe. Lancet Psychiatry. 2017;4(8):634–42.

12. Pulmanis T, Pelne, A, Taube, M. Mental Health in Latvia in 2013: a thematic report 2014. https://spkc.gov.lv/upload/Petijumi%20un%20zinojumi/Sabiedribas%20veselibas%20petijumi/psihiska_veseliba_lv_2013.pdf. Accessed June 2018.

13. Vrublevska J, Trapencieris M, Snikere S, Grinberga D, Velika B, Pudule I, et al. The 12-month prevalence of depression and health care utilization in the general population of Latvia. J Affect Disord. 2017;210:204–10.

14. Screening for Depression in Adults. US preventive services task force recommendation statement. Ann Intern Med. 2009;151(11):784–W.256. https://static1.squarespace.com/static/54d4ea02e4b0b004cf66dba6/t/564b6e58e4b0defb2f78d64f/1447784024456/us_preventative_services_task_force_recommendation.pdf. Accessed June 2018.

15. Pignone MP, Gaynes BN, Rushton JL, Burchell CM, Orleans CT, Mulrow CD, et al. Screening for depression in adults: a summary of the evidence for the US preventive services task force. Ann Intern Med. 2002;136(10):765–76.

16. Joffres M, Jaramillo A, Dickinson J, Lewin G, Pottie K, Shaw E, et al. Recommendations on screening for depression in adults. CMAJ. 2013;185(9):775–82.

17. Mokkink LB, Terwee CB, Patrick DL, Alonso J, Stratford PW, Knol DL, et al. The COSMIN study reached international consensus on taxonomy, terminology, and definitions of measurement properties for health-related patient-reported outcomes. J Clin Epidemiol. 2010;63(7):737–45.

18. El-Den S, Chen TF, Gan Y-L, Wong E, O'Reilly CL. The psychometric properties of depression screening tools in primary healthcare settings: a systematic review. J Affect Disord. 2018;225:503–22.

19. Gilbody S, Richards D, Brealey S, Hewitt C. Screening for depression in medical settings with the Patient Health Questionnaire (PHQ): a diagnostic meta-analysis. J Gen Intern Med. 2007;22(11):1596–602.

20. Spitzer RL, Kroenke K, Williams JB. Validation and utility of a self-report version of PRIME-MD: the PHQ primary care study. Primary Care Evaluation of Mental Disorders. Patient Health Questionnaire. JAMA. 1999;282(18):1737–44.

21. Kroenke K, Spitzer RL, Williams JB. The PHQ-9: validity of a brief depression severity measure. Gen Intern Med. 2001;16(9):606–13.

22. Kroenke K, Spitzer RL, Williams JBW, Löwe B. The Patient Health questionnaire somatic, anxiety, and depressive symptom scales: a systematic review. Gen Hosp Psychiatry. 2010;32(4):345–59.

23. McGuire AW, Eastwood J-A, Macabasco-O'Connell A, Hays RD, Doering LV. Depression screening: utility of the patient health questionnaire in patients with acute coronary syndrome. Am J Crit Care. 2013;22(1):12–9.

24. Navinés R, Castellví P, Moreno-España J, Gimenez D, Udina M, Cañizares S, et al. Depressive and anxiety disorders in chronic hepatitis C patients: reliability and validity of the Patient Health Questionnaire. J Affect Disord. 2012;138(3):343–51.

25. Hyphantis T, Kotsis K, Voulgari PV, Tsifetaki N, Creed F, Drosos AA. Diagnostic accuracy, internal consistency, and convergent validity of the Greek version of the patient health questionnaire 9 in diagnosing depression in rheumatologic disorders. Arthritis Care Res. 2011;63(9):1313–21.

26. Gelaye B, Tadesse MG, Williams MA, Fann JR, Vander Stoep A, Andrew Zhou X-H. Assessing validity of a depression screening instrument in the absence of a gold standard. Ann Epidemiol. 2014;24(7):527–31.

27. Kiely KM, Butterworth P. Validation of four measures of mental health against depression and generalized anxiety in a community based sample. Psychiatry Res. 2015;225(3):291–8.

28. Kocalevent R-D, Hinz A, Brähler E. Standardization of the depression screener Patient Health Questionnaire (PHQ-9) in the general population. Gen Hosp Psychiatry. 2013;35(5):551–5.

29. Alonso J, Angermeyer MC, Bernert S, Bruffaerts R, Brugha TS, Bryson H, et al. Prevalence of mental disorders in Europe: results from the European Study of the Epidemiology of Mental Disorders (ESEMeD) project. Acta Psychiatr Scand Suppl. 2004;420:21–7.

30. Inoue T, Tanaka T, Nakagawa S, Nakato Y, Kameyama R, Boku S, et al. Utility and limitations of PHQ-9 in a clinic specializing in psychiatric care. BMC Psychiatry. 2012;12:73.

31. Pilkonis PA, Lan Y, Dodds NE, Johnston KL, Maihoefer CC, Lawrence SM. Validation of the depression item bank from the Patient-Reported Outcomes Measurement Information System (PROMIS®) in a 3-month observational study. J Psychiatr Res. 2014;56:112–9.

32. Ryan TA, Bailey A, Fearon P, King J. Factorial invariance of the Patient Health Questionnaire and Generalized Anxiety Disorder Questionnaire. Br J Clin Psychol. 2013;52(4):438–49.

33. Titov N, Dear BF, McMillan D, Anderson T, Zou J, Sunderland M. Psychometric comparison of the PHQ-9 and BDI-II for measuring response during treatment of depression. Cogn Behav Ther. 2011;40(2):126–36.

34. Beard C, Hsu KJ, Rifkin LS, Busch AB, Björgvinsson T. Validation of the PHQ-9 in a psychiatric sample. J Affect Disord Suppl. 2016;193(C):267–73.

35. Kroenke K, Spitzer RL, Williams JBW. The Patient Health Questionnaire-2: validity of a two-item depression screener. Med Care. 2003;41(11):1284–92.

36. Arroll B, Goodyear-Smith F, Kerse N, Fishman T, Gunn J. Effect of the addition of a "help" question to two screening questions on specificity for diagnosis of depression in general practice: diagnostic validity study. BMJ. 2005;331(7521):884–6.

37. Löwe B, Kroenke K, Gräfe K. Detecting and monitoring depression with a two-item questionnaire (PHQ-2). J Psychosom Res. 2005;58(2):163–71.

38. Arroll B, Khin N, Kerse N. Screening for depression in primary care with two verbally asked questions: cross sectional study. BMJ. 2003;327(7424):1144–6.

39. Cazard F, Ferreri F. Bipolar disorders and comorbid anxiety: prognostic impact and therapeutic challenges. Encephale. 2013;39(1):66–74.

40. Central Statistical Bureau of Latvia. http://www.csb.gov.lv/sites/default/files/skoleniem/iedzivotaji/etniskais_sastavs.pdf. Accessed June 2018.

41. Rancans E, Vrublevska J, Snikere S, Koroleva I, Trapencieris M. The point prevalence of depression and associated sociodemographic correlates in the general population of Latvia. J Affect Disord. 2014;156:104–10.

42. Vrublevska J, Trapencieris M, Rancans E. Adaptation and validation of the Patient Health Questionnaire-9 to evaluate major depression in a primary care sample in Latvia. Nord J Psychiatry. 2017;72:1–7.

43. Sheehan DV, Lecrubier Y, Sheehan KH, Amorim P, Janavs J, Weiller E, et al. The Mini-International Neuropsychiatric Interview (MINI): the development and validation of a structured diagnostic psychiatric interview for DSM-IV and ICD-10. J Clin Psychiatry. 1998;59(Suppl 20):22–33.

44. Pinninti NR, Madison H, Musser E, Rissmiller D. MINI international neuropsychiatric schedule: clinical utility and patient acceptance. Eur Psychiatry. 2003;18(7):361–4.

45. Duburcq A, Blin P, Charpak Y, Blachier C, Allicar MP, Bouhassira M, et al. Use of a structured diagnostic interview to identify depressive episodes in an epidemiologic study: a posteriori internal validation. Rev Epidemiol Sante Publique. 1999;47(5):455–63.

46. Heckman CJ, Cohen-Filipic J, Darlow S, Kloss JD, Manne SL, Munshi T. Psychiatric and addictive symptoms of young adult female indoor tanners. Am J Health Promot. 2014;28(3):168–74.

47. Nease DE Jr, Maloin JM. Depression screening: a practical strategy. J Fam Pract. 2003;52(2):118–24.

48. Manea L, Gilbody S, McMillan D. Optimal cut-off score for diagnosing depression with the Patient Health Questionnaire (PHQ-9): a meta-analysis. CMAJ. 2012;184(3):E191–6.

49. Lamers F, Jonkers CCM, Bosma H, Penninx BWJH, Knottnerus JA, van Eijk JTM. Summed score of the Patient Health Questionnaire-9 was a reliable and valid method for depression screening in chronically ill elderly patients. J Clin Epidemiol. 2008;61(7):679–87.

50. Robins LN, Wing J, Wittchen HU, Helzer JE, Babor TF, Burke J, et al. The composite international diagnostic interview. An epidemiologic Instrument suitable for use in conjunction with different diagnostic systems and in different cultures. Arch Gen Psychiatry. 1988;45(12):1069–77.

51. Stafford L, Berk M, Jackson HJ. Validity of the Hospital Anxiety and Depression Scale and Patient Health Questionnaire-9 to screen for depression in patients with coronary artery disease. Gen Hosp Psychiatry. 2007;29(5):417–24.

52. Streiner DL, Norman GR. Scaling responses. 2nd ed., Health Measurement Scales: a practical guide to their development and useOxford: Oxford University Press; 1995.

53. Huang FY, Chung H, Kroenke K, Delucchi KL, Spitzer RL. Using the Patient Health Questionnaire-9 to measure depression among racially and ethnically diverse primary care patients. J Gen Intern Med. 2006;21(6):547–52.

54. Lee PW, Schulberg HC, Raue PJ, Kroenke K. Concordance between the PHQ-9 and the HSCL-20 in depressed primary care patients. J Affect Disord. 2007;99(1–3):139–45.

55. Arroll B, Goodyear-Smith F, Crengle S, Gunn J, Kerse N, Fishman T, et al. Validation of PHQ-2 and PHQ-9 to screen for major depression in the primary care population. Ann Fam Med. 2010;8(4):348–53.

56. Li C, Friedman B, Conwell Y, Fiscella K. Validity of the Patient Health Questionnaire 2 (PHQ-2) in identifying major depression in older people. J Am Geriatr. 2007;55(4):596–602.

57. Rice DB, Thombs BD. Risk of bias from inclusion of currently diagnosed or treated patients in studies of depression screening tool accuracy: a cross-sectional analysis of recently published primary studies and meta-analyses. PLoS ONE. 2016;11(2):e0150067.

27

Chewing khat and risky sexual behavior among residents of Bahir Dar City administration, Northwest Ethiopia

Andargie Abate[*], Minale Tareke, Mulat Tirfie, Ayele Semachew, Desalegne Amare and Emiru Ayalew

Abstract

Introduction: Khat is a well-known natural stimulant and is widely used in Ethiopia, particularly in Bahir Dar city. Khat chewing is linked with risky sexual behaviors.

Objective: The study was aimed to determine the prevalence of chewing khat and its relation with risky sexual behaviors among residents of Bahir Dar City administration, Northwest Ethiopia.

Methods: A community based cross-sectional study was conducted from January to February, 2016. The data were collected using an interviewer administered structured questionnaire. Logistic regression analysis was applied to assess association between dependent and explanatory variables.

Results: The proportion of lifetime and current chewing khat among the study participants were 25.7 and 19.5%, respectively. Males (AOR 5.0; 95% CI 3.0–8.2) than females, merchants (AOR 4.9; 95% CI 2.6–9.3) than government employees, and those with average monthly income of ≥ 3001 Ethiopian birr (AOR 2.4; 95% CI 1.2–4.8) than ≤ 1000 had an increased current chewing khat prevalence. Having lifetime history of chewing khat was significantly associated with ever had sexual intercourse, having extra sexual partners, watching pornographic film and self-reported sexually transmitted infections.

Conclusion: Chewing khat is associated with increment of having risky sexual behaviors and self-reported sexually transmitted infections. Harm reduction measures are needed to prevent the community from engaging in khat use and risky sexual behaviors.

Keywords: Khat chewing, Risky sexual behavior, Bahir Dar, Ethiopia

Introduction

Khat is a natural stimulant from the *Catha edulis* plant which is grown in southern Arabia and Eastern Africa, and primarily in the countries of Ethiopia, Somalia, Kenya and Yemen [1–3]. It is a bushy plant whose leaves are chewed for social and psychological reasons due to the active psycho-stimulant substance known as cathinone which affects central nervous system (CNS) like amphetamine. The leaves are freshly stripped from the trees at dawn and rapidly distributed in regions where

Khat chewing is widespread since cathinone can be found only in fresh *Catha edulis* leaves [1, 2, 4].

An estimated 10 million people worldwide chew khat, and commonly found and consumed in the southwestern part of Arabian Peninsula and East Africa, and immigrant communities living in Europe and North America [3, 5, 6]. Similarly, Ethiopia is hardly hit by khat consumption. Both institution and community based studies done in Jimma have indicated the high prevalence of khat use seeing that 46 and 37.8%, respectively, chewed khat at least once in their lifetime [7, 8]. Previously, khat was mainly cultivated and chewed in limited, particularly eastern, part of the country. Nowadays, however, it is grown and consumed in all parts of the country including Amhara region [2, 9].

*Correspondence: Andargie_abate@yahoo.com
College of Medicine and Health Science, Bahir Dar University, Bahir Dar, Ethiopia

The recent sharp increment in khat consumption brings socio-economic, psychological and physical health sequelae of individuals involved. Though chewing khat is reported to induce a state of elation and feelings of increased alertness and arousal, at the end of a khat session, users may experience a depressed mood, irritability, loss of appetite, gastritis and peptic ulcer disease and difficulty sleeping [3, 10].

In addition, different studies in Ethiopia have revealed that the habit of chewing khat leads to a fragment of family, and multiple sexual practices. The habit, thus, could fuel spread of sexually transmitted infections (STIs) due to the associated risky sexual behaviors like having casual sex, unprotected sex and early initiation of sexual activity reported among chewers [11–15].

The number of khat users has increased in Ethiopia during recent decades and the habit has become popular in all sections of the society. Although khat is a legal substance in the country, it can be an entry point to the use of other illicit drugs, and risky sexual practices. This has to be made aware to local governmental officials and other concerned bodies to reduce its consequences. However, despite the prevalence of khat use and its effects were studied at institution basis, still, there is limited knowledge on khat chewing and its relation with risky sexual behaviors at the community level. Therefore, it is imperative to do this research determining the prevalence of lifetime and current chewing khat and its relation to risky sexual behaviors among residents of Bahir Dar City administration, Northwest Ethiopia. The findings will assist health care providers and program planners focusing their approach in the management of health problems related to khat consumption.

Methodology
Study design and period
A community based cross-sectional study was conducted to assess the level of chewing khat and its relation to risky sexual behaviors among residents of Bahir Dar city administration, Northwest Ethiopia from February to March 2016.

Study area and population
The study was conducted in Bahir Dar city administration which is the capital city of Amhara national regional state. The city is located in Northwest Ethiopia around 565 km from Addis Ababa, the capital city of Ethiopia. The city is divided into 9 sub cities and 17 kebeles, and Tisabay, Zege, and Meshenti kebeles are currently under the city administration. In the city and around it, most of the farmers substitute their crop farm with khat cultivation to increase their income [16]. This availability of substance may precipitate community to use khat for

people who live in the city and out of the city throughout the country. All populations aged 18 years and above who were invited for interview from selected kebeles of Bahir Dar City administration were study population.

Inclusion and exclusion criteria
All people aged 18 years and above who lived for at least 6 months in selected kebeles during the study period and volunteer was included for the interview. However, relatives who came and family members who were not present during the study period were excluded. Those who were unable to communicate and seriously ill were excluded from the interview.

Sample size determination
The sample size was determined using a formula for estimating a single population proportion. Considering 95% confidence interval (CI) ($Z\alpha/2 = 1.96$), 5% margin of error and 37.8% proportion of khat chewing taken from a previous study [8] generated a minimum sample size of 361. After adjusting with 10% as non-response rate and two as design effect, a total of 794 respondents were recruited in the study.

Sampling technique and procedure
The representative sample size was selected using multistage sampling technique. Ten kebeles out of total 20 were selected randomly using lottery method. Certain villages from each kebele were randomly selected. Therefore, a total of 794 households were distributed proportionally to the size of households in the selected kebeles, and villages based on a number of houses in selected kebeles and villages, respectively, referred from recent kebele registration. The shared households for each village were divided by a total number of households in a given village to determine a sampling interval and then households were selected by systematic random sampling technique. One individual was selected randomly from members of the household aged 18 years and above.

Data collection and quality control
The pretested interviewer administered structured questionnaire was used to collect the data. The designed questionnaire was initially developed in English and translated first into the local language (Amharic) and then back to English with expertise to ensure its consistency. The questionnaire was pretested on 5% of total sample size in one non-selected Kebele, and modification and correction were done 1 week before data collection. The respondents were interviewed in their own language (Amharic). Three data collectors (BSc Nurse) and one supervisor (experienced public health officer) were selected and 2-day training was given to orient them on

the tools to be used, the purpose of the study and how to approach respondents and obtain consent. The filled questionnaires were checked for completeness and consistency by supervisors. Incomplete questionnaires were returned to data collectors on the following day for the correction by revisiting the households.

The operational definitions used in this study were (a) lifetime chewer: an individual is considered an ever chewer even if he/she had chewed only once in his/her lifetime; (b) current user: individuals who were chewing khat within 3 months preceding the study; (c) having extra sexual partner: an individual is considered as having extra sexual partner if ever married individual had sexual partner in addition to his/her spouse; (d) ever had sexual intercourse: an individual is considered as an ever had sexual intercourse if a single individual had history of having sexual intercourse even only once in his/her lifetime; (e) inconsistent condom use: rarely, never and occasionally use of condoms during sexual contact other than always; (f) sexual behavior: an individual is considered as having risky sexual behavior if he/she reported having penetrative vaginal sex without using condom or inconsistently use with any partner rather than regular partner, having multiple sexual partners, having extra sexual partners, starting sexual intercourse before 18 years, watching pornographic film and sex with causal or commercial sex worker. In this study, respondents who engaged in at least one of the above behavior were considered as having risky sexual behavior.

Data processing and analysis

The data was entered into computers using Epi-data version 3.1 and exported to SPSS version 20 for analysis. Percentage, frequency, and mean were used to describe the study participants in relation to relevant variables using tables. Chi-square ($\times 2$) and/or Fisher's exact test were applied to assess associations between variables. Logistic regression was performed to assess the association between outcomes and different explanatory variables. The strength of association was interpreted using odds ratio and 95% confidence interval. P value < 0.05 was considered statistically significant in this study.

Results

Socio-demographic characteristics of the study participants

All of the recruited study participants were interviewed yielding response rate of 100%; off them, 99.6% were urban dwelling and the remaining were from rural area. Majorities 457 (57.6%) of study participants were male and 408 (51.4%) were married. Of the total study participants, 249 (39.3%) were in age group of 25–34 years old, 253 (31.9%) grade 9–12 by education, and 384 (48.4%)

had an average monthly income of ≤ 1000 Ethiopian Birr. Seven hundred eighty-three (98.6%) participants were Amhara by ethnicity and 623 (78.5%) were orthodox Tewahedo followers (Table 1).

Prevalence of khat chewing

Of the total 794 study participants, 204 (25.7%) had a history of chewing khat at least once in their life; of them, 79.9% had the history of chewing in the last 12 months. About 95 percent of those who chewed in the last 12 months practiced khat chewing within last 3 months. When the total 794 study participants were considered,

Table 1 Socio-demographic characteristics of study participants, Bahir Dar City administration, Northwest Ethiopia, 2017

Variables	Category	Frequency (%)
Sex	Male	457 (57.6)
	Female	337 (42.4)
Age	18–24	249 (31.4)
	25–34	312 (39.3)
	35–44	114 (14.4)
	≥ 45	119 (15.0)
Residence (Sub city)	Abay Mado	182 (22.9)
	Belay Zeleke	222 (28.0)
	Fasilo	129 (16.2)
	Meshenti (satellite kebele)	25 (3.1)
	Shum Abo	163 (20.5)
	Zenzelima (satellite kebele)	73 (9.2)
Occupation	Government employ	213 (26.8)
	Merchant	254 (32.0)
	Daily laborer	126 (15.9)
	Student	96 (12.1)
	Farmer/housewife/private	105 (13.2)
Education	No formal education	165 (20.8)
	1–8 grade	134 (16.9)
	9–12 grade	253 (31.9)
	Diploma and above	242 (30.5)
Religion	Orthodox Tewahedo	623 (78.5)
	Muslim	147 (18.5)
	Others	24 (3)
Ethnicity	Amhara	783 (98.6)
	Others	11 (1.4)
Marital status	Married	408 (51.4)
	Single	351 (44.2)
	Widowed/separated	35 (4.4)
Average monthly income	< 1000 EBR	384 (48.4)
	1001–2000 EBR	223 (28.1)
	2001–3000 EBR	102 (12.8)
	≥ 3001 EBR	85 (10.7)

163 (20.5%) and 155 (19.5%) of participants chewed khat within last twelve and 3 months, respectively. Among 155 study participants who were practicing khat chewing currently (within last 3 months), 68 (43.9%) chewed weekly followed by 66 (42.6%) daily, 16 (10.3%) occasionally and 5 (3.2%) monthly (Data not shown in table).

Reasons for practicing khat chewing
The study participants stated a number of ideas to be considered as reasons for practicing khat chewing. These included fighting depressed mood and getting concentration were mentioned by 56.9 and 45.6% of study participants, respectively (Table 2).

Problems encountered on khat chewers
The study participants mentioned several problems which are occurred due to their khat chewing practice. The participants thought that they lost money to get khat as stated by 67 (32.8%) of the total 204 chewers. Khat chewing also influenced their social relationships with their friends and parents as mentioned by 45 (22.1%) of chewers. Moreover, they were also exposed to physical health problems like injury and engagement in unprotected sex (Table 3).

Risky sexual behaviors
Of the total 443 married/divorced/separated/widowed participants, 44 (9.93%) had extra sexual partners. Fifteen (34.1%) of those who had extra sexual partners had more than one extra sexual partners. Near to 56 percent of the total 351 single study participants had a history of sexual intercourse at least once in their life. Of these, 161 (82.1%) had experienced sexual intercourse within the last 12 months before the study. Out of the total 195 study participants who had a history of sexual intercourse

Table 2 Reasons stated by study participants for practicing khat chewing, Bahir Dar City administration, Northwest Ethiopia, 2017

Variables	Category	Khat chewing (%)
To get concentration	Yes	93 (45.6)
	No	111 (54.4)
Relieving emotional problems	Yes	57 (27.9)
	No	147 (72.1)
Desiring experiment	Yes	43 (21.1)
	No	161 (78.9)
Easily availability of khat	Yes	29 (14.2)
	No	175 (85.8)
Fighting depressed mood	Yes	116 (56.9)
	No	88 (43.1)
Religious purpose	Yes	78 (38.2)
	No	126 (61.8)
Availability of excess pocket money	Yes	7 (3.4)
	No	197 (96.6)
Socialization	Yes	52 (25.5)
	No	152 (74.5)
Getting acceptance by others	Yes	27 (13.2)
	No	177 (86.8)
Passing time	Yes	65 (31.9)
	No	139 (68.1)
Getting personal pleasure	Yes	81 (39.7)
	No	123 (60.3)
Peer pressure	Yes	69 (33.8)
	No	135 (66.2)
Lack of job	Yes	27 (13.2)
	No	177 (86.8)

Table 3 Problems encountered by study participants due to khat chewing, Bahir Dar City administration, Northwest Ethiopia, 2017

Variables	Category	Khat chewing (%)
Accident or injury	Yes	13 (6.4)
	No	191 (93.6)
Losses money	Yes	67 (32.8)
	No	137 (67.2)
Damage to objects or clothing	Yes	13 (6.4)
	No	191 (93.6)
Problem on relation with families	Yes	45 (22.1)
	No	159 (77.9)
Problem on relation with friends	Yes	18 (8.8)
	No	186 (91.2)
Problem on relation with others	Yes	12 (5.9)
	No	192 (94.1)
Poor performance at work	Yes	19 (9.3)
	No	185 (90.7)
Victim by robbery or theft	Yes	11 (5.4)
	No	193 (94.6)
Trouble with police	Yes	11 (5.4)
	No	193 (94.6)
Hospitalized at emergency	Yes	8 (3.9)
	No	196 (96.1)
Engaged in sex they regretted next day	Yes	12 (5.9)
	No	192 (94.1)
Engaged in unprotected sex	Yes	13 (6.4)
	No	191 (93.6)
Blackouts or flashbacks	Yes	15 (7.4)
	No	189 (92.6)
Other medical problems	Yes	11 (5.4)
	No	193 (94.6)
Quarrel/fight/scuffle	Yes	43 (21.1)
	No	161 (78.9)

Table 4 Determinant factors associated with the prevalence of khat chewing among study participants, Bahir Dar City administration, Northwest Ethiopia, 2017

Variables	Category	Khat chewing		COR (95%CI)	AOR (95%CI)
		No	Yes		
Sex	Male	284 (62.1)	173 (37.9)	*6.0 (4.–9.1)*	*6.2 (4–9.7)*
	Female	306 (90.8)	31 (9.2)	1.00	1.00
Age	18–24	196 (78.7)	53 (21.3)	1.00	1.00
	25–34	215 (68.9)	97 (31.1)	*1.7 (1.1–2.5)*	*2.1 (1.3–3.5)*
	35–44	90 (78.9)	24 (21.1)	1.0 (0.6–1.7)	1.7 (0.8–3.4)
	≥ 45	89 (74.8)	30 (25.2)	1.3 (0.8–2.1)	*2.0 (1.0–4.3)*
Marital status	Married	313 (76.7)	95 (23.3)	1.00	1.00
	Single	247 (70.4)	104 (29.6)	*1.4 (1.0–1.9)*	*1.7 (1.1–2.7)*
	Widowed/separated	30 (85.7)	5 (14.3)	0.6 (0.2–1.5)	1.0 (0.3–2.9)
Education	No formal education	132 (80.0)	33 (20)	1.00	1.00
	1–8 grade	90 (67.2)	44 (32.8)	*2.0 (1.2–3.3)*	*1.8 (1.0–3.4)*
	9–12 grade	180 (71.1)	73 (28.9)	*1.6 (1.0–2.6)*	1.3 (0.7–2.5)
	Diploma and above	188 (77.7)	54 (22.3)	1.2 (0.7–1.9)	1.0 (0.5–2.1)
Occupation	Government employ	177 (83.1)	36 (16.9)	1.00	1.00
	Merchant	162 (63.8)	92 (36.2)	*2.8 (1.8–4.3)*	*3.3 (1.9–5.9)*
	Daily laborer	101 (80.2)	25 (19.8)	1.2 (0.7–2.1)	1.9 (0.9–4.1)
	Student	74 (77.1)	22 (22.9)	1.5 (0.8–2.7)	*3.3 (1.4–7.5)*
	Farmer/housewife/private	76 (72.4)	29 (27.6)	*1.9 (1.1–3.3)*	*4.3 (2.0–9.1)*
Average monthly income	≤ 1000 EBR	308 (80.2)	76 (19.8)	1.00	1.00
	1001–2000 EBR	160 (71.7)	63 (28.3)	*1.6 (1.1–2.3)*	*1.8 (1.1–2.9)*
	2001–3000 EBR	68 (66.7)	34 (33.3)	*2.0 (1.3–3.3)*	*2.3 (1.3–4.3)*
	≥ 3001 EBR	54 (63.5)	31 (36.5)	*2.3 (1.4–3.9)*	*2.2 (1.2–4.3)*

NB: Italic indicates significant value

COR crude odds ratio; *AOR* adjusted odds ratio; *95%CI* 95% confidence interval

at least once in life, 95 (48.7%) experienced sexual intercourse with causal partners and/or commercial sex workers and the remaining 100 (51.3%) practiced with regular partners.

In addition, 113 (70.8%) of 161 participants who had experienced sexual intercourse used a condom during their sexual activity with a condition of consistent (59.3%) and inconsistent (40.7%) usage. Regarding their self-reported sexually transmitted infections (STIs), 68 (8.6%) of the total participants had the history of STIs within last 12 months before this study. Moreover, 2.5% the total participants watched pornographic film (data not shown in table).

Determinant factors associated with the prevalence of khat chewing

Results from the bivariate analysis have shown that sex, age, marital status, educational level, occupational status and average monthly income had statistically significant association with the prevalence of khat chewing. All these six variables were considered for the multiple logistic regression analysis. Except for educational status,

the remaining five variables were retained as significantly associated factors of khat chewing among participants. The results confirmed that males had five times higher odds for chewing khat compared to females (AOR 5.0; 95% CI 3.0–8.2). Similarly, participants aged 25–34 years had 2.4 times higher odds for khat chewing compared to participants aged 18–24 years (AOR 2.4; 95% CI 1.4–4.1). Moreover, merchant study participants were near to five times more likely to chew khat than government employs (AOR 4.9; 95% CI 2.6–9.3). Likewise, those study participants who had more than three thousands average monthly income were 2.4 times more likely to chew khat than those who had less than one thousand average monthly income (AOR 2.4; 95% CI 1.2–4.8) (Table 4).

Risky sexual behaviors and their relation to khat chewing practice

The association of at least once in life khat chewing and alcohol drinking practice with risky sexual behaviors were analyzed using bivariate logistic regression. And then, those variables that fulfilled P-value < 0.2 were entered into multiple logistic regressions for further analysis. Furthermore, the association of those variables with

Table 5 Relation of khat chewing with risky sexual behaviors among study participants, Bahir Dar City administration, Northwest Ethiopia, 2017

Variables	Category	Having extra sexual partner (married)	ever had sexual intercourse (single)	Having sexual intercourse within last 12 months (single)	sexual partners	No condom use	Inconsistent condom use	Pornographic film watching	Self-reported STIs
Sex	Male	2.0 (1.0–3.8)	0.8 (0.5–1.3)	1.5 (0.7–3.1)	2.1 (1.2–3.8)		0.6 (0.3–1.2)	0.25**	2.8 (1.6–5.1)
	Female	1.00	1.00	1.00	1.00	1.00	1.00		1.00
Age	18–24	1.00	1.00	1.00	1.00	1.00	1.00	0.37**	1.00
	25–34	1.0 (0.4–2.5)	3.2 (2.0–5.1)	1.6 (0.8–3.5)	1.1 (0.6–2.0)	0.8 (0.4–1.6)	1.1 (0.6–2.3)		1.7 (0.9–3.1)
	≥35	0.8 (0.3–2.1)	4.4 (1.7–11.5)	1.2 (0.4–3.8)	4.1 (1.5–11.2)	0.6 (0.2–1.4)	0.6 (0.2–2.0)		1.4 (0.7–2.7)
Chewing khat	Yes	2.2 (1.1–4.2)	2.0 (1.2–3.2)	1.5 (0.7–3.1)	1.2 (0.7–2.0)	0.9 (0.5–1.6)	1.1 (0.6–2.2)	3.9 (1.3–12.3)	8.1 (4.7–14.0)
	No	1.00	1.00	1.00	1.00	1.00	1.00		1.00
Alcohol use	Yes	2.1 (1.1–3.9)	3.0 (1.9–4.6)	1.5 (0.8–3.0)	1.2 (0.7–2.0)	1.7 (0.9–3.0)	1.1 (0.5–2.1)	4.4 (1.2–15.5)	2.2 (1.3–3.7)
	No	1.00	1.00	1.00	1.00	1.00	1.00		1.00
Sex*	Male	1.4 (0.7–2.9)	0.4 (0.2–0.7)	NA	2.4 (1.2–4.8)	1.6 (0.8–3.0)	NA	NA	1.2 (0.6–2.3)
	Female	1.00	1.00		1.00	1.00			1.00
Age*	18–24	1.00	1.00		1.00	1.00			1.00
	25–34	0.7 (0.3–2.0)	3.1 (1.9–5.0)	NA	1.0 (0.6–1.9)	0.8 (0.4–1.5)	NA	NA	1.2 (0.6–2.4)
	≥35	0.7 (0.3–1.9)	3.4 (1.3–9.3)		4.0 (1.4–11.2)	0.5 (0.2–1.3)			1.5 (0.7–3.1)
Chewing khat*	Yes	2.2 (1.1–4.6)	2.5 (1.4–4.3)	NA	0.8 (0.4–1.6)	NA	NA	4.0 (1.3–12.8)	8.3 (4.6–15.1)
	No	1.00	1.00		1.00				1.00
Alcohol use*	Yes	2.1 (1.1–4.2)	3.2 (2.0–5.3)	NA	0.9 (0.5–1.7)	1.5 (0.8–2.9)	NA	4.5 (1.2–16.1)	2.6 (1.4–4.5)
	No	1.00	1.00		1.00	1.00			1.00

NB: *Italic* indicates significant value

NA not applicable

* Adjusted OR (95% CI)

** Fisher's Exact Test

less than five observation was analyzed using only cross-tabulation and Fisher's Exact Test. Table 5 has shown the relationships of khat chewing practice with some risky sexual behaviors suggesting that khat chewing has significantly increased the odds of having extra sexual partners for married (AOR: 2.2; 95% CI 1.1–4.6); ever had sexual intercourse for single (AOR 2.5; 95% CI 1.1–4.3); pornographic film watching(AOR 4.0; 95% CI 1.3–12.8) and self-reported STIs (AOR 8.3; 95% CI 4.6–15.1) by 2.2, 2.5,4.0 and 8.3 times, respectively, when compared to those not chewing khat.

Alcohol drinkers had an increased odds of having extra sexual partners (AOR 2.1; 95% CI 1.1–4.2); ever had sexual intercourse (AOR 3.2; 95% CI 2.0–5.3); watching pornographic film (AOR 4.5; 95% CI 1.2–16.1), and self-reported STIs (AOR 2.6; 95% CI 1.4–4.5) by more than two times when compared to those who did not drink (Table 5).

Discussion

The increment in the number of khat chewers globally needs a better understanding of the local burden and most common influencing factors and its relation to risky sexual behaviors. This paper has found that life time and current prevalence of chewing khat were 25.7 and 19.5%, respectively. The life time prevalence of the current study is in line with the findings in Eastern Ethiopia (24.2%) [17] and Ethiopian University students (24%) [18]. Nevertheless, this study has revealed relatively higher lifetime and current chewing khat prevalence than the result from Jimma, Ataye, Lalibela, Gondar and Dera parts of Ethiopia (14.3–17.9% and 13.3–14.2%, respectively) [19–22].

The higher prevalence of khat chewing in the current study and Eastern Ethiopia might be due to the fact that these two sites cultivate the substance leading availability of khat with least cost. Easily accessibility of substance and its low cost exposes the community to develop habits of chewing [16, 18, 23].

The lifetime (42.0%) and current (32.5%) prevalence of chewing khat in Gondar town Northwest Ethiopia [24] were higher than 25.7 and 19.5%, respectively, from the current study. The difference might be due to the difference in the study participants. The study done in Gondar consisted only college students, but the current study included both students and other participants in the community. According to the similar study, students who perceived that khat helps to study better were more likely to chew khat than those who did not perceive [18]. This has shown that students were expected to use khat to enhance their academic performance which is kept in a report from Kenya [25]. This is also supported by the current study indicating that being students increased the habit of chewing khat compared to government employees.

In this study, the most commonly mentioned reasons for chewing khat are fighting depressed mood (56.9%) followed by getting concentration (45.6%). Similar findings were also documented from the study done in Gondar town northwest Ethiopia where concentration during the study and getting entertainment and relaxation were reported by 62.3 and 36.9% of participants, respectively [24]. In addition, religious purpose, peer pressure, passing time and socialization were also mentioned as reasons of chewing khat in the current and previous studies done in University of Gondar and Dera district [9, 18].

The present study showed that males had around six times more probability of chewing khat than females which is consistent with studies in Ethiopia and Saudi Arabia [9, 17, 20, 22, 26, 27]. This might be due to the fact that the number of substance users is high among males than females, and it is accepted to use substances among males in different parts of the world including Ethiopia. In other words, this could be due to the culture which discourages the habit of chewing khat among females. This is also supported by the study done in Kenya showing that respondents strongly agreed on luxuriated habit of Khat chewing more boys than girls [25].

Likewise, occupation, marital status, and average monthly income were the most important parameters either to increase or hinder the chance of chewing khat in this study which is in line with other study done elsewhere [28]. Merchants and students practiced the habit near to five times more than government employees. The students might use the substance for getting concentration during the study and due to peer pressure since students pass their time with their friends. Students used chewing khat to study better than not used [18]. Having friends with khat chewing and peer pressure were confirmed as they scupper the people for a habit of chewing. More than half of respondents under the influence of their peer used substances [29]. The current study has also revealed that merchants were more likely to chew khat than government employees which is in line with the report from Dera district, Ethiopia [9].

The study participants with higher incomes in this study were more likely for chewing khat than to those with relatively lower incomes. This thought has concurred with the study done in Yemen [30] and University students of Ethiopia [17]. Furthermore, study participants with highest family socio-economic status were more prone to substance use [22]. This might be due to lack/shortage of money to buy khat since diversion of income for purchase of khat results in neglecting the family needs leading to family conflicts and discords. Thus, participants with low income will be restricted from chewing khat.

Khat chewing brings socio-economic and physical health problem on chewers. The current study participants mentioned that they lost their money performed their work poorly and damaged their objects to get khat which is in coherent with results reported from northwest Ethiopia [31, 32]. Moreover, khat chewing influenced their social relationships with their friends, parents, and others. This might be due to the reason that they lost their time on chewing khat resulting in a shortage of time to participate in any social related activities. For instance, chewers lost an average of three and half hours for single chewing practice without considering the time lost for buying and preparation according to this study. In addition, this study found that the chewers' physical health including exposure to STIs is also damaged due to their practice.

This study has revealed that chewing khat has a significant association to increase odds of developing risky sexual behaviors which are endorsed by other study done in Dilla University, Ethiopia [33]. Studies were done in the United Kingdom and Ghana have shown the increased impact of substance use on taking of risky sexual behaviors though they assessed the effect of other substances rather than khat [26, 34]. These risky sexual behaviors included having extramarital sexual partners; ever had sexual intercourse; and self-reported STIs. The significant relation of initiation of sexual intercourse and chewing khat was similarly reported in Dilla University, Ethiopia [33]. Moreover, those substance users were actively engaged with multiple sexual partners according to the study done in Ghana among homeless children and adolescents [26]. Chewing khat and alcohol drinking habit could also place the married individuals to have extramarital sexual relationships according to the present result which may facilitate the transmission of STIs. Similar findings reported from Bahir Dar University, Ethiopia resulting in having multiple sexual partners and sex with commercial sex workers, and sexual intercourse for money generation [35].

The self-reported STIs might be due to their inconsistent use of condoms during their sexual activity which was documented in the current study reporting that near to six percent of the participants engaged in unprotected sex. Similarly, another study conducted in Ghana [26] is in line with the present study. Although the study was not done on khat chewers, the finding from Sao Paulo Brazil has supported the effect of substance use on inconsistent utilization of condom [36]. The current study also documented not using of condom among alcohol drinkers during their last sexual activity that may increase the prevalence of self-reported STIs since alcohol drinking increased risky sexual behavior as affirmed by a study in Pawe District and Bahir Dar University, Ethiopia [35, 37]. It is not statistically significant; however, khat chewers have shown slightly increased odds of having sexual intercourse within last 12 months and inconsistent use of a condom.

In general, the discussion, implication, and conclusion of this study were performed by considering the limitation of the study. The relation of khat chewing with risky sexual behaviors was not possible to make clear cause-effect relationship since the study design was cross-sectional. In addition, the data were collected using questionnaires adopted and adapted by reviewing different published articles indicating not assessed by a standard tool which was another limitation. Psychological morbidity was not screened suggesting that the paper did not address the effect of chewing khat on psychological health.

Conclusion

Khat chewing is relatively prevalent among community residents in the study area which is significantly associated with male gender, being a merchant, student and having an average of more than 1001 EBR monthly income. This study also examined that khat use was found to be a risk factor for the development of risky sexual behaviors exposing them at risk for acquisition and transmission of STIs. Therefore, creating community awareness to address the problem of khat chewing and related consequences was recommended to health professionals and volunteer community health workers. The result demands an integrated strategy to effectively control both khat use and related STIs. In addition, further studies are needed using longitudinal study design to explore the actual interactions between khat use and risky sexual behaviors among community residents.

Authors' contributions
AA is the primary investigator responsible for the overall research project. AA and MT have conceptualized and designed the study. AA, MT, MT, AS, DA and EA have involved in the data analysis, interpretation of findings, and writing and revision of the manuscript. All authors read and approved the final manuscript.

Acknowledgements
The authors are grateful to Bahir Dar University, college of medicine and health sciences for financial and facilities support of the study. We would also like to thank Bahir Dar City administration health office for provision of the necessary information and technical support. The study participants are duly acknowledged for voluntarily responding to the questionnaire. We are grateful to data collectors, supervisors and kebele leaders for their cooperation during the field work.

Competing interests
The authors declare that they have no competing interests.

Consent for publication
Not applicable.

Funding
This research work is funded by Bahir Dar University, college of medicine and health sciences.

References
1. Cox G, Rampes H. Adverse effects of khat: a review. Adv Psychiatr Treat. 2003;9:456–63.
2. ECDD. Assessment of khat (Catha edulis Forsk): The World Health Organization (WHO) Expert Committee on Drug Dependence. Expert Committee on Drug Dependence. 2006.
3. NIDA. Drug facts: Khat. www.drugabuse.gov. National Institute on Drug Abuse (NIDA). 2013. Accessed Jan 2017.
4. Dhaifalah I, Santavy J. Khat habit and its health effect. A natural amphetamine. Biomed Paps. 2004;148(1):11–5.
5. Al-Motarreba A, Al-Haborib M, Broadleyc KJ. Khat chewing, cardiovascular diseases and other internal medical problems: The current situation and directions for future research, review. J Ethnopharmacol. 2010;132(3):540–8.
6. Balint EE. Khat (*Catha Edulis*) a controversial plant: blessing or curse? Szeged University. Ph.D. Thesis. 2010.
7. Gelaw Y, Haile-Amlak A. Khat chewing and its socio-demographic correlates among the staff of Jimma University. Ethiop J Health Dev. 2004;18:179–84.
8. Damena T, Mossie A, Tesfaye M. Khat chewing and mental distress: a community based study, in Jimma city, Southwestern Ethiopia. Ethiop J Health Sci. 2011;21(1):37–46.
9. Zeleke A, Awoke W, Gebeyehu E, Fentie A. Khat chewing practice and its perceived health effects among communities of Dera Woreda, Amhara region, Ethiopia. Open J Epidemiol. 2013;3:160–8.
10. Numan N. The Green Leaf: Khat. World J Med Sci. 2012;7(4):210–23.
11. Abebe D, Debella A, Dejene A, Degefa A, Abebe A, Urga K, Ketema L. Khat chewing habit as a possible risk behaviour for HIV infection: a case-control study. Ethiop J Health Dev. 2005;19(3):174–81.
12. Derese A, Seme A, Misganaw C. Assessment of substance use and risky sexual behaviour among Haramaya University Students, Ethiopia. Sci J Public Health. 2014;2(2):102–10.
13. Fentahun N, Mamo A. Risky sexual behaviors and associated factors among male and female students in Jimma zone preparatory schools, Southwest Ethiopia: comparative study. Ethiop J Health Sci. 2014;24(1):59–68.
14. Malaju MT, Asale GA. Association of Khat and alcohol use with HIV infection and age at first sexual initiation among youths visiting HIV testing and counseling centers in Gamo-Gofa Zone, South West Ethiopia. BMC Int Health Hum Rights. 2013;13:10.

15. Tilahun M, Ayele G. Factors associated with age at first sexual initiation among youths in Gamo Gofa, South West Ethiopia: a cross sectional study. BMC Public Health. 2013;13:622.

16. Gebiresilus AG, Gebresilus BG, Yizengaw SS, Sewasew DT, Mengesha TZ. Khat use prevalence, causes and its effect on mental health, Bahir-Dar, north west Ethiopia. Eur Sci J. 2014;10(23):234–53.

17. Reda AA, Moges A, Biadgilign S, Wondmagegn BY. Prevalence and determinants of khat (catha edulis) chewing among high school students in Eastern Ethiopia: a cross-sectional study. PLoS ONE. 2012;7(3):e33946.

18. Gebrehanna E, Berhane Y, Worku A. Khat chewing among Ethiopian University students—a growing concern. BMC Public Health. 2014;14:1198.

19. Dachew BA, Bifftu BB, Tiruneh BT. Khat use and its determinants among university students in Northwest Ethiopia: a multivariable analysis. Int J Med Sci Public Health. 2015;4(3):319–23.

20. Desale AY, Argaw MD, Yalew AW. Prevalence and associated factors of risky sexual behaviours among in-school youth in Lalibela town, north wollo zone, Amhara regional sate, Ethiopia: a cross-sectional study design. Sci J Public Health. 2016;4(1):57–64.

21. Dires E, Soboka M, Kerebih H, Feyissa GT. Factors associated with khat chewing among high school students in Jimma Town Southwest Ethiopia. J Psychiatry. 2016;19(4):372.

22. Lakew A, Tariku B, Deyessa N, Reta Y. Prevalence of catha edulis (khat) chewing and its associated factors among ataye secondary school students in northern shoa, Ethiopia. Adv Appl Sociol. 2014;4:225–33.

23. Patrick ME, Wightman P, Schoeni RF, Schulenberg AE. Socioeconomic status and substance use among young adults: a comparison across constructs and drugs. J Stud Alcohol Drugs. 2012;73:772–82.

24. Teni FS, Surur AS, Hailemariam A, Aye A, Gurmu AE, Tessema B. Prevalence, reasons, and perceived effects of Khat chewing among students of a college in Gondar town, Northwestern Ethiopia: a cross-sectional study. Ann Med Health Sci Res. 2015;5(6):454–60.

25. Ngeranwa DJN. Impact of khat cultivation on educational performance among upper primary schools pupils in Gachoka division, Embu County, Kenya. M.Sc. Thesis. 2013.

26. Asante KO, Meyer-Weitz A, Petersen I. Substance use and risky sexual behaviours among street connected children and youth in Accra, Ghana. Subst Abuse Treat Prev Policy. 2014;9:45.

27. Mahfouz MS, Rahim BEA, Solan YMH, Makeen AM, Alsanosy RM. Khat chewing habits in the population of the Jazan Region, Saudi Arabia: prevalence and associated factors. PLoS ONE. 2015;10(8):e0134545.

28. Haile D, Lakew Y. Khat chewing practice and associated factors among adults in Ethiopia: further analysis using the 2011 demographic and health survey. PLoS ONE. 2015;10(6):e0130460.

29. Damte A. Negative peer pressure among adolescent students in selected secondary and preparatory schools of Addis Ababa. M.Sc. Thesis. 2014.

30. Al-Abed AAA, Sutan R, Al-Dubai SAR, Aljunid SM. Family context and Khat chewing among adult yemeni women: a cross-sectional study. BioMed Res Int. 2014. https://doi.org/10.1155/2014/505474.

31. Baynesagne M, Ayele D, Weldegerima B. Prevalence, attitude and associated problems of Khat use among Bahir Dar university students, Northwestern Ethiopia. Pharmacol online. 2009;1:157–65.

32. Genene B, Haniko N, Weldegerima B. Prevalence, factors and consequences of Khat chewing among high school students of Gondar town, Northwestern Ethiopia. Pharmacol online. 2009;3:387–97.

33. Tadesse M. Substance abuse and sexual HIV-risk behaviour among Dilla University students, Ethiopia. Educ Res. 2014;5(9):368–74.

34. Jackson C, Sweeting H, Haw S. Clustering of substance use and sexual risk behavior in adolescence: analysis of two cohort studies. BMJ Open. 2012;2:e000661.

35. Mulu W, Yimer M, Abera B. Sexual behaviours and associated factors among students at Bahir Dar University: a cross sectional study. Reprod Health. 2014;11:84.

36. Reis RK, Melo ES, Gir E. Factors associated with inconsistent condom use among people living with HIV/Aids. Rev Bras Enferm. 2016;69(1):40–6.

37. Agajie M, Belachew T, Tilahun T, Amentie M. Risky sexual behavior and associated factors among high school youth in Pawe Woreda Benishangul Gumuz Region. Sci J Clin Med. 2015;4(4):67–75.

28

Association between an angiotensin-converting enzyme gene polymorphism and Alzheimer's disease in a Tunisian population

Najiba Fekih-Mrissa[1*], Ines Bedoui[2], Aycha Sayeh[1], Hajer Derbali[2], Meriem Mrad[1], Ridha Mrissa[2] and Brahim Nsiri[1]

Abstract

Background: The angiotensin-converting enzyme gene (ACE) insertion/deletion (I/D or indel) polymorphism has long been linked to Alzheimer's disease (AD), but the interpretation of established data remains controversial. The aim of this study was to determine whether the angiotensin-converting enzyme is associated with the risk of Alzheimer's disease in Tunisian patients.

Methods: We analyzed the genotype and allele frequency distribution of the ACE I/D gene polymorphism in 60 Tunisian AD patients and 120 healthy controls.

Results: There is a significantly increased risk of AD in carriers of the D/D genotype (51.67% in patients vs. 31.67% in controls; $p = .008$, OR = 2.32). The D allele was also more frequently found in patients compared with controls (71.67% vs. 56.25%; $p = .003$, OR = 2.0). Moreover, as assessed by the Mini-Mental State Examination, patient D/D carriers were more frequently found to score in the severe category of dementia (65%) as compared to the moderate category (32%) or mild category (3%).

Conclusions: The D/D genotype and D allele of the ACE I/D polymorphism were associated with an increased risk in the development of AD in a Tunisian population. Furthermore, at the time of patient evaluation (average age 75 years), patients suffering with severe dementia were found predominantly in D/D carriers and, conversely, the D/D genotype and D allele were more frequently found in AD patients with severe dementia. These preliminary exploratory results should be confirmed in larger studies and further work is required to explore and interpret possible alternative findings in diverse populations.

Keywords: Angiotensin-converting enzyme gene, Alzheimer's disease

Background

Alzheimer's disease (AD) is a common cause of morbidity and mortality among the elderly and is characterized by progressive memory loss and cognitive dysfunction [1]. The brains of AD patients are essentially characterized by neuronal and synaptic loss, extracellular plaques composed of amyloid-β peptides, and intra-neuronal neurofibrillary tangles. Senile plaques composed mainly of amyloid-β (Aβ) are particularly important in the pathology of AD [2]. Among the Aβ-related genes, angiotensin-converting enzyme gene (ACE) is closely related to the production and degradation of Aβ [3]. However, ACE also catalyzes the formation of the vasoconstrictor angiotensin II (Ang II) from angiotensin I. The actions of Ang II within the central nervous system are also of increasing interest in the context of Alzheimer's disease

*Correspondence: fnajiba@yahoo.fr
[1] Laboratory of Molecular Biology, Department of Hematology, Military Hospital of Tunisia, Mont Fleury, 1008 Tunis, Tunisia
Full list of author information is available at the end of the article

(AD). Ang II inhibits the release of acetylcholine (ACh) and has a pro-inflammatory effect [4].

The ACE gene is located on chromosome 17q23. The most common polymorphism of the ACE gene is the insertion/deletion (I/D) variant of 287 base pairs in intron 16. This polymorphism has been suggested to be associated with serum ACE protein levels [5], the specific activity of the ACE protein domain [6], and the transcriptional activity of the ACE gene promoter region [7]. Furthermore, ACE may lower amyloid-β levels by promoting its degradation and, thereby, reinforce the hypothesis of the role of ACE in the pathogenesis of AD [8]. However, a more nuanced hypothesis supposes divergent roles of ACE in the degradation of Aβ. ACE may first mediate a short-term neuroprotective action but the production of Ang II then may lead to longer term and more wide-ranging deleterious consequences (i.e., hypertension, damage to the blood–brain barrier, reduced cerebral blood flow, Aβ deposition, inflammation, and reduced cholinergic activity) [4]. Therefore, in either explanation of pathogenesis, the ACE I/D polymorphism becomes an important consideration as a risk factor for AD susceptibility. Perhaps because of these diverse actions of ACE, potential associations with AD have been examined in a great number of studies worldwide but have generated equivocal results [9–11].

This current study examined the genetic polymorphism (I/D) of the ACE gene in a group of AD individuals and controls. The purpose was to determine the nature of the relationship between the ACE gene and the risk of AD in Tunisian subjects.

Methods
Study population
We studied 60 patients with AD (20 female, 40 male) recruited from the Department of Neurology at the Military Hospital of Tunis. The mean age was 75.18 years ± 5.31 (SD). The diagnoses of probable AD were based upon the National Institute of Neurological and Communicative Diseases and Stroke/Alzheimer's Disease and Related Disorders Association (NINCDS–ADRDA) clinical diagnostic criteria and Diagnostic and Statistical Manual of Mental Disorders (DSM IV) criteria with no clinical or laboratory evidence of a cause other than AD for dementia [12, 13]. All participants underwent a complete clinical investigation that included medical history, neurological and neuropsychological examinations (Mini Mental State Examination (MMSE) [14], clock-drawing tests, the 5-word test, auditory verbal learning test, and Frontal Assessment Battery), screening laboratory tests, and neuro-imaging consisting of CT-scan and/or magnetic resonance imaging (MRI). MRI scans displayed substantial reduction in the volume of

the medial temporal lobe and hippocampus in patients with Alzheimer's disease as compared to controls.

Additionally, the control group consisted of 120 age- and gender-matched subjects (46 female, 74 male) with diverse Tunisian origin similar to that of the patients and chosen based on their medical history and physical examination. Their cognitive function was assessed using the MMSE examination [14] with all scores exceeding 26. Further, the controls did not exhibit any signs of dementia and reported no family history of AD or dementia.

All participants (or their guardians) in this study gave their fully informed consent. The study protocol was approved by the Ethics Committee of the Military Hospital of Tunisia and has therefore been performed in accordance with the ethical standards laid down in the 1964 Declaration of Helsinki and its later amendments.

Laboratory methods
Genomic DNA was extracted from peripheral blood leukocytes with a DNA extraction kit (QIAmp blood kit, Qiagen GmbH [Hilden, Germany]) according to the manufacturer's protocol. ACE genotyping was carried out by polymerase chain reaction using oligonucleotide sense primer 5′-CTG GAG ACC ACT CCC ATC CTT TCT-3′, and the antisense primer 5′-GAT GTG GCC ATC ACA TTC GTC AGA T-3′. DNA samples (100 ng) were subjected to 35 cycles of PCR amplification under the following conditions: initial denaturation at 94 °C for 5 min (min), denaturation at 94 °C for 45 s (s), annealing at 58 °C for 1 min, extension at 72 °C for 45 s, and final extension at 72 °C for 7 min. The PCR products were electrophoresed on a 2% agarose gel stained with ethidium bromide to visualize three patterns: I/I (a 490-bp fragment), D/D (a 190-bp fragment), and I/D (both 490- and 190-bp fragments) (Fig. 1).

Statistical analysis
All analyses related to the case–control study were performed using the Statistical Package for the Social Sciences v.16 (IBM, Armonk, NY USA). Data on quantitative

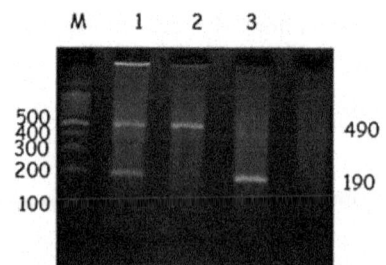

Fig. 1 Agarose gel electrophoresis of PCR amplified products of the ACE (I/D) gene polymorphism. M represents 100-bp DNA ladder; lane 3 as DD genotype (190 bp); lane 2, as II genotype (490 bp) and lane 1, as ID genotypes (490 and 190 bp) of the ACE gene

characteristics are expressed as mean ± SD. Differences between cases and controls were evaluated by using the Chi-square test or Fisher's exact test for qualitative variables. The Chi-square goodness-of-fit test was used to assess the genotype and allele frequencies for deviations from Hardy–Weinberg equilibrium. The Chi-square test of independence was used to ascertain possible dependences between MMSE scores of patients and genotypes. In addition, the odds ratio (OR) and 95% confidence intervals (CI) were calculated with two-by-two contingency table methods to measure the strength of associations (effect sizes). The ACE gene I/D polymorphism and the clinical characteristics of patients were compared to controls using Chi-square or Fisher exact tests (when cell frequencies were small). Probability values (p values) less than .05 were considered statistically significant.

Results

The demographic data for all subjects are presented in Table 1. The mean ages (± SD) of the cases and controls were 75.18 years (± 5.31) and 72.94 years ± (5.0). There were no significant differences in any of the mean values regarding blood chemistry, including triglycerides and cholesterol, between the AD and control groups. MMSE scores, however, differed significantly between patients with AD and controls ($p < .001$). Both the case and control groups were in Hardy–Weinberg equilibrium ($\chi^2 = .014$, $p = .90$; $\chi^2 < 10^{-3}$, $p = .99$; respectively). The ACE gene I/D genotype distributions and allele frequencies of the study groups are presented in Table 2. The analysis of genotype frequencies revealed an over-representation of the D/D genotype among patients compared to that of the control group (51.67% vs. 31.67%, respectively). This observation indicates an increased susceptibility of the D/D genotype carriers to AD ($p = .008$, OR = 2.32). However, the difference of the I/D genotype frequencies between patients and controls was not significant ($p = .24$). The I/I genotype was observed among

Table 1 Comparison of clinical variables in Alzheimer patients and controls

Clinical variable	Patients (N = 60) n (%)	Controls (N = 120) n (%)	p value
Gender F/M	20 (33.3)/40 (66.6)	46 (38.3)/74 (61.6)	–
Age years ± SD	75.18 ± 5.31	72.94 ± 5.0	–
Age of onset years ± SD	69 ± 4.48	–	–
MMSE	14 (6–22)	28 (> 26)	< 10^{-3}
Tobacco use	12 (20)	30 (25)	.45
Diabetes	13 (21.6)	18 (15)	.26
Hypertension	15 (25)	20 (16.6)	.18

Significant p values in italics

Table 2 Genotype and allele frequencies of the ACE polymorphism in AD patients and controls

ACE I/D	Patients N = 60 n (%)	Controls N = 120 n (%)	χ^2	OR [CI 95%]	p value
II	5 (8.33)	23 (19.17)	3.57	.38 (.13–1.06)	.06
ID	24 (40.00)	59 (49.17)	1.35	.69 (.37–1.28)	.24
DD	31 (51.67)	38 (31.67)	6.7	2.32 (1.21–4.34)	.008
I	34 (28.33)	105 (43.75)	8.02	.5 (.30–.80)	.003
D	86 (71.67)	135 (56.25)		2 (1.25–3.33)	

CI confidence interval, OR odds ratio, p value probability value

Significant p values are in italics

5 patients (8.33%) and 23 controls (19.17%) ($p = .06$). The ACE allele frequencies revealed that the D allele was found to be predominant among the AD group (71.67%) while the I allele was predominant among the control subjects (43.75%) with a statistically significant difference ($p = .003$, OR = 2.0). The D allele is statistically associated with an increased risk of AD in our population.

In an effort to discern any relationship between genotypes (alleles) and the severity of dementia, Table 3 details the allocation of patient genotypes and alleles among three categories of Mini-Mental State Examination (MMSE) scores. The Chi-square test of independence broadly indicates that these MMSE categories are dependent upon genotypes ($\chi^2_{df = 4} = 18.1$, $p = .001$) and alleles ($\chi^2_{df = 2} = 18.1$, $p < 10^{-3}$). In particular, the D/D genotype appears in 65% of patients with severe dementia, in 32% with moderate dementia, and in only 3% of those with mild dementia (as measured by the MMSE). Conversely, there are 26 patients with severe dementia and, of them, 77% are D/D carriers, 23% are I/D carriers, and there are no I/I carriers. Although there is a scant number of patients (5) who are I/I carriers (8.3% of all patients), nevertheless 3 (60%) have mild dementia, whereas none have severe symptoms. Conversely, patients in the top scoring MMSE category (mild dementia) are more likely to be I/D carriers (67%) followed by I/I carriers (25%). However, only 1 patient is a D/D carrier suffering with mild dementia. The effects are significant: The odds are 4 times larger for suffering severe versus moderate symptoms ($p = .04$) and 37 times larger for suffering severe versus mild symptoms ($p < 10^{-3}$) for AD patient D/D carriers as compared to non-D/D carriers. The analysis of the alleles reveals a similar trend. Patient carriers of the D allele are predominantly sufferers of severe dementia (53%), 35% have moderate dementia, whereas 12% have mild dementia. Conversely, 88% of those with severe dementia are D carriers. Overall, the odds are 3.6 times higher for scoring in the lowest MMSE

Table 3 MMSE severity by ACE I/D genotypes and alleles in Alzheimer's patients

ACE I/D genotype and alleles n (%) N = 60	MMSE ranges n% (C, R, T)			Severe vs. moderate Severe vs. mild	
	0–9 (severe) N = 26	10–18 (moderate) N = 22	19–23 (mild) N = 12	OR [CI 95%]	p values
II 5 (8)	0 (0, 0, 0)	2 (9, 40, 3)	3 (25, 60, 5)	– 96 [3.2–2800] (*)	.13 .002
ID 24 (40)	6 (23, 25, 10)	10 (45, 42, 17)	8 (67, 33, 13)	3.3 [.94–12] 27 [2.8–260]	.07 $< 10^{-3}$
II + ID 29 (48)	6 (23, 21, 10)	12 (55, 41, 20)	11 (92, 38, 18)	4 [1.2–14] 37 [3.9–340	.04 $< 10^{-3}$
DD 31 (52)	20 (77, 65, 33)	10 (45, 32, 17)	1 (8, 3, 2)	– –	– –
I 34 (28)	6 (12, 18, 5)	14 (32, 41, 12)	14 (58, 41, 12)	3.6 [1.2–10] 11 [3.3–35]	.02 $< 10^{-3}$
D 86 (72)	46 (88, 53, 38)	30 (68, 35, 25)	10 (42, 12, 8)	– –	

DD versus II, ID, and I* genotypes; Statistics calculated using Fisher's exact test; (*) Haldane's correction used; CI confidence interval, % (C, R, T) column %, row %, % of total (all % rounded to nearest whole percentage point), OR odds ratio, p value probability value

Significant p values are in italics

category (severe dementia) as compared to the moderate category ($p = .02$) for D carriers. The odds are 11 times higher for scoring in the lowest MMSE score category as compared to the highest score category, i.e., those with mild dementia ($p < 10^{-3}$). Given the patients in this study, with an average age at AD diagnosis of 69 years and evaluated at an average age of 75 years, those suffering severe dementia are statistically more likely to be D/D carriers (or D allele carriers) and, conversely, D/D (or D carriers) are statistically more likely to suffer severe dementia.

Discussion

This study analyzed the frequencies of the ACE I/D polymorphism in AD patients in comparison with a control group. The D/D genotype ($p = .008$, OR = 2.32) and D allele ($p = .003$, OR = 2.0) were found to be risk factors for AD. The inheritance of the homozygous I/I genotype was marginally associated ($p = .06$) with a reduced risk for AD and the ACE I/D heterozygotes showed no statistical differences in frequencies between subjects and controls ($p = .24$).

Moreover, given the particular demographics of our patient group, D/D carriers were more likely to score in the lowest category of MMSE scores (severe dementia) as compared with I/* carriers. Additionally, there were only 8 I/I carriers of whom none suffered from severe dementia as measured by the MMSE.

The ACE insertion–deletion polymorphism has been frequently studied as a genetic risk factor for AD but the results detailing the relationship between ACE indel and AD are inconsistent. Conflicting results prompt questions as to whether the polymorphism is a risk factor at all and, when answered in the affirmative, lead to

further disagreements as to which genotype(s) is (are) the responsible risk factor(s).

Several studies have failed to find any association implicating the I/D polymorphism as a risk factor for AD [15–18]. In fact, a recently conducted meta-analysis suggested that the ACE I/D polymorphism is unlikely to be a major determining factor in the development of AD [10].

In contrast, however, other studies have determined the ACE indel polymorphism to be a risk factor for AD but they disagree as to which allele and genotype(s) are the responsible factor(s). For example, several studies have revealed associations of the I allele (and/or I/D genotype) with an increased risk of AD and, conversely, the D/D genotype with a lower risk of AD [19–26]; whereas, there are studies in diametric opposition that implicate the ACE D allele as a risk factor [27–30].

Here, our findings demonstrated that the ACE D allele frequency was significantly increased in the AD group as compared to controls. In particular, our results are in agreement with similar research conducted with a Tunisian population where the authors reported an increased risk of AD in D/D genotype carriers [31].

The lack of coherency among ACE-AD investigations may be explained by the differing genetic backgrounds among ethnicities or, in some cases, possibly intra-population heterogeneities. A meta-analysis that included three ethnic groups (North European, South Caucasian, and East Asian subjects) addressing the relationship between the ACE indel polymorphism and AD has shown ethnic-dependent results. Although all groups revealed that the D homozygotes were at reduced risk of AD, there was no overlap whatsoever in allelic frequencies among the three groups. Heterozygotes were at increased risk in

North Europeans, whereas I homozygotes were at higher risk in East Asians [9]. There is evidence, however, that ethnicity alone, in a genetically heterogeneous population, may not prove to be sufficient to explain conflicting results. For example, a study from Japan found that the ACE I/I genotype is associated with an increased prevalence of AD, only to be contradicted by other Japanese studies [22, 32].

The present study with Tunisian subjects benefits from the determination that populations of the Maghreb show a substantial degree of genetic homogeneity, regardless of culture and geography [33, 34]. This is corroborated, in part, by the only other ACE-AD study to date with Tunisian subjects that also report commensurate genotype frequencies with those subjects of the present study [31].

The mechanism whereby the ACE I/D polymorphism could contribute to the development of AD pathology remains contentious. In general, explanations can first be parsed into two main categories that depend on the dual character of ACE.

Serum ACE levels have been found to be associated with ACE I/D, with the highest serum ACE levels in subjects with ACE genotype D/D and the lowest serum ACE levels in subjects with genotype I/I [5, 18, 35, 36]. ACE promotes the formation of angiotensin II from angiotensin I and inactivates the vasodilator bradykinin; the net result is vasopressin activity [37, 38]. Such a perturbation in vasoconstriction for the regulation of blood pressure may likely influence normal cell function in many different tissues, such as in vascular endothelia which, in turn, may cause neural cell degeneration and contribute to the development of dementia. Increasingly, the actions of ACE and, therefore, angiotensin II within the central nervous system are of increasing interest in the context of Alzheimer's disease [4, 35, 39].

Another proposed mechanism for AD development is explained via the amyloid hypothesis which suggests that the deposition of beta-amyloid (Aβ) is a primary event in the pathological cascade for AD. Research indicates that ACE cleaves amyloid-β (Aβ) and, therefore, inhibits amyloid-β peptide aggregation and thus plaque formation [8, 40, 41].

The alteration of activity of this enzyme in the central nervous system (CNS) may have an impact upon the Aβ accumulation thereby resulting in senile plaque which is central to the pathogenesis of Alzheimer's disease. The research implicating the I allele as a risk factor and the D allele as protective in AD [15, 17–22, 35] is consistent with this hypothesis given that ACE activity is highest in D homozygotes [5, 36].

There have been proposed several hypotheses that attempt to reconcile the trichotomous associations of the ACE I/D polymorphism with AD (no association versus D versus I as risk factors) given the dual activities of ACE (cleavage of Aβ versus possible vascular dysfunction via endothelia damage). The proposals include a theory of homeostasis disruption whereby increased levels of ACE mediate short-term Aβ clearance but that up-regulation of Ang II in turn causes hypertension, damage to the blood–brain barrier, reduced cerebral blood flow results in de novo Aβ deposition, inflammation, regional white matter volume changes, and reduced cholinergic activity [35, 42–44]. Another explanation advanced to explain the findings of contrary associations between ACE I/D and AD is that this polymorphism is in varying linkage disequilibrium, depending on ethnic group, to other single nucleotide polymorphisms (e.g., rs4343, rs4335, and rs4291) that have stronger associations with AD [31, 38, 43, 45, 46]. Yet other research, while at times finding ACE I/D-AD associations and in other instances finding no independent ACE I/D-AD association, has nevertheless found associations or more pronounced effects when gene–gene interactions (e.g., ACE I/D-apolipoprotein E) were considered [18, 35, 46]. This suggests that the ACE I/D polymorphism may be, at a minimum, an effect modifier in the etiology of AD.

The present research also found an association of ACE D/D carriers with the lowest MMSE scores as compared with I carriers. Other researchers have also investigated this association with varying results. Yip et al. did not find any association between ACE I/D and AD [47]. Similarly, a Danish study failed to find an association between ACE genotypes and cognitive decline [48]. However, Richard et al. found that DD carriers had the lowest cognitive scores and that cognitive decline was more prevalent in these subjects when compared with I/D subjects as a reference class (Moreover, they report that the combined effect of the presence of at least one APOE ε4 allele and D homozygosity was a risk factor for cognitive decline) [49]. A Greek study reported that subjects who were double homozygous [ACE DD and TNF GG (tumor necrosis factor)] presented with significantly decreased MMSE scores as compared to other double genotypes [50]. Similarly, a study involving an African–Caribbean population found an association between increased age and cognitive decline was significantly stronger in people with the ACE DD genotype [51]. In contrast, however, a study by Chou et al. found that AD patients, homozygous for the I allele, presented with a more rapid AD deterioration than did those who had other ACE genotypes as measured by the MMSE [52].

It is notable that the debate between the association of ACE I/D and AD and the corresponding debate between the opposing natures of ACE (and Ang II) on the central nervous system is mirrored in the current debate over the clinical use of ACE inhibitors (ACE-Is) in AD beyond their role as a treatment for hypertension. While some research indicates that the use of ACE-Is (or angiotensin receptor blockers) in older adults with AD is associated with a slower rate of cognitive decline [42, 53–55], other research cautions in the use of ACE inhibitors as they may interfere with Aβ clearance [40, 56, 57].

Currently, only the APOE ε4 allele is widely accepted as a risk factor for AD. However, approximately 42% of persons with late-onset AD are not APOE ε4 carriers. Thus, the absence of the APOE ε4 allele does not rule out an AD diagnosis [58]. Research has also found ACE to be over-expressed in the hippocampus, frontal cortex, and caudate nucleus of patients with AD [55]. Consequently, study of the ACE I/D polymorphism has become a subject of interest in the etiology of AD.

The present research would have benefited from a larger sample size to increase the power of the results. A larger sample would also allow stratification by AD subtypes and allow a more detailed study of the association of genotypes with MMSE scores regressed upon age, sex, and duration of disease. Future research directions should include investigations of variants in linkage disequilibrium with ACE I/D, examining associations between ACE I/D genotypes and ACE levels (peripheral and in the central nervous system), study of gene–gene interactions (e.g., ACE I/D with APOE), and longitudinal, genotype association studies of MMSE score progression and the study of disease evolution among ACE inhibitor cohorts.

Conclusions

In summary, our study shows an association of the ACE gene I/D polymorphism with AD in a Tunisian population. The D/D genotype confers significant susceptibility for AD and is associated with lower MMSE scores among AD patients as compared to other genotypes in the Tunisian population. These preliminary exploratory results should be confirmed in a larger study and further work is required to discern among possible differing findings in diverse populations.

Abbreviations

ACE: angiotensin-converting enzyme; Ach: acetylcholine; Ang II: angiotensin II; AD: Alzheimer's disease; Aβ: amyloid-β; APOE: apolipoprotein E; CI: confidence intervals; I/D: insertion/deletion; MMSE: Mini-Mental State Examination; MRI: magnetic resonance imaging; NINCDS–ADRDA: National Institute of Neurological and Communicative Diseases and Stroke/Alzheimer's Disease and Related Disorders Association; OR: odds ratio.

Authors' contributions

NFM wrote the first draft of the manuscript and contributed to the editing of the final manuscript. IB and HD contributed to the sample collection and data recording. AS and MM contributed to the study design, statistical analyses, and interpretation of data. RM and BN contributed to the study design and review of the manuscript. All authors read and approved the final manuscript.

Author details

[1] Laboratory of Molecular Biology, Department of Hematology, Military Hospital of Tunisia, Mont Fleury, 1008 Tunis, Tunisia. [2] Department of Neurology, Military Hospital of Tunisia, Montfleury, Tunis 1008, Tunisia.

Acknowledgements

We would like to thank Dr. Christian Winchell for his precious help in correcting this manuscript.

Competing interests

The authors declare that they have no competing interests.

Consent for publication

Written informed consent form was obtained from all participants.

Funding

This research did not receive any specific grant from funding agencies in the public, commercial, or not-for-profit sectors.

References

1. Mucke L. Neuroscience: Alzheimer's disease. Nature. 2009;461(7266):895–7.
2. Selkoe DJ. Biochemistry and molecular biology of amyloid beta-protein and the mechanism of Alzheimer's disease. Handb Clin Neurol. 2008;89:245–60.
3. Kehoe PG, Miners S, Love S. Angiotensins in Alzheimer's disease-friend or foe? Trends Neurosci. 2009;32(12):619–28.
4. Miners JS, van Helmond Z, Raiker M, Love S, Kehoe PG. ACE variants and association with brain Abeta levels in Alzheimer's disease. Am J Transl Res. 2010;3(1):73–80.
5. Biller H, Zissel G, Ruprecht B, Nauck M, Busse Grawitz A, Muller-Quernheim J. Genotype-corrected reference values for serum angiotensin-converting enzyme. Eur Respir J. 2006;28(6):1085–90.
6. van Esch JH, van Gool JM, de Bruin RJ, Payne JR, Montgomery HE, Hectors M, et al. Different contributions of the angiotensin-converting enzyme C-domain and N-domain in subjects with the angiotensin-converting enzyme II and DD genotype. J Hypertens. 2008;26(4):706–13.
7. Wu SJ, Hsieh TJ, Kuo MC, Tsai ML, Tsai KL, Chen CH, et al. Functional regulation of Alu element of human angiotensin-converting enzyme gene in neuron cells. Neurobiol Aging. 2013;34(7):1921.
8. Baughman RP, Teirstein AS, Judson MA, Rossman MD, Yeager H Jr, Bresnitz EA, et al. Clinical characteristics of patients in a case control study of sarcoidosis. Am J Respir Crit Care Med. 2001;164(10 Pt 1):1885–9.
9. Lehmann DJ, Cortina-Borja M, Warden DR, Smith AD, Sleegers K, Prince JA, et al. Large meta-analysis establishes the ACE insertion–deletion polymorphism as a marker of Alzheimer's disease. Am J Epidemiol. 2005;162(4):305–17.
10. Wang XB, Cui NH, Yang J, Qiu XP, Gao JJ, Yang N, et al. Angiotensin-converting enzyme insertion/deletion polymorphism is not a major determining factor in the development of sporadic Alzheimer disease: evidence from an updated meta-analysis. PLoS ONE. 2014;9(10):e111406.
11. Wang XB, Cui NH, Gao JJ, Qiu XP, Yang N, Zheng F. Angiotensin-converting enzyme gene polymorphisms and risk for sporadic Alzheimer's disease: a meta-analysis. J Neural Transm (Vienna). 2015;122(2):211–24.
12. McKhann G, Drachman D, Folstein M, Katzman R, Price D, Stadlan EM. Clinical diagnosis of Alzheimer's disease: report of the NINCDS–ADRDA Work Group under the auspices of Department of Health and Human Services Task Force on Alzheimer's Disease. Neurology. 1984;34(7):939–44.
13. Gmitrowicz A, Kucharska A. Developmental disorders in the fourth edition of the American classification: diagnostic and statistical manual of mental disorders (DSM IV-optional book). Psychiatr Pol. 1994;28(5):509–21.
14. Folstein MF, Folstein SE, McHugh PR. "Mini-mental state". A practical method for grading the cognitive state of patients for the clinician. J Psychiatr Res. 1975;12(3):189–98.
15. Panza F, Solfrizzi V, D'Introno A, Colacicco AM, Capurso C, Capurso A, et al. Shifts in angiotensin I converting enzyme insertion allele frequency

across Europe: implications for Alzheimer's disease risk. J Neurol Neurosurg Psychiatry. 2003;74(8):1159–61.

16. Seripa D, Forno GD, Matera MG, Gravina C, Margaglione M, Palermo MT, et al. Methylenetetrahydrofolate reductase and angiotensin converting enzyme gene polymorphisms in two genetically and diagnostically distinct cohort of Alzheimer patients. Neurobiol Aging. 2003;24(7):933–9.

17. Nacmias B, Bagnoli S, Tedde A, Cellini E, Bessi V, Guarnieri B, et al. Angiotensin converting enzyme insertion/deletion polymorphism in sporadic and familial Alzheimer's disease and longevity. Arch Gerontol Geriatr. 2007;45(2):201–6.

18. Trebunova M, Slaba E, Habalova V, Gdovinova Z. ACE I/D polymorphism in Alzheimer's disease. Cent Eur J Biol. 2008;3(1):49–54.

19. Narain Y, Yip A, Murphy T, Brayne C, Easton D, Evans JG, et al. The ACE gene and Alzheimer's disease susceptibility. J Med Genet. 2000;37(9):695–7.

20. Kehoe PG, Russ C, McIlory S, Williams H, Holmans P, Holmes C, et al. Variation in DCP1, encoding ACE, is associated with susceptibility to Alzheimer disease. Nat Genet. 1999;21(1):71–2.

21. Alvarez R, Alvarez V, Lahoz CH, Martinez C, Pena J, Sanchez JM, et al. Angiotensin converting enzyme and endothelial nitric oxide synthase DNA polymorphisms and late onset Alzheimer's disease. J Neurol Neurosurg Psychiatry. 1999;67(6):733–6.

22. Hu J, Miyatake F, Aizu Y, Nakagawa H, Nakamura S, Tamaoka A, et al. Angiotensin-converting enzyme genotype is associated with Alzheimer disease in the Japanese population. Neurosci Lett. 1999;277(1):65–7.

23. Elkins JS, Douglas VC, Johnston SC. Alzheimer disease risk and genetic variation in ACE: a meta-analysis. Neurology. 2004;62(3):363–8.

24. Mattila KM, Rinne JO, Roytta M, Laippala P, Pietila T, Kalimo H, et al. Dipeptidyl carboxypeptidase 1 (DCP1) and butyrylcholinesterase (BCHE) gene interactions with the apolipoprotein E epsilon4 allele as risk factors in Alzheimer's disease and in Parkinson's disease with coexisting Alzheimer pathology. J Med Genet. 2000;37(10):766–70.

25. Zhang JW, Li XQ, Zhang ZX, Chen D, Zhao HL, Wu YN, et al. Association between angiotensin-converting enzyme gene polymorphism and Alzheimer's disease in a Chinese population. Dement Geriatr Cogn Disord. 2005;20(1):52–6.

26. Hassanin OM, Moustafa M, El Masry TM. Association of insertion–deletion polymorphism of ACE gene and Alzheimer's disease in Egyptian patients. Egypt J Med Human Genet. 2014;15(4):355–60.

27. Farrer LA, Sherbatich T, Keryanov SA, Korovaitseva GI, Rogaeva EA, Petruk S, et al. Association between angiotensin-converting enzyme and Alzheimer disease. Arch Neurol. 2000;57(2):210–4.

28. Isbir T, Agachan B, Yilmaz H, Aydin M, Kara I, Eker D, et al. Interaction between apolipoprotein-E and angiotensin-converting enzyme genotype in Alzheimer's disease. Am J Alzheimers Dis Other Demen. 2001;16(4):205–10.

29. Palumbo B, Cadini D, Nocentini G, Filipponi E, Fravolini ML, Senin U. Angiotensin converting enzyme deletion allele in different kinds of dementia disorders. Neurosci Lett. 1999;267(2):97–100.

30. Richard F, Fromentin-David I, Ricolfi F, Ducimetiere P, Di Menza C, Amouyel P, et al. The angiotensin I converting enzyme gene as a susceptibility factor for dementia. Neurology. 2001;56(11):1593–5.

31. Achouri-Rassas A, Ali NB, Cherif A, Fray S, Siala H, Zakraoui NO, et al. Association between ACE polymorphism, cognitive phenotype and APOE E4 allele in a Tunisian population with Alzheimer disease. J Neural Transm (Vienna). 2016;123(3):317–21.

32. Wakutani Y, Kowa H, Kusumi M, Yamagata K, Wada-Isoe K, Adachi Y, et al. Genetic analysis of vascular factors in Alzheimer's disease. Ann N Y Acad Sci. 2002;977:232–8.

33. Bahri R, Esteban E, Moral P, Chaabani H. New insights into the genetic history of Tunisians: data from Alu insertion and apolipoprotein E gene polymorphisms. Ann Hum Biol. 2008;35(1):22–33.

34. El Moncer W, Esteban E, Bahri R, Gaya-Vidal M, Carreras-Torres R, Athanasiadis G, et al. Mixed origin of the current Tunisian population from the analysis of Alu and Alu/STR compound systems. J Hum Genet. 2010;55(12):827–33.

35. Tian J, Shi J, Bailey K, Harris JM, Pritchard A, Lambert JC, et al. A polymorphism in the angiotensin 1-converting enzyme gene is associated with damage to cerebral cortical white matter in Alzheimer's disease. Neurosci Lett. 2004;354(2):103–6.

36. Rigat B, Hubert C, Alhenc-Gelas F, Cambien F, Corvol P, Soubrier F. An insertion/deletion polymorphism in the angiotensin I-converting enzyme gene accounting for half the variance of serum enzyme levels. J Clin Investig. 1990;86(4):1343–6.

37. Erdos EG, Skidgel RA. The angiotensin I-converting enzyme. Lab Invest. 1987;56(4):345–8.

38. Sayed-Tabatabaei FA, Oostra BA, Isaacs A, van Duijn CM, Witteman JC. ACE polymorphisms. Circ Res. 2006;98(9):1123–33.

39. Kakinuma Y, Hama H, Sugiyama F, Yagami K, Goto K, Murakami K, et al. Impaired blood–brain barrier function in angiotensinogen-deficient mice. Nat Med. 1998;4(9):1078–80.

40. Hemming ML, Selkoe DJ. Amyloid beta-protein is degraded by cellular angiotensin-converting enzyme (ACE) and elevated by an ACE inhibitor. J Biol Chem. 2005;280(45):37644–50.

41. Oba R, Igarashi A, Kamata M, Nagata K, Takano S, Nakagawa H. The N-terminal active centre of human angiotensin-converting enzyme degrades Alzheimer amyloid beta-peptide. Eur J Neurosci. 2005;21(3):733–40.

42. Soto ME, van Kan GA, Nourhashemi F, Gillette-Guyonnet S, Cesari M, Cantet C, et al. Angiotensin-converting enzyme inhibitors and Alzheimer's disease progression in older adults: results from the Reseau sur la Maladie d'Alzheimer Francais cohort. J Am Geriatr Soc. 2013;61(9):1482–8.

43. Lucatelli JF, Barros AC, Silva VK, Machado Fda S, Constantin PC, Dias AA, et al. Genetic influences on Alzheimer's disease: evidence of interactions between the genes APOE, APOC1 and ACE in a sample population from the South of Brazil. Neurochem Res. 2011;36(8):1533–9.

44. Hou Z, Yuan Y, Zhang Z, Hou G, You J, Bai F. The D-allele of ACE insertion/deletion polymorphism is associated with regional white matter volume changes and cognitive impairment in remitted geriatric depression. Neurosci Lett. 2010;479(3):262–6.

45. Zhang Z, Deng L, Yu H, Shi Y, Bai F, Xie C, et al. Association of angiotensin-converting enzyme functional gene I/D polymorphism with amnestic mild cognitive impairment. Neurosci Lett. 2012;514(1):131–5.

46. Kehoe PG, Katzov H, Feuk L, Bennet AM, Johansson B, Wiman B, et al. Haplotypes extending across ACE are associated with Alzheimer's disease. Hum Mol Genet. 2003;12(8):859–67.

47. Yip AG, Brayne C, Easton D, Rubinsztein DC. An investigation of ACE as a risk factor for dementia and cognitive decline in the general population. J Med Genet. 2002;39(6):403–6.

48. Frederiksen H, Gaist D, Bathum L, Andersen K, McGue M, Vaupel JW, et al. Angiotensin I-converting enzyme (ACE) gene polymorphism in relation to physical performance, cognition and survival—a follow-up study of elderly Danish twins. Ann Epidemiol. 2003;13(1):57–65.

49. Richard F, Berr C, Amant C, Helbecque N, Amouyel P, Alperovitch A. Effect of the angiotensin I-converting enzyme I/D polymorphism on cognitive decline. The EVA Study Group. Neurobiol Aging. 2000;21(1):75–80.

50. Georgiopoulos G, Chrysohoou C, Errigo A, Pes G, Metaxa V, Zaromytidou M, et al. Arterial aging mediates the effect of TNF-a and ACE polymorphisms on mental health in elderly individuals. Insights from IKARIA study. QJM: monthly journal of the Association of Physicians; 2017.

51. Stewart R, Powell J, Prince M, Mann A. ACE genotype and cognitive decline in an African–Caribbean population. Neurobiol Aging. 2004;25(10):1369–75.

52. Chou PS, Wu MN, Chou MC, Chien I, Yang YH. Angiotensin-converting enzyme insertion/deletion polymorphism and the longitudinal progression of Alzheimer's disease. Geriatr Gerontol Int. 2017;17(10):1544–50.

53. Nelson L, Tabet N, Richardson C, Gard P. Antihypertensives, angiotensin, glucose and Alzheimer's disease. Expert Rev Neurother. 2013;13(5):477–82.

54. Li NC, Lee A, Whitmer RA, Kivipelto M, Lawler E, Kazis LE, et al. Use of angiotensin receptor blockers and risk of dementia in a predominantly male population: prospective cohort analysis. BMJ (Clinical research ed). 2010;340:b5465.

55. Ohrui T, Tomita N, Sato-Nakagawa T, Matsui T, Maruyama M, Niwa K, et al. Effects of brain-penetrating ACE inhibitors on Alzheimer disease progression. Neurology. 2004;63(7):1324–5.

56. Jochemsen HM, Teunissen CE, Ashby EL, van der Flier WM, Jones RE, Geerlings MI, et al. The association of angiotensin-converting enzyme with biomarkers for Alzheimer's disease. Alzheimer's Res Ther. 2014;6(3):27.

29

Amygdala functional connectivity in female patients with major depressive disorder with and without suicidal ideation

Shengnan Wei[1,2], Miao Chang[2], Ran Zhang[3], Xiaowei Jiang[1,2], Fei Wang[1,2,3] and Yanqing Tang[1,3,4*]

Abstract

Background: Major depressive disorder (MDD) is a known major risk factor for suicide and is one of the most common mental disorders. Meanwhile, gender differences in suicidal behavior have long been recognized including the finding that women have higher rates of suicidal ideation and/or suicidal behavior than men. The mechanism underlying suicide ideation in female patients with MDD remains poorly understood. The aim of the present study was to examine possible suicidal behavior-related neural circuitry in female MDD.

Methods: In this study, 15 female participants with the first-episode MDD with suicidal ideation and 24 participants with the first-episode MDD without suicidal ideation as well as 39 female participants in a healthy control (HC) group, ranging in age from 18 to 50 years, underwent resting-state functional magnetic resonance imaging. The whole-brain amygdala resting-state functional connectivity (rsFC) was compared among these three groups.

Results: Compared with female participants with the first-episode MDD without suicidal ideation and those in the HC group, female participants with the first-episode MDD with suicidal ideation showed a significant difference in rsFC between the amygdala and precuneus/cuneus ($p < 0.05$, corrected). No significant difference in amygdala–precuneus/cuneus rsFC was observed between female patients with the first-episode MDD without suicidal ideation and the HC group ($p < 0.05$, corrected).

Conclusions: Our findings suggest that suicidal ideation in female patients with the first-episode MDD may be related to an abnormality in amygdala neural circuitry. The abnormality in amygdala–precuneus/cuneus functional connectivity might present the trait feature for suicide in women with the first-episode MDD. The precuneus/cuneus may be an important region related to suicide and require future study.

Keywords: First episode, Female, Depressive, Suicidal ideation, Amygdala, Functional connectivity

Background

Suicide is an important health problem worldwide. WHO (World Health Organization) reported that suicide is the 20th leading cause of death worldwide. Major depressive disorder (MDD) is a known major risk factor for suicide and is one of the most common mental disorders [1], with a lifetime incidence of 17.1% [2]. Chen and Angst et al. reported that around 15% patients with MDD

ultimately die by suicide [3, 4]. The recent study reported that 25% adolescent with MDD had a lifetime history of suicide attempt [5]. Meanwhile, gender is also a strong sociodemographic correlate and has been associated strongly with suicidal behavior. Gender differences in suicidal behavior have long been recognized [6], including the finding that women have higher rates of suicidal ideation and nonfatal suicidal behavior than men [7]. Therefore, the studies of women with MDD are important for identifying factors associated with suicidal behavior.

Structural magnetic resonance imaging (MRI) [8–12] and functional MRI [13] studies have demonstrated brain abnormalities in people with MDD who exhibit suicidal

*Correspondence: yanqingtang@163.com
[3] Department of Psychiatry, First Affiliated Hospital, China Medical University, Shenyang 110001, Liaoning, People's Republic of China
Full list of author information is available at the end of the article

behavior. The amygdala is the key brain region involved in emotional and cognitive processing. The amygdala's role in processing emotional stimuli has been demonstrated in animal and human research [14–16], and it also has been implicated centrally in people with MDD [17–23]. First, the previous studies also have shown that abnormalities of volume and connectivity of amygdala were associated with the mechanisms of suicide in people with MDD [24, 25]. Second, one study also showed an association between amygdala-middle temporal area connectivity and suicidal ideas in suicide attempters [26]. It was found that suicide attempters showed significantly increased resting-state functional connectivity (rsFC) of the left amygdala with the right insula and left superior orbitofrontal area, and those with MDD showed increased rsFC of the right amygdala with the left middle temporal area [26]. However, the previous study also showed a negative result of amygdala morphometric difference in suicidal patients [27] and another study is the lack of correlation between suicidal ideation and amygdala–precuneus RSFC in adolescents [28].

The mechanism underlying suicide in patients with MDD remains poorly understood. There is little study of the relationship between women with first-episode MDD and suicide. In our study, we performed a seed-based analysis of the amygdala rsFC in female patients with first-episode MDD with suicidal ideation and without suicidal ideation, and healthy control (HC) participants, ranging in age from 18 to 50 years. The goal of the present study was to examine the amygdala rsFC of female patients with first-episode MDD with suicidal ideation and without suicidal ideation.

Methods

Participants

The study included 39 participants with first-episode MDD and 39 HC participants between the ages of 18 and 50 years. The first-episode MDD participants were recruited from the outpatient clinics at the Department of Psychiatry, First Affiliated Hospital of China Medical University, Shenyang, China. The HC participants were recruited from Shenyang, China, using community advertisement. The presence or absence of Axis I diagnoses was independently determined by two trained psychiatrists using the Structured Clinical Interview for DSM-IV Axis I Disorders (SCID) in participants 18 years old or older.

The first-episode MDD initially was diagnosed in participants with MDD who had not presented with a manic episode within the 1-year follow-up study. These participants did not present with or have a history of other Axis I disorders, including substance abuse or dependence.

HC participants did not have any first-degree relatives with Axis I disorders.

Suicidal ideation, defined as thoughts of engaging in behavior intended to end one's life, has been identified as an important precursor of both attempted and completed suicide [29–31]. In our study, we used the Beck 19-item Scale for Suicide Ideation [32] to assess whether there has the suicidal ideation. According to our previous research of epidemiology of suicide [33], the presence of suicidal ideation was the outcome variable based on the Beck 19-item Scale for Suicide Ideation; we used the item about suicidal ideation found in the Beck 19-item Scale for Suicide Ideation to stratify our patients. The depressed patients divided into groups with suicidal ideation and without suicidal ideation. We obtained symptom measures using the Hamilton Depression Rating Scale (HAMD).

For all three groups, individuals were excluded if any of the following were present: (1) any MRI contraindications; (2) history of head trauma with loss of consciousness for 5 min or more, or any neurological disorder; (3) any concomitant major medical disorder. All participants were right-handed and scanned within 24 h of the initial contact with the research team. All participants provided written informed consent after reading a detailed description of the study. The Institutional Review Board of China Medical University approved the study.

MRI data acquisition

We acquired data using a GE (Boston, MA) MR Signa HDx 3.0T MRI scanner at the First Affiliated Hospital, China Medical University, Shenyang, China. Head motion was minimized with restraining foam pads. We used a standard head coil for radio-frequency transmission and reception of the nuclear magnetic resonance signal. The participants were asked to keep their eyes closed but remain awake during the scan. We acquired fMRI images using a spin echo planar imaging (EPI) sequence, parallel to the anterior–posterior commissure plane with the following scan parameters: repetition time (TR) = 2000 ms; echo time (TE) = 40 ms; image matrix = 64×64; field of view (FOV) = 24×24 cm^2; 35 contiguous slices of 3 mm without gap; scan time = 6 min 40 s (the 6 min 40 s scans included a total of 200 volumes). We acquired a high-resolution structural image using a three-dimensional fast spoiled gradient-echo T1-weighted sequence: TR = 7.1 ms, TE = 3.2 ms, FOV = 24 cm $\times$ 24 cm, matrix = 240×240, slice thickness = 1.0 mm without gap, and 176 slices.

Functional connectivity processing

We conducted resting-state fMRI data preprocessing using SPM8 (http://www.fil.ion.ucl.ac.uk/spm/softw

are/spm8) and the Resting-State fMRI Data Analysis Toolkit (REST; http://www.restfmri.net). The first ten images were deleted, and then, the data underwent further preprocessing, which included slice timing correction, head motion correction, spatial normalization, and smoothing. We computed head motion parameters by estimating translation in each direction and angular rotation about each axis for each volume. We excluded data sets if head motion was more than 3 mm maximum displacement in any of the x-, y-, or z-directions or more than 3° of any angular motion throughout the course of the scan. To assess the head motion confound, we compared the mean framewise displacement [34] among the three groups. The results showed no significant differences in head motion when comparing the three groups ($p = 0.81$). We performed spatial normalization using a standard EPI template from the Montreal Neurological Institute (MNI). The voxel size was resampled to $3 \times 3 \times 3$ mm^3. We performed spatial smoothing with an 8-mm full-width at half maximum Gaussian filter. To remove low-frequency drifts and physiological high-frequency noise, we performed linear detrending and temporal bandpass (0.01–0.08 Hz) filtering. To remove the effects of nuisance covariates, we performed linear regression of head motion parameters, global mean signal, white matter signal, and cerebrospinal fluid signal [35–37].

Definition of region of interest
The amygdala was selected as the region of interest (ROI). We defined the bilateral amygdala ROI according to the automated anatomical labeling template [38] contained in REST, which had been resampled to $3 \times 3 \times 3$ mm^3. We averaged the blood oxygen-level-dependent (BOLD) time series of the voxels within the ROI to generate the reference time series for the ROI.

Functional connectivity and statistical analysis
We analyzed demographic and clinical characteristics using IBM SPSS Statistics for Windows, Version 21.0 (Armonk, New York).

We performed functional connectivity analysis using correlation analysis between the seed bilateral amygdala ROI and a gray matter mask in a voxel-wise manner using Data Processing and Analysis for Brain Imaging software (DPABI; DPABI_V1.2_141101, http://rfmri.org/dpabi). We then transformed the correlation coefficients to Z values using the Fisher's r-to-z transformation.

We used one-way analysis of variance (ANOVA) to compare rsFC among the three groups. Statistical significance was set at corrected $p < 0.05$ (uncorrected $p < 0.01$) using Gaussian random field correction, which we performed using the DPABI software. We extracted Z values from the gray matter mask showing significant differences among the three groups. Post hoc, we performed two-sample t tests of the Z values between each pair of groups (HC vs. female patients with MDD with suicidal ideation, HC vs. female patients with MDD without suicidal ideation, and female patients with MDD with suicidal ideation vs. without suicidal ideation) using SPSS ($p < 0.05$).

Results
Demographics and clinical characteristics
Following the Beck 19-item Scale for Suicide Ideation, we identified 15 female participants with suicidal ideation and 24 female participants without suicidal ideation. A comparison of demographic characteristics for each group is shown in Table 1. We did not identify significant differences among the three groups in age or education, but we did observe significant differences in HAMD scores ($p < 0.001$) among the three groups by analysis of one-way ANOVA. Post hoc analyses showed higher HAMD scores in female participants in the MDD with suicidal ideation and MDD without suicidal ideation groups compared with HAMD scores in the HC group

Table 1 Demographics and clinical data of female participants

	MDD with suicidal ideation (n = 15)	MDD without suicidal ideation (n = 24)	HC (n = 39)	F/χ²	p
Age (years)[a]	32.47 ± 11.39	33.50 ± 6.70	29.15 ± 9.33	1.91	0.16
Education (years)[a]	13.67 ± 2.55	13.54 ± 3.02	13.10 ± 2.60	0.32	0.77
HAMD score[a]	22.40 ± 8.62	17.21 ± 8.97	1.26 ± 2.02	72.58	0.000
Lifetime suicide attempts[b]	3 (20%)	3 (12.5%)	0	0.39*	0.53*

HC healthy controls, HAMD Hamilton Depression Rating Scale

* Compared between patient groups

[a] Data are presented as mean ± SD (standard deviation)

[b] Data are presented as n (%)

($p < 0.001$); however, we did not observe significant differences in HAMD scores between female participants in the MDD with suicidal ideation and MDD without suicidal ideation groups ($p = 0.06$).

Group differences in amygdala rsFC
The results of one-way ANOVA showed that there were significant differences in amygdala–precuneus/cuneus rsFC in a comparison of the three groups ($p < 0.05$, corrected). Brain regions showed significant changes in functional connectivity from bilateral amygdala to bilateral precuneus/cuneus (MNI coordinates for the maximal point of difference: $x = -6$ mm, $y = -63$ mm, $z = 63$ mm, 628 voxels, $T = 11.57$, $p < 0.05$, corrected; Fig. 1).

Female patients with first-episode MDD with suicidal ideation showed greater (positive) amygdala–precuneus/cuneus rsFC in contrast to negative amygdala precuneus rsFC in female patients with first-episode MDD

without suicidal ideation and in HC participants. Post hoc pairwise comparisons indicated that the amygdala–precuneus/cuneus rsFC were increased significantly in female patients with first-episode MDD with suicidal ideation separately compared with female patients with first-episode MDD without suicidal ideation or the HC group ($p < 0.05$, corrected). We did not observe significant differences in amygdala–precuneus/cuneus rsFC between female patients with first-episode MDD without suicidal ideation and the HC group (Fig. 2).

Clinical variables
Exploratory analyses did not reveal any significant correlations between rsFC in regions showing significant group differences and scores on HAMD in women with first-episode MDD with suicidal ideation and women with first-episode MDD without suicidal ideation.

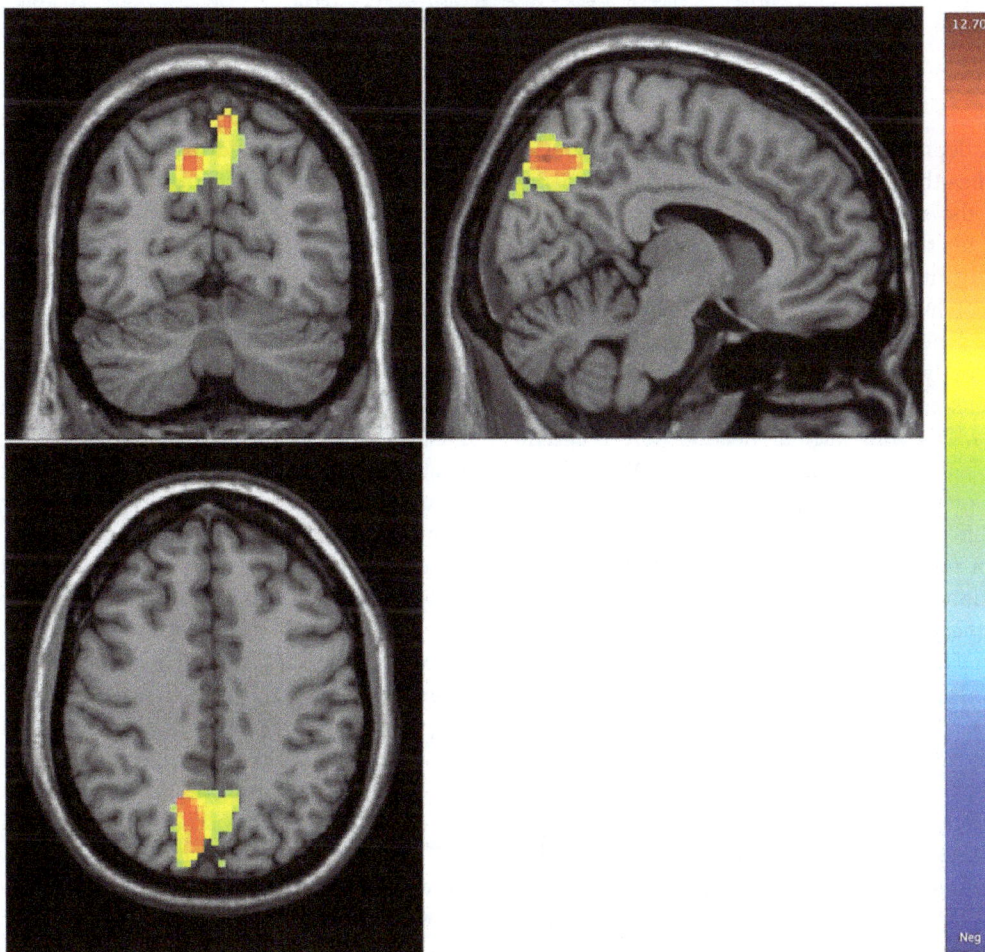

Fig. 1 Results of one-way ANOVA showing abnormalities in amygdala–precuneus/cuneus resting-state functional connectivity in a comparison of the three groups

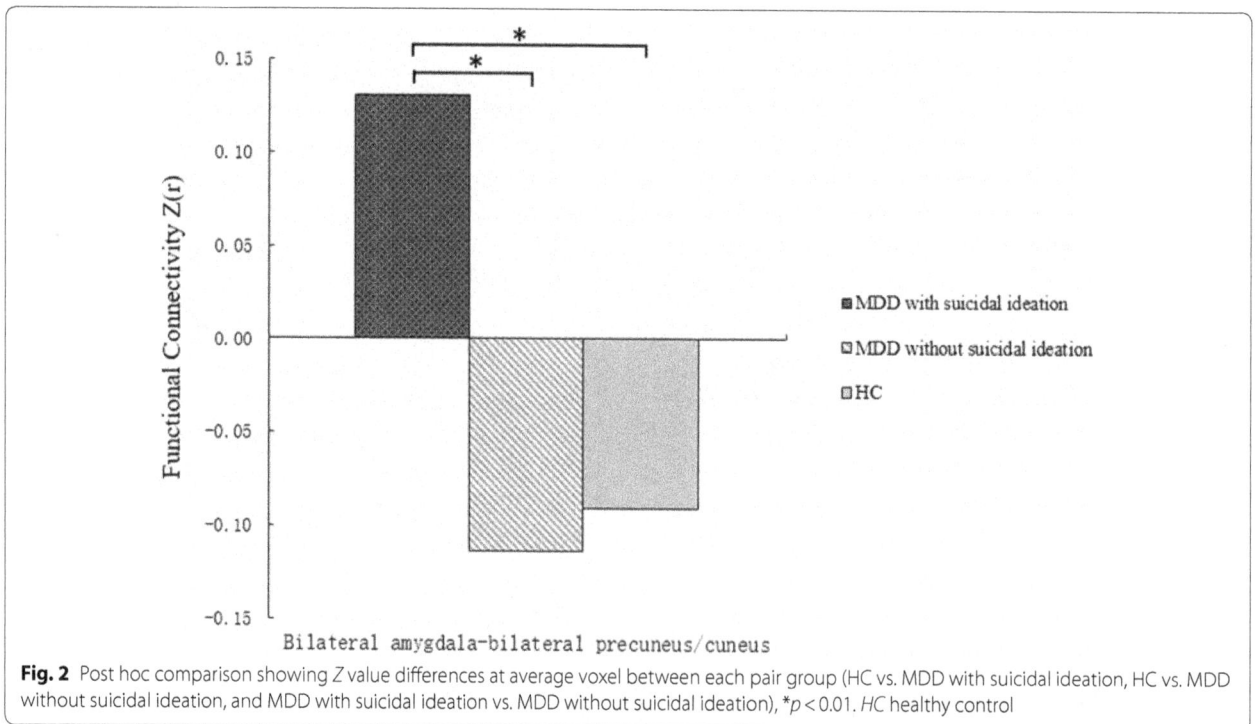

Fig. 2 Post hoc comparison showing Z value differences at average voxel between each pair group (HC vs. MDD with suicidal ideation, HC vs. MDD without suicidal ideation, and MDD with suicidal ideation vs. MDD without suicidal ideation), *$p < 0.01$. *HC* healthy control

Discussion

In this study, depression severity in patients groups was higher than health control group. There may be deeply related with the disease of MDD itself. However, our results suggested that the depression severity was not significantly different between two patients groups, which is consistent with the another study of brain structures in suicidal and nonsuicidal female patients with MDD [24]. In our study, we reported that changes in amygdala–precuneus/cuneus rsFC in female patients with first-episode MDD with suicidal ideation were different from female patients with first-episode MDD without suicidal ideation and HC group. However, there were not significant differences in amygdala–precuneus/cuneus rsFC between patients with first-episode MDD without suicidal ideation and the HC group. These findings also suggest that the mechanism underlying suicidal ideation may be related to an abnormality in amygdala–precuneus/cuneus neural circuitry in female patients with first-episode MDD.

Interestingly, two key brain regions underlying suicidal ideation, the amygdala and precuneus, have been strongly implicated in female patients with first-episode MDD. As stated in preface, the amygdala may be a brain region related to the mechanisms of suicidal behavior with MDD. The previous study reported that impulsivity in patients with MDD with a history of suicide attempts was associated with an altered paralimbic (precuneus) encoding of value differences during

intertemporal choice [9]. A study of the structural brain found that, among suicide attempters with psychotic disorders, a history of high-lethality attempts was associated with significantly smaller volumes of gray matter in the right cuneus [39]. Studies of fMRI showed that past suicidal behavior in people with the early course psychotic MDD was associated with lower activity in midline parietal regions, including the cuneus and precuneus, when performing cognitive control tasks [40], and the correlation between BOLD signal and relief was greater in nonsuicidal, self-injury patients in areas associated with reward or pain and addiction, including the anterior precuneus [41]. Why precuneus/cuneus may be related to suicide due to its own functions. The previous fMRI studies showed that the precuneus may be related significantly to emotion processing [42–45]. For example, one study of neural correlates of intentional and incidental self-processing suggested that self-processing involves distinct processes and can occur in areas, including the left precuneus, previously implicated in self-awareness [42]. The same regions including the precuneus constitute a functional network of reflective self-awareness that is thought to be a core function of consciousness [43]. The precuneus is associated with mentalizing, self-reference, and autobiographic information [44]. A review of the precuneus functional anatomy and behavioral correlates showed that recent functional imaging findings in healthy subjects suggest a central role for the precuneus in a wide spectrum of highly integrated tasks, including visuospatial imagery, episodic memory retrieval, and self-processing operations—namely, first-person perspective taking and an experience of agency [45]. Therefore, we hypothesize that the precuneus/cuneus may be also associated with the patients with MDD with suicidal behavior.

The circuit of the amygdala–precuneus has been highlighted in MDD, because a recent study reported that adolescents with MDD had positive rsFC between the amygdala and precuneus in contrast to healthy adolescents who showed negative rsFC in this circuit [28], whether this circuit is related to suicide is unclear in this study. From the above studies, those findings do confirm our results that an abnormality in the neural circuitry of the amygdala–precuneus/cuneus may be an important mechanism in suicidal ideation in patients with first-episode MDD. We speculated that the functional connectivity between the amygdala and precuneus could be very important to MDD with suicidal behavior. Thus far, no detailed studies of gender differences have been conducted in amygdala–precuneus/cuneus functional connectivity in MDD with suicidal behavior. Therefore, our results need to be proved by future research. The present study provided evidence that the abnormalities in amygdala–precuneus/cuneus functional connectivity might present the trait feature for female in MDD with suicidal ideation. Moreover, they may indicate potential differentiating markers may improve the early prevention in female in MDD with suicidal ideation. In addition, the clinicians could treat patients in MDD with suicidal ideation using physical therapy-related brain regions. The first limitation in this study is that the assessments of Axis I disorders were performed according to the DSM-IV, not the DSM-V, which could affect the accuracy of the diagnoses. Then, we only investigated the abnormalities of neural circuitry in females with MDD, and did not study males with MDD. Another limitation is the small sample size of the MDD with suicidal ideation group.

Conclusions

Our findings suggest that suicidal ideation in female patients with first-episode MDD may be related to an abnormality in the amygdala neural circuitry. The abnormality in amygdala–precuneus/cuneus functional connectivity might present the trait feature for suicide in women with first-episode MDD. The precuneus/cuneus may be an important region related to suicide and thus requires future study.

Abbreviations

MDD: major depressive disorder; HC: healthy controls; fMRI: functional magnetic resonance imaging; rsFC: resting-state functional connectivity; SCID: the Structured Clinical Interview for DSM-IV Axis I Disorders; HAMD: the Hamilton Depression Rating Scale.

Authors' contributions

YT and SW designed the experiment. MC and RZ acquired the data. RZ and XJ analyzed the data. YT, FW, and SW wrote the manuscript. All authors read and approved the final manuscript.

Author details

[1] Brain Function Research Section, First Affiliated Hospital, China Medical University, Shenyang, Liaoning, People's Republic of China. [2] Department of Radiology, First Affiliated Hospital, China Medical University, Shenyang, Liaoning, People's Republic of China. [3] Department of Psychiatry, First Affiliated Hospital, China Medical University, Shenyang 110001, Liaoning, People's Republic of China. [4] Department of Geriatric Medicine, First Affiliated Hospital, China Medical University, Shenyang, Liaoning, People's Republic of China.

Acknowledgements

We would like to thank the patients and family members who contributed so much to this study and the First Affiliated Hospital of China Medical University for its active support of the project.

Competing interests

The authors declare that they have no competing interests.

Consent for publication

Not applicable.

Funding

This work was supported by Grants from the National Natural Science Foundation of China (81701336 to Shengnan Wei, 81271499 and 81571311 to Yanqing Tang, and 81571331 to Fei Wang), the Liaoning Education Foundation (L2015591 to Shengnan Wei), Liaoning Pandeng Scholar (to Fei Wang), National Key Research and Development Program (2016YFC0904300 to Fei Wang), National High Tech Development Plan (863) (2015AA020513 to Fei Wang), and National Key Research and Development Program (2016YFC1306900 to Yanqing Tang).

References

1. Kessler RC, Chiu WT, Demler O, Merikangas KR, Walters EE. Prevalence, severity, and comorbidity of 12-month DSM-IV disorders in the National Comorbidity Survey Replication. Arch Gen Psychiatry. 2005;62(6):617–27.
2. Kessler RC, McGonagle KA, Swartz M, Blazer DG, Nelson CB. Sex and depression in the National Comorbidity Survey. I: lifetime prevalence, chronicity and recurrence. J Affect Disord. 1993;29(2–3):85–96.
3. Chen YW, Dilsaver SC. Lifetime rates of suicide attempts among subjects with bipolar and unipolar disorders relative to subjects with other Axis I disorders. Biol Psychiat. 1996;39(10):896–9.
4. Angst J, Hengartner MP, Gamma A, von Zerssen D, Angst F. Mortality of 403 patients with mood disorders 48 to 52 years after their psychiatric hospitalisation. Eur Arch Psychiatry Clin Neurosci. 2013;263(5):425–34.
5. Blanco C, Hoertel N, Franco S, Olfson M, He JP, Lopez S, Gonzalez-Pinto A, Limosin F, Merikangas KR. Generalizability of clinical trial results for adolescent major depressive disorder. Pediatrics. 2017;140(6):e20161701.
6. Zhang J, McKeown RE, Hussey JR, Thompson SJ, Woods JR. Gender differences in risk factors for attempted suicide among young adults: findings from the Third National Health and Nutrition Examination Survey. Ann Epidemiol. 2005;15(2):167–74.
7. Henderson JP, Mellin C, Patel F. Suicide—a statistical analysis by age, sex and method. J Clin For Med. 2005;12(6):305–9.
8. Jia Z, Huang X, Wu Q, Zhang T, Lui S, Zhang J, Amatya N, Kuang W, Chan RC, Kemp GJ, et al. High-field magnetic resonance imaging of suicidality in patients with major depressive disorder. Am J Psychiatry. 2010;167(11):1381–90.
9. Wagner G, Schultz CC, Koch K, Schachtzabel C, Sauer H, Schlosser RG. Pre frontal cortical thickness in depressed patients with high-risk for suicidal behavior. J Psychiatr Res. 2012;46(11):1449–55.
10. Peng H, Wu K, Li J, Qi H, Guo S, Chi M, Wu X, Guo Y, Yang Y, Ning Y. Increased suicide attempts in young depressed patients with abnormal temporal–parietal–limbic gray matter volume. J Affect Disord. 2014;165:69–73.

11. Lee YJ, Kim S, Gwak AR, Kim SJ, Kang SG, Na KS, Son YD, Park J. Decreased regional gray matter volume in suicide attempters compared to suicide non-attempters with major depressive disorders. Compr Psychiatry. 2016;67:59–65.

12. Jia Z, Wang Y, Huang X, Kuang W, Wu Q, Lui S, Sweeney JA, Gong Q. Impaired frontothalamic circuitry in suicidal patients with depression revealed by diffusion tensor imaging at 3.0 T. J Psychiatry Neurosci. 2014;39(3):170–7.

13. Fan T, Wu X, Yao L, Dong J. Abnormal baseline brain activity in suicidal and non-suicidal patients with major depressive disorder. Neurosci Lett. 2013;534:35–40.

14. LeDoux JE. Brain mechanisms of emotion and emotional learning. Curr Opin Neurobiol. 1992;2(2):191–7.

15. Lebowitz BD, Pearson JL, Schneider LS, Reynolds CF 3rd, Alexopoulos GS, Bruce ML, Conwell Y, Katz IR, Meyers BS, Morrison MF, et al. Diagnosis and treatment of depression in late life. Consensus statement update. Jama. 1997;278(14):1186–90.

16. Costafreda SG, Brammer MJ, David AS, Fu CH. Predictors of amygdala activation during the processing of emotional stimuli: a meta-analysis of 385 PET and fMRI studies. Brain Res Rev. 2008;58(1):57–70.

17. van Eijndhoven P, van Wingen G, van Oijen K, Rijpkema M, Goraj B, Jan Verkes R, Oude Voshaar R, Fernandez G, Buitelaar J, Tendolkar I. Amygdala volume marks the acute state in the early course of depression. Biol Psychiat. 2009;65(9):812–8.

18. Weniger G, Lange C, Irle E. Abnormal size of the amygdala predicts impaired emotional memory in major depressive disorder. J Affect Disord. 2006;94(1–3):219–29.

19. Kronenberg G, van Elst LT, Regen F, Deuschle M, Heuser I, Colla M. Reduced amygdala volume in newly admitted psychiatric in-patients with unipolar major depression. J Psychiatr Res. 2009;43(13):1112–7.

20. Tang Y, Wang F, Xie G, Liu J, Li L, Su L, Liu Y, Hu X, He Z, Blumberg HP. Reduced ventral anterior cingulate and amygdala volumes in medication-naive females with major depressive disorder: a voxel-based morphometric magnetic resonance imaging study. Psychiatry Res. 2007;156(1):83–6.

21. Lee HY, Tae WS, Yoon HK, Lee BT, Paik JW, Son KR, Oh YW, Lee MS, Ham BJ. Demonstration of decreased gray matter concentration in the midbrain encompassing the dorsal raphe nucleus and the limbic subcortical regions in major depressive disorder: an optimized voxel-based morphometry study. J Affect Disord. 2011;133(1–2):128–36.

22. Anand A, Li Y, Wang Y, Wu J, Gao S, Bukhari L, Mathews VP, Kalnin A, Lowe MJ. Activity and connectivity of brain mood regulating circuit in depression: a functional magnetic resonance study. Biol Psychiat. 2005;57(10):1079–88.

23. Arnone D, McKie S, Elliott R, Thomas EJ, Downey D, Juhasz G, Williams SR, Deakin JF, Anderson IM. Increased amygdala responses to sad but not fearful faces in major depression: relation to mood state and pharmacological treatment. Am J Psychiatry. 2012;169(8):841–50.

24. Monkul ES, Hatch JP, Nicoletti MA, Spence S, Brambilla P, Lacerda AL, Sassi RB, Mallinger AG, Keshavan MS, Soares JC. Fronto-limbic brain structures in suicidal and non-suicidal female patients with major depressive disorder. Mol Psychiatry. 2007;12(4):360–6.

25. Wagner G, Koch K, Schachtzabel C, Schultz CC, Sauer H, Schlosser RG. Structural brain alterations in patients with major depressive disorder and high risk for suicide: evidence for a distinct neurobiological entity? NeuroImage. 2011;54(2):1607–14.

26. Kang SG, Na KS, Choi JW, Kim JH, Son YD, Lee YJ. Resting-state functional connectivity of the amygdala in suicide attempters with major depressive disorder. Prog Neuropsychopharmacol Biol Psychiatry. 2017;77:222–7.

27. Gifuni AJ, Ding Y, Olie E, Lawrence N, Cyprien F, Le Bars E, Bonafe A, Phillips ML, Courtet P, Jollant F. Subcortical nuclei volumes in suicidal behavior: nucleus accumbens may modulate the lethality of acts. Brain Imaging Behav. 2016;10(1):96–104.

28. Cullen KR, Westlund MK, Klimes-Dougan B, Mueller BA, Houri A, Eberly LE, Lim KO. Abnormal amygdala resting-state functional connectivity in adolescent depression. JAMA Psychiatry. 2014;71(10):1138–47.

29. Brown GK, Beck AT, Steer RA, Grisham JR. Risk factors for suicide in psychiatric outpatients: a 20-year prospective study. J Consult Clin Psychol. 2000;68(3):371–7.

30. Crandall C, Fullerton-Gleason L, Aguero R, LaValley J. Subsequent suicide mortality among emergency department patients seen for suicidal behavior. Acad Emerg Med. 2006;13(4):435–42.

31. Kuo WH, Gallo JJ, Tien AY. Incidence of suicide ideation and attempts in adults: the 13-year follow-up of a community sample in Baltimore, Maryland. Psychol Med. 2001;31(7):1181–91.

32. Beck AT, Kovacs M, Weissman A. Assessment of suicidal intention: the scale for suicide ideation. J Consult Clin Psychol. 1979;47(2):343–52.

33. Wei S, Li H, Hou J, Chen W, Tan S, Chen X, Qin X. Comparing characteristics of suicide attempters with suicidal ideation and those without suicidal ideation treated in the emergency departments of general hospitals in China. Psychiatry Res. 2018;262:78–83.

34. Yan CG, Cheung B, Kelly C, Colcombe S, Craddock RC, Di Martino A, Li Q, Zuo XN, Castellanos FX, Milham MP. A comprehensive assessment of regional variation in the impact of head micromovements on functional connectomics. NeuroImage. 2013;76:183–201.

35. Erdogan SB, Tong Y, Hocke LM, Lindsey KP, Frederick BB. Correcting for blood arrival time in global mean regression enhances functional connectivity analysis of resting state fMRI-BOLD signals. Front Hum Neurosci. 2016;10:311.

36. Greicius MD, Krasnow B, Reiss AL, Menon V. Functional connectivity in the resting brain: a network analysis of the default mode hypothesis. Proc Natl Acad Sci USA. 2003;100(1):253–8.

37. Fox MD, Snyder AZ, Vincent JL, Corbetta M, Van Essen DC, Raichle ME. The human brain is intrinsically organized into dynamic, anticorrelated functional networks. Proc Natl Acad Sci USA. 2005;102(27):9673–8.

38. Tzourio-Mazoyer N, Landeau B, Papathanassiou D, Crivello F, Etard O, Delcroix N, Mazoyer B, Joliot M. Automated anatomical labeling of activations in SPM using a macroscopic anatomical parcellation of the MNI MRI single-subject brain. NeuroImage. 2002;15(1):273–89.

39. Giakoumatos CI, Tandon N, Shah J, Mathew IT, Brady RO, Clementz BA, Pearlson GD, Thaker GK, Tamminga CA, Sweeney JA, et al. Are structural brain abnormalities associated with suicidal behavior in patients with psychotic disorders? J Psychiatr Res. 2013;47(10):1389–95.

40. Minzenberg MJ, Lesh TA, Niendam TA, Yoon JH, Cheng Y, Rhoades RN, Carter CS. Control-related frontal–striatal function is associated with past suicidal ideation and behavior in patients with recent-onset psychotic major mood disorders. J Affect Disord. 2015;188:202–9.

41. Osuch E, Ford K, Wrath A, Bartha R, Neufeld R. Functional MRI of pain application in youth who engaged in repetitive non-suicidal self-injury vs. psychiatric controls. Psychiatry Res. 2014;223(2):104–12.

42. Kircher TT, Brammer M, Bullmore E, Simmons A, Bartels M, David AS. The neural correlates of intentional and incidental self processing. Neuropsychologia. 2002;40(6):683–92.

43. Kjaer TW, Nowak M, Lou HC. Reflective self-awareness and conscious states: PET evidence for a common midline parietofrontal core. NeuroImage. 2002;17(2):1080–6.

44. Amft M, Bzdok D, Laird AR, Fox PT, Schilbach L, Eickhoff SB. Definition and characterization of an extended social-affective default network. Brain Struct Func. 2015;220(2):1031–49.

45. Cavanna AE, Trimble MR. The precuneus: a review of its functional anatomy and behavioural correlates. Brain. 2006;129(Pt 3):564–83.

30

Relationship of Internet gaming disorder with dissociative experience in Italian university students

Concetta De Pasquale[1*], Carmela Dinaro[2] and Federica Sciacca[1]

Abstract

The purpose of this study was twofold: (a) to investigate the prevalence of Internet gaming disorder (IGD) among Italian university students and (b) to explore the associations between the former and dissociative phenomena. The sample included 221 college students, 93 males and 128 females, aged between 18 and 25 ($M = 21.56$; SD $= 1.42$). They were asked to state their favourite games choice and were administered a demographic questionnaire, the APA symptom checklist based on the diagnostic criteria of IGD in the DSM-5, the Internet Gaming Disorder Scale Short Form (IGD9-SF) and the Italian version of dissociative experience scale for adolescents and young adults. The different game types used are distributed as follows: Massively Multiplayer Online Role-Playing Game (30%), flash games (26%), multiplayer games (24%), and online gambling (23%). The results of the study showed a high incidence of Internet gaming disorder risk in college students (84.61%). Specifically, our data confirmed the literature on the incidence of the male gender bias among online players ($M = 28.034$; SD $= 2.213$). Thirty-three subjects (31 male and 2 female) on 221 (14.9%) matched five or more criteria for clinical diagnosis of IGD. The data showed a positive correlation between Internet gaming disorder risk and some dissociative experiences: depersonalisation and derealisation (AbII/item6 $r = .311$; DD/item6 $r = .322$); absorption and imaginative involvement (AbII/item2 $r = .319$; AbII/item8 $r = .403$) and passive influence (PI/item3 $r = .304$; PI/item4 $r = .366$; PI/item9 $r = .386$). This study shedded light on psychopathological aspects that preceded the spread of IGD and encourages the implementation of a programmatic plan of preventative interventions by Italian public institutions, to prevent and tame the spreading of such addictive behaviours.

Keywords: Addiction, Dissociative experience, Young adults, Internet gaming disorder

Introduction

The online game in contemporary society is a problem that should not be underestimated. Selnow stated that video games are a sort of "electronic friend" that provide the company and satisfy the relational needs of an individual [1].

The game has been a human life's constant since the past times. Callois revised the anthropological concept of game, describing it as a free and voluntary activity, source of joy and fun that can have a negative aspect; if the game goes beyond its limits, if it loses its free character and

separated from reality, it can only produce "derived" and "corrupted" forms [2].

The widespread diffusion of technological devices has affected the gaming practices as well. Indeed, in recent times, digital and online gaming became a common form of entertainment, growing in popularity. This definition encompasses games requiring a connection, on multiple platforms and a variety of interactions with other players. Online gaming differs from its offline version in the central role given to a nonhuman entity setting out the rules and deciding upon players' state in the game. According to the last report of the Entertainment Software Association (ESA), 31% of gamers are under the age of 18 and 60% are male [3].

Massively Multiplayer Online Role-Playing Game (MMORPG), multiplayer games, flash games, and online

*Correspondence: depasqua@unict.it
[1] Department of Education Science, University of Catania, Via Teatro Greco, 84, Catania, Italy
Full list of author information is available at the end of the article

gambling (especially online poker) are the most consumed categories of games played online worldwide.

MMORPG are online role-playing games, themed mainly around fantasy narratives or conflict scenarios. They involve the creation of a digital avatar, defining its identity and appearance, and taking place in virtual worlds where players interact with each other. The multiplayer dimension is realized through the hosted connection of multiple individual machines to a server, be it consoles, personal computers or mobile devices.

Depending on the case, participation may be simultaneous, with all players in action at the same time, or asynchronous, when players' interaction is not contemporaneous.

Flash games are played directly from the browser without the need to download additional programs.

Online gambling games are digital transpositions of traditional gambling; their novelty comes from the monetary dimension attached to games, intertwined with risk and prediction of uncertain outcome.

To form a conceptual framework, it is useful to refer to Griffith [4], who suggests considering online gaming addiction in the same light as drugs and other addictive substances. Indeed, subsequent research confirmed that engrossed players' brain shares similar features with that of drug addicts.

Along this similarity, the technological addictions are characterized by the central role of a technological device in thoughts and affections of the individual, by its ability to swing mood tone towards positive and rewarding experiences [5, 6]. In more detail, the neurobiological bases of gaming addiction are similar to those of the chemicals' addiction [7, 8]. In the gaming addict, as well as in the drug addict, it is possible to notice the high levels of dopamine, norepinephrine and a high presence of endorphins [9]. Holden [10] has also verified that pathological videogames players show changes of brain activity in the limbic and frontal systems similar to those occurring in cocaine addicts, namely a significant reduction of white substance in the orbitofrontal and inferior fronto occipital area. According to recent psychiatric nosography, the Internet gaming disorder (IGD) appears in the DSM-5 in Section III as a condition that is not yet classified as a formal disorder, but requires further research and clinical investigation [11].

DSM-5 proposes nine criteria to diagnose IGD: (1) Preoccupation with Internet games: the individual thinks intensively about previous gaming activity or anticipates playing the next game as Internet gaming becomes the dominant activity in daily life; (2) Withdrawal symptoms when Internet gaming is absent (typically described as irritability, anxiety, or sadness, but there are no physical signs of pharmacological withdrawal.); (3) Tolerance:

the need to spend increasing amounts of time engaged in Internet games; (4) Unsuccessful attempts to control the participation in Internet games; (5) Loss of interests in previous hobbies and entertainment as a result of, and with the exception of, Internet games; (6) Continued excessive use of Internet games despite knowledge of psychosocial problems; (7) Has deceived family members, therapists, or others regarding the amount of Internet gaming; (8) Use of Internet games to escape or relieve a negative mood (i.e. feelings of helplessness, guilt, anxiety); (9) Has jeopardized or lost a significant relationship, job, or educational or career opportunity because of participation in Internet games.

A strand of the literature highlights the association between psychiatric disorders and Internet gaming disorder, showing a correlation between IGD, dissociation and mood disorders (depression, anxiety) [12–18].

Starting from these premises, the purpose of this study was twofold: (a) to investigate the prevalence of Internet gaming disorder (IGD) among Italian university students and (b) to explore the associations between the former and dissociative phenomena.

Materials and methods
Study sample
The sample consisted of 240 university students recruited from different departments of University of Catania (Italy) over the period from March 2017 to December 2017.

All students gave written informed consent before being included in the study.

Data were collected in two separate sessions. In the first stage, students were administered the demographic questionnaire, asked their favourite games choice, and administered the Symptom Checklist-90 Revised (SCL-90 R). Derogatis' Symptom Checklist (SCL-90R) was applied to screen for psychopathological syndromes and to seize the students' clinical level of distress. In the second stage, we conducted a diagnostic interview following the diagnostic criteria of IGD in the DSM-5 and students were administered the Internet Gaming Disorder Scale Short Form (IGD9-SF) alongside with the Italian version of dissociative experience scale for adolescents and young adults (A-DES).

The Symptom Checklist-90 Revised (SCL-90 R) [19] questionnaire shows that 19 participants display clear psychopathological conditions, such as depression and psychosis. Hence, we excluded them from the sample to avoid pollution of group-level results. The final sample of the study includes 221 college students, 93 males and 128 females, aged between 18 and 25 ($M = 21.56$; DS = 1.42). The sample was drawn from the following departments: Architecture = 6%, Education Sciences = 28%,

Engineering = 18%, Physics = 11%, Psychology = 32%, Agricultural Sciences = 5%.

Measures and procedure

The protocol we employed consists of a demographic questionnaire gaming preferences, the IGD9-SF, a diagnostic interview targeting IGD as of the DSM-5 criteria, and the Italian version of dissociative experience scale for A-DES.

The IGD9-SF [20] was a short psychometric instrument that defines the nine basic criteria according to the DSM-5 [11], developed by Orsolya Kiraly and Zsolt Demetrovics, of the Institute of Psychology Eotvos Lorand University, and Halley M. Pontes and Mark D. Griffiths, of the University of Nottingham. The answers to the nine questions composed this test are structured in a Likert scale of five points: 1 "never", 2 "rarely", 3 "sometimes", 4 "often", 5 "very often".

The IGD9-SF allowed the evaluation of the disorder severity by summing the gamers' answers. This score can range from 9 to 45, with higher scores pointing to higher degrees of gaming disorder. In addition, the scale allowed a more granular classification: we define disordered gamers as those falling in the bin from 36 to 45 points, while non-disordered gamers belong in the remaining score range, from 9 to 35 [21]. We evaluated the instrument reliability using Cronbach's alpha ($\alpha = .87$).

To diagnose the presence of IGD, we administered the APA symptom checklist containing the nine IGD criteria in "yes/no" format [21]. The disorder was diagnosed when more than five symptoms out of nine are self-reported, in line with the DSM-5 [11]. We ranked the Internet gaming disorder effects according to its disruption on normal activities, from mild, to moderate, to severe. Individuals reporting severe Internet gaming disorder spend more hours on the computer and reported losses or lack of interest in social activities.

The Italian version of dissociative experience scale for A-DES consisted of 30 questions on everyday life experiences [22]. Participants are asked to state the frequency of experiencing a specific situation (from 0 = never to 10 = always). This version was an adaptation of the one developed at the University of Arkansas [23]. The A-DES is divided into four subscales: Dissociative amnesia (DA), absorption and imaginative involvement (AbII), depersonalization and derealisation (DD), and passive influence (PI). Dissociative amnesia (DA) was characterized by one or more episodes of inability to remember important personal information, usually too relevant to be explained with ordinary forgetfulness. Absorption and imaginative involvement (AbII) concerned an involvement, leading to neglecting the surrounding environment. Depersonalization–derealisation (DD) disorder

occurred when the subject persistently or repeatedly feels as a disembodied observer of her activities or lacks confidence in the actual reality of her environment, or any combination of the former symptoms. Passive influence (PI) has been defined as the tendency to feel dispossessed of one own feelings, thought and behaviours, as if these were forcedly imposed by an external source [11].

We reported A-DES reliability using Cronbach's alpha ($\alpha = .95$). In addition, the reliability of the individual subscales was the following: DA = .76, AbII = .66, DD = .85, PI = .74, while split-half correlation is DA = .63, AbII = .48, DD = .67, PI = .57 [22].

Statistical analyses

We ran a set of statistical analyses on our data, namely t test on group differentials, factors correlation, and multivariate linear regression and instruments reliability was assessed with Cronbach's alpha. We employed SPSS 24 in this study.

Results

The descriptive analysis showed that the 73% of sample declared to be a player and use more than one type of game. The different game types used are distributed as follows: MMORPG (30%), flash games (26%), multiplayer games (24%), online gambling (23%).

The APA symptoms checklist identified that 33 out of 221 subjects reported at least 5 of the aforementioned IGD symptoms, corresponding to 14.9% of the whole sample: this subset was largely composed by men, 31 out of 33.

Our sample presented a dominant share of high scores in the IGDS9-SF test (84.61%), suggesting the presence of relevant IDG risks. The total scores in the IGD9-SF (compared with the normative cut-offs previously described in the "Measures and procedure" section) showed relevant gender differences towards gaming. In comparison with women, men showed a significantly higher risk of IGD, as shown in the last line of Table 1, which summarizes the most relevant results of the IGD risk gender differences.

Specifically, men showed significant differences in item 1 ($p = .0178$), 3 ($p = .001$) and 4 ($p = .000$) which is related to the expression of alertness and apprehension, the difficulty of controlling gaming activity and growing need to play to achieve satisfaction and pleasure.

Concerning the results obtained in A-DES, the descriptive analysis of our sample showed a significant presence ($p < .05$) of dissociative experiences in men ($M = 50.15$; SD = 35.25) resulting from the sum of the underlying subscales: AbII ($M = 14.5699$; SD = 9.65536), DD ($M = 14.8280$; SD = 13.23338), PI ($M = 9.6667$; SD = 8.18845), as shown in Table 2.

Table 1 Comparison of male and female subsamples on internet gaming disorder (IGD9-SF test)

IGD9-SF	University students ($N=221$)					
	Male		Female		t	p
	M	SD	M	SD		
1. Do you feel preoccupied with your gaming behaviour?	3.0860	.40796	3.0000	.00000	2.3870	.0178
2. Do you feel more irritability, anxiety or even sadness when you try to either reduce or stop your gaming activity?	3.0645	.35528	3.0156	.17678	1.3455	.1799
3. Do you feel the need to spend increasing amount of time engaged gaming in order to achieve satisfaction or pleasure?	3.1935	.59450	3.0156	.17678	3.1989	.0016
4. Do you systematically fail when trying to control or cease your gaming activity?	3.1613	.53751	3.0000	.00000	3.3980	.0008
5. Have you lost interests in previous hobbies and other entertainment activities as result of your engagement with the game?	3.0430	.29170	3.0156	.17678	.8664	.3872
6. Have you continued your gaming activity despite knowing it was causing problems between you and other people?	3.0430	.29170	3.0156	.17678	.8664	.3872
7. Have you deceived any of your family members, therapists or others because the amount of your gaming activity?	3.0217	.20851	3.0000	.00000	1.1785	.2399
8. Do you play in order to temporarily escape or relieve a negative mood?	3.3656	.77719	3.2188	.62667	1.5527	.1219
9. Have you jeopardized or lost an important relationship, job or an educational or career opportunity because of your gaming activity?	3.0860	.40796	3.0156	.17678	1.7413	.0830
Total score	28.034	2.2138	27.293	.7566	3.5124	.0005

IGD9-SF: Internet Gaming Disorder Scale Short Form; N: sample number; t: t test statistic; p: probability value; M: mean; SD: standard deviation

Table 2 Comparison of male and female subsamples on dissociative experience (A-DES)

A-DES	University students ($N=221$)					
	Male		Female		t	p
	M	SD	M	SD		
DA	11.0860	9.78537	8.8189	9.45534	1.7340	.0843
AbII	14.5699	9.65536	10.9375	8.36072	2.9862	.0031
DD	14.8280	13.23338	10.2756	13.37712	2.5089	.0128
PI	9.6667	8.18845	6.8898	7.11161	2.6878	.0077
Total score	50.1505	35.25927	36.9764	34.36440	2.7829	.0059

A-DES: dissociative experience scale for adolescent and young adult; N: sample number; DA: dissociative amnesia; AbII: absorption and imaginative involvement; DD: depersonalization and derealisation; PI: passive influence; t: t test statistic; p: probability value; M: mean; SD standard deviation

Table 3 reported the Pearson correlations between A-DES subscales scores and IGD9-SF test. Specifically, the increasing time spent playing, the loss of control, and daily activities impairment correlated with loss of awareness of the surrounding environment (AbII/item3 $r=.446$; AbII/item4 $r=.314$; AbII/item9 $r=.341$; DD/item9 $r=.293$), with a sense of foreignness from their feelings, thoughts and behaviours (PI/item3 $r=.304$; PI/item4 $r=.366$; PI/item9 $r=.386$) and with episodes of amnesia (DA/item3 $r=.264$; DA/item4 $r=.323$). Moreover, relational difficulties due to the game correlated significantly with experiences of depersonalisation and derealisation (AbII/item6 $r=.311$; DD/item6 $r=.322$), with episodes of dissociative amnesia up to the moments of extraneousness towards oneself (DA/item6 $r=.281$; PI/item6 $r=.277$). Absorption and imaginative involvement episodes correlate with states of anxiety, irritability and emotional fragility, when trying to reduce or stop playing (AbII/item2 $r=.319$; AbII/item8 $r=.403$). Furthermore, weaker but equally interesting correlations have been highlighted. Specifically, loss of interest in previous hobbies and other entertainment activities and the temporarily need to escape or relieve a negative mood correlated with episodes of dissociative amnesia for past or newly acquired events (DA/item5 $r=.245$; DA/item8 $r=.267$), with sense of foreignness from own feelings and behaviours and loss of awareness of the surrounding environment (AbII/item5 $r=.228$; PI/item5 $r=.271$; DD/item5 $r=.267$; PI/item8 $r=.273$).

Table 3 Correlations (Pearson r) between A-DES scores and IGD9-SF scores

A-DES	University students (N = 221)								
	IGD9-SF								
	Item 1	Item 2	Item 3	Item 4	Item 5	Item 6	Item 7	Item 8	Item 9
DA	.083	.165	.264**	.323**	.245**	.281**	.170	.267**	.299
AbII	.288**	.319**	.446**	.314**	.228**	.311**	.234**	.403**	.341**
PI	.138	.206	.304**	.366**	.271**	.277**	.151	.273**	.386**
DD	.003	.150	.164	.230**	.267**	.322**	.177	.158	.293**

N: sample number; A-DES: dissociative experience scale for adolescent and young adult; DA: dissociative amnesia; AbII: absorption and imaginative involvement; PI: passive influence; DD: depersonalization and derealisation; IGD9-SF: Internet Gaming Disorder Scale Short Form

** $p < .05$

Discussion and conclusions

This study shedded light on the high incidence of Internet gaming disorder risk in college students assessed in our research (84.61%). Specifically, our data were in line with the literature consensus on the male gender bias among online players.

Sport, physical combat competitive spirit, and the challenge are the fundamental features of online games and are, therefore, the elective choice of male students. Men are especially prone to the charm of power and sublimated conflict [24] that these kinds of games allow: it might be considered as a symbolic way to test one's skills and capacity. While many other reasons concur in the explanation of gaming addiction, it is clear that some applications make this addiction more likely.

The high significance displayed by items 1, 3, and 4 of the IGD9-SF test leads us to point out how online players misperceive their activity. In fact, what they consider central and crucial in their life is nothing more than a pastime: this misconception prevents them from realizing their drift away from other activities, as much as their enormous use of network traffic.

They do not cultivate hobbies, sports, and grow ever farther away from consolidated friendships in the actual world. These are replaced by those established online, gradually implementing a sort of oblivion from the surrounding world. Testing and showing off their personal skills is a twofold activity. On one hand, online players value it as a pleasant experience and, on the other hand, this might lead to a gradual and unconscious disconnection from reality, replaced by a fictive self that gains relevance in one's personality. This latter phenomenon eventually leads to a more fragile control over the individual's life and her self-awareness. The correlation between Internet gaming disorder risk and some dissociative experiences that emerge from our study supports this hypothesis. As shown by the correlations with items 5, 6, 8 and 9 of IGD0-SF if the immersion of the online player in the virtual world becomes predominant, it can turn into a mode of alienation, losing awareness of the surrounding environment, with disconnection from one's feelings, thoughts and behaviours and with experiences of amnesia. Vulnerable people presenting disorders of affective and emotional regulation are obviously more exposed to the risk of Internet gaming disorder, as with other addictions. These subjects are more prone to crave for increasing levels of pleasure and involvement experienced within the gaming environment, which serves a playful and cathartic function at once. Online gaming becomes a device to handle anxiety and tension generated by the existential circumstances, to cope with isolation, social withdrawal, frustration, and life dissatisfaction [25–28].

Until recently, the literature formed a growing consensus on the interactions of comorbidity (including depression, anxiety and psychopathology in general), with Internet gaming disorder risk. These factors suggestively contribute to increase the vulnerability towards a problematic use of Internet [12].

We believe that this study provides interesting insights into aspects to be addressed as the first signs of a severe psychopathological condition [29].

Based on these results, we encourage the implementation of a programmatic prevention plan by Italian public health and education institutions to anticipate and limit the spread of online gaming addiction.

The educational, healthy, use of the Web may be taught as a school subject in itself, having a strong transdisciplinary connotation.

These interventions gain their effectiveness when they spur a search for authentic, real-life experiences enriching one's identity through genuine interaction with other people, tight daily and weekly scheduling of activities. The latter permit to steer away from detrimental habits like disproportionate consumption of videogames and technological devices, like smartphones or tables. It is necessary to balance the activities of the online gaming with studying, reading and social activities.

It is important to support a preventive education that should involve family members, public institutions and the society as a whole to promote a culture of desire keeping contact with the real "principle of duty".

However, a viable psycho-pedagogical process should be modelled ad hoc for groups of young adults, with the objective of developing cognitive behavioural strategies aimed at removing those risky thoughts and actions, which prevent these individuals from operating positive changes in their life [30, 31].

Authors' contributions
CDP conceived the study, participated in its design and coordination, helped to draft the manuscript and performed the statistical analysis of the study. FS participated in the design of the study, administered the questionnaires, helped to draft the manuscript, and performed the statistical analysis of the study. CD participated in the design of the study, administered the questionnaires and helped to draft the manuscript. All authors read and approved the final manuscript.

Author details
[1] Department of Education Science, University of Catania, Via Teatro Greco, 84, Catania, Italy. [2] Drug Addiction Health Service, SER.T-ASP3 in Catania, Via Fabio, 1, Acireale (CT), Italy.

Acknowledgements
The authors gratefully thank all the university students who participated in this study.

Competing interests
The authors declare that they have no competing interests.

Consent for publication
The material was collected anonymously after obtaining the consent of the student.

References
1. Selnow GW. Playing videogames: the electronic friend. J Commun. 1984;34(2):148–56.
2. Callois R. Man play and games. Urbana: University of Illinois Press; 2001 **(translated from the French by Barash M.)**.
3. Sales, Demographic and Usage Data, Essential Facts About the Computer and Video Game Industry, ESA Entertainment Software Association. 2017. http://www.theesa.com/wp-content/uploads/2017/04/EF2017_FinalDigital.pdf. Accessed Apr 2017.
4. Griffiths MD. Technological addiction, vol. 76., Clinical psychology forum 1995. p. 14–9.
5. Gross JJ, Yip SW, Ma SS, Shi XH, Liu L, et al. Is neural processing of negative stimuli altered in addiction independent of drug effects? Findings from drug-naïve youth with internet gaming disorder. Neuropsychopharmacology. 2018;43(6):1364–72. https://doi.org/10.1038/npp.2017.283.
6. Yen JY, Ko CH, Yen CF, Chen SH, Chung WL, Chen CC. Psychiatric symptoms in adolescents with Internet addiction: comparison with substance use. Psychiatry Clin Neurosci. 2008;62(1):9–16.
7. Dong G, Zhou H, Zhao X. Impulse inhibition in people with Internet addiction disorder: electrophysiological evidence from a Go/NoGo study. Neurosci Lett. 2010;485(2):138–42. https://doi.org/10.1016/j.neulet.2010.09.002.
8. Han DH, Bolo N, Daniels MA, Arenella L, Lyoo IK, Renshaw PF. Brain activity and desire for internet video game play. Compr Psychiatry. 2011;52(1):88–95. https://doi.org/10.1016/j.comppsych.2010.04.004.
9. Volkow ND, Wang GJ, Fowler JS, Tomasi D, Telang F. Addiction: beyond dopamine reward circuitry. Proc Natl Acad Sci USA. 2011;108(37):15037–42. https://doi.org/10.1073/pnas.1010654108.
10. Holden C. Behavioral addictions: do they exist? Science. 2001;294(5544):980–2. https://doi.org/10.1126/science.294.5544.980.
11. American Psychiatric Association. Diagnostic and statistical manual of mental disorders. 5th ed. Washington, DC: American Psychiatric Press; 2013.
12. Bernardi S, Pallanti S. Internet addiction: a descriptive clinical study focusing on comorbidities and dissociative symptoms. Compr Psychiatry. 2009;50(6):510–6.
13. Ha JH, Yoo HJ, Cho IH, Chin B, Shin D, Kim JH. Psychiatric comorbidity assessed in Korean children and adolescents who screen positive for Internet addiction. J Clin Psychiatry. 2006;67(5):821–6.
14. Kim K, Ryu E, Chon MY, Yeun EJ, Choi SY, Seo JS, et al. Internet addiction in Korean adolescents and its relation to depression and suicidal ideation: a questionnaire survey. Int J Nurs Stud. 2006;43(2):185–92.
15. Yen JY, Ko CH, Yen CF, Wu HY, Yang MJ. The comorbid psychiatric symptoms of Internet addiction: attention deficit and hyperactivity disorder [ADHD], depression, social phobia, and hostility. J Adolesc Health. 2007;41(1):93–8.
16. Choi K, Son H, Park M, Han J, Kim K, Lee B, et al. Internet overuse and excessive daytime sleepiness in adolescents. Psychiatry Clin Neurosci. 2009;63(4):455–62.
17. De Berardis D, D'Albenzio A, Gambi F, Sepede G, Valchera A, Conti CM, et al. Alexithymia and its relationships with dissociative experiences and Internet addiction in a nonclinical sample. Cyberpsychol Behav. 2009;12(1):67–9.
18. Shepherd RM, Edelmann RJ. Reasons for Internet use and social anxiety. Pers Individ Diff. 2005;39(5):949–58.
19. Derogatis LR, Unger R. Symptom checklist-90-revised. Corsini Encyclopedia of Psychology. New Jersey: Wiley; 2010. p. 1–2. https://doi.org/10.1002/9780470479216.corpsy0970.
20. Pontes HM, Griffiths MD. Measuring DSM-5 Internet gaming disorder: development and validation of a short psychometric scale. Comput Hum Behav. 2015;4(5):137–43.
21. Ko CH, Yen JY, Wang PW, Chen CS, Yen CF. Corrigendum to "Evaluation of the diagnostic criteria of Internet gaming disorder in the DSM-5 among young adults in Taiwan". J Psychiatr Res. 2014;57:185.
22. De Pasquale C, Sciacca F, Hichy Z. Validation of the italian version of the dissociative experience scale for adolescents and young adults. Ann Gen Psychiatry. 2016;15:31.
23. Bernstein EM, Putnam FW. Development, reliability, and validity of a dissociation scale. J Nerv Ment Dis. 1986;174(12):727–35.
24. Kuss DJ, Griffiths MD, Karila L, Billieux J. Internet addiction: a systematic review of epidemiological research for the last decade. Curr Pharm Des. 2014;20(25):4026–52.
25. Li D, Liau A, Khoo A. Examining the influence of actual-ideal self-discrepancies, depression, and escapism, on pathological gaming among massively multiplayer online adolescent gamers. Cyberpsychol Behav Soc Netw. 2011;14(9):535–9.
26. Grüsser SM, Thalemann R, Griffiths MD. Excessive computer game playing: evidence for addiction and aggression? Cyberpsychol Behav. 2007;10(2):290–2.
27. Vorderer P, Bryant J. Playing video games: motives, responses, and consequences. Mahwah: Lawrence Erlbaum Associates Publishers; 2006. p. 480.
28. Fornaro M, Ventriglio A, De Pasquale C, Pistorio ML, De Berardis D, Cattaneo CI, et al. Sensation seeking in major depressive patients: relationship to sub-threshold bipolarity and cyclothymic temperament. J Affect Disord. 2013;148(2–3):375–83.
29. Müller KW, Janikian M, Dreier M, Wölfling K, Beutel ME, Tzavara C, Richardson C, Tsitsika A. Regular gaming behavior and internet gaming disorder in European adolescents: results from a cross-national representative survey of prevalence, predictors, and psychopathological correlates. Eur Child Adolesc Psychiatry. 2015;24(5):565–74. https://doi.org/10.1007/s00787-014-0611-2.
30. King DL, Delfabbro PH, Doh YY, Wu AMS, Kuss DJ, Pallesen S, et al. Policy and prevention approaches for disordered and hazardous gaming and internet use: an international perspective. Prev Sci. 2018;19(2):233–49. https://doi.org/10.1007/s11121-017-0813-1.
31. Bonnaire C, Phan O. Negative perceptions of the risks associated with gaming in young adolescents: an exploratory study to help thinking about a prevention program. Arch Pediatr. 2017;24(7):607–17. https://doi.org/10.1016/j.arcped.2017.04.006.

31

Prevalence and associated factors of depression among patients with HIV/AIDS in Hawassa, Ethiopia

Bereket Duko[1]* ⓘ, Epherem Geja[1], Mahlet Zewude[2] and Semere Mekonen[2]

Abstract

Background: Globally, 350 million people are affected by depression and 800,000 people die due to suicide every year due to depression. People living with HIV/AIDS face different challenges, including HIV-related perceived stigma, lack of social support and also depression. This study aimed to assess prevalence and factors associated with depressive symptom among people living with HIV/AIDS attending Hawassa University Comprehensive Specialized Hospital, Hawassa, Ethiopia.

Methods: Hospital-based cross-sectional study was implemented in 2016. A total of 401 HIV-positive patients who had regular visit at Hawassa University Comprehensive Specialized Hospital, Hawassa, Ethiopia were included in the study. Systematic random sampling technique was used to recruit study participants. Patient Health Questionnaire item nine (PHQ-9) was used to assess depressive symptoms. In addition to this, Oslo social support scale and HIV perceived stigma scale were used to assess social support and HIV-related perceived stigma, respectively.

Results: A total of 401 study participants were included in the study, giving a response rate of 96.2%. The mean age of the respondents was 38 years (SD ± 10.23). This study revealed that 48.6% of HIV-positive patients had depression. Patients who had poor social support [AOR = 2.53, (95% CI 1.70, 9.13)], HIV-related perceived stigma [AOR = 2.83, (95% CI 1.78, 4.48)] and CD4 cell count < 200 [AOR = 3.89, (95% CI 1.02, 14.83)] were more likely to have depression as compared to individuals who had good social support, no perceived HIV stigma and CD4 cell count > 200, respectively.

Conclusion: Having poor social support, HIV-related perceived stigma and low CD4 cell count (< 200) had statistically significant association with depressive symptom. Training of health workers in ART clinics and availing manuals on assessing mental health issues is useful to screen and treat depression among HIV patients.

Keywords: Depressive symptom, Perceived stigma, Social support, HIV, Ethiopia, Prevalence, Associated factors, Depression, Hawassa, South Ethiopia

Background

HIV/AIDS is one of a chronic disease which affects human immune systems and it increases vulnerability to infections and other immunological disorders [1]. Globally, different studies in 2013 revealed that an estimated 35 million people were living with HIV/AIDS, of which 24.7 million are living in Sub-Saharan Africa and 1.6 million people died related to HIV/AIDS [2]. In developing countries, 9.5 million people were receiving HIV treatment in 2012 [3].

According to the WHO 2015 report, 350 million people were affected by depression worldwide. Due to this problem, over 800,000 people die by suicide every year globally [4]. WHO estimated that the incidence of suicide related to depression will reach approximately 1.53 million people by the year 2020. Based on finding from general population study, the life-time risk of depression is one in five women and one in ten men in their lifetime [5].

*Correspondence: berkole.dad@gmail.com
[1] Faculty of Health Sciences, College of Medicine and Health Sciences, Hawassa University, P. O. Box 1560, Hawassa, Ethiopia
Full list of author information is available at the end of the article

Findings from different studies show that 121 million people living with HIV/ADIS are affected by depression globally [6]. Studies conducted in different countries on prevalence of depression among HIV patients showed 58.75% in Delhi (India) [7], 29.4% in Brazil [8], 54.4% in Italy [9], 37% in United States [10], 25.4% in South Africa [6, 11], 25.3% of women and 31.4% of men in Botswana [12], 47% in Uganda [13], 43.9% in Mekele, Ethiopia [14], 45.8% in Harar, Ethiopia [15] and 38.94% in Debrebirhan, Ethiopia [16].

Depressive symptom among HIV-positive clients is associated with low income, widowed, being female, non-adherence of ART, having frequent of schedule for clinical visit in a month, low educational status, being female, age category (40–49), and having stage III and Stage IV HIV-related symptom [16, 17].

Being mentally impaired has been linked with an impaired adherence to ART and poor treatment outcome, decrease in CD4 count and increase in viral load. In addition, depression has been associated with high-risk behaviors like engaging in unsafe sex [11, 15, 17].

Based on different study findings, the magnitude of depressive symptom among people living with HIV/AIDS is high. Though it has a great impact on their treatment outcome, it was not assessed at Hawassa University Comprehensive Specialized Hospital. Therefore, this study aims to assess the prevalence and factors of depressive symptom among people living with HIV attending Hawassa University Comprehensive Specialized Hospital, ART clinic, South Ethiopia.

Methods
Study setting and population
Hospital-based cross-sectional study design was implemented from April to May 2016 at Hawassa University Comprehensive Specialized Hospital, Hawassa, Ethiopia. Among 1440 HIV patients who had regular follow-up at ART clinics, 417 study participants were recruited for the study; those unable to communicate because of their illness and those who need intensive care were excluded from the study. Study participants were included using systematic random sampling technique, $K = 3$. Sixteen patients were refused to participate in the study.

Data collection
Trained and experienced nurses had collected the data using pretested interviewer administered questionnaire. The data collection tool includes socio-demographic characteristics (age, education, occupation, marital status and others). Oslo 3-item social support scale has the sum score scale ranging from 3 to 14 with three broad categories: "poor support" 3–8, "moderate support" 9–11 and

"strong support" 12–14 [18]. It was reliable in our study (Cronbach's $\alpha = 0.88$). HIV-related perceived stigma was collected by an 11-item HIV stigma scale. It consisted of four-point Likert scale (strongly disagree, disagree, agree, strongly agree) questions concerning perceived isolation, shame, guilt and disclosure of the HIV status. The item scores of the stigma questions were summed to construct a single stigma variable. Our study participants were classified as having or not having perceived stigma using the mean of the stigma variable as cutoff point [19, 20]. The instrument was adopted and translated to Amharic language and back to English and highly reliable in the study (Cronbach's $\alpha = 0.92$). The presence of depression was assessed by patient health questionnaires item nine (PHQ-9). It is a 9-item questionnaire, commonly used to screen for symptoms of depression in primary health care and in outpatients and validated in Ethiopia with sensitivity $= 86\%$ and specificity $= 67\%$. The scales use a cutoff score for depression of greater than or equal to 5 [21].

Data processing and analyses
SPSS version 20 was used to analyze the data. The association of each independent variable with the outcome variable was seen by bivariate analysis. In order to identify potential confounders, binary logistic regression model was used. A p value of less than 0.05 was considered statistically significant and adjusted odds ratio with 95% CI was calculated to determine association.

Results
Socio-demographic characteristics of the study participants
A total of 401 study participants were included in the study, giving a response rate of 96.2%. The mean ($\pm SD$) age of the respondents was 38 years (± 10.228). Among the study participants, 149 (38.9%) were in age range between 35 and 44 years, 193 (50.4%) were orthodox religion followers, 178 (46.5%) were married, 138 (36%) were attended primary education, 96 (25.1%) were house wife, and 340 (88.8%) were living in urban. The median monthly income of the respondents was 875 Ethiopian birr (31.45 USD) (Table 1).

Clinical and psychosocial characteristics of the study participants
Among respondents, the maximum CD4 cell count was 1622 with a mean of 541.08. 330 (86.2%) of the study participants had CD4 cell counts ranges between 200 and 1000. 357, (93.2%) of respondents were on ART, 162 (42.3%) were found in stage II HIV/AIDS, 259 (67.6%) had poor social support, 168 (43.9%) had perceived stigma and 72 (18.8%) were current substance (khat, alcohol, cigarette) users (Table 2).

Table 1 Distribution of people living with HIV/AIDS at Hawassa University Comprehensive Specialized Hospital, Hawassa, Ethiopia, 2016/2017

Characteristics	Category	Frequency	Percent (%)
Sex	Male	129	29
	Female	272	71
Age	18–34	141	36.8
	35–44	149	38.9
	45–54	62	16.2
	>54	31	8.1
Residence	Urban	340	88.8
	Rural	43	11.2
Religion	Protestant	160	41.8
	Orthodox	193	50.4
	Muslim	29	7.6
Educational level	Unable to write and read	68	17.8
	Primary education (grade 1–8)	138	36
	Secondary education (grade 9–12)	110	28.7
	Tertiary education (college and above)	67	17.5
Ethnicity	Sidama	48	12.5
	Oromo	88	23.0
	Amhara	93	24.3
	Wolaita	102	26.6
	Gurage	32	8.4
	Other	20	5.2
Marital status	Single	69	18.0
	Married	178	46.5
	Separated	19	5.0
	Divorced	45	11.7
	Widowed/widower	72	18.8
Occupation status	Merchant	76	19.8
	Government employee	65	17.0
	Privet employee	71	18.5
	Day laborer	33	8.6
	Student	17	4.4
	House wife	96	25.1
	Jobless	25	6.5
Monthly income	<735ETB per month	199	52.0
	735–1176ETBper month	49	12.8
	>1176ETB per month	135	35.2

Prevalence of depressive symptom among the study participants

Depressive symptom was found using PHQ-9 scale. Based on the cutoff point ≥ 11, 48.6% of the HIV clients had depression.

Factors associated with depressive Symptoms

Binary logistic regression analysis revealed that poor social support, CD4 count (<200) and perceived HIV stigma were associated with depressive symptom (Table 3).

Discussion

Institution-based cross-sectional study was conducted to assess the prevalence and factors associated with depression among patients HIV/AIDS at Hawassa University Comprehensive specialized hospital using PHQ9. The finding of this study (48.6%) was higher than studies in rural South Africa 42.4% [6, 11], in Malawi 18.9% [22], and in Ethiopia 43.9%, 45.8%, 38.94% in Mekele, Harar and Debreberihan, respectively [14–16]. On the other side, the study finding was lower than studies done in Delhi (India) 58.75% [7], North Central Nigeria 56.7%

Table 2 Description of clinical and psychosocial factors among people living with HIV/AIDS at Hawassa University Comprehensive Specialized Hospital, Hawassa, Ethiopia, 2016/2017

Variables	Category	Frequency	Percent %
CD4 cell count	< 200	33	8.6
	200–1000	330	86.2
	≥ 1000	20	5.2
Started ART taking	Yes	357	93.2
	No	26	6.8
Perceived stigma	Yes	168	43.9
	No	215	56.1
Current substance	Yes	72	18.8
	No	311	81.2
HIV/AIDS stages	Stage I	150	39.2
	Stage II	162	42.3
	Stage III	58	15.1
	Stage IV	13	3.4
Social support	Poor social support	259	67.6
	Moderate social support	110	28.7
	Strong social support	14	3.7

[23], in Cameroon 63% [24] and in Ethiopia [25]. The difference might be related to study design, data collection tool, sample size and study participant's variation.

HIV-related perceived stigma had significant association with depressive symptom. The finding is similar to the study done in Botswana [12], in Ethiopia [14–16, 25]. Having HIV, which is one of the chronic life-long diseases and which is prone to high levels of stigma, they may find it easier to be alone to avoid stigma or discrimination, or they may not have the energy to be socially engaged [26].

Clients who had poor social support were 2.5 times more likely to have depressive symptom when compared to clients who had strong social support (AOR = 2.53, 95% CI 1.70, 9.13). The finding was similar to the study conducted in Delhi (India) [7], in Nigeria in 2008 [27], and in North Central Nigeria in 2013 [23]. This might be due to the fact that social isolation reduces social support, which can have a negative impact on mental and physical well-being [28].

Individuals who had < 200 CD4 cell count had significant association with depressive symptom. This was similar to the study conducted in Malawi [22], and Debrebirhan, Ethiopia [16]. This might be due to severe immune depression and HIV illness is underlining causes of depression [29].

Table 3 Factors associated with depression among people living with HIV/AIDS at Hawassa University Comprehensive Specialized Hospital, Hawassa, Ethiopia, 2016/2017

Characteristics	Depression Yes	Depression No	COR (95% CI)	AOR (95% CI)
Sex				
Female	140	132	1.49 (0.96, 2.34)	1.44 (0.82, 2.52)
Male	46	65	1	1
Age				
18–34	74	67	1.34 (0.61, 2.92)	1.31 (0.51,3.38)
35–44	62	87	0.86 (0.397, 1.885)	0.86 (0.34,2.14)
45–54	36	26	1.68 (0.71, 4.01)	1.59 (0.61, 4.18)
>54	14	17	1	1
Educational level				
Unable to read and write	34	34	1.23 (0.63, 2.43)	
Primary education	74	64	1.43 (0.79, 2.26)	
Secondary education	48	62	0.96 (0.52, 1.76)	
Tertiary education	30	37	1	1
Marital status				
Married	88	90	1.52 (0.86, 2.67)	1.76 (0.89, 3.46)
Separated	7	12	0.91 (0.32, 2.59)	0.83 (0.24,2.87)
Divorced	22	23	1.48 (0.69, 3.17)	1.28 (0.52, 3.15)
Widowed/widower	42	30	2.17 (1.11, 4.27)	1.78 (0.72,4.38)
Single	27	42	1	1
Monthly income				
<735 ETB	105	94	1.67 (1.07, 2.60)	1.60 (0.95, 2.68)
735–1176	27	22	1.84 (0.95, 3.56)	1.40 (0.67,2.95)
>1176	54	81	1	1
Substance use				
Yes	37	35	1.13 (0.68,1.92)	
No	149	162	1	1
ART taking				
Yes	173	184	0.940 (0.42, 2.08)	
No	13	13	1	1
HIV/AIDS stages				
Stage II	74	88	0.94 (0.59, 1.46)	0.77 (0.46, 1.29)
Stage III	31	27	1.27 (0.69, 2.35)	1.02 (0.49, 2.10)
Stage IV	10	3	3.71 (0.98, 14.02)	2.79 (0.64, 12.09)
Stage I	71	79	1	1
Perceived stigma				
Yes	108	60	3.16 (2.08, 4.82)	2.83 (1.78, 4.48)**
No	78	137	1	1
Social support				
Poor	104	155	1.21 (0.39, 3.71)	2.53 (1.70, 9.13)**
Moderate	77	33	4.20 (1.31,13.48)	7.09 (1.91, 26.29)*
Strong	5	9	1	1

Table 3 (continued)

Characteristics	Depression		COR (95% CI)	AOR (95% CI)
	Yes	No		
CD4				
< 200	23	10	2.30 (0.73, 7.25)	3.89 (1.02, 14.83)*
200–1000	153	177	0.86 (0.35, 2.13)	1.27 (0.47, 3.47)
≥ 1000	10	10	1	*1*

Depression (Yes)-PHQ ≥ 11, * significant association (*p*-value < 0.05) ** significant association (*p*-value < 0.01)

Italic values represent references of the variable

Unlike other study, being female sex, being divorced and unmarried and those using substance had no statistically significant association with depression.

Conclusion

Depressive symptom was high (48.6%) among the current study population. Perceived HIV-related stigma, poor social support and CD4 count (< 200) had significant association with depressive symptom. Hence, depression is highly prevalent among HIV-positive patients, still underdiagnosed and undertreated but it needs further research. Therefore, Ministry of Health should give more emphasis to those clients with depressive symptoms. Further research on risk factors of depression should be conducted to strengthen and broaden the current findings.

Limitation of the study

We did not do detailed validation study for perceived HIV-related stigma scale and Oslo 3-item social support scale.

Authors' contributions
BD conceived the study and was involved in the study design, reviewed the article, analysis, report writing and drafted the manuscript. EG, MZ and SM were involved in the study design and analysis. All authors read and approved the final manuscript.

Author details
[1] Faculty of Health Sciences, College of Medicine and Health Sciences, Hawassa University, P. O. Box 1560, Hawassa, Ethiopia. [2] Hawassa University Comprehensive Specialized Hospital, Hawassa University, Hawassa, Ethiopia.

Acknowledgements
The authors appreciate the respective study institution for their help and the study participants for their cooperation in providing all necessary information.

Competing interests
The authors declare that they have no competing interests.

Consent for publication
Not applicable.

University. Permission letter was obtained and submitted to Hawassa University Comprehensive Specialized Hospital. Study participants were informed about their rights to interrupt the interview at any time and written informed consent was obtained from each study participants. Confidentiality was maintained at all levels of the study. HIV-positive subjects who were found to have moderate to severe depressive symptoms had poor social support and perceived HIV-related stigma was referred to psychiatry clinics for further investigations.

Funding
No funding source.

References
1. WHO. HIV/AIDS and mental health. Geneva: Switzerland; 2008.
2. United Nation Aquired Immunodefeciency Syndrom (UNAIDS). The global AIDS epidemic. Geneva: UNAIDS; 2013.
3. United Nation. The millennium development goals report. New York: Nations EaSAotU; 2014.
4. WHO. 2012. http://www.who.int/mental_health/management/depression/who_paper_depression_wfm.
5. WHO. 2012 https://www.who.int/mental_health/suicide-prevention/en/.
6. Pappin M, Edwin Wouters E, Booysen F. Anxiety and depression amongst patients enrolled in a public sector anti retroviral treatment programme in South Africa: a cross-sectional study. BMC Public Health. 2012;12:244.
7. Bhatia MS, Munjal S. Prevalence of depression in people living with HIV/AIDS undergoing ART and factors associated with it. J Clin Diagn Res Jcdr. 2014;8:WC01.
8. Castrighini C, Gir E, Neves L, Reis R, Galva ˜o M, Hayashido M. Depression and self-esteem of patients positive for HIV/AIDS in an inland city of Brazil. Retro Virol. 2010;7:P66.
9. Goulet JL, Molde S, Constantino SJ, Gaughan D, Selwyn PA. Psychiatric comorbidity and the long-term care of people with aids. J Urban Health. 2000;77(2):213–21.
10. Asch SM, Kilbourne AM, Gifford AL, et al. Underdiagnosis of depression in hiv: who are we missing? J Gen Intern Med. 2003;18(6):450–60.
11. Prince M, Patel V, Saxena S, Maj M, Maselko J, et al. No health without mental health. Lancet. 2007;370:859–77.
12. Gupta R, Dandu M, Packel L, Rutherford G, Leiter K, Phaladze N, et al. Depression and HIV in Botswana: a population-based study on gender-specific socio economic and behavioral correlates. PLoS ONE. 2010;5:e14252.
13. Kaharuza FM, Bunnell R, Moss S, Purcell DW, Bikaako-Kajura W, et al. Depression and CD4 cell count among persons with HIV infection in Uganda. AIDS Behav. 2006;10:105–11.
14. Berhe H, Bayray A. Prevalence of depression and associated factors among people living with HIV/AIDSI in Tigray, Ethiopia. North Ethiopia: a cross sectional hospital based study. IJPSR. 2013;4(2):765–75.
15. Mohammed M, Mengistie B, Dessie Y, Godana W. Prevalence of depression and associated factors among HIV patients seeking treatments in ART clinics at Harar Town, Eastern Ethiopia. J AIDS Clin Res. 2015;6:474.
16. Eshetu DA, Woldeyohannes SM, Alemayehu M, Techane GN, Tegegne MT, Dagne K. Prevalence of depression and associated factors among HIV/AIDS Patients attending ART Clinic at Debrebirhan referral hospital, North Showa, Amhara Region, Ethiopia. Am J Community Psychol. 2014;2(6):101–8.
17. Berg CJ, Michelson SE, Safren SA. Behavioral aspects of HIV care: adherence, depression, substance use, and HIV transmission behaviors. Infect Dis Clin North Am. 2007;21(1):181–200.
18. Dalgard OS, Dowrick C, Lehtinen V, Vazquez-Barquero JL, Casey P, Wilkinson G, et al. Negative life events, social support and gender difference in depression. Soc Psychiatry Psychiatr Epidemiol. 2006;41(6):444–51.
19. Van Rie A, Sengupta S, Pungrassami P, Balthip Q, Choonuan S, Kasetjaroen Y, et al. Measuring stigma associated with tuberculosis and HIV/AIDS in southern Thailand: exploratory and confirmatory factor analyses of two new scales. Trop Med Int Health. 2008;13(1):21–30.
20. Franke MF, Muñoz M, Finnegan K, Zeladita J, Sebastian JL, Bayona JN, Shin SS. Validation and abbreviation of an HIV stigma scale in an adult spanish-speaking population in urban Peru. AIDS Behav. 2010;14:189–99.
21. Gelaye B, Williams MA, Lemma S, et al. Validity of the patient health questionnaire-9 for depression screening and diagnosis in East Africa. Psychiatry Res. 2013;210(2):653–61.
22. Kim MH, Mazenga AC, Yu X, Devandra A, Nguyen C, Ahmed S, Kazembe PN, Sharp C. Factors associated with depression among adolescents living with HIV in Malawi. BMC Psychiatry. 2015;15(1):264.
23. Shittu RO, et al. Prevalence and correlates of depressive disorders among people living with HIV/AIDS, in North Central Nigeria. J AIDS Clin Res. 2013;4:251.

24. L'akoa RM, Noubiap JJ, Fang Y, Ntone FE, Kuaban C. Prevalence and correlates of depressive symptoms in HIV-positive patients: a cross-sectional study among newly diagnosed patients in Yaoundé, Cameroon. BMC psychiatry 2013;13:228

25. Endeshaw MM. Stigma: a contributing factor to depressive symptoms in people with HIV seeking Treatment at Gondar University Hospital, Master's thesis, 2012. https://digital.lib.washington.edu/researchworks/bitstream/handle/1773/20694/Endeshaw_washington_0250O_10536.pdf?sequence=1&isAllowed=n

26. Wallach I, Brotman S. Ageing with HIV/AIDS: a scoping study among people aged 50 and over living in Quebec. Ageing Soc. 2013;33:1212–42.

27. Sale S, Gadanya M. Prevalence and factors associated with depression in HIV/AIDS patients aged 15–25 years at Aminu Kano Teaching Hospital, Nigeria. J Child Adolesc Ment Health. 2008;20:95–9.

28. Greysen SR, Horwitz LI, Covinsky KE, et al. Does social isolation predict hospitalization and mortality among HIVь and uninfected older veterans? J Am Geriatr Soc. 2013;61:1456–63.

29. Freeman M, Nkomo N, Kafaar Z, Kelly K. Factors associated with prevalence of mental disorder in people living with HIV/AIDS in South Africa. AIDS Care. 2007;19:1201–9.

32

Variation in admission rates between psychiatrists on call in a university teaching hospital

Jay Moss[1]*[ID], Dippy Nauranga[1], Doyoung Kim[2], Michael Rosen[2], Karen Wang[1] and Krista Lanctot[1,2]

Abstract

Background: Hospital-based physicians must routinely decide whether patients receiving care in the emergency room require admission to an acute care bed. We endeavoured to understand clinician-related factors that influence the decision to admit.

Methods: We retrospectively examined data collected between August 1, 2013 and July 31, 2015 for patients triaged as mental health assessments in the emergency department of a university teaching hospital. We identified 1530 unique cases who had been reviewed by the staff psychiatrist for a decision on whether to admit to an acute care bed. Patient and physician characteristics were analyzed by standard descriptive methods, comparative statistics (Chi square and analysis of variance) and regression analyses using SPSS version 24.0 (IBM Corp. Armonk, NY, USA).

Results: There were no differences in patient characteristics in the clinical encounters reviewed by different staff psychiatrists. The physician factor found significant in deciding whether to admit the patient was assignment to PES (psychiatric emergency services). This appeared to be the only physician variable impacting the decision to admit a patient with PES psychiatrists admitting less often than their colleagues ($p = 0.018$, Table 3). The effect size of the variable in terms of odds ratio was 0.592.

Interpretation: Training and practice in emergency psychiatry lead to lower admission rates when these clinicians are on call. Training in emergency psychiatry for all psychiatrists participating in a call pool may result in lowered admission rates.

Background

The decision to admit a patient from a teaching hospital emergency department is generally at the discretion of the consultant specialist following a referral from the emergency room (ER) physician. The patient is usually first assessed by the specialty resident on call before reviewing the patient with the specialty consultant on call. This arrangement is fairly standard across North American teaching hospitals with some variation at different locations. For the most part, the decision to admit a patient to hospital is at the discretion of the specialist consultant with input from the resident.

Previous studies looking at admissions to psychiatry have examined patient factors that tend to predict admission. These factors include, but are not limited to, elevated suicide risk, specific diagnosis (schizophrenia and affective disorders) and a history of poor impulse control reflected in suicide attempts, self-harm behaviours, and substance abuse [1, 2]. External and service factors that may influence disposition such as timeliness of access to community-based treatments also influence the decision to admit [3]. There have also been efforts to study the decision-making process that determines whether a patient is admitted to psychiatry.

The psychiatric emergency service (PES) has evolved over the past 25 years as a dedicated program embedded in the emergency rooms of many North American teaching hospitals. The psychiatry resident training program at

*Correspondence: jay.moss@sunnybrook.ca
[1] Department of Psychiatry, Sunnybrook Health Sciences Centre, Toronto, Canada
Full list of author information is available at the end of the article

the University of Toronto requires every second year psychiatry resident to complete a 5 weeks rotation on a PES. The rotation combines supervised clinical encounters with PES staff i n addition to didactic and small group l earning in emergency psychiatry. Psychiatry residents are required to participate in on-call duties over the course of their 5 years residency. This training model has been evaluated by resident performance in clinical and examination settings as well as the acquisition of core competencies considered essential in the emergency psychiatry setting.

There is general consensus that the decision-making process is complex with variability between psychiatrists depending on what clinical criteria are applied in arriving at the decision to admit [4, 5]. There have been few studies examining inter-rater reliability between PES providers and disposition decisions. Consensus between clinicians on the decision to admit was found to be poor [6]. One possible factor that may contribute to this variability is clinician experience. In support of this, an educational program offered to second year psychiatry residents was effective in reducing admission to the level of more senior residents [7]. However, other factors contributing to the decision to admit have not been elucidated.

We performed a retrospective review of admissions to psychiatry by on-call staff at a large university affiliated general hospital to determine whether there were differences in rates of admission between staff psychiatrists with the goal of identifying factors associated with these differences.

Setting

Sunnybrook Health Sciences Centre is a large teaching hospital affiliated with the University of Toronto located in Toronto, Ontario, Canada with identified priority programs in a number of clinical areas including Brain Sciences. The emergency department provides triage and clinical assessment by the ER physician for all patients. The ER physician decides whether to refer the patient to the PES for urgent assessment. During weekday hours (8:30 a.m. to 4:30 p.m.), there is a dedicated PES team comprised of an RN, psychiatry resident, and staff psychiatrist. Outside of these hours, the PES RN is available until 11:00 p.m. with the on-call psychiatry resident and staff psychiatrist (most of whom do not work in PES) providing overnight and weekend coverage. The ER physician may refer to the PES RN for advice on management and disposition. Alternatively, the ER physician may refer the patient to the psychiatry resident on call who will assess the patient and then review (usually by phone) with the psychiatry staff on call who then decides whether the patient is admitted to psychiatry. All departmental staff psychiatrists working greater or equal to 0.6

full-time equivalents are required to participate in call. Of the 32 staff psychiatrists participating in the call pool, 4 were members of the PES team and shared weekday coverage allocated by a dedicated schedule.

Method

We retrospectively collected data from the period between August 1, 2013 and July 31, 2015. During this period, there were a total of 115,050 patient visits registered in the emergency department. From this total, 6428 (5.6%) were triaged as "Mental Health Assessment".

Following an examination by the ER physician, 778 (12%) of these patients were referred to the PES RN who met with the patient and reviewed their findings and recommendations with the ER physician before discharge. The ER physicians referred 1574 (25%) for a consultation with the on-call psychiatry resident. The patients seen by the psychiatry resident were either admitted to psychiatry or discharged. In general, the ER physician would refer high risk and complex patients to the on-call psychiatry resident. At the time of referral, the patient may be voluntary or detained under the Mental Health Act (MHA) of Ontario for a psychiatric assessment. Voluntary patients may choose to leave the hospital before the psychiatric assessment is completed. Upon completion of the assessment, patient disposition options include discharge from the ER (often with outpatient follow-up), admission to the acute psychiatry inpatient unit as a voluntary patient or admission as an involuntary patient. The focus for this study w as the binary outcome of admission or non-admission and we did not account for voluntary or involuntary status. Out of the 1574 referrals, encounters were excluded if there was no staff psychiatrist identified, the patient was reviewed by a staff psychiatrist who saw a very minimal number of patients (defined as < 8 patients during the study season), or the encounter resulted in an admission other than the psychiatric inpatient unit such as a surgical unit or the critical care unit (CCU). All other encounters were included in the database.

Towards the end of the study period, a survey of call experience was circulated to all psychiatrists participating in the call pool. Each psychiatrist received a survey the day following call and was asked to consider their most recent call experience. The survey enlisted a Likert scale to quantify subjective perceptions of confidence levels and opportunities for learning while on call. Anchor points ranged from 1 (strongly disagree) to 5 (strongly agree). Twenty-eight of 31 (90%) psychiatrists completed the survey.

Statistical analysis

Analysis of data was completed by standard descriptive methods, comparative statistics (Chi square and analysis of variance, ANOVA) and regression analyses using SPSS version 24.0 (IBM Corp. Armonk, NY, USA). Patient and clinician factors in those admitted versus not were compared using the Pearson Chi squared test for categorical variables and ANOVA for continuous variables to identify factors significantly associated with admission to psychiatry.

Patient factors collected included sex, age, age category [youth (ages 14–21 inclusive), general or geriatric (65 and older)], multiple visits during the study timeframe and previous admission experience within the study timeframe. Patient diagnosis categories were based on International Classification of Disease (ICD-10-CM) and included dementia, delirium, substance-related disorders, schizophrenic and other psychotic disorders, bipolar and related disorders, depression, anxiety, obsessive compulsive and related disorders, trauma and stress related disorders, dissociative disorders, somatic disorders, eating disorders, personality disorders, neurodevelopmental disorders and other miscellaneous diagnoses. Clinician characteristics observed were affiliation with age related division (youth, geriatric, or general), gender, practice in a specialty (psycho-oncology, mood and anxiety disorders, consultation liaison, psychiatric emergency services, and women's mental health) versus general psychiatry, years of practice, and primary type of care practice (inpatient or outpatient). Another Pearson Chi squared test was performed to compare the disposition of the groups of those with specialty match (i.e., youth patients seen by youth specialties, and geriatric patients by geriatric specialties) and those who were not matched.

Informed by the comparative statistics, we looked at the four significantly different physician factors plus two factors from the survey results (perceived competency while on-call survey scores [1 strongly disagree to 5 strongly agree] and opportunities for learning, while on-call survey scores [1 strongly disagree to 5 strongly agree]) completed by the physicians to assess their impact on admissions while controlling for significant patient factors determined from the previous comparative statistics. This was completed using multivariate logistic regression (Enter method), following the multicollinearity test of all variables. 95% confidence interval (95% CI), and p value were reported for regression analyses.

Results

Of the 1574 referrals for a psychiatry consultation with the on-call resident, 1530 cases met inclusion criteria. In total, 31 physicians saw these encounters with a mean of 49.4 encounters per physician (range 13–103 encounters per physician). Physician and patient characteristics for the 1530 encounters are shown in Table 1. Patients were more commonly female (61.2%) with a mean age

of 37.3 ± 18.6 years. In addition, the emergency visits were mostly composed of general age groups (64.7%). Physicians were typically male (71.3%) with a mean of 14.3 ± 8.7 years of practice and typically practiced outpatient care (74.4%). A small proportion of the visits were specialty-matched (8.2%).

Comparative statistics resulting in patients admitted versus not are shown in Table 2. Patient factors that differed significantly between the groups were patient age, geriatric patients, previous admission, and those with diagnosis of dementia, SCZ, BPD, anxiety, trauma/stress, and other MISC disorders. The relatively low number of geriatric patients (8.9%) is likely due to a number of factors. There is a well-established community-based psychogeriatric program at Sunnybrook that provides long-term follow-up and likely reduces the hospitalization rate for this population. Geriatric patients in the Sunnybook ER who present with Delirium a referred to General Internal Medicine with psychiatry providing a consultative role. Geriatric patients with Dementia are referred to the social work program for optimization of community resources as well as rapid access to long-term care placement. Patients with Dementia in the ER are also seen by Geriatric Psychiatry in a consultative role to optimize medication management. Additional patient characteristics such as income, housing status, cultural identity, and other demographic factors were not included in this study as the focus was on clinician variables influencing the decision to admit. There were no differences in patient characteristics in the clinical encounters reviewed by staff psychiatrists. Significantly different clinician factors were clinicians' gender, PES training status, practice in specialty or general, and those with the specialty in Psycho-Oncology, and Inpatient Care.

Multivariate regression analysis examined the four physician factors (years of practice in psychiatry, practice in general or specialty, practice in PES or other, specialty in outpatient or inpatient), which were determined to be significantly different between the groups of the patients admitted and not, plus the two survey results (subjective ratings on competency and learned-something-new surveys) involved in the decision to admit the patient, adjusted by significantly different patient factors shown in comparative statistics analysis (Table 2). Prior to multivariate logistic regression, all variables in the model passed the multicollinearity test (all above the tolerance level of 0.4).

Patient and environmental factors associated with a greater likelihood of admission include previous admissions ($\text{Exp}(B) = 1.64$, $p = 0.002$), geriatric patients ($\text{Exp}(B) = 1.69$, $p = 0.016$), diagnosis of schizophrenia ($\text{Exp}(B) = 3.41$, $p < 0.0005$), bipolar disorder

Table 1 Clinician and patient factors

	Total $n = 1530$
Patient factors	
Male (%)	593 (38.8)
Age (years ± SD)	37.3 ± 18.6
Youth (14–21) (%)	400 (26.1)
General (22–64) (%)	990 (64.7)
Geriatrics (65+) (%)	136 (8.9)
Others (< 14) (%)	4 (0.3)
Diagnoses (ICD-10-CM category)	
Dementia and delirium (%)	21 (1.4)
Substance-related disorders (%)	99 (6.5)
Schizophrenia and other psychotic disorders (%)	241 (15.8)
Bipolar and related disorders (%)	129 (8.4)
Depressive disorders (%)	350 (22.9)
Anxiety disorders (%)	107 (7.0)
Obsessive compulsive and related disorders (%)	12 (0.8)
Trauma and stress-related disorders (%)	71 (4.6)
Dissociative disorders (%)	3 (0.2)
Somatic symptom and related disorders (%)	3 (0.2)
Eating disorders (%)	1 (0.1)
Personality disorders (%)	27 (1.8)
Neurodevelopmental disorders (%)	1 (0.1)
Miscellaneous diagnoses (%)	465 (30.4)
Multiple visits	449 (29.3)
With previous admission (%)	247 (16.1)
Specialty match (%)	125 (8.2)

	Total $n = 1530$
Physician factors	
Male (%)	1091 (71.3)
Years of practice (mean ± SD)	14.3 ± 8.7
PES training (%)	308 (20.1)
Specialist/highly specialized (%)	247 (16.1)
Sub-division of primary specialty area (%)	
Youth	395 (25.8)
Geriatric	143 (9.3)
General	753 (49.2)
PES	308 (20.1)
Inpatient	240 (15.7)
Outpatient	166 (10.8)
Consultation liaison	39 (2.5)
Women's Mental Health	91 (5.9)
Oncology	48 (3.1)
OCD	43 (2.8)
CBT	42 (2.7)
Neuropsych	15 (1.0)
Other	239 (15.6)
Frequent care practice type (%)	
Outpatient	1139 (74.4)
Inpatient	391 (25.6)

($\mathrm{Exp}(B) = 2.86$, $p < 0.0005$), or related disorders. On the other hand, patients with a diagnosis of anxiety, trauma or stress related disorders were less likely to be admitted ($\mathrm{Exp}(B) = 0.28$, $p < 0.0005$; $\mathrm{Exp}(B) = 0.46$, $p = 0.009$, respectively, Table 3).

The physician factor found significant in deciding whether to admit the patient was assignment to PES. This appeared to be the only physician variable impacting the decision to admit a patient with PES psychiatrists admitting less often than their colleagues ($p = 0.018$, Table 3). The effect size of the variable in terms of odds ratio (OR) was 0.592.

A subanalysis within the PES psychiatrists examined whether greater clinical coverage had an impact on admission rates. Within the PES staff complement, weekday coverage was stratified with one psychiatrist providing 40% of the weekday coverage, one providing 30%, one providing 20% and one providing 10% of the weekday coverage. The differing amount of coverage by PES psychiatrists did not impact the proportion of patients admitted ($X^2 = 2.75$, $df = 3$, $p = 0.432$).

Discussion

Previous studies have focused on patient and systems factors that influence the decision to admit a patient seen in the emergency department to the psychiatry inpatient unit [8]. There has been some consideration of clinician factors that influence the decision to admit but little is known about these variables [9]. In addition to clinician variables, efforts to integrate input from patients and their families add additional variables into an already complex process of decision making [10].

We reviewed consecutive patient encounters in the emergency department of a large teaching hospital to measure and understand differences in the admission rates between on-call psychiatrists. Before the decision to admit, the patient would have been seen by a succession of clinicians including the ER triage RN, ER physician, and the psychiatry resident on call. In addition, collateral information may have been obtained from a family member or other person known to the patient. Following a telephone review and discussion between the psychiatry resident and staff psychiatrist on call, the staff psychiatrist would ultimately decide whether to admit the patient.

Psychiatrists who spend a portion of their clinical duties in PES were less likely to admit. In this study, there was a compliment of 4 psychiatrists providing PES coverage during weekday hours (8:30 to 4:30) from a total complement of 32 staff. After hours, call (weeknights and weekends) was shared equally between all staff psychiatrists including those working in PES.

Table 2 Admission rates for each factor

	Number admitted (n = 780)	Percent admittance (%)	x^2 or $F(df)$	p value
Clinician factors				
Gender				
Female	243	55.4	4.7 (1)	0.030
Male	537	49.2		
Years of practice			2.3 (1)	0.126
PES training	126	40.9	15.7 (1)	< 0.0005
Specialist/highly specialized	153	61.9	14.2 (1)	< 0.0005
Specialty area				
Youth	192	48.6	1.2 (1)	0.273
Geriatric	75	52.4	0.1 (1)	0.712
Inpatient	140	58.3	6.2 (1)	0.013
Outpatient	81	48.8	0.4 (1)	0.551
Consultation liaison	20	51.3	0.0 (1)	0.970
Women's mental health	52	57.1	1.5 (1)	0.225
Psycho-oncology	34	70.8	7.8 (1)	0.005
OCD	24	55.8	0.4 (1)	0.520
CBT	26	61.9	2.1 (1)	0.151
Neuropsych	10	66.7	1.5 (1)	0.222
Frequent care practice type among all physicians				
Outpatient	566	49.7	3.0 (1)	0.085
Inpatient	214	54.7		
Patient factors				
Gender				
Female	484	51.5	0.3 (1)	0.577
Male	297	50.1		
Age			6.3 (1)	0.012
Age groups				
Youth (14–21)	193	48.3	1.6 (1)	0.204
General (22–64)	501	50.6	0.2 (1)	0.692
Geriatrics (65+)	85	62.5	7.9 (1)	0.005
Diagnoses (ICD-10-CM category)				
Dementia and delirium	16	76.2	5.4 (1)	0.020
Substance-related disorders	44	44.4	1.8 (1)	0.179
Schizophrenia and other psychotic disorders	179	74.3	62.1 (1)	< 0.0005
Bipolar and related disorders	94	72.9	27.0 (1)	< 0.0005
Depressive disorders	168	48.0	1.6(1)	0.204
Anxiety disorders	21	19.6	45.3 (1)	< 0.0005
Obsessive compulsive and related disorders	5	41.7	0.4 (1)	0.517
Trauma and stress-related disorders	19	26.8	17.5 (1)	< 0.0005
Dissociative disorders	2	66.7	0.3 (1)	0.586
Somatic symptom and related disorders	0	0.0	3.1 (1)	0.077
Eating disorders	0	0.0	1.0 (1)	0.308
Personality disorders	15	55.6	0.2 (1)	0.631
Neurodevelopmental disorders	1	100	1.0 (1)	0.327
Miscellaneous diagnoses	216	46.5	5.5 (1)	0.019
Multiple visits	244	54.3	2.9 (1)	0.090
Previous admission	150	60.7	11.2 (1)	0.001
Specialty match				
Yes	81	51.3	0.0 (1)	0.940
No	699	50.9		

Table 3 Multivariate logistic regression analysis

	Exp(B)	95% CI for Exp(B)		df	p value
		Lower	Upper		
Patient factors					
Previous admittance	1.639	1.200	2.238	1	0.002
Geriatric group of patients	1.688	1.104	2.582	1	0.016
Dementia and delirium	2.568	0.873	7.558	1	0.087
Schizophrenia or psychotic disorders	3.414	2.373	4.911	1	<0.0005
Bipolar or related disorders	2.859	1.818	4.494	1	<0.0005
Anxiety disorder	0.283	0.166	0.482	1	<0.0005
Stress or trauma	0.459	0.255	0.824	1	0.009
Miscellaneous diagnoses	1.022	0.778	1.343	1	0.876
Psychiatrist factors					
Years of practice	0.992	0.978	1.006	1	0.268
Learned _Something_new survey score of 2 relative to score of 1	1.078	0.500	2.324	1	0.848
Learned _Something_new survey score of 3 relative to score of 1	0.955	0.556	1.641	1	0.868
Learned _Something_new survey score of 4 relative to score of 1	1.027	0.693	1.523	1	0.893
Learned _Something_new survey score of 5 relative to score of 1	1.125	0.708	1.788	1	0.619
Competency survey score of 4 relative to score of 3	1.075	0.641	1.805	1	0.784
Competency survey score of 5 relative to score of 3	0.923	0.540	1.577	1	0.769
Specialty in inpatient versus outpatient	1.061	0.746	1.509	1	0.743
Practice in specialty versus general	0.890	0.642	1.233	1	0.484
Specialty in PES versus other	0.592	0.384	0.913	1	0.018

These results appear both predictable and surprising. Psychiatrists working in the specialized area of PES would have more experience with the patient population that attends care in the emergency department. This may lead to a greater risk tolerance for discharging a patient with a severe mental illness. However, psychiatrists working in an inpatient setting would also be familiar with this population. Inpatient psychiatrists may apply an inherent bias towards admission based on their observations of the beneficial effects of admission and possibly to reinforce the value of their work. There may also be a financial incentive to admit patients if beds are not optimally utilized.

Challenging the variation in admission rates is the fact that all staff psychiatrists had undergone resident training in emergency psychiatry and would have logged many hours on call during residency with exposure to the same population they would be overseeing as a staff psychiatrist. These skills and practices should be enduring.

In the model of clinical care provided in a university teaching hospital, the interface between psychiatry resident and staff may also be worth examining to determine relative influences. Ultimately, it is the staff psychiatrist who decides whether to admit but this decision may be influenced by the experience and attitude of the resident providing the information. Given similarities in training and workplace cultures, it is not surprising that concordance in diagnosis between psychiatric residents and staff is strong [11]. A more complex dynamic is the unique relationship between resident and staff psychiatrist. In addition to the "power" imbalance, there may be subtle relational factors that influence outcome. For instance, a confident and outspoken resident may have a significant influence on the staff psychiatrist. Our study did not examine relational factors between residents and staff psychiatrists and how they may have influenced decision making.

This study did not evaluate outcomes of the decision to admit. Nearly, one-third of the study population had multiple visits to the ER during the study period. Slightly more than half (54%) of these patients were admitted. Although reasons for admission were not evaluated, multiple visits may represent a failure to meet patient needs. This subpopulation warrants further study. On the surface, lower admission rates may appear preferable with respect to inpatient bed utilization, but may not result in better patient outcomes. It is possible that patients who were not admitted suffered worse outcomes ranging from eventual admission to another facility to catastrophically, suicide. Future research must incorporate meaningful outcome measures to determine whether the decision to admit or discharge was the "right" decision.

If lower admission rates are considered a preferred outcome, these results may be instructive. Educational programs offered by PES staff to the staff psychiatrist call pool may impact outcomes. This educational model was shown to be effective in reducing admission rates for junior psychiatry residents [7]. Perhaps, all staff psychiatrists participating in the call pool should take regular weekday shifts in PES to increase exposure to this decision-making practice. Of course, this would expand the PES staff psychiatrist complement and dilute the experience resulting in an overall increase in admission rates.

Although this study examined admissions to psychiatry, the results may be generalizable to other specialties such as general internal medicine, where a subset of the call pool has additional experience in consultations to the emergency department.

Considering the value of inpatient beds in our health care systems, it is important to examine potentially modifiable factors influencing the decision to admit as well as patient outcomes related to these decisions.

Authors' contributions
JM and DN conceived the study; DN, MR and KW participated in the data collection; DK, MR and KL performed the statistical analysis; JM drafted the manuscript; JM, DN, DK, MR, KW and KL reviewed and edited the manuscript. All authors read and approved the final manuscript.

Author details
[1] Department of Psychiatry, Sunnybrook Health Sciences Centre, Toronto, Canada. [2] Department of Psychiatry and Neuropsychopharmacology Research Program, Sunnybrook Health Sciences Centre, Toronto, Canada.

Acknowledgements
None.

Competing interests
The authors declare that they have no competing interests.

Consent for publication
Consent for publication has been provided.

Funding
No Funding.

References
1. Way BB, Banks S. Clinical factors related to admission and release decisions in psychiatric emergency services. Psychiatr Serv. 2001;52:214–8.
2. Goldberg JF, Ernst CL, Bird S. Predicting hospitalization versus discharge in suicidal patients presenting to a psychiatric emergency service. Psychiatr Serv. 2007;58:561–5.
3. Feigelson EB, Davis EB, Mackinnon R, et al. The decision to hospitalize. Am J Psychiatry. 1978;135(3):354–7.
4. Baca-Garcia E, Diaz-Sastre C, Garcia Resa E, et al. Variables associated with hospitalization decisions by emergency psychiatrists after a patient's suicide attempt. Psychiatr Serv. 2004;55:792–7.
5. Apsler R, Bassuk E. Differences among clinicians in the decision to admit. Arch Gen Psychiatry. 1983;40:1133–7.
6. Way BB, Allen MH, Mumpower JL, et al. Interrater agreement among psychiatrist in psychiatric emergency assessments. Am J Psychiatry. 1988;155(10):1423–8.
7. Meyerson AT, Moss JZ, Belville R, et al. Influence of experience on major clinical decisions. Arch Gen Psychiatry. 1979;36:423–7.
8. Marson D, McGovern M, Pomp H. Psychiatric decision making in the emergency room: a research overview. Am J Psychiatry. 1988;145(8):918–25.
9. Rabinowitz J, Mark M, Slyuzberg M. How individual clinicians make admission decisions in psychiatric emergency rooms. J Psychiatr Res. 1994;28(5):475–82.
10. Charles C, Gafni A, Whelan T. Decision-making in the physician encounter: revisiting the shared treatment decision-making model. Soc Sci Med. 1999;49:651–61.
11. Warner MD, Peabody CA. Reliability of diagnosis made by psychiatric residents in a general emergency department. Psychiatr Serv. 1995;46(12):1284–6.

Permissions

The contributors of this book come from diverse backgrounds, making this book a truly international effort. This book will bring forth new frontiers with its revolutionizing research information and detailed analysis of the nascent developments around the world.

We would like to thank all the contributing authors for lending their expertise to make the book truly unique. They have played a crucial role in the development of this book. Without their invaluable contributions this book wouldn't have been possible. They have made vital efforts to compile up to date information on the varied aspects of this subject to make this book a valuable addition to the collection of many professionals and students.

This book was conceptualized with the vision of imparting up-to-date information and advanced data in this field. To ensure the same, a matchless editorial board was set up. Every individual on the board went through rigorous rounds of assessment to prove their worth. After which they invested a large part of their time researching and compiling the most relevant data for our readers.

The editorial board has been involved in producing this book since its inception. They have spent rigorous hours researching and exploring the diverse topics which have resulted in the successful publishing of this book. They have passed on their knowledge of decades through this book. To expedite this challenging task, the publisher supported the team at every step. A small team of assistant editors was also appointed to further simplify the editing procedure and attain best results for the readers.

Apart from the editorial board, the designing team has also invested a significant amount of their time in understanding the subject and creating the most relevant covers. They scrutinized every image to scout for the most suitable representation of the subject and create an appropriate cover for the book.

The publishing team has been an ardent support to the editorial, designing and production team. Their endless efforts to recruit the best for this project, has resulted in the accomplishment of this book. They are a veteran in the field of academics and their pool of knowledge is as vast as their experience in printing. Their expertise and guidance has proved useful at every step. Their uncompromising quality standards have made this book an exceptional effort. Their encouragement from time to time has been an inspiration for everyone.

The publisher and the editorial board hope that this book will prove to be a valuable piece of knowledge for researchers, students, practitioners and scholars across the globe.

List of Contributors

Jonathan M. Meyer
Department of Psychiatry, University of California, San Diego, California, USA

Daisy S. Ng-Mak and Krithika Rajagopalan
Sunovion Pharmaceuticals Inc., 84 Waterford Drive, Marlborough, MA 01752, USA

Chien-Chia Chuang
Vertex Pharmaceuticals, Cambridge, MA, USA

Antony Loebel
Sunovion Pharmaceuticals Inc., Fort Lee, NJ, USA

Nana Xiong, Jing Wei, Xia Hong, Tao Li and Jing Jiang
Department of Psychological Medicine, Peking Union Medical College Hospital, Chinese Academy of Medical Sciences and Peking Union Medical College, Beijing 100730, People's Republic of China

Kurt Fritzsche
Department of Psychosomatic Medicine and Psychotherapy, University Medical Centre Freiburg, Freiburg, Germany

Rainer Leonhart
Institute of Psychology, University of Freiburg, Freiburg, Germany

Liming Zhu
Department of Gastroenterology, Peking Union Medical College Hospital, Chinese Academy of Medical Sciences and Peking Union Medical College, Beijing, China

Guoqing Tian
Department of Traditional Chinese Medicine, Peking Union Medical College Hospital, Chinese Academy of Medical Sciences and Peking Union Medical College, Beijing, China

Xudong Zhao
Department of Psychosomatic Medicine, Dongfang Hospital, School of Medicine, Tongji University, Shanghai, China

Lan Zhang
Mental Health Centre, West China Hospital, Sichuan University, Chengdu, Sichuan, China

Rainer Schaefert
Department of General Internal Medicine and Psychosomatics, University Hospital Heidelberg, Heidelberg, Germany

Ahmad N. AlHadi
Department of Psychiatry, College of Medicine, King Saud University, King Saud University Medical City, Riyadh 11322, Saudi Arabia
SABIC Psychological Health Research and Applications Chair (SPHRAC), College of Medicine, King Saud University, King Saud University Medical City, Riyadh 11322, Saudi Arabia

Fahad M. AlShahrani
Family Medicine Department, King Abdulaziz Medical City, National Guard, Riyadh, Saudi Arabia
College of Medicine, King Saud bin Abdulaziz University for Health Sciences, Riyadh, Saudi Arabia

Ali A. Alshaqrawi
Department of Psychiatry, King Saud University Medical City, Riyadh, Saudi Arabia

Mohanned A. Sharefi
Department of Emergency Medicine, Prince Sultan Military Medical City, Riyadh, Saudi Arabia

Saud M. Almousa
Department of Internal Medicine, King Fahad Medical City, Riyadh, Saudi Arabia

Habte Belete
Psychiatry Department, College of Medicine and Health Science, Bahir Dar University, Bahir Dar, Ethiopia

Ahmad N. AlHadi and Deemah A. AlAteeq
Department of Psychiatry, College of Medicine, King Saud University, Riyadh, Saudi Arabia
SABIC Psychological Health Research and Applications Chair (SPHRAC), College of Medicine, King Saud University, Riyadh 11322, Saudi Arabia

Eman Al-Sharif, Hamdah M. Bawazeer and Hasan Alanazi
College of Medicine, King Saud University, Riyadh, Saudi Arabia

Abdulaziz T. AlShomrani
College of Medicine, Al Imam Mohammad Ibn Saud Islamic University, Riyadh, Saudi Arabia
SABIC Psychological Health Research and Applications Chair (SPHRAC), College of Medicine, King Saud University, Riyadh 11322, Saudi Arabia

Raafat M. Shuqdar
College of Medicine, Taibah University, Madinah, Saudi Arabia
SABIC Psychological Health Research and Applications Chair (SPHRAC), College of Medicine, King Saud University, Riyadh 11322, Saudi Arabia

Reem AlOwaybil
SABIC Psychological Health Research and Applications Chair (SPHRAC), College of Medicine, King Saud University, Riyadh 11322, Saudi Arabia

Concetta De Pasquale
Department of Medical Surgeon Science and Applied Technology. GF
Ingrassia, University of Catania, Catania, Italy

Federica Sciacca
Department of Education Science, University of Catania, Via Teatro Greco, 84, Catania, Italy

Zira Hichy
Department of Education of Education Science, University of Catania, Via Teatro Greco, 84, Catania, Italy

Getinet Ayano, Dawit Assefa, Kibrom Haile, Asrat Chaka, Haddish Solomon, Petros Hagos, Zegeye Yohannis, Kelemua Haile, Lulu Bekana, Melkamu Agidew, Seife Demise, Belachew Tsegaye and Melat Solomon
Research and Training Department, Amanuel Mental Specialized Hospital, Addis Ababa, Ethiopia

Ahmed Mhalla, Bochra Ben Mohamed, Badii Amamou, Anouar Mechri and Lotfi Gaha
Psychiatry Department, Fattouma Bourguiba Hospital, 5000 Monastir, Tunisia

Faculty of Medicine of Monastir, University of Monastir, Monastir, Tunisia

Christoph U. Correll
Department of Psychiatry, The Zucker Hillside Hospital, Glen Oaks, NY, USA.
Department of Psychiatry and Molecular Medicine, Hofstra Northwell School of Medicine, Hempstead, NY, USA.
Center for Psychiatric Neuroscience, Feinstein Institute for Medical Research, Manhasset, NY, USA

Helen Lazaratou and Dimitris Dikeos
National and Kapodistrian University of Athens, Vas Sofias 72, 11528 Athens, Greece

Vasilis Stavropoulos
National and Kapodistrian University of Athens, Vas Sofias 72, 11528 Athens, Greece
Federation University Australia, Mount Helen, Ballarat, VIC, Australia

Kathleen A. Moore and Rapson Gomez
Federation University Australia, Mount Helen, Ballarat, VIC, Australia

A. Messaoud, A. Mrad, A. Mhalla, B. Amemou and L. Gaha
Research Laboratory 'Vulnerability to psychotic disorders LR 05 ES 10', Department of Psychiatry, Monastir University Hospital, University of Monastir, Monastir, Tunisia

R. Mensi I. Azizi and W. Douki
Research Laboratory 'Vulnerability to psychotic disorders LR 05 ES 10', Department of Psychiatry, Monastir University Hospital, University of Monastir, Monastir, Tunisia
Laboratory of Biochemistry-Toxicology, Monastir University Hospital, University of Monastir, Monastir, Tunisia

M. F. Najjar
Laboratory of Biochemistry-Toxicology, Monastir University Hospital, University of Monastir, Monastir, Tunisia

I. Trabelsi and M. H. Grissa
Department of Emergency, Monastir University Hospital, University of Monastir, Monastir, Tunisia

N. Haj Salem and A. Chadly
Department of Forensic Medicine, Monastir University Hospital, University of Monastir, Monastir, Tunisia

Monika Elemery, Gabor Faludi and Judit Lazary
Department of Psychiatry and Psychotherapy, Semmelweis University, Budapest, Hungary

Iren Csala
Department of Psychiatry and Psychotherapy, Semmelweis University, Budapest, Hungary
Institute of Behavioral Sciences, Semmelweis University, Budapest, Hungary

Peter Dome
Department of Psychiatry and Psychotherapy, Semmelweis University, Budapest, Hungary
National Institute of Psychiatry and Addiction, Budapest, Hungary

Fruzsina Martinovszky Imola Sandor Zsuzsa Gyorffy and Emma Birkas
Institute of Behavioral Sciences, Semmelweis University, Budapest, Hungary

Balazs Dome
Department of Tumor Biology, National Koranyi Institute of Pulmonology, Budapest, Hungary.
Department of Thoracic Surgery, Medical University of Vienna, Vienna, Austria
Department of Thoracic Surgery, National Institute of Oncology and Semmelweis University, Budapest, Hungary
Division of Molecular and Gender Imaging, Department of Biomedical Imaging and Image-guided Therapy, Medical University of Vienna, Vienna, Austria

Soo-Hyun Paik, Mi Ran Choi, Su Min Kwak, Sol Hee Bang, Ji-Won Chun, Jin-Young Kim, Jihye Choi, Hyun Cho, Jo-Eun Jeong and Dai-Jin Kim
Department of Psychiatry, Seoul St. Mary's Hospital, The Catholic University of Korea College of Medicine, Seoul, 222, Banpo-daero, Seocho-gu, Seoul 06591, South Korea

T. K. Grimholt and D. Jacobsen
Department of Acute Medicine, Oslo University Hospital, Nydalen, Pb 4950, Oslo, Norway

O. R. Haavet
Department of General Practice, Institute of Health and Society, University of Oslo, Oslo, Norway

Ø. Ekeberg
Division of Mental Health and Addiction, Oslo University Hospital, Oslo, Norway

Department of Behavioural Sciences in Medicine, Institute of Basic Medical Sciences, Faculty of Medicine, University of Oslo, Oslo, Norway

Ahmed Mhallah Walid Haj Salah and Lotfi Gaha
Research Laboratory "Vulnerability to Psychotic Disorders LR05ES10", Faculty of Medicine, University of Monastir, 5012 Monastir, Tunisia
Department of Psychiatry, University Hospital in Monastir, Monastir, Tunisia

Rym Mensi, Amal Messaoud, Islem Azizi and Wahiba Douki
Research Laboratory "Vulnerability to Psychotic Disorders LR05ES10", Faculty of Medicine, University of Monastir, 5012 Monastir, Tunisia
Clinical Biochemistry and Toxicology Laboratory, University Hospital in Monastir, Monastir, Tunisia

Mohamed Fadhel Najjar
Clinical Biochemistry and Toxicology Laboratory, University Hospital in Monastir, Monastir, Tunisia

Hsiu-Hung Wang
College of Nursing, Kaohsiung Medical University, Kaohsiung, Taiwan

Shu-Ching Ma
College of Nursing, Kaohsiung Medical University, Kaohsiung, Taiwan.
Nursing Department, Chi-Mei Medical Center, Tainan, Taiwan
Bachelor Program of Senior Services, Southern Taiwan University of Science and Technology, Tainan, Taiwan

Tsair-Wei Chien
Research Department, Chi-Mei Medical Center, 901 Chung Hwa Road, Yung Kung Dist., Tainan 710, Taiwan
Department of Hospital and Health Care Administration, Chia-Nan University of Pharmacy and Science, Tainan, Taiwan

Adrian Heald
Department of Medicine, Leighton Hospital, Crewe CW1 4QJ, Cheshire, UK
The School of Medicine and Manchester Academic Health Sciences Centre, University of Manchester, Manchester M13 9PT, UK

Martin Gibson
The School of Medicine and Manchester Academic Health Sciences Centre, University of Manchester, Manchester M13 9PT, UK

John Pendlebury Vinesh Narayan and Peter Haddad
Greater Manchester West Mental Health NHS Foundation Trust, Greater Manchester, UK

Simon Anderson
Institute of Cardiovascular Sciences, University of Manchester, Manchester, UK

Mark Guy
Department of Clinical Biochemistry, Salford Royal Hospital, Salford M6 8HD, UK

Mark Livingston
Department of Blood Sciences, Walsall Manor Hospital, Walsall WS2 9PS, UK

Rajnish Mago
Simple and Practical Mental Health, Philadelphia, PA, USA
210 W Rittenhouse Square Suite 404, Philadelphia, PA 19103, USA

Andrea Fagiolini
University of Siena Medical Center, Siena, Italy

Emmanuelle Weiller
H. Lundbeck A/S, Valby, Denmark

Catherine Weiss
Otsuka Pharmaceutical Development and Commercialization, Inc, Princeton, NJ, USA

Elham Baharzadeh, Fereydoun Siassi and Gity Sotoudeh
Department of Community Nutrition, School of Nutritional Sciences and Dietetics, Tehran University of Medical Sciences, Hojatdost Street, Naderi Street, KeshavarzBlv., Tehran, Iran

Mostafa Qorbani
Non-communicable Diseases Research Center, Alborz University of Medical Sciences, Karaj, Iran

Fariba Koohdani
Department of Cellular, Molecular Nutrition, School of Nutritional Sciences and Dietetics, Tehran University of Medical Sciences, Tehran, Iran

Neda Pak
Shariati Hospital, School of Medicine, Tehran University of Medical Sciences, Tehran, Iran
Children Hospital of Excellence, School of Medicine, Tehran University of Medical Sciences, Tehran, Iran

Yang-Whan Jeon, Sang-Ick Han and E. Jin Park
Department of Psychiatry, College of Medicine, Incheon St. Mary's
Hospital, The Catholic University of Korea, 56 Dongsu-ro, Bupyeong-gu, Incheon 21431, South Korea

Anna Adam and Grigoris Abatzoglou
School of Medicine, Service of Child and Adolescent Psychiatry, AHEPA Hospital, Third Psychiatric Clinic, Aristotle University of Thessaloniki, Thessaloniki, Greece

Grigoris Kiosseoglou and Zaira Papaligoura
School of Psychology, Aristotle University of Thessaloniki, Thessaloniki, Greece

Waleed M. Sweileh
Department of Physiology and Pharmacology/ Toxicology, College of Medicine and Health Sciences, Nablus, Palestine

Asrat Chaka, Zegeye Yohannis and Getinet Ayano
Department of Psychiatry, Amanuel Mental Specialized Hospital, Addis Ababa, Ethiopia

Tadesse Awoke
Department of Epidemiology and Biostatistics, University of Gondar, Gondar, Ethiopia

Minale Tareke and Andargie Abate
College of Medicine and Health Science, Bahir Dar University, Bahir Dar, Ethiopia

Mulugeta Nega
College of Medicine and Health Science, Haramaya University, Harer, Ethiopia

Gaizhi Li
Shanxi Medical University, The First Hospital of Shanxi Medical University, Taiyuan, China
Department of Child and Adolescent Psychiatry, Shanghai Mental Health Center, Shanghai
Jiao Tong University School of Medicine, No 600 Wanping Nan Road, Xuhui, Shanghai 200030, China

Kathryn Rossbach
NCSP, Greater Atlanta area, Atlanta, USA

Wenqing Jiang and Yasong Du
Department of Child and Adolescent Psychiatry, Shanghai Mental Health Center, Shanghai
Jiao Tong University School of Medicine, No 600 Wanping Nan Road, Xuhui, Shanghai 200030, China

Temesgen Ergetie and Minale Tareke
Department of Psychiatry, College of Medicine and Health Sciences, Bahir Dar University, Bahir Dar, Ethiopia

Zegeye Yohanes and Wubit Demeke
Amanuel Specialized Mental Hospital, Addis Ababa, Ethiopia

Biksegn Asrat
Department of Psychiatry, College of Medicine and Health Sciences, Gondar University, Gondar, Ethiopia

Andargie Abate
College of Medicine and Health Sciences, Bahir Dar University, Bahir Dar, Ethiopia

Farshid Shamsaei
Behavioural Disorders and Substance Abuse Research Centre, Hamadan
University of Medical Sciences, Hamadan, Iran

Fatemeh Nazari
Department of Nursing and Midwifery, Hamadan University of Medical Sciences, Hamadan, Iran

Efat Sadeghian
Chronic Diseases (Home Care) Research Centre, School of Nursing and Midwifery, Hamadan University of Medical Sciences, Hamadan, Iran

Elmars Rancans, Rolands Ivanovs and Jelena Vrublevska
Department of Psychiatry and Narcology, Riga Stradins University, Tvaika Street 2, Riga 1005, Latvia

Marcis Trapencieris
Institute of Philosophy and Sociology, University of Latvia, Kalpaka bulv. 4, Riga, Latvia

Andargie Abate, Minale Tareke, Mulat Tirfie, Ayele Semachew, Desalegne Amare and Emiru Ayalew
College of Medicine and Health Science, Bahir Dar University, Bahir Dar, Ethiopia

Najiba Fekih-Mrissa, Aycha Sayeh, Meriem Mrad and Brahim Nsiri
Laboratory of Molecular Biology, Department of Hematology, Military Hospital of Tunisia, Mont Fleury, 1008 Tunis, Tunisia

Ridha Mrissa, Ines Bedoui and Hajer Derbali
Department of Neurology, Military Hospital of Tunisia, Montfleury, Tunis 1008, Tunisia

Shengnan Wei and Xiaowei Jiang
Brain Function Research Section, First Affiliated Hospital, China Medical University, Shenyang, Liaoning, People's Republic of China.
Department of Radiology, First Affiliated Hospital, China Medical University, Shenyang, Liaoning, People's Republic of China

Fei Wang
Brain Function Research Section, First Affiliated Hospital, China Medical University, Shenyang, Liaoning, People's Republic of China.
Department of Radiology, First Affiliated Hospital, China Medical University, Shenyang, Liaoning, People's Republic of China
Department of Psychiatry, First Affiliated Hospital, China Medical University, Shenyang 110001, Liaoning, People's Republic of China

Yanqing Tang
Brain Function Research Section, First Affiliated Hospital, China Medical University, Shenyang, Liaoning, People's Republic of China.
Department of Psychiatry, First Affiliated Hospital, China Medical University, Shenyang 110001, Liaoning, People's Republic of China
Department of Geriatric Medicine, First Affiliated Hospital, China Medical University, Shenyang, Liaoning, People's Republic of China

Miao Chang
Department of Radiology, First Affiliated Hospital, China Medical University, Shenyang, Liaoning, People's Republic of China

Ran Zhang
Department of Psychiatry, First Affiliated Hospital, China Medical University, Shenyang 110001, Liaoning, People's Republic of China

Concetta De Pasquale and Federica Sciacca
Department of Education Science, University of Catania, Via Teatro Greco, 84, Catania, Italy

Carmela Dinaro
Drug Addiction Health Service, SER.T-ASP3 in Catania, Via Fabio, 1, Acireale (CT), Italy

Bereket Duko and Epherem Geja
Faculty of Health Sciences, College of Medicine and Health Sciences, Hawassa University, Hawassa, Ethiopia

Mahlet Zewude and Semere Mekonen
Hawassa University Comprehensive Specialized Hospital, Hawassa University, Hawassa, Ethiopia

Jay Moss, Dippy Nauranga and Karen Wang
Department of Psychiatry, Sunnybrook Health Sciences Centre, Toronto, Canada

Krista Lanctot
Department of Psychiatry, Sunnybrook Health Sciences Centre, Toronto, Canada
Department of Psychiatry and Neuropsychopharmacology Research Program, Sunnybrook Health Sciences Centre, Toronto, Canada

Doyoung Kim and Michael Rosen
Department of Psychiatry and Neuropsychopharmacology Research Program, Sunnybrook Health Sciences Centre, Toronto, Canada

Index

Nicotine Dependence, 84-86, 88-89

O

Obsessive Compulsive Symptoms (OCS), 64

Olanzapine, 1-2, 4-5, 8-9

P

Patient Health Questionnaire, 12, 18-19, 36, 43-44, 179, 183, 204-205, 209-211, 241, 245

Perceived Stigma, 178-179, 181-182, 191-197, 241-242, 244

Phq-15, 10, 12-13, 15-16, 18-19, 40-42

Psychometric Testing, 45-46

Q

Quetiapine, 1-5, 8-9

R

Rasch Measurement, 116, 119, 123

Resting-state Functional Magnetic Resonance Imaging, 184, 190, 228

Risperidone, 1-5, 8-9

S

Schizophrenia, 1-9, 20, 29, 34, 50-53, 55-57, 59-60, 62-63, 83, 97, 107-115, 122, 125-126, 129-131, 134, 151, 164, 190, 193-194, 197-198, 200, 202-203, 247, 250-252

Sds, 133-135

Selective Serotonin Reuptake Inhibitor, 150, 156

Somatic Distress, 10-17

Suicidal Ideation, 39, 41, 55, 77-79, 82, 99, 102, 165-166, 171, 228-234

T

Taq1a Ankk1, 91, 94, 96

Triglycerides, 76-83, 107-108, 111-114, 223

Tunisian, 37, 40, 56-57, 76-77, 82, 107, 113-114, 221-222, 225-227

W

Wisc-iii, 158-161, 163

Z

Ziprasidone, 1-3, 8-9

www.ingramcontent.com/pod-product-compliance
Lightning Source LLC
Chambersburg PA
CBHW061312190326
41458CB00011B/3781